Handbook of Clinical Urology

Handbook of Clinical Urology

Editor: Timothy Lawson

AMERICAN
MEDICAL PUBLISHERS
www.americanmedicalpublishers.com

AMERICAN
MEDICAL PUBLISHERS
www.americanmedicalpublishers.com

Cataloging-in-Publication Data

Handbook of clinical urology / edited by Timothy Lawson.
p. cm.
Includes bibliographical references and index.
ISBN 978-1-63927-994-4
1. Urinary organs--Diseases. 2. Genitourinary organs--Diseases.
3. Urinary organs--Diseases--Diagnosis. 4. Urinary organs--Diseases--Treatment.
5. Urology. I. Lawson, Timothy.
RC900 .H36 2023
616.6--dc23

American Medical Publishers,
41 Flatbush Avenue,
1st Floor, New York,
NY 11217, USA

ISBN 978-1-63927-994-4 (Hardback)

Contents

Preface

Urology is a medical specialty that focuses on the disorders affecting the female and male urinary tract systems. The main organs of the urinary tract are the bladder, kidneys and ureters. This discipline is also concerned with the male organs that are capable of producing children, such as scrotum, penis, prostate and testes. Urology is connected with a wide range of medical diseases ranging from urinary control to cancer. Kidney stones, prostate issues, urinary tract infections and issues with bladder control are a few examples of urologic disorders. Some of these disorders are temporary while others are chronic. Urology includes the treatment of disorders like prostate or bladder cancer, congenital anomalies, stress incontinence, kidney stones and traumatic injury through surgery. It also includes the clinical management of disorders like benign prostatic hyperplasia and urinary-tract infections. This book aims to understand the clinical perspectives of urology. It will provide significant information of this discipline to help develop a good understanding of clinical management of urologic disorders. The readers would gain knowledge that would broaden their perspective in this area of medicine.

This book is a result of research of several months to collate the most relevant data in the field.

When I was approached with the idea of this book and the proposal to edit it, I was overwhelmed. It gave me an opportunity to reach out to all those who share a common interest with me in this field. I had 3 main parameters for editing this text:

1. Accuracy – The data and information provided in this book should be up-to-date and valuable to the readers.

2. Structure – The data must be presented in a structured format for easy understanding and better grasping of the readers.

3. Universal Approach – This book not only targets students but also experts and innovators in the field, thus my aim was to present topics which are of use to all.

Thus, it took me a couple of months to finish the editing of this book.

I would like to make a special mention of my publisher who considered me worthy of this opportunity and also supported me throughout the editing process. I would also like to thank the editing team at the back-end who extended their help whenever required.

Editor

1

A Review of Outcomes and Technique for the Robotic-Assisted Laparoscopic Retroperitoneal Lymph Node Dissection for Testicular Cancer

Zeyad R. Schwen, Mohit Gupta, and Phillip M. Pierorazio

Department of Urology, James Buchanan Brady Urological Institute, Johns Hopkins University School of Medicine, Baltimore, MD, USA

Correspondence should be addressed to Zeyad R. Schwen; zschwen21@gmail.com

Academic Editor: Timothy A. Masterson

Objectives. The robotic-assisted laparoscopic retroperitoneal lymph node dissection (R-RPLND) represents a new frontier in the surgical management of testicular cancer in the realm of minimally invasive urologic oncology. We aimed to review the early outcomes as compared to the laparoscopic and open approaches as well as describe the operative technique for the R-RPLND. *Materials and Methods.* We reviewed all the literature related to the R-RPLND based on an electronic PubMed search up until July 2017. *Results and Discussion.* Encouraged by favorable early oncologic and safety outcomes for treatment of clinical stage (CS) I nonseminomatous germ cell tumor (NSGCT), the R-RPLND affords the same recovery advantages as the laparoscopic retroperitoneal lymph node dissection (L-RPLND) while offering greater dexterity, superior visualization, and a theoretically shorter learning curve for the surgeon. While R-RPLND has a promising future in the management of patients with primary and-postchemotherapy NSGCT, larger and more vigorous prospective studies are needed before supplanting the open RPLND as the gold standard approach for primary low-stage NSGCT or becoming an equivalent surgical modality in the postchemotherapy setting.

1. Introduction

Testicular germ cell tumor (GCT) is the most common solid tumor in men between the ages of 20–44. Men diagnosed with GCT have excellent survival rates due to advances in the multimodal treatment paradigm of chemotherapy, radiation therapy, and surgery [1]. Retroperitoneal lymph node dissection (RPLND) remains an established treatment option for nonseminomatous GCT in the primary setting for low-stage (clinical stages (CSs) I and II) diseases and residual masses after chemotherapy [1]. Due to the excellent survival outcome, with a 5-year overall survival rate of 98%, there has been a greater emphasis on reducing morbidity and long-term toxicity for testicular cancer survivors. Open RPLND (O-RPLND) remains the gold standard approach for surgical management of the retroperitoneum for GCTs. It is, however, maximally invasive and can result in significant postoperative morbidity and prolonged hospitalizations [2–4].

For primary CS I and CS II NSGCT, minimally invasive RPLND has become a less morbid alternative to the O-RPLND while touting favorable early oncologic outcomes [5, 6]. Laparoscopic RPLND (L-RPLND), first reported in 1992, offered a reduced recovery time, less blood loss, and lower complication rates compared to O-RPLND [5, 7]. However, the operation had a very steep learning curve [8], a lower lymph node yield [9], and critics have pointed out that the L-RPLND's long-term oncologic outcomes have not been studied as rigorously as O-RPLND, which is partly related to the high rate of adjuvant chemotherapy given to patients with positive lymph nodes [10].

The natural evolution of minimally invasive urologic oncology from laparoscopy to robotics laid the foundation for the first robotic-assisted laparoscopic RPLND (R-RPLND) to be performed in 2006 by Davol et al. [11]. The advantages of R-RPLND over L-RPLND were similar to other urologic operations that transitioned to a robotic approach: a reduced learning curve, three-dimensional visualization, and greater instrument dexterity from the wristed instruments. Boosted by early results demonstrating equivalence in oncologic and safety measures compared to open and laparoscopic approaches, the R-RPLND has become an excellent option for the treatment of CS I and CS II nonseminomatous GST (NSGCT) and is emerging as a feasible approach for postchemotherapy RPLND [12]. In this article, we will review the technique and early outcomes of R-RPLND as compared to both O-RPLND and L-RPLND for the management of primary low-stage nonseminomatous and postchemotherapy GCT.

2. Materials and Methods

We performed an electronic PubMed search for all relevant publications regarding the outcomes and technique of the R-RPLND up until July 2017. We used the keywords robotic, retroperitoneal lymph node dissection, and testicular cancer, which resulted a total of 36 papers. All single and multi-institutional R-RPLND studies in adults with testicular cancer were included and reviewed in addition to studies investigating outcomes associated with O-RPLND and L-RPLND.

3. Results and Discussion

3.1. Primary Low-Stage Nonseminomatous Testicular Cancer

3.1.1. Role of RPLND in the Guideline-Directed Management of Low-Stage NSGCT. Patients diagnosed with CS I NSGCT, based on NCCN guidelines, have the option of active surveillance, platinum-based chemotherapy, or RPLND [1]. While each treatment option offers an excellent survival rate, each has its own respective drawbacks as well. Active surveillance offers the best opportunity to avoid unnecessary treatment and is the preferred treatment based on NCCN guidelines for CS IA disease; however, patients with recurrence are often subject to three or four cycles of platinum-based chemotherapy, and not all patients are willing to accept the anxieties associated with surveillance [13]. Adjuvant chemotherapy offers the best cure rate as a single modality, approaching 97%; however, it will overtreat a significant number of men and subject them to the known and unknown long-term toxicities of platinum-based chemotherapy [14]. These long-term toxicities include secondary malignancy, early cardiovascular disease, and a number of single-organ toxicities, including nephrotoxicity, pulmonary toxicity, ototoxicity, neurotoxicity, and hypogonadism [15]. Primary RPLND offers the ability to accurately stage the extent of disease while avoiding the significant toxicity of chemotherapy [16, 17] or the high relapse rate that is observed in 20–30% of patients who choose surveillance [13, 18]. While RPLND for CS I NSGCT may result in overtreatment for some patients, 25–35% of patients will harbor metastatic disease on presentation without radiographic evidence of pathologic retroperitoneal lymph nodes [19]. When RPLND is performed at a high-volume institution, the risk of recurrence is low (2%) with survival rates exceeding 95% [20]. From the open experience, RPLND alone is curative in 80–90% of patients with pN1 disease discovered in the retroperitoneum [21]. The disadvantages of RPLND are the risk of complications, which include ejaculatory dysfunction, blood loss, visceral injuries, ileus, and chylous ascites [4]. In the phase III randomized study of primary chemotherapy versus RPLND, the recurrence rate was higher in the RPLND group (8% versus 0.5%), but 37% of patients undergoing chemotherapy experienced a grade III or IV toxicity, compared to only 9% of RPLND patients [22].

4. Outcomes

4.1. Oncologic Outcomes. While the first use of the L-RPLND was for the purpose of staging alone, the intent of the R-RPLND is to match the oncologic efficacy of O-RPLND while providing the benefits of a minimally invasive approach. The largest R-RPLND series to date, a multi-institutional study of 47 CS I and 5 CS II patients which includes our patient experience, reported an excellent 2-year recurrence-free survival of 97% in the entire cohort [6]. Stepanian et al., with a median follow-up of 49 months, reported no retroperitoneal or distant recurrences in 19 patients undergoing robotic RPLND [23]. These results are summarized in Table 1. Impressively, 75% (6/8) of patients with positive retroperitoneal lymph nodes received no additional therapy while two patients with elements of embryonal carcinoma in their retroperitoneum on final pathology received chemotherapy. It is worth noting that three of these patients had teratoma who were definitively treated with surgery alone and were not candidates for chemotherapy. Pearce et al. reported that 62% (5/8) of patients with positive lymph nodes received chemotherapy with a single out-of-template recurrence of teratoma after chemotherapy [6]. These oncologic results compare favorably to O-RPLND and L-RPLND which, based on the findings from a large meta-analysis of >800 patients, experience recurrence-free rates of 92.5% and 95.4%, respectively [9]. While the results are promising, the low rates of positive lymph nodes in these series, ranging from 17% to 42%, and the use of adjuvant chemotherapy for node-positive patients make drawing conclusions, regarding comparative efficacy to O-RPLND and L-RPLND, a challenge. Furthermore, the majority of these studies investigating R-RPLND have short follow-up and varying surgical techniques, which further complicates their collective analysis.

Lymph node yield, a correlate for the extent of node dissection, can provide valuable information regarding the staging and therapeutic benefit of R-RPLND. Importantly, their reported median lymph node yield (LNY) of 26 nodes (IQR 18-32) outperformed the LNY reported in a contemporary meta-analysis of L-RPLND, which reported a median of 16 lymph nodes [9]. R-RPLND, however, appears to be similar to LNY observed in O-RPLND, which ranges from 28–33 [24, 25]. Conversely, in a separate head-to-head comparison from our institution of 16 R-RPLNDs and 21 L-RPLNDs from a single-surgeon experience, no difference

Table 1: Summary of perioperative outcomes from notable series for primary and postchemotherapy R-RPLND.

Primary RPLND													
Group	Year	*N*	CS I	CS II	Operative time (mins)	EBL (ml)	Lymph node yield	LOS (days)	Complication rate (%)	Positive lymph nodes (%)	Recurrence-free rate (%)	Antegrade ejaculation (%)	Follow-up (months)
Harris et al. [26]	2015	16	16	0	294	75	22	—	6.3	12.5	—	100	13.5
Cheney et al. [32]	2015	10	9	1	311	100	22	2.75	—	30	80	91	22
Stepanian et al. [23]	2016	16	11	5	293	50	19.5	1	5	38	100	90	49
Pearce et al. [6]	2017	47	42	5	235	50	26	1	14	17	97	96	16
Postchemo RPLND													
Group	Year	*N*	CS I	CS II	Operative time (mins)	EBL (ml)	Lymph node yield	LOS (days)	Complication rate (%)	Positive lymph nodes (%)	Recurrence-free rate (%)	Antegrade ejaculation (%)	Follow-up (months)
Cheney et al. [32]	2015	8	7	1	369	313	18	2.2	—	62.5	100	—	22
Stepanian et al. [23]	2016	4	1	3	324	150	22	1.5	—	50	100	100	41
Kamel et al. [12]	2016	12	6	6	312	475	22	3	25	50	100	66.7	31

LOS = length of stay; EBL = estimated blood loss; CS = clinical stage.

in the LNY was found [26]. To date, no prospective R-RPLND series has been published, and long-term oncologic and survival outcomes have yet to be reported in a large series. While the early results are promising and appear to suggest favorable recurrence rates and LNY compared to L-RPLND and O-RPLND in the hands of experienced robotic surgeons, determining oncologic equivalency to O-RPLND and L-RPLND will require larger, prospective series with longer follow-up.

Furthermore, though the oncologic outcomes of the primary RPLND for the management of low-stage NSGCT are often deliberated, there is considerable agreement that RPLNDs should be performed exclusively by experienced high-volume surgeons at experienced institutions, which result in fewer complications and superior oncologic outcomes [20, 27]. The early published oncologic outcomes of the R-RPLND, it is worth noting, are from experienced robotic surgeons in high-volume academic centers.

4.2. Perioperative Outcomes. As in other minimally invasive surgeries in urologic oncology, the R-RPLND affords a reduced blood loss and shorter recovery time, both of which translate into shorter hospital stays [28]. Blood loss is minimized for R-RPLND primarily due to the tamponading effects of pneumoperitoneum on venous bleeding. For R-RPLND, Harris et al. demonstrated equivalent blood loss (75 mL, IQR 50–100 mL) and operative time (270.5 minutes (mins), IQR 236–299 mins) compared to L-RPLND [26]. Similarly, two other series reported a median blood loss of 50 mL [6, 23], significantly less than the reported 184–450 mL blood loss for open primary RPLND [4, 29–31].

Perhaps, the most significant advantage that is afforded by the R-RPLND is the shorter recovery time compared to O-RPLND that translates into a shorter hospital length of stay (LOS). Pearce et al. and Stepanian et al. both reported a median LOS of 1 day which was far superior to both L-RPLND and O-RPLND (3.3 days and 6.6 days, resp.) [6, 9, 23]. Cheney et al., in a smaller series of 10 patients with low-stage NSGCT who received a R-RPLND, experienced a similarly short 2.7 day LOS [32]. Some O-RPLND series at experienced high-volume centers, however, have managed to reduce the difference in LOS compared to minimally invasive approaches. Syan-Bhanvadia et al. via the extraperitoneal open approach and Beck et al. of Indiana University have reported a mean LOS of 2.8 to 3 days [30, 31]. The dramatically reduced hospitalization of R-RPLND is likely explained by both the less morbid incision compared to O-RPLND and the lower rates of postoperative ileus. Together, this translates into a shorter convalescence due to less pain, earlier ambulation, and earlier return of bowel function.

Minimally invasive approaches for RPLND, however, are limited by a greater operative time compared to O-RPLND, which persists even beyond the learning curve [9]. In a large meta-analysis, L-RPLND performed by experienced surgeons had significantly greater operative time compared with O-RPLND (204 mins versus 186 mins) [9]. A similar trend applies to R-RPLND, reporting greater operative times ranging from 239 to 311 minutes [6, 26, 32]. While there are no studies investigating costs associated with R-RPLND, prior studies have demonstrated that the reduced LOS associated with L-RPLND drove its reduced cost relative to O-RPLND [33]. While the cost of robotic technology may be high relative to laparoscopy, cost savings for R-RPLND may be achieved through shorter length of stays and reduced complication rates, as was shown for laparoscopic versus robotic partial nephrectomy [34].

4.3. Complications. As part of the rationale for primary RPLND to avoid the long-term toxicities of chemotherapy, surgical complications need to be minimized at all costs. O-RPLND, however, has traditionally experienced relatively high intraoperative and postoperative complication rates at 5–7% and 24–33%, respectively [2, 4]. More contemporary O-RPLND series, however, report lower overall complication rates as low as 7% for primary RPLND [35]. The majority of serious intraoperative complications represent visceral injury or bleeding from lumbar veins or the great vessels which may require transfusions or, rarely, open conversion. Pearce et al. reported only two (4.3%) intraoperative complications, one of which was due to an aortic injury requiring open conversion for vascular repair. Conversion rates reported in the literature for L-RPLND are similarly rare (3.7%, range 1–5.4%) [9].

Postoperative complication rates are similarly low for R-RPLND compared to open and laparoscopic approaches. Pearce et al. reported only two Clavien Grade 1 complications and two Clavien Grade 3 complications for a postoperative complication rate of 8.5% [6]. While making direct comparisons is challenging, it appears that postoperative complications for R-RPLND are congruent to large series of L-RPLND and O-RPLND, reporting complication rates of 15.5% [9] and 7–33% [4, 35], respectively. Of note, R-RPLND experienced dramatically fewer instances of postoperative ileus compared to open series (2% versus 18%) [4, 6]. This is likely related to differences in the technique of bowel mobilization. Interestingly, two of four complications reported by Pearce et al. were chylous ascites (4.3%), which is significantly greater than the 0.4%–1.7% rate reported in a primary open series [4, 9, 36]. This complication includes only two patients and may represent a statistical anomaly due to the small cohort size or the early learning curve; however, it cannot be ignored and it warrants further consideration in future R-RPLND series. The rate of chylous ascites for R-RPLND, however, appears to be an improvement over L-RPLND, which has published rates as high as 6.6% [9, 37]. Proponents of R-RPLND believe that the improved dexterity and visualization facilitates superior ligation of lymphatics relative to L-RPLND.

The vast majority of low-stage NSGCT patients should obtain a nerve-sparing procedure to preserve antegrade ejaculation for reducing the morbidity of long-term sexual dysfunction. Pearce et al. reported 100% preservation of antegrade ejaculation [6]. Similar excellent functional outcomes are reported in the smaller R-RPLND series. In a comparative series to L-RPLND, 11% of patients who underwent a laparoscopic procedure experienced ejaculatory dysfunction compared to 0% in the robotic cohort [26]. Cheney et al. also reported a preservation of antegrade ejaculation in 10 of 11 patients [32].

5. Primary RPLND Technique

5.1. Intraoperative Technique. R-RPLND for primary CS I NSGCT involves a transperitoneal approach with the patient typically positioned in the modified flank position with a slightly flexed table. After pneumoperitoneum is achieved with a Veress needle, a 12 mm camera port and three 8 mm robotic ports are placed in a standard linear fashion to triangulate the retroperitoneum. Typically, a 12 mm AirSeal and a 5 mm blunt assistant port are also placed. Others have described a supine or dorsal lithotomy positioning with the patient placed in Trendelenburg and robotic docking occurring over the patient's left shoulder for the daVinci Si or alongside the patient for the daVinci Xi using a four-port linear configuration [23]. A major advantage to supine positioning is a more convenient shift to a bilateral template without repositioning the patient upon either identifying positive LNs on frozen sectioning for primary RPLNDs or in the postchemotherapy setting. A modified node template dissection, including nerve sparing, is performed as previously described [38–40]. A unilateral template may be performed for CS I disease, and a bilateral template is recommended for CS II disease [41]. After reflection of the ipsilateral colon to reveal the retroperitoneum, dissection is performed following boundaries of the renal vein superiorly, the ureter laterally, and the iliac bifurcation inferiorly. The gonadal vein is identified and ligated at the level of its origin, and the remaining portion of the ipsilateral spermatic cord is dissected free from the inguinal ring. For a left-sided template, lymph node packets are removed from the left common iliac nodes, preaortic, paraaortic, and retroaortic areas. Right sided-templates include lymph nodes from the paracaval, interaortocaval, and preaortic spaces. The sympathetic chain and postganglionic nerve fibers are identified and preserved. Hem-o-lok clips are placed on lymph node packets for preventing postoperative lymphatic leak as well as for control of lumbar vessels. Retrocaval and retroaortic lymph node packets can be more challenging to manage and require special consideration to ensure a complete lymph node dissection. Lumbar vessels are ligated using a variety of techniques, including surgical clips, ties, or suture ligation. The dexterity of robotic instruments allows for complete control of the great vessel to ensure dissection of all retrocaval or retroaortic tissue. In addition, the magnified view facilitates nerve dissection and preservation; the camera angle often allows a unique view of retrocaval and retroaortic structures. After hemostasis is achieved, a fibrin sealant may be applied to the lymphatic beds to prevent lymphatic leaks. A drain is typically not placed.

5.2. Postoperative Care. Patients are transferred to the floor where their diet is advanced from clear liquids on the night of surgery to a fat-free regular diet on the day after surgery. It is our practice to follow a low-fat diet that is regularly advanced over four weeks to minimize the risk of chyle leak. There is a paucity of data regarding the efficacy of this approach; however, we have not experienced a chyle leak in our institutional experience with minimally invasive RPLND following this protocol. Patients receive education from a nutritionist regarding a low-fat diet (≤20 g fat/day), which they will continue for 4 weeks postoperatively. Patients are usually discharged home on postoperative day 1 after they are tolerating a regular diet and have successfully ambulated and voided with adequate pain control. Patients usually return to school or work within 2 weeks.

6. Postchemotherapy RPLND

Postchemotherapy RPLND (PC-RPLND) for patients with residual tumors after chemotherapy represents a far more challenging surgery compared to the primary RPLND setting. Desmoplasia from the therapeutic action of chemotherapy can fuse normal tissue planes and add complexity to dissection of tissues and, if needed, repair of vascular injuries. The risk-benefit ratio of cancer cure and morbidity of surgery makes justification of an investigational, minimally invasive technique more challenging. However, select surgeons and centers report perioperative outcomes supporting minimally invasive PC-RPLND as a safe surgery. In addition, perioperative outcomes and complications, including the preservation of antegrade ejaculation, are significantly worse due to the need for a bilateral template and the treatment effect of chemotherapy on the retroperitoneal tissue [3, 4]. Based on the favorable outcomes of L-RPLND in the postchemotherapy setting [42], the natural evolution of the R-RPLND has included attempts by experienced robotic surgeons to perform postchemotherapy R-RPLND (PC-RPLND) in selected patients. To date, only two smaller series have demonstrated early feasibility [12, 32]. The Mayo Clinic R-RPLND experience included nine patients who were postchemotherapy. Notably, their median LNY (18 nodes), blood loss (313 mL), and LOS (2.2 days) were not significantly different from their primary R-RPLND patients; however, their PC-RPLND patients experienced significantly greater operative time (369 mins versus 311 mins, $p = 0.03$). Notably, two patients required open conversion in the postchemotherapy group, which represents a conversion rate of 22.3%. At a median follow-up of 22 months, there were no retroperitoneal recurrences. Kamel et al., in a series of 12 patients, experienced a 91.7% completion rate with only a single open conversion due to what the author considered poor patient selection [12]. It is also worth mentioning that Stepanian et al. included four robotic PC-RPLNDs with no conversions [23]. At a median follow-up of 31 months, there were no recurrences. Currently, the literature on robotic PC-RPLND outcomes is immature and requires larger series before conclusions regarding oncologic and safety performance can be made. From these smaller series, we can conclude that R-RPLND in the postchemotherapy setting is feasible with an understandably higher rate of open conversion. Postchemotherapy RPLND has inherent objectives that are different from the primary RPLND setting, and incomplete control of the retroperitoneum or an incomplete resection during RPLND is a predictor of worse survival in the postchemotherapy setting [43]. Therefore, it is our position that oncologic outcomes remain the priority in the postchemotherapy setting, and oncologic outcomes should not be leveraged against perioperative outcomes. As larger, multi-institutional cohorts are published, we can hopefully better evaluate the merits and technique of a robotic PC-RPLND.

7. Conclusion

The first L-RPLND performed in 1992 and the first R-RPLND performed in 2006 marked the beginnings of a minimally invasive era to reduce the treatment morbidity for testicular cancer survivors. Early results from expert robotic surgeons at high-volume academic institutions have demonstrated both feasibility as well as favorable early oncologic outcomes and complication rates in the primary RPLND setting compared to O-RPLND and L-RPLND. Larger, prospective studies are required to better evaluate long-term oncologic outcomes and complication rates in both the primary and postchemotherapy settings.

References

[1] R. J. Motzer, E. Jonasch, N. Agarwal et al., "Testicular cancer, version 2.2015," *Journal of the National Comprehensive Cancer Network*, vol. 13, no. 6, pp. 772–799, 2015.

[2] C. Cary, T. A. Masterson, R. Bihrle, and R. S. Foster, "Contemporary trends in postchemotherapy retroperitoneal lymph node dissection: additional procedures and perioperative complications," *Urologic Oncology*, vol. 33, no. 9, pp. 389 e15–389 e21, 2015.

[3] L. C. Macleod, S. Rajanahally, J. G. Nayak et al., "Characterizing the morbidity of postchemotherapy retroperitoneal lymph node dissection for testis cancer in a national cohort of privately insured patients," *Urology*, vol. 91, pp. 70–76, 2016.

[4] V. S. Subramanian, C. T. Nguyen, A. J. Stephenson, and E. A. Klein, "Complications of open primary and postchemotherapy retroperitoneal lymph node dissection for testicular cancer," *Urologic Oncology*, vol. 28, no. 5, pp. 504–509, 2010.

[5] S. B. Bhayani, A. Ong, W. K. Oh, P. W. Kantoff, and L. R. Kavoussi, "Laparoscopic retroperitoneal lymph node dissection for clinical stage I nonseminomatous germ cell testicular cancer: a long-term update," *Urology*, vol. 62, no. 2, pp. 324–327, 2003.

[6] S. M. Pearce, "Safety and early oncologic effectiveness of primary robotic retroperitoneal lymph node dissection for nonseminomatous germ cell testicular cancer," *European Urology*, vol. 71, no. 3, pp. 476–482, 2017.

[7] G. S. Gerber, N. K. Bissada, J. C. Hulbert et al., "Laparoscopic retroperitoneal lymphadenectomy: multi-institutional analysis," *Journal of Urology*, vol. 152, no. 4, pp. 1188–1191, 1994.

[8] G. Janetschek, R. Peschel, A. Hobisch, and G. Bartsch, "Laparoscopic retroperitoneal lymph node dissection," *Journal of Endourology*, vol. 15, no. 4, pp. 449–453, 2001.

[9] J. J. Rassweiler, W. Scheitlin, A. Heidenreich, M. P. Laguna, and G. Janetschek, "Laparoscopic retroperitoneal lymph node dissection: does it still have a role in the management of clinical stage I nonseminomatous testis cancer? A European perspective," *European Urology*, vol. 54, no. 5, pp. 1004–1015, 2008.

[10] J. Sheinfeld and T. A. Masterson, "A Laparoscopic approach is best for retroperitoneal lymph node dissection," *Journal of Urology*, vol. 197, no. 6, pp. 1384–1386, 2017.

[11] P. Davol, J. Sumfest, and D. Rukstalis, "Robotic-assisted laparoscopic retroperitoneal lymph node dissection," *Urology*, vol. 67, no. 1, p. 199, 2006.

[12] M. H. Kamel, N. Littlejohn, M. Cox, E. A. Eltahawy, and R. Davis, "Post-chemotherapy robotic retroperitoneal lymph node dissection: institutional experience," *Journal of Endourology*, vol. 30, no. 5, pp. 510–519, 2016.

[13] C. Kollmannsberger, T. Tandstad, P. L. Bedard et al., "Patterns of relapse in patients with clinical stage I testicular cancer managed with active surveillance," *Journal of Clinical Oncology*, vol. 33, no. 1, pp. 51–57, 2015.

[14] T. Tandstad, O. Stahl, U. Hakansson et al., "One course of adjuvant BEP in clinical stage I nonseminoma mature and expanded results from the SWENOTECA group," *Annals of Oncology*, vol. 25, no. 11, pp. 2167–2172, 2014.

[15] H. S. Haugnes, G. J. Bosl, H. Boer et al., "Long-term and late effects of germ cell testicular cancer treatment and implications for follow-up," *Journal of Clinical Oncology*, vol. 30, no. 30, pp. 3752–3763, 2012.

[16] S. D. Fossa, N. Aass, M. Winderen, O. P. Börmer, and D. R. Olsen, "Long-term renal function after treatment for malignant germ-cell tumours," *Annals of Oncology*, vol. 13, no. 2, pp. 222–228, 2002.

[17] R. A. Huddart, A. Norman, M. Shahidi et al., "Cardiovascular disease as a long-term complication of treatment for testicular cancer," *Journal of Clinical Oncology*, vol. 21, no. 8, pp. 1513–1523, 2003.

[18] R. de Wit, "Optimal management of clinical stage I nonseminoma: new data for patients to consider," *Journal of Clinical Oncology*, vol. 32, no. 34, pp. 3792-3793, 2014.

[19] E. B. Fernandez, J. W. Moul, J. P. Foley, E. Colon, and D. G. McLeod, "Retroperitoneal imaging with third and fourth generation computed axial tomography in clinical stage I nonseminomatous germ cell tumors," *Urology*, vol. 44, no. 4, pp. 548–552, 1994.

[20] A. J. Stephenson, G. J. Bosl, R. J. Motzer et al., "Retroperitoneal lymph node dissection for nonseminomatous germ cell testicular cancer: impact of patient selection factors on outcome," *Journal of Clinical Oncology*, vol. 23, no. 12, pp. 2781–2788, 2005.

[21] A. J. Stephenson and J. Sheinfeld, "The role of retroperitoneal lymph node dissection in the management of testicular cancer," *Urologic Oncology*, vol. 22, no. 3, pp. 225–233, 2004.

[22] P. Albers, R. Siener, S. Krege et al., "Randomized phase III trial comparing retroperitoneal lymph node dissection with one course of bleomycin and etoposide plus cisplatin chemotherapy in the adjuvant treatment of clinical stage I Nonseminomatous testicular germ cell tumors: AUO trial AH 01/94 by the German Testicular Cancer Study Group," *Journal of Clinical Oncology*, vol. 26, no. 18, pp. 2966–2972, 2008.

[23] S. Stepanian, M. Patel, and J. Porter, "Robot-assisted laparoscopic retroperitoneal lymph node dissection for testicular cancer: evolution of the technique," *European Urology*, vol. 70, no. 4, pp. 661–667, 2016.

[24] K. F. Abdel-Aziz, J. K. Anderson, R. Svatek, V. Margulis, A. I. Sagalowsky, and J. A. Cadeddu, "Laparoscopic and open retroperitoneal lymph-node dissection for clinical stage I nonseminomatous germ-cell testis tumors," *Journal of Endourology*, vol. 20, no. 9, pp. 627–631, 2006.

[25] M. Nayan, M. A. S. Jewett, J. Sweet et al., "Lymph node yield in primary retroperitoneal lymph node dissection for non-seminoma germ cell tumors," *Journal of Urology*, vol. 194, no. 2, pp. 386–391, 2015.

[26] K. T. Harris, M. A. Gorin, M. W. Ball, P. M. Pierorazio, and M. E. Allaf, "A comparative analysis of robotic vs laparoscopic retroperitoneal lymph node dissection for testicular cancer," *BJU International*, vol. 116, no. 6, pp. 920–923, 2015.

[27] H. Y. Yu, N. D. Hevelone, S. Patel, S. R. Lipsitz, and J. C. Hu, "Hospital surgical volume, utilization, costs and outcomes of retroperitoneal lymph node dissection for testis cancer," *Advances in Urology*, vol. 2012, Article ID 189823, 8 pages, 2012.

[28] V. Ficarra, G. Novara, W. Artibani et al., "Retropubic, laparoscopic, and robot-assisted radical prostatectomy: a systematic review and cumulative analysis of comparative studies," *European Urology*, vol. 55, no. 5, pp. 1037–1063, 2009.

[29] S. B. Williams, D. W. McDermott, D. Winston et al., "Morbidity of open retroperitoneal lymph node dissection for testicular cancer: contemporary perioperative data," *BJU International*, vol. 105, no. 7, pp. 918–921, 2010.

[30] S. D. Beck, M. D. Peterson, R. Bihrle, J. P. Donohue, and R. S. Foster, "Short-term morbidity of primary retroperitoneal lymph node dissection in a contemporary group of patients," *Journal of Urology*, vol. 178, no. 2, pp. 504–506, 2007.

[31] S. Syan-Bhanvadia, S. T. Bazargani, T. G. Clifford, J. Cai, G. Miranda, and S. Daneshmand, "Midline extraperitoneal approach to retroperitoneal lymph node dissection in testicular cancer: minimizing surgical morbidity," *European Urology*, vol. 72, no. 5, pp. 814–820, 2017.

[32] S. M. Cheney, P. E. Andrews, B. C. Leibovich, and E. P. Castle, "Robot-assisted retroperitoneal lymph node dissection: technique and initial case series of 18 patients," *BJU International*, vol. 115, no. 1, pp. 114–120, 2015.

[33] R. E. Link, M. E. Allaf, R. Pili, and L. R. Kavoussi, "Modeling the cost of management options for stage I nonseminomatous germ cell tumors: a decision tree analysis," *Journal of Clinical Oncology*, vol. 23, no. 24, pp. 5762–5773, 2005.

[34] M. Kates, M. W. Ball, H. D. Patel et al., "The financial impact of robotic technology for partial and radical nephrectomy," *Journal of Endourology*, vol. 29, no. 3, pp. 317–322, 2015.

[35] V. Poulakis, K. Skriapas, R. de Vries et al., "Quality of life after laparoscopic and open retroperitoneal lymph node dissection in clinical Stage I nonseminomatous germ cell tumor: a comparison study," *Urology*, vol. 68, no. 1, pp. 154–160, 2006.

[36] P. A. Kenney and I. A. Tuerk, "Complications of laparoscopic retroperitoneal lymph node dissection in testicular cancer," *World Journal of Urology*, vol. 26, no. 6, pp. 561–569, 2008.

[37] M. Neyer, R. Peschel, T. Akkad et al., "Long-term results of laparoscopic retroperitoneal lymph-node dissection for clinical stage I nonseminomatous germ-cell testicular cancer," *Journal of Endourology*, vol. 21, no. 2, pp. 180–183, 2007.

[38] J. P. Donohue, J. A. Thornhill, R. S. Foster, R. G. Rowland, and R. Bihrle, "Retroperitoneal lymphadenectomy for clinical stage A testis cancer (1965 to 1989): modifications of technique and impact on ejaculation," *Journal of Urology*, vol. 149, no. 2, pp. 237–243, 1993.

[39] G. Janetschek, A. Reissigl, R. Peschel, A. Hobisch, and G. Bartsch, "Laparoscopic retroperitoneal lymph node dissection for clinical stage I nonseminomatous testicular tumor," *Urology*, vol. 44, no. 3, pp. 382–391, 1994.

[40] L. Weissbach and E. A. Boedefeld, "Localization of solitary and multiple metastases in stage II nonseminomatous testis tumor as basis for a modified staging lymph node dissection in stage I," *Journal of Urology*, vol. 138, no. 1, pp. 77–82, 1987.

[41] A. J. Stephenson and E. A. Klein, "Surgical management of low-stage nonseminomatous germ cell testicular cancer," *BJU International*, vol. 104, no. 9, pp. 1362–1368, 2009.

[42] H. Steiner, N. Leonhartsberger, B. Stoehr, R. Peschel, and R. Pichler, "Postchemotherapy laparoscopic retroperitoneal lymph node dissection for low-volume, stage II, nonseminomatous germ cell tumor: first 100 patients," *European Urology*, vol. 63, no. 6, pp. 1013–1017, 2013.

[43] B. S. Carver, B. Shayegan, S. Eggener et al., "Incidence of metastatic nonseminomatous germ cell tumor outside the boundaries of a modified postchemotherapy retroperitoneal lymph node dissection," *Journal of Clinical Oncology*, vol. 25, no. 28, pp. 4365–4369, 2007.

2

Congenital Bladder and Urethral Agenesis: Two Case Reports and Management

Salahaddin Delshad,[1,2] **Hadith Rastad,**[3] **and Parham Mardi**[4]

[1]*Department of Pediatric Surgery, School of Medicine, Iran University of Medical Sciences, Tehran, Iran*
[2]*Department of Pediatric Surgery, Maryam Hospital, Karaj, Iran*
[3]*Non-Communicable Diseases Research Center, Alborz University of Medical Sciences, Karaj, Iran*
[4]*Student Research Committee, Alborz University of Medical Sciences, Karaj, Iran*

Correspondence should be addressed to Salahaddin Delshad; salaheddin.delshad1@gmail.com

Academic Editor: Miroslav Djordjevic

Background. Agenesis of the bladder and urethra is a rare congenital anomaly, with a very few living cases reported in the literature so far. *Case Presentation.* We are reporting two female patients (3 and 6 years old) with bladder and urethral agenesis who presented with urinary incontinence. In both patients, magnetic resonant imaging (MRI) revealed a case of bladder and urethral agenesis with normal ureters draining into the vagina. Patients underwent a neobladder and conduit creation surgery. The neobladder was constructed from the whole cecum and a part of the ascending colon, followed by an anastomose of the ureters into the neobladder in a nonrefluxing fashion; the appendix was used simultaneously as a continent catheterizable conduit. The two patients attained urinary continence postoperatively. *Conclusion.* We reported two cases of bladder agenesis, and for the first time, we have performed neobladder creation surgery using the cecum and ascending colon. One-year follow-up did not reveal any complications.

1. Background

While urological anomalies are among the most common congenital defects [1], bladder agenesis is an extremely rare congenital anomaly, with approximately 74 cases described with only 25 cases of live birth reported in the literature written in English until 2020 [2]. The live-birth patients are often diagnosed in infancy or early childhood, presenting with other anomalies, urinary incontinence, and recurrent urinary tract infection (UTI) [3]. Here, we have reported two cases of bladder and urethral agenesis with the bilateral ectopic ureteral opening into the vagina.

2. Case Presentation

2.1. Case 1. A 3-year-old girl with a history of urinary incontinence, fecal incontinence, and imperforated anus who previously underwent colostomy was referred to our clinic for possible surgical correction. She is the only child in the family of nonconsanguineous parents and was born full-term with spontaneous vaginal delivery and normal birth weight. The mother's age was 25 years at the time of pregnancy.

Physical examination of the external genitalia demonstrated the normal appearance of the vulva, and ureteral orifices were not visible in the vagina, but we noted vaginal leakage of urine. Routine blood tests, including serum creatinine and urine tests, were normal. The absence of the bladder was noted on genitourinary ultrasonography. For further examination, IVP with contrast was performed, showing bilateral ectopic ureters opening directly into the vagina in the absence of the urinary bladder and urethra (Figure 1). MRI confirmed our diagnosis of bladder agenesis. It also identified a hypoplastic sacrum. Initially, the patient underwent a successful anorectoplasty after performing an EMG showing a normal functioning anal sphincter. One month later, colostomy was closed, and the patient achieved fecal continence despite having severe hypoplasia of the sacrum. After 14 months, when the patient was four years old, she underwent a successful neobladder and continent catheterizable stoma creation surgery. The stoma opens to the abdominal wall superior to the left anterior superior iliac spine. After surgery, the patient had both fecal and urinary continence.

2.2. Case 2. A 6-year-old girl with a history of urinary incontinence came to our clinic. The patient was fecal continent. She was born full-term with normal vaginal delivery of nonrelated parents and had two other healthy siblings. The external genitalia was normal on physical examination. At presentation, serum creatinine, blood urea nitrogen, and urea analysis tests were all normal. Bladder and urethral agenesis with bilateral ectopic ureters opening into the vagina was detected on IVP with contrast followed by abdominal and pelvic MRI. She had no other congenital anomalies. She underwent a successful creation of a neobladder when she was six years old, using the whole cecum, a part of the ascending colon, and a continent catheterizable stoma that opens to the abdominal wall superior to the anterior superior iliac spine. After surgery, the patient had both fecal and urinary continence.

2.3. Surgical Procedure. In both cases, we opted for a single-stage definitive method of procedure as explained below.

Initially, the cecum and ascending colon were investigated using barium enema to detect any abnormalities. The volume of an absent vesicle was estimated at 300 mL. The reservoir will expand with time. The whole cecum and a part of the ascending colon were dissected off to make a urinary reservoir (neobladder), and the appendix was dissected with careful preservation of mesentery and blood vessels and used as a conduit. The tip of the appendix was anastomosed to the taeniae coli of the cecum by a flap-valve antireflux mechanism (Figure 2). The base was opened to the skin at RLQ; a catheter was passed into the conduit. Ureters were dissected from the vagina and attached by an antireflux mechanism (Figure 3). Then, two catheters were inserted into the ureters passing from the skin through an abdominal orifice 3 cm superior to the iliac crest. The neobladder was fixed posterior to the pubic bone. About 300 mL of normal saline was passed through the conduit after closing catheters of ureters to check for leakage.

At postoperative follow-up, both patients' urine analysis only showed RBC cast until day five after surgery. On day 7, ureter catheters were removed. Finally, contrast radiography did not detect any leakage or reflux, and patients were discharged on the eighth postoperative day, while the two patients attained urinary continence. Patients' parents were trained to drain the bladder using a catheter, at least eight times a day (intermittent self-catheterization). Patients were followed up for a year after surgery. In the following year after surgery, the patient was followed up by multiple contrast radiography and did not show any signs of stricture or prolapse. No other complications, such as UTI, were observed. The patients' parents did not give consent to scintigraphy.

3. Discussion

We presented two rare cases of bladder agenesis and ureteral opening into the vagina. Our cases both underwent successful neobladder creation.

Bladder agenesis is life noncompatible in the case of ureter obstruction. In live-birth cases like our cases, drainage of urine to the amniotic fluid through ectopic ureters preserves the renal function during the fetal period. [4] However, these patients will suffer from urinary incontinence after birth.

The etiology of bladder agenesis is unclear. In patients with bladder agenesis and hindgut abnormalities, as seen in our first case, the abnormal division of the cloaca is a more probable hypothesis rather than other raised hypotheses such as a primary developmental failure or secondary atrophy of the urogenital sinus [5]. Diagnosis of bladder agenesis is challenging. In order to diagnose bladder agenesis, it is essential to verify clinical findings and physical examinations with imaging studies. In this case, we have used both IVP with contrast and MRI. Although MRI is more informative for the diagnosis, IVP findings are necessary for the planning of the surgery [6].

The management of bladder agenesis is based on the severity and extent of the anomaly; previous literature has reported additional considerations and different adjunctive procedures in the management course due to a variety of concomitant anomalies [7].

Urinary reconstruction for bladder agenesis is accomplished by urinary diversions, such as ureterosigmoidostomy, stoma of ureters to the skin, or umbilicus [8]. The complications such as ureter necrosis, urinary incontinence, skin irritation, and ascites were frequent in these procedures. Although in this procedure the ileocecal valve is removed and hydroelectrolytic loss and malnutrition are expected, none of our patients shows gastrointestinal or malnutrition signs.

In both cases, we made a neobladder from the whole cecum and a part of the ascending colon, followed by anastomose of ureters into a neobladder using an antireflux mechanism. Then, we implanted the appendix as a catheterizable conduit into the urinary reservoir in a nonrefluxing mechanism. There is a controversy in the literature over the outcome of the antireflux mechanism. The antireflux mechanism showed a lower risk of pyelonephritis and bacteriuria [9, 10] but higher risk of the stone formation and stricture [11]. However, one randomized trial showed no difference between refluxing or antireflux anastomosis in terms of renal outcomes [12].

During the literature review, we found few other publications that addressed lower urinary tract reconstruction and attained continence in patients with bladder agenesis; Kasat et al. [3] managed a case of a five-year-old child with bladder agenesis and ectopic ureter opening into the vestibule using a continent ileocecal pouch (Penn pouch) with the Mitrofanoff principle [3].

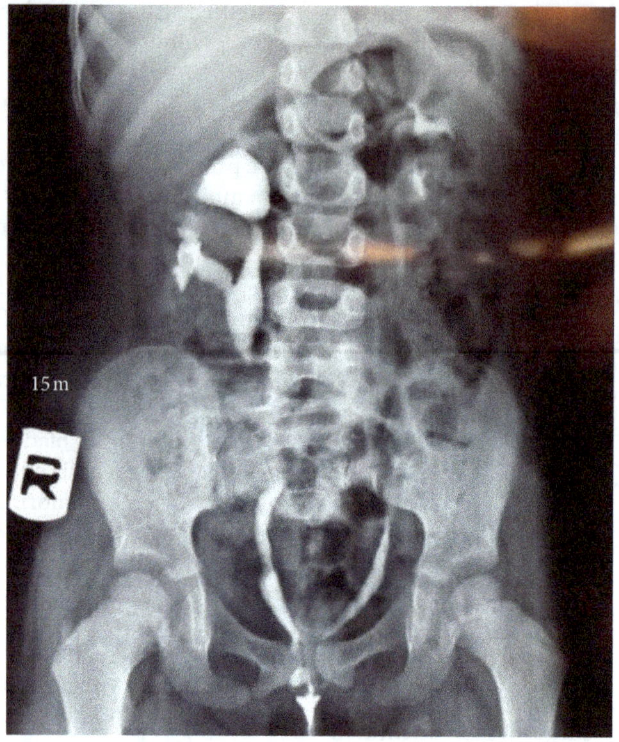

FIGURE 1: IVP with contrast showing agenesis of the bladder and ureters opening to the vagina.

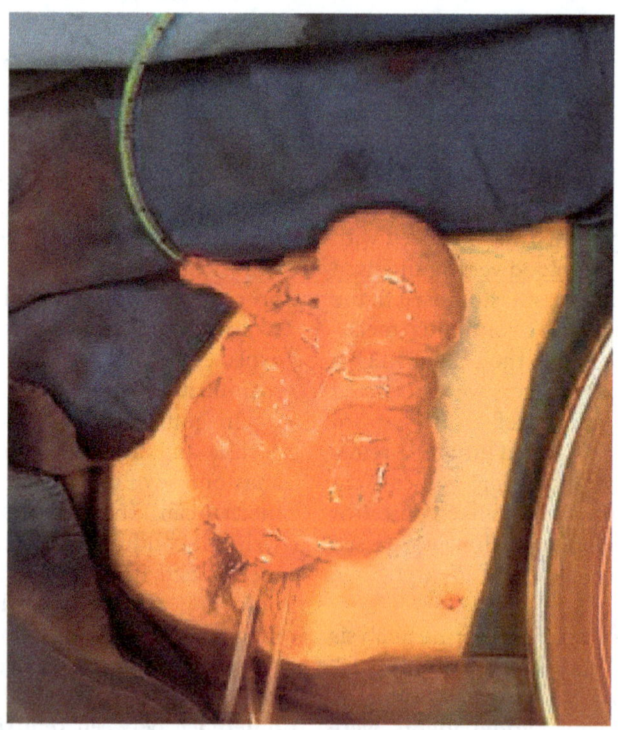

FIGURE 2: Normal saline passing through the conduit (appendix) after closing catheters of ureters.

More recently, Nazim and Zaidi [13] for an eight-year-old girl with a triad of complete agenesis of the bladder and urethra, solitary functioning left kidney, and an ectopic ureter opening into the vagina used both the sigmoid colon and ileum to made an orthotopic urinary reservoir, and the appendix was used as a catheterizable Mitrofanoff stoma [13].

Indiana pouch surgery is another option in these patients. In this procedure, the reservoir is created out of the ascending colon and the ileum. As ileum has a considerable amount of mucus secretion, electrolyte imbalances are expected in Indiana pouch surgery. Theoretically, using the ascending colon and cecum is associated with a lower risk of electrolyte imbalances [14].

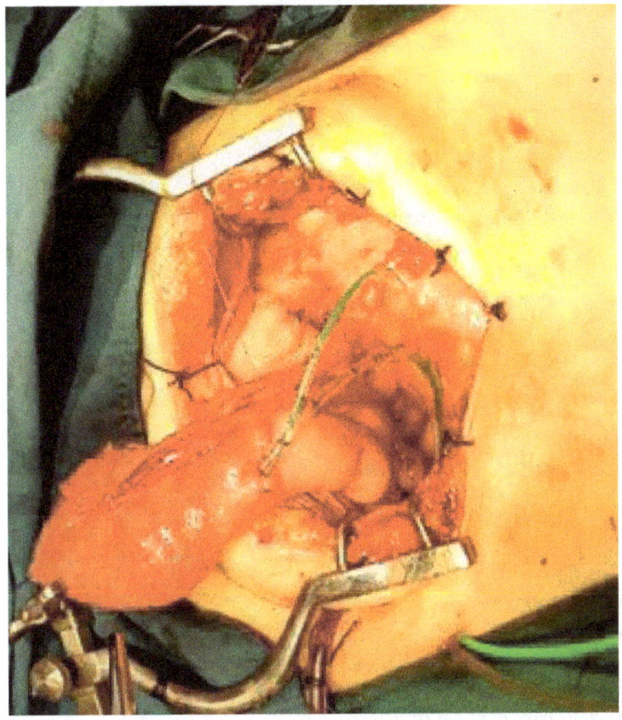

Figure 3: Neobladder creation surgery using the cecum and a part of the ascending colon.

The advantages of the urinary continent and antireflux mechanisms inherent to this procedure have been well documented. The use of the appendix as the continent catheterizable conduit is common in the treatment of patients who need lower urinary reconstruction due to its availability and independent blood supply [15].

4. Conclusion

Urinary bladder agenesis is a very rare congenital condition that is associated with multiple anomalies. It should be considered in patients with unexplained or atypical UTIs because early diagnosis and neobladder creation surgery can prevent or delay the progression to chronic kidney disease. We discussed two successful neobladder creation with the attainment of urinary continence in our patients with bladder agenesis.

Abbreviations

UTI: Urinary tract infection
IVP: Intravenous pyelogram
MRI: Magnetic resonance imaging
EMG: Electromyography
RLQ: Right lower quadrant (of the abdomen)
RBC: Red blood cells
CCC: Continent catheterizable conduit.

Ethical Approval

The present case reports were confirmed by the Alborz University of Medical Science's ethical committee (IR.ABZUMS.REC.1398.081) (June 13, 2019).

Consent

Detailed written informed consent was obtained from the parents. A copy is provided to the journal.

Authors' Contributions

SD did the surgical interventions, reviewed surgical aspects, and participated in preparing the manuscript. PM and HR substantially drafted the manuscript and revised it critically. All authors read and approved the final version of the manuscript.

Acknowledgments

The authors thank the parents of the patients for permitting them to use the medical information for this publication.

References

[1] S. Moorthie, H. Blencowe, H. Blencowe et al., "Estimating the birth prevalence and pregnancy outcomes of congenital

malformations worldwide," *Journal of Community Genetics*, vol. 9, no. 4, pp. 387–396, 2018.
[2] V. Indiran, K. Chokkappan, and E. Gunaseelan, "Rare case of urinary bladder agenesis-Multislice CT abdomen imaging," *Journal of Radiology Case Reports*, vol. 7, no. 2, pp. 44–49, 2013.
[3] L. S. Kasat, S. S. Borwankar, A. Naregal, M. Jain, R. P. Sakalkale, and R. Bajaj, "Bladder agenesis with urometrocolpos," *Pediatric Surgery International*, vol. 15, no. 5-6, pp. 415-416, 1999.
[4] M. A. Fahmy, "Urinary bladder," in *Rare Congenital Genitourinary Anomalies*, pp. 85–104, Springer Berlin Heidelberg, Heidelberg, Germany, 2015.
[5] C. L. Krull, C. F. Heyns, and D. P. Klerk, "Agenesis of the bladder and urethra: a case report," *Journal of Urology*, vol. 140, no. 4, pp. 793-794, 1988.
[6] C. E. Bayne and C. A. Peters, "Congenital infundibulopelvic stenosis: indications for intervention, surgical technique, and review of literature," *Journal of Pediatric Urology*, vol. 12, no. 6, pp. 389.e1–389.e5, 2016.
[7] K. Sarica and S. Küpeli, "Agenesis of bladder associated with multiple organ anomalies," *International Urology and Nephrology*, vol. 27, no. 6, pp. 697–703, 1995.
[8] S. C. Gopal, A. N. Gangopadhyay, S. P. Sharma, and S. K. Pandit, "Membranous atresia of the lower oesophagus," *Pediatric Surgery International*, vol. 8, no. 2, pp. 140-141, 1993.
[9] A. Kristjansson, H. Abol-Enein MD, P. Alm et al., "Long-term renal morphology and function following enterocystoplasty (refluxing or anti-reflux anastomosis): an experimental study," *BJU International*, vol. 78, no. 6, pp. 840–846, 1996.
[10] A. Minervini, G. Boni, G. Salinitri, G. Mariani, and R. Minervini, "Evaluation of renal function and upper urinary tract morphology in the ileal orthotopic neobladder with no antireflux mechanism," *Journal of Urology*, vol. 173, no. 1, pp. 144–147, 2005.
[11] A. A. Shaaban, M. Abdel-latif, A. Mosbah et al., "A randomized study comparing an antireflux system with a direct ureteric anastomosis in patients with orthotopic ileal neobladders," *BJU International*, vol. 97, no. 5, pp. 1057–1062, 2006.
[12] A. Kristjánsson, L. Wallin, and W. Månsson, "Renal function up to 16 years after conduit (refluxing or anti-reflux anastomosis) or continent urinary diversion. 1. Glomerular filtration rate and patency of uretero-intestinal anastomosis," *British Journal of Urology*, vol. 76, no. 5, pp. 539–545, 1995.
[13] S. M. Nazim and Z. Zaidi, "Bilateral ectopic ureters with bladder agenesis," *JPMA. The Journal of the Pakistan Medical Association*, vol. 62, no. 10, pp. 1086–1089, 2012.
[14] D. G. Holmes, J. B. Thrasher, G. Y. Park, D. C. Kueker, and J. W. Weigel, "Long-term complications related to the modified Indiana pouch," *Urology*, vol. 60, no. 4, pp. 603–606, 2002.
[15] H. F. McAndrew and P. S. Malone, "Continent catheterizable conduits: which stoma, which conduit and which reservoir?" *BJU International*, vol. 89, no. 1, pp. 86–89, 2002.

3

Kidney Stone Disease: An Update on Current Concepts

Tilahun Alelign[1,2] and Beyene Petros[1]

[1]Department of Microbial, Cellular and Molecular Biology, College of Natural Sciences, Addis Ababa University, P.O. Box 1176, Addis Ababa, Ethiopia
[2]Department of Biology, Debre Birhan University, P.O. Box 445, Debre Birhan, Ethiopia

Correspondence should be addressed to Tilahun Alelign; tilalewa@gmail.com

Academic Editor: Mohammad H. Ather

Kidney stone disease is a crystal concretion formed usually within the kidneys. It is an increasing urological disorder of human health, affecting about 12% of the world population. It has been associated with an increased risk of end-stage renal failure. The etiology of kidney stone is multifactorial. The most common type of kidney stone is calcium oxalate formed at Randall's plaque on the renal papillary surfaces. The mechanism of stone formation is a complex process which results from several physicochemical events including supersaturation, nucleation, growth, aggregation, and retention of urinary stone constituents within tubular cells. These steps are modulated by an imbalance between factors that promote or inhibit urinary crystallization. It is also noted that cellular injury promotes retention of particles on renal papillary surfaces. The exposure of renal epithelial cells to oxalate causes a signaling cascade which leads to apoptosis by p38 mitogen-activated protein kinase pathways. Currently, there is no satisfactory drug to cure and/or prevent kidney stone recurrences. Thus, further understanding of the pathophysiology of kidney stone formation is a research area to manage urolithiasis using new drugs. Therefore, this review has intended to provide a compiled up-to-date information on kidney stone etiology, pathogenesis, and prevention approaches.

1. Introduction

1.1. Overview of Kidney Stones. Kidney stones are mainly lodged in the kidney(s) [1]. Mankind has been afflicted by urinary stones since centuries dating back to 4000 B.C. [2], and it is the most common disease of the urinary tract. The prevention of renal stone recurrence remains to be a serious problem in human health [3]. The prevention of stone recurrence requires better understanding of the mechanisms involved in stone formation [4]. Kidney stones have been associated with an increased risk of chronic kidney diseases [5], end-stage renal failure [3, 6], cardiovascular diseases [7, 8], diabetes, and hypertension [9]. It has been suggested that kidney stone may be a systemic disorder linked to the metabolic syndrome. Nephrolithiasis is responsible for 2 to 3% of end-stage renal cases if it is associated with nephrocalcinosis [10].

The symptoms of kidney stone are related to their location whether it is in the kidney, ureter, or urinary bladder [11]. Initially, stone formation does not cause any symptom. Later, signs and symptoms of the stone disease consist of renal colic (intense cramping pain), flank pain (pain in the back side), hematuria (bloody urine), obstructive uropathy (urinary tract disease), urinary tract infections, blockage of urine flow, and hydronephrosis (dilation of the kidney). These conditions may result in nausea and vomiting with associated suffering from the stone event [12]. Thus, the treatment and time lost from work involves substantial cost imposing an impact on the quality of life and nation's economy.

1.2. Epidemiology of Kidney Stones. Globally, kidney stone disease prevalence and recurrence rates are increasing [13], with limited options of effective drugs. Urolithiasis affects about 12% of the world population at some stage in their lifetime [14]. It affects all ages, sexes, and races [15, 16] but occurs more frequently in men than in women within the age of 20–49 years [17]. If patients do not apply metaphylaxis, the

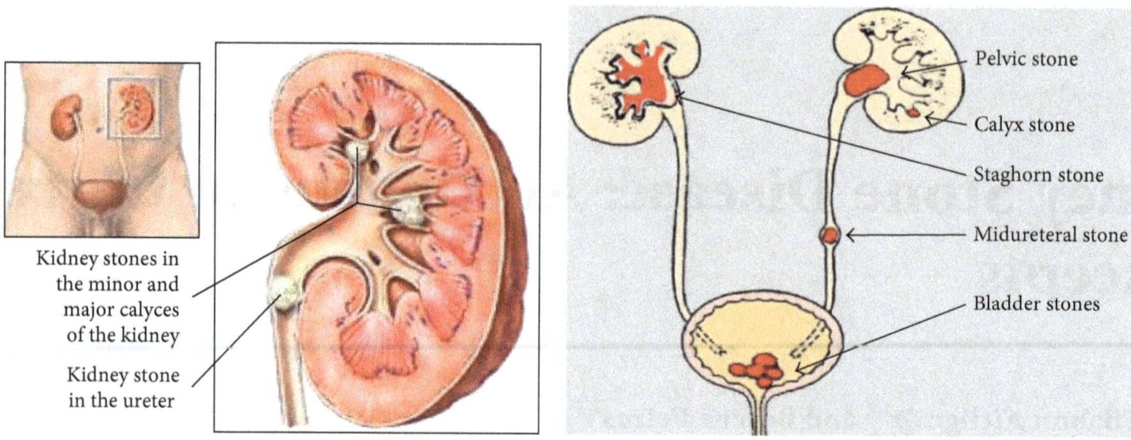

(a) (b)

FIGURE 1: Kidney stone locations in the urinary system. (a) Adopted from [25]. (b) Adopted from [26].

relapsing rate of secondary stone formations is estimated to be 10–23% per year, 50% in 5–10 years, and 75% in 20 years of the patient [15]. However, lifetime recurrence rate is higher in males, although the incidence of nephrolithiasis is growing among females [18]. Therefore, prophylactic management is of great importance to manage urolithiasis.

Recent studies have reported that the prevalence of urolithiasis has been increasing in the past decades in both developed and developing countries. This growing trend is believed to be associated with changes in lifestyle modifications such as lack of physical activity and dietary habits [19–21] and global warming [16]. In the United States, kidney stone affects 1 in 11 people [22], and it is estimated that 600,000 Americans suffer from urinary stones every year. In Indian population, about 12% of them are expected to have urinary stones and out of which 50% may end up with loss of kidney functions [23].

2. The Urinary System and Stones

The urinary filtrate is formed in the glomerulus and passes into the tubules where the volume and content are altered by reabsorption or secretions. Most solute reabsorption occurs in the proximal tubules, whereas fine adjustments to urine composition take place in the distal tubule and collecting ducts. The loop of Henle serves to concentrate urine composed of 95% water, 2.5% urea, 2.5% mixture of minerals, salts, hormones, and enzymes. In the proximal tubules, glucose, sodium, chloride, and water are reabsorbed and returned to the blood stream along with essential nutrients such as amino acids, proteins, bicarbonate, calcium, phosphate, and potassium. In the distal tubule, the salt and acid-base balance of blood is regulated [24]. The location of stones may vary as indicated in Figure 1.

3. Types of Kidney Stones

The chemical composition of kidney stones depends on the abnormalities in urine composition of various chemicals. Stones differ in size, shape, and chemical compositions (mineralogy) [27]. Based on variations in mineral composition and pathogenesis, kidney stones are commonly classified into five types as follows [28].

3.1. Calcium Stones: Calcium Oxalate and Calcium Phosphate. Calcium stones are predominant renal stones comprising about 80% of all urinary calculi [29]. The proportion of calcium stones may account for pure calcium oxalate (CaOx) (50%), calcium phosphate (CaP, termed as apatite) (5%), and a mixture of both (45%) [30]. The main constituent of calcium stones is brushite (calcium hydrogen phosphate) or hydroxyapatite [31, 32]. Calcium oxalate is found in the majority of kidney stones and exists in the form of CaOx monohydrate (COM, termed as mineral names: whewellite, $CaC_2O_4{\cdot}H_2O$), and CaOx dihydrate (COD, weddellite, $CaC_2O_4{\cdot}2H_2O$), or as a combination of both which accounts for greater than 60% [33]. COM is the most thermodynamically stable form of stone. COM is more frequently observed than COD in clinical stones [34].

Many factors contribute to CaOx stone formation such as hypercalciuria (resorptive, renal leak, absorptive, and metabolic diseases), hyperuricosuria, hyperoxaluria, hypocitraturia, hypomagnesuria, and hypercystinuria [35]. Mostly, urinary pH of 5.0 to 6.5 promotes CaOx stones [36], whereas calcium phosphate stones occur when pH is greater than 7.5 [11]. The recurrence of calcium stone is greater than other types of kidney stones.

3.2. Struvite or Magnesium Ammonium Phosphate Stones. Struvite stones occur to the extent of 10–15% and have also been referred to as infection stones and triple phosphate stones. It occurs among patients with chronic urinary tract infections that produce urease, the most common being *Proteus mirabilis* and less common pathogens include *Klebsiella pneumonia*, *Pseudomonas aeruginosa*, and *Enterobacter* [1, 28, 29]. Urease is necessary to split/cleave urea to ammonia and CO_2, making urine more alkaline which elevates pH (typically > 7). Phosphate is less soluble at alkaline versus acidic pH, so phosphate precipitates on to the insoluble ammonium products, yielding to a large staghorn stone formation [37]. Women's are likely to develop this type of stone than the male. *Escherichia coli* is not capable of splitting urea and is not associated with struvite stones [38].

3.3. Uric Acid Stones or Urate. This accounts approximately for 3–10% of all stone types [1, 29]. Diets high in purines especially those containing animal protein diet such as meat and fish, results in hyperuricosuria, low urine volume, and low urinary pH ($pH < 5.05$) exacerbates uric acid stone formation [11, 28, 39]. Peoples with gouty arthritis may form stones in the kidney(s). The most prevalent cause of uric acid nephrolithiasis is idiopathic [38], and uric acid stones are more common in men than in women.

3.4. Cystine Stones. These stones comprise less than 2% of all stone types. It is a genetic disorder of the transport of an amino acid and cystine. It results in an excess of cystinuria in urinary excretions [1, 29], which is an autosomal recessive disorder caused by a defect in the rBAT gene on chromosome 2 [40], resulting in impaired renal tubular absorption of cystine or leaking cystine into urine. It does not dissolve in urine and leads to cystine stone formation [11]. People who are homozygous for cystinuria excrete more than 600 millimole insoluble cystine per day [28]. The development of urinary cystine is the only clinical manifestation of this cystine stone disease [40].

3.5. Drug-Induced Stones. This accounts for about 1% of all stone types [1]. Drugs such as guaifenesin, triamterene, atazanavir, and sulfa drugs induce these stones. For instance, people who take the protease inhibitor indinavir sulphate, a drug used to treat HIV infection, are at risk of developing kidney stones [28]. Such lithogenic drugs or its metabolites may deposit to form a nidus or on renal calculi already present. On the other hand, these drugs may induce the formation of calculi through its metabolic action by interfering with calcium oxalate or purine metabolisms [38].

4. Kidney Stone Compositions

The chemical compositions of urinary stones include crystals and noncrystalline phases or the organic material (the matrix). The organic matrix of urinary stones consists of macromolecules such as glycosaminoglycans (GAG's), lipids, carbohydrates, and proteins. These molecules play a significant role by promoting or inhibiting the processes of kidney stone development (Table 1). The main components of the stone matrix are proteins (64%), nonamino sugars (9.6%), hexosamine as glucosamine (5%), water (10%), and inorganic ash (10.4%). The matrix acts as a template participating in the assembly of kidney stones. The matrix of all stones contains phospholipids (8.6%) of the total lipid, which in turn represents about 10.3% of stone matrix. Cell membrane phospholipids, as part of organic matrix, promote the formation of calcium oxalate and calcium phosphate stones [41]. Albumin is the major component of the matrix of all stone types [42].

Brushite stone is a hard phosphate mineral with an increasing incidence rate, and a quarter of calcium phosphate (CaP) patients form stones containing brushite [43]. In the urinary tract, CaP may be present in the form of hydroxyapatite, carbonate apatite, or brushite (calcium monohydrogen phosphate dihydrate, $CaHPO4{\cdot}2H2O$). Brushite is resistant to shock wave and ultrasonic lithotripsy treatment [44].

4.1. Etiology of Kidney Stones. Formation of kidney stones (calculogenesis) is a complex and multifactorial process including intrinsic (such as age, sex, and heredity) and extrinsic factors such as geography, climate, dietary, mineral composition, and water intake [15]. A summary of possible causes of kidney stone formation is shown in Table 2.

5. Mechanisms of Renal Stone Formation

The pathogenesis of kidney stone or biomineralization is a complex biochemical process which remains incompletely understood [41]. Renal stone formation is a biological process that involves physicochemical changes and supersaturation of urine. Supersaturated solution refers to a solution that contains more of dissolved material than could be dissolved by the solvent under normal circumstances [34]. As a result of supersaturation, solutes precipitate in urine leads to nucleation and then crystal concretions are formed. That is, crystallization occurs when the concentration of two ions exceeds their saturation point in the solution [55]. The transformation of a liquid to a solid phase is influenced by pH and specific concentrations of excess substances. The level of urinary saturation with respect to the stone-forming constituents like calcium, phosphorus, uric acid, oxalate, cystine, and low urine volume are risk factors for crystallization [1, 56]. Thus, crystallization process depends on the thermodynamics (that leads to nucleation) and kinetics (which comprises the rates of nucleation or crystal growth) of a supersaturated solution [57]. Therefore, lithiasis can be prevented by avoiding supersaturation.

However, it should be noted that stone formation is usually dependent on the level of imbalance between urinary inhibitors and promoters of crystallization. All stones share similar events with respect to the mineral phase of stone formation. But, the sequence of events leading to stone formation differs depending on the type of stone and urine chemistry. For instance, crystallization of calcium-based stones (calcium oxalate or calcium phosphate) occurs in supersaturated urine if it is with low concentrations of inhibitors. Uric acid interferes the solubility of calcium oxalate and promotes CaOx stone formation. In healthy controls, crystallization process is opposed by inhibitory substances and gets safe [1]. The sequence of events that trigger stone formation includes nucleation, growth, aggregation, and retention of crystals within the kidneys [27, 58].

5.1. Crystal Nucleation. The first step in the formation of kidney stone begins by the formation of nucleus (termed as nidus) from supersaturated urine retained inside the kidneys [11, 42]. In a supersaturated liquid, free atoms, ions, or molecules start forming microscopic clusters that precipitate

Table 1: Urinary stone matrix protein modulators of crystallization in nephrolithiasis [34, 41].

Serial Number	Name of protein	Role in crystallization			
		Nucleation	Growth	Aggregation	Cell adherence
1	Nephrocalcin (NC)	I	I	I	—
2	Tamm–Horsfall protein (THP)	P	—	I/P	—
3	Osteopontin/uropontin (OPN)	I	I	I	I/P
4	Albumin	P	—	I	—
5	Urinary prothrombin fragment-1 (UPTF1)	I	I	I	—
6	Alpha-1-microglobulin	—	—	I	—
7	S100A	—	I	I	—
8	Inter-alpha-inhibitor	I	I	I	I
9	Bikunin	I	I	I	I
10	Renal lithostathine	—	I	—	—
11	Alpha defensin	—	P	P	—
12	Human phosphatecytidylyl transferase 1, choline, beta	—	I	—	—
13	Myeloperoxidase	—	P	P	—
14	Nucleolin	—	—	—	P
15	Histone-lysine N methyltransferase	—	I	I	—
16	Inward rectifier K channel	—	I	I	—
17	Protein Wnt-2	—	I	I	—
18	Alpha-2HS glycoprotein	P	I	—	—
19	Crystal adhesion inhibitor (CAI)	—	—	—	I
20	Hyaluronic acid (HA)	—	—	—	P
21	Chondroitin sulphate	—	I	I	—
22	Heparin sulphate (HS)	—	I	—	—
23	Human urinary trefoil factor 1(THF1)	—	I	—	—
24	Monocyte chemoattractant protein-1 (MCP 1)	—	—	—	P
25	Annexin II	—	—	—	P
26	CD44	—	—	—	P
27	Matrix Gla protein (MGP)	—	I	—	I
28	Histone H1B	—	P	—	—
29	Fibronectin	—	—	I	I
30	Collagen	P	—	—	—
31	Glycosaminoglycans	I	I	I	I
32	Citrate	—	I	—	—
33	Pyrophosphate	—	I	—	—
34	Magnesium	—	I	—	—

I: inhibitor; P: promoter; "—": no effect.

when the bulk free energy of the cluster is less than that of the liquid. For example, charged soluble molecules such as calcium and oxalate combine to form calcium oxalate crystals and become insoluble [34]. Nucleation may be formed in the kidney through free particle or fixed particle mechanism [26, 34]. In supersaturated solutions, if promoters exceed that of inhibitors, nucleation starts [34].

Once a nucleus is created (and/or if it is anchored), crystallization can occur at lower chemical pressure than required for the formation of the initial nucleus. Existing epithelial cells, urinary casts, RBCs, and other crystals in urine can act as nucleating centers in the process of nuclei formation termed as heterogeneous nucleation [41]. The organic matrix, mucopolysaccharide acts as a binding agent by increasing heterogeneous nucleation and crystal aggregation [59]. On the other hand, nanobacteria is claimed to form apatite structures serving as a crystallization center for stone formation [60]. The whole process potentiates stone formation. The role of oxalate-degrading bacteria, such as *Oxalobacter formigenes*, in CaOx stone formation is a subject of current research [61]. Thus, treatment which targets the process of nucleation intervention is one of the best approaches to control kidney stone.

5.2. Crystal Growth. Crystals in urine stick together to form a small hard mass of stone referred as crystal growth. Stone growth is accomplished through aggregation of preformed

Table 2: Risk factors associated with kidney stone formations.

Number	Risk factors	References
1	*Lifestyle habits and dietary/nutritional factors*: such as excessive intake of animal proteins and salt and deficiencies of chelating agents like citrate, fiber, and alkali foods	[9, 13, 19, 45]
2	*Metabolic disorders*: such as hypercalciuria, hypocitraturia, hyperoxaluria, hyperuricosuria, and history of gout (defective metabolism of uric acid)	[38, 46–48]
3	*Hypercalcemic disorders*: primary hyperparathyroidism and other disturbances of calcium metabolism	[49]
4	*Urine composition*: excessive excretion of promoters of urinary crystallization and reduced excretion of inhibitors (urine deficient in inhibitory substances)	[1, 45, 49]
5	*Low urine volume*: inadequate water intake (dehydration and supersaturated urine)	[45, 49, 50]
6	*Recurrent urinary tract infections*: abnormalities of urinary pH and alkalinization of urine by bacterial urease (such as *Proteus mirabilis*)	[38, 49]
7	*Genetic predisposition/inherited disorders*: family history of stones (*genetic* susceptibility); genetic monogenic diseases (single abnormal gene disorders on the autosomes); renal tubular acidosis	[1, 9, 48, 49, 51]
8	*Anatomical abnormalities*: factors such as defects in medullary sponge kidney, ureteropelvic junction stenosis, pyeloureteral duplication, polycystic renal disease, and horseshoe kidney	[1, 48, 49, 52]
9	*Hypertension*	[46]
10	*Obesity*	[46–48]
11	*Climate change* (global warming), occupation, geographic conditions, and seasonal variations (higher in summer than winter)	[1, 49]
12	*Inflammatory bowel disease* and other intestinal malabsorption or associated disease states	[9, 49]
13	Absence of intestinal *oxalate-degrading bacteria*	[53, 54]
14	*Lithogenic drugs*: such as indinavir (Crixivan), a protease inhibitor, sulfonamides (sulfadiazine), uricosuric agents, which have low solubility andpromotes the formation of calculi, and ceftriaxone (high dose on long terms)	[28, 38, 49, 50]

crystals or secondary nucleation of crystal on the matrix-coated surface [62]. Once a nidus has achieved, the overall free energy is decreased by adding new crystal components to its surface. The total free energy of the cluster is increased by the surface energy. The process of stone growth is slow and requires longer time to obstruct the renal tubules [34]. From organic matrix, mainly Tamm–Horsfall protein and osteopontin are promoters of CaOx stone formation [13]. Under in vitro study, crystals induced in human urine demonstrated an intimate association between calcium-containing crystals and organic matrix (lipids and proteins). Lipids of cellular membranes are basically believed to involve in nucleation of crystals [63].

5.3. Crystal Aggregation. The process whereby a small hard mass of a crystal in solution sticks together to form a larger stone is called aggregation. All models of CaOx urolithiasis concede that crystal aggregation is probably involved in crystal retention within the kidneys [41]. Crystal aggregation is considered to be the most critical step in stone formation.

5.4. Crystal-Cell Interaction. The attachment of grown crystals with the renal tubule lining of epithelial cells is termed as crystal retention or crystal-cell interaction [41, 64]. In individuals with hyperoxaluria, renal tubular epithelial cells were injured due to exposure to high oxalate concentrations or sharp calcium oxalate monohydrate (COM) crystals [10, 65, 66]. Crystal-cell interaction results in the movement of crystals from basolateral side of cells to the basement membrane [10]. Then, crystals could be taken into cells and anchored to the basement membrane of the kidneys [66]. The interaction of COM crystals with the surface of renal epithelial cells could be a critical initiating event in nephrolithiasis. An increased retention force between the crystal and injured renal tubule epithelium cells promotes CaOx crystallization [67]. Most of the crystals attached to epithelial cells are thought to be digested by macrophages and/or lysosomes inside cells and then discharged with urine [66].

Following renal tubular cell injury, cellular degradation produces numerous membrane vesicles which are nucleators of calcium crystals as supported by in vitro and in vivo studies [41]. Injured cells release substances like renal prothrombin fragment-1 or other anionic proteins which induce COM crystal agglomeration [68]. Reactive oxygen species is thought to be one of the factors involved in renal cell injury [69]. Thus, reduction of renal oxidative stress could be an effective treatment option.

Injured cells potentiate to invert its cell membrane which is anionic to the urinary environment and acts as site of crystal adherence. COM crystals have stronger affinity of attachment towards the inverted anionic membrane [69], than calcium oxalate dihydrate (COD) crystals [70]. On the other hand, deposition of COM crystal was observed in Madin–Darby canine kidney epithelial cells (MDCK cells), than at proximal tubular epithelial cells derived from pig kidney (LLC-PK1 cells) study models [71]. This preferential difference may be due to the presence of a binding molecule such as hyaluronan on Madin–Darby canine kidney epithelial cells for COM crystal attachment [67]. Although the detailed mechanisms of crystal-cell interaction remain unexplored, one of the best ways to treat urolithiasis is to control crystal-cell retentions.

5.5. Endocytosis of CaOx Crystals. Endocytosis or engulfment of crystals by renal tubular cells is the earliest process in the formation of kidney stones. Studies on tissue culture crystal-cell interactions indicated that COM crystals rapidly adhere to microvilli on the cell surface and subsequently internalized. Polyanion molecules present in tubular fluid/urine such as glycosaminoglycans, glycoproteins, and citrate may coat crystals and inhibit the binding of COM crystals to cell membrane [41]. For example, Tamm–Horsfall glycoproteins (THP) have a dual biological role in stone formation. Lieske et al. [72] reported that THP may promote renal stone formation by initiating the interaction of COM crystals with distal tubular cells of the nephron. Another study revealed that, upon lowering pH and raising ionic strength, THP's viscosity increases which exhibits high tendency of polymerization and fails to inhibit crystallization. Moreover, THP becomes a strong promoter of crystallization in the presence of additional calcium ions [73]. In contrast, THP is thought to protect against COM stone formation by inhibiting COM aggregation when it is at high pH and low ionic strength as reported by Hess [73]. COM aggregation assays revealed that desialylated THP promoted COM aggregation, while normal THP inhibited aggregation [74]. Similar reports revealed that THP may inhibit calcium oxalate crystal aggregation, whereas uromodulin may promote aggregation [75]. Inactivating the THP gene in mouse embryonic stem cells results in spontaneous formation of calcium crystals in adult kidneys. This is a convincing evidence that THP is a critical urinary inhibitor of human nephrolithiasis [76].

Various cellular and extracellular events are involved during stone formation. Modulators targeting the steps from supersaturation to crystal retention may be a potential means to block stone formation. Similarly, the blockage of crystal binding molecules (such as osteopontin, hyaluronic acid, sialic acid, and monocyte chemoattractant protein-1) expressed on epithelial cell membranes may be an alternative approach to prevent stone formation [41]. Experimental findings demonstrated that stone calcification is triggered by reactive oxygen species (ROS) and the development of oxidative stress [77]. In vitro [78, 79] and in vivo [80, 81] studies have demonstrated that CaOx crystals are toxic for renal epithelial cells that produce injury and renal cell death. Similarly, an exposure to hypercalciuria produces cellular injury and ROS-induced lipid peroxidation which stimulates calcium oxalate deposition [82]. The pathophysiology of urinary stone formation is incompletely understood. A summary of the various steps involved in stone formation is shown below (Figure 2).

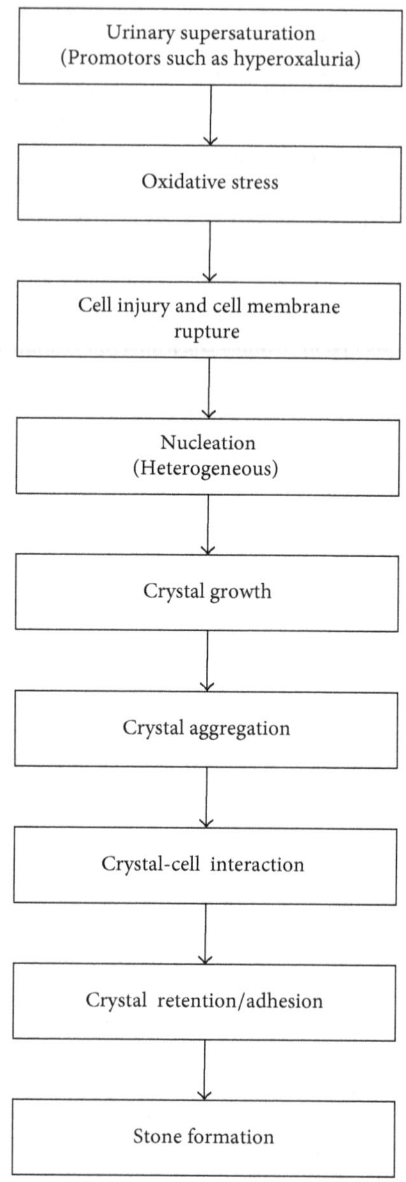

Figure 2: Schematic representation of the various events of kidney stone formation.

5.6. Cell Injury and Apoptosis. Exposure to high levels of oxalate or CaOx crystals induces epithelial cellular injury, which is a predisposing factor to subsequent stone formation [83, 84]. CaOx crystal depositions in the kidneys upregulate the expression and synthesis of macromolecules that can promote inflammation [85]. Crystals may be endocytosed by cells or transported to the interstitium. It has been suggested that injured cells develop a nidus which promotes the retention of particles on the renal papillary surface [86]. In individuals with severe primary hyperoxaluria, renal tubular cells are injured and crystals become attached to them [66]. The addition of CaOx crystals onto Madin–Darby canine kidney (MDCK) cell lines showed an increase in the release of lysosomal enzymes, prostaglandin E2, and cytosolic enzymes [87]. A study on animal models also revealed that the administration of high concentrations of CaOx crystals or oxalate ions appears to be toxic causing renal tubular cell damage [41]. It has been suggested that oxalate increases the availability of free radicals by inhibiting enzymes responsible for their degradation. For instance, reactive oxygen species can damage the mitochondrial membrane and reduce its transmembrane potential. These events are known features of early process in apoptotic pathways [88].

The activation of p38 mitogen-activated protein kinase (p38 MAPK) signaling pathway regulates the expression of cellular proteins. The various extracellular stimuli or stresses like ultraviolet radiation and proinflammatory cytokines may activate p38 MAPK which results in phosphorylation and activation of transcription factors [89]. The exposure of renal cells to oxalate increases an altered gene expression that induces apoptosis signaling cascades [88]. A study revealed that the exposure of HK-2 cells to increased oxalate levels results in an increased transcriptional activation of IL-2R beta mRNA and consequently increases IL-2R beta protein levels which drive cellular changes like induction of inflammation. Oxalate-induced activation may trigger p38 MAPK signaling by acting on cell membranes, although the exact mechanisms have not been established [90].

Apoptosis at the level of renal tubular cells may lead to stone formation through cellular demise and postapoptotic necrosis which could promote calcium crystal aggregation and growth. This fact has been supported by in vitro study on MDCK cells being exposed to oxalate ions [91]. However, it has to be noted that some cells did not respond to oxalate injury. This may be due to the fact that changes in gene expression could protect from apoptosis and then inhibit from lithiasis [35]. These findings highlight the need for future studies clarifying novel biochemical targets of kidney stone formation and the utility of p38 MAPK inhibitors in preventing stone formation.

5.7. Genetic Basis of Kidney Stone Formation. Environmental factors interacting with underlying genetic factors cause rare stone disease [92]. The production of promoters and inhibitors of crystallization depends on proper functioning of the renal epithelial cells. Cellular dysfunction affects the supersaturation of urinary excretion by influencing ions such as calcium, oxalate, and citrate [93]. Some genetic defects which lead to stone formation are shown in Table 3.

5.8. Randall's Plaques. Randall's plaques appear to be the precursor's origin of urinary stone development although it is unclear whether it involves in all stone types or not [62]. Moreover, the pathogenesis of Randall's plaque itself is not clearly known [94]. The majority of CaOx stones are found to be attached with renal papillae at the sites of Randall's plaque [26]. It is located at the interstitial basement membrane in loop of Henle [95, 96]. Calcium phosphate (apatite), and purine crystal compositions were identified in plaques, whereas apatite is dominant [97]. Initially, calcium phosphate crystals and organic matrix are deposited along the basement membranes of the thin loops of Henle and extend further into the interstitial space to the urothelium, constituting the so-called Randall plaques. Evidence suggests that a primary interstitial apatite crystal formation secondarily leads to CaOx stone formation [13]. In supersaturated urine, crystals adhere to the urothelium which may enhance subsequent stone growth [98].

Due to renal cell injury, plaque is exposed to supersaturated urine. Renal epithelial cell damage (degradation) products promote heterogeneous nucleation and promotes crystal adherence in renal cells. Randall plaque calcification is triggered by oxidative stress. Cells may express molecules at distal and collecting tubules which act as crystal binding sites such as phosphatidylserine, CD44, osteopontin, and hyaluronan [27, 99]. Renal epithelial cells of the loop of Henle or collecting ducts produce membrane vesicles at the basal side which leads to plague formation [77]. Thus, apatite crystal deposits have been proposed to act as nidus for CaOx stone formation by attachment on further matrix molecules [13, 77]. However, the driving forces in plaque formation and the involved matrix molecules remain elusive.

Kidney stones are either attached to the renal papillae or found freely [100]. According to the fixed particle pathway, the beginning of calcium phosphate (CaP) deposition in the interstitium establishes a nucleus for CaOx formation. CaP formed in the basement membrane of the loops of Henle, the inner medullary collecting ducts, and ducts of Bellini serves as an attachment site for stone development. Idiopathic stone formers develop CaOx attached to fixed sites of interstitial plaque [26]. Stones of the distal tubular acidosis attach to plugs protruding from dilated ducts of Bellini, whereas cystinuria stones do not attach to the renal plagues (found freely) [26]. CaP, uric acid, or cystine crystals formed in the renal tubules plug at the terminal collecting ducts. When mineralization reaches the renal papillary surface, plaques rupture exposing CaP crystals to the pelvic urine. Then, urinary macromolecules deposit over the exposed CaP crystals and promote CaOx deposition on CaP [4].

5.9. Kidney Stone Inhibitors and Promoters. Inhibitors are substances which decrease the initiation of supersaturation, nucleation, crystal growth, rate of aggregation, or any other processes required to stone formation [34]. Normally, urine contains chemicals that prevent crystal formation. Inhibitors in urine includes small organic anions such as citrate, small inorganic anions such as pyrophosphates, multivalent metallic cations such as magnesium, or macromolecules such as osteopontin, glycosaminoglycans, glycoproteins, urinary prothrombin fragment-1, and Tamm–Horsfall proteins [41, 62]. These inhibitors do not seem to work equally for everyone; therefore, some people form stones. But, if crystals formed remain tiny, usually it travels through the urinary tract and passes out from the body with urine splash without being noticed. Inhibitors may act either directly by interacting with crystal or indirectly by influencing the urinary environment [42]. When inhibitory compounds adsorb onto the surface of the crystal, it inhibits nucleation, crystal growth, aggregation, or crystal-cell adherence.

In contrast, promoters are substances which facilitate stone formation by various mechanisms [62]. Some of the promoters include cell membrane lipids (phospholipids, cholesterol, and glycolipids) [42], calcitriol hormone enhancement via parathyroid hormone stimulation [101], oxalate, calcium, sodium, cystine, and low urine volume [34]. Among recurrent stone formers, urinary oxalate excretion was found to be higher, whereas citrate excretion was lower [102]. Studies indicated that oxalate can increase chloride, sodium, and water reabsorption in the proximal tubule and activate multiple signaling pathways in renal epithelial cells [103]. In general, an imbalance between urinary stone inhibitors and promoters has been suggested

Table 3: Gene involved in hypercalciuria, gene products, and renal phenotype [93].

Gene	Gene product/function	Renal phenotype
VDR	Vitamin D receptor	Decreased calcium reabsorption leading to hypercalciuria and nephrocalcinosis
CLCNS	Cl/H antiporter	Inactivating mutation causes hypercalciuria, hyperphosphaturia, low molecular weight proteinuria, nephrocalcinosis, stone
CASR	Calcium sensing receptor	Gain of function mutation produces hypercalciuria, nephrocalcinosis, stone
CLDN16	Tight junction protein	Hypercalciuria, magnesium wasting, nephrocalcinosis, stone
NPT2a/c	Sodium phosphate cotransporter	Hypercalciuria, hypophosphatemia, phosphate wasting, nephrocalcinosis, stone
TRPV5	Calcium selective transient receptor potential channel	Hypercalciuria, hyperphosphaturia
sAC	Soluble adenylate cyclase/bicarbonate exchanger/	Hypercalciuria, stones
KLOTHO	Aging suppression protein/regulator of calcium homeostasis	Hypercalciuria

to be the cause for stone formation [34]. A list of substances generally considered to inhibit or promote stone formation process is shown in Table 1.

6. Preventive Options for Urolithiasis

Effective kidney stone prevention depends upon addressing the cause of stone formation. Generally, to prevent the first episodes of kidney stone formation or its secondary episodes, proper management of diet and the use of medications is required. Primary prevention of kidney stone disease via dietary intervention is low-cost public health initiative with massive societal implications. Thus, nutritional management is the best preventive strategy against urolithiasis [104].

Regardless of the underlying etiology and drug treatment of the stone disease, patients should be instructed to increase their water intake in order to maintain a urine output of at least 2 liter per day [49]. A simple and most important lifestyle change to prevent stone disease is to drink more water/liquids. Enough fluid intake reduces urinary saturation and dilutes promoters of CaOx crystallization. Dietary recommendations should be adjusted based on individual metabolic abnormalities. For absorptive hyperoxaluria, low oxalate diet and increased dietary calcium intake are recommended [61].

A high sodium intake boosts stone risk by reducing renal tubular calcium reabsorption and increasing urinary calcium [105]. Restriction of animal proteins is also encouraged since animal proteins provide an increased acid load because of its high content of sulfur-containing amino acids. Thus, high protein intake reduces urine pH and the level of citrate and enhances urinary calcium excretion via bone reabsorption. Therefore, if you have very acidic urine, you may need to eat less meat, fish, and poultry and avoid food with vitamin D [106]. Instead, an increase intake of fruits and vegetables rich in potassium is recommended [49].

People who form calcium stones used to be told to avoid dairy products and other foods with high calcium content. However, persons with a tendency of kidney stone formation should not be advised to restrict calcium intake unless it has been known that he/she has an excessive use of calcium [107]. A reduced intake of calcium leads to an increased intestinal absorption of oxalate, which itself may account for an increased risk of stone formation. Calcium supplements may reduce oxalate absorption because the calcium binds dietary oxalate in the gut lumen. However, the benefit of taking calcium pills is controversial. Vitamin C has been implicated in stone formation because of in vivo conversion of ascorbic acid to oxalate. Therefore, a limitation of vitamin C supplementation is recommended [105].

For prevention of calcium oxalate, cystine, and uric acid stones, urine should be alkalinized by eating a diet high in fruits and vegetables, taking supplemental or prescription citrate, or drinking alkaline mineral waters. For uric acid stone formers, gout needs to be controlled, and for cystine stone formers, sodium and protein intakes need to restricted. For prevention of calcium phosphate and struvite stones, urine should be acidified. For struvite stones, acidifying the urine is the single most important step [108]. Patients must receive careful follow-up to be sure that the infection has cleared. However, the current treatment modalities are not efficient to prevent urolithiasis, and further research is required.

7. Conclusion

Despite considerable improvements in the development of new therapies for the management of urinary stones, the incidence of urolithiasis is increasing worldwide. Many aspects of renal stone formation remain unclear. However, it is certain that renal cell injury, crystal retention, cell apoptosis, Randall's plaque, and associated stone inhibitors or promoters play important roles for kidney stone formation. These seem to be critical targets that lead to developing a novel strategy to prevent kidney stone disease and drugs against kidney stones. In addition, the identification of novel treatment targets on the basis of molecular and cellular alterations in relation to stone formation will help develop better drugs. Moreover, better understanding of the mechanisms of urolithiasis associated with stone inhibitors or promoters will be critical for stone-removing medications. Furthermore, understanding the underlying pathophysiology, pathogenesis, and genetic basis of kidney stone formation will hopefully lead to discover novel drugs and strategies to manage urolithiasis in the near future.

References

[1] L. Giannossi and V. Summa, "A review of pathological biomineral analysis techniques and classification schemes," in *An Introduction to the Study of Mineralogy*, C. Aydinalp, Ed., InTechOpen, InTech, IMAA-CNR, Italy, 2012, http://www.intechopen.com/books/.

[2] M. Lopez and B. Hoppe, "History, epidemiology and regional diversities of urolithiasis," *Pediatric Nephrology*, vol. 25, no. 1, pp. 49–59, 2008.

[3] K. Mikawlrawng, S. Kumar, and R. Vandana, "Current scenario of urolithiasis and the use of medicinal plants as antiurolithiatic agents in Manipur (North East India): a review," *International Journal of Herbal Medicine*, vol. 2, no. 1, pp. 1–12, 2014.

[4] S. R. Khan, M. S. Pearle, W. G. Robertson et al., "Kidney stones," *Nature Reviews Disease Primers*, vol. 2, p. 16008, 2016.

[5] V. K. Sigurjonsdottir, H. L.Runolfsdottir, O. S. Indridason et al., "Impact of nephrolithiasis on kidney function," *BMC Nephrology*, vol. 16, no. 1, p. 149, 2015.

[6] Z. M. El-Zoghby, J. C. Lieske, R. N. Foley et al., "Urolithiasis and the risk of ESRD," *Clinical Journal of the American Society of Nephrology*, vol. 7, no. 9, pp. 1409–1415, 2012.

[7] A. D. Rule, V. L. Roger, L. J. Melton et al., "Kidney stones associate with increased risk for myocardial infarction," *Journal of the American Society of Nephrology*, vol. 21, no. 10, pp. 1641–1644, 2010.

[8] E. M. Worcester and F. L. Coe, "Nephrolithiasis," *Primary Care*, vol. 35, no. 2, pp. 369–391, 2008.

[9] E. N. Taylor, M. J. Stampfer, and G. C. Curhan, "Obesity, weight gain and the risk of kidney stones," *Journal of the American Medical Association*, vol. 293, no. 4, pp. 455–462, 2005.

[10] M. Courbebaisse, C. Prot-Bertoye, J. Bertocchio et al., "Nephrolithiasis of adult: from mechanisms to preventive medical treatment," *Revue Medicale Internationale*, vol. 38, no. 1, pp. 44–52, 2017.

[11] S. B. N. Kumar, K. G. Kumar, V. Srinivasa, and S. Bilal, "A review on urolithiasis," *International Journal of Universal Pharmacy and Life Sciences*, vol. 2, no. 2, pp. 269–280, 2012.

[12] J. M. Teichman and M. H. Joel, "Acute renal colic from ureteral calculus," *New England Journal of Medicine*, vol. 350, no. 7, pp. 684–693, 2004.

[13] T. Knoll, "Epidemiology, pathogenesis and pathophysiology of urolithiasis," *European Urology Supplements*, vol. 9, no. 12, pp. 802–806, 2010.

[14] C. K. Chauhan, M. J. Joshi, and A. D. B. Vaidya, "Growth inhibition of struvite crystals in the presence of herbal extract *Commiphora wightii*," *Journal of Materials Science*, vol. 20, no. 1, pp. 85–92, 2008.

[15] O. W. Moe, "Kidney stones: pathophysiology and medical management," *The Lancet*, vol. 367, no. 9507, pp. 333–344, 2006.

[16] V. Romero, H. Akpinar, and D. G. Assimos, "Kidney stones: a global picture of prevalence, incidence, and associated risk factors," *Reviews in Urology*, vol. 12, no. 2-3, pp. e86–e96, 2010.

[17] V. O. Edvardsson, O. S. Indridason, G. Haraldsson, O. Kjartansson, and R. Palsson, "Temporal trends in the incidence of kidney stone disease," *Kidney International*, vol. 83, no. 1, pp. 146–152, 2013.

[18] B. Afsar, M. C. Kiremit, A. A. Sag et al., "The role of sodium intake in nephrolithiasis: epidemiology, pathogenesis, and future directions," *European Journal of Internal Medicine*, vol. 35, pp. 16–19, 2016.

[19] W. G. Robertson, P. J. Heyburn, M. Peacock, F. A. Hanes, and R. Swaminathan, "The effect of high animal protein intake on the risk of calcium stone-formation in the urinary tract," *Clinical Science*, vol. 57, no. 3, pp. 285–288, 1979.

[20] K. B. Singh and S. Sailo, "Understanding epidemiology and etiologic factors of urolithiasis: an overview," *Scientific Visualization*, vol. 13, no. 4, pp. 169–174, 2013.

[21] N. H. Sofia and T. M. Walter, "Prevalence and risk factors of kidney stone," *Global Journal For Research Analysis*, vol. 5, 2016.

[22] C. D. Scales, A. C. Smith, J. M. Hanley, and C. S. Saigal, "Prevalence of kidney stones in the United States," *European Urology*, vol. 62, no. 1, pp. 160–165, 2012.

[23] K. C. Joseph, B. Bharat, H. Parek, and M. J. Joshi, "Inhibition of growth of urinary type calcium hydrogen phosphate dihydrate crystals by tartaric acid and tamarind," *Current Science*, vol. 88, pp. 1232–1238, 2005.

[24] C. O'Callaghan, Edited by P. V. Yangkul and L. Ammi Visnaga, Eds., Blackwell Publishing Ltd., Oxford, UK, 2006.

[25] I. H. Zahid, A. S. Bawazir, and R. Naser, "Plant based native therapy for the treatment of Kidney stones in Aurangabad (M.S)," *Journal of Pharmacognosy and Phytochemistry*, vol. 1, no. 6, pp. 189–193, 2013.

[26] A. P. Evan, "Physiopathology and Etiology of stone formation in the kidney and the urinary tract," *Pediatric Nephrology*, vol. 25, no. 5, pp. 831–841, 2010.

[27] N. Chhiber, M. Sharma, T. Kaur, and S. Singla, "Mineralization in health and mechanism of kidney stone formation," *International Journal of Pharmaceutical Science Invention*, vol. 3, pp. 25–31, 2014.

[28] C. Barbasa, A. Garciaa, L. Saavedraa, and M. Muros, "Urinary analysis of nephrolithiasis markers," *Journal of Chromatography B*, vol. 781, no. 1-2, pp. 433–455, 2002.

[29] F. L. Coe, A. Evan, and E. Worcester, "Kidney stone disease," *Journal of Clinical Investigation*, vol. 115, no. 10, pp. 2598–2608, 2005.

[30] A. Chaudhary, S. K. Singla, and C. Tandon, "In vitro evaluation of *Terminalia arjuna* on calcium phosphate and calcium oxalate crystallization," *Indian Journal of Pharmaceutical Sciences*, vol. 72, no. 3, pp. 340–345, 2010.

[31] F. L. Coe, J. H. Parks, and J. R. Asplin, "The pathogenesis and treatment of kidney stones," *New England Journal of Medicine*, vol. 327, no. 16, pp. 1141–1152, 1992.

[32] A. Skolarikos, M. Straub, T. Knoll et al., "Metabolic evaluation and recurrence prevention for urinary stone patients: EAU guidelines," *European Urology*, vol. 67, no. 4, pp. 750–763, 2015.

[33] A. Bensatal and M. R. Ouahrani, "Inhibition of crystallization of calcium oxalate by the extraction of *Tamarix gallica* L," *Urological Research*, vol. 36, no. 6, pp. 283–287, 2008.
[34] D. R. Basavaraj, C. S. Biyani, A. J. Browning, and J. J. Cartledge, "The role of urinary kidney stone inhibitors and promoters in the pathogenesis of calcium containing renal stones," *EAU-EBU Update Series*, vol. 5, no. 3, pp. 126–136, 2007.
[35] F. Dal-Moro, M. Mancini, I. M. Tavolini, V. De Marco, and P. Bassi, "Cellular and molecular gateways to urolithiasis: a new insight," *Urologia Internationalis*, vol. 74, pp. 193–197, 2005.
[36] D. V. Kishore, F. Moosavi, and D. R. K. Varma, "Effect of ethanolic extract of *Portulaca oleracea* linn. on ethylene glycol and ammonium chloride induced urolithiasis," *International Journal of Pharmacy and Pharmaceutical Sciences*, vol. 5, no. 2, pp. 134–140, 2013.
[37] D. P. Griffith, "Struvite stones," *Kidney International*, vol. 13, no. 5, pp. 372–382, 1978.
[38] M. Dursun, A. Otunctemur, and E. Ozbek, "Kidney stones and ceftriaxone," *European Medical Journal of Urology*, vol. 3, no. 1, pp. 68–74, 2015.
[39] T. C. Ngo and D. G. Assimos, "Uric acid nephrolithiasis: recent progress and future directions," *Reviews in Urology*, vol. 9, pp. 17–27, 2007.
[40] K. Ahmed, P. Dasgupta, and M. S. Khan, "Cystine calculi: challenging group of stones," *Postgraduate Medical Journal*, vol. 82, no. 974, pp. 799–801, 2006.
[41] K. P. Aggarwal, S. Narula, M. Kakkar, and C. Tandon, "Nephrolithiasis: molecular mechanism of renal stone formation and the critical role played by modulators," *BioMed Research International*, vol. 2013, Article ID 292953, 21 pages, 2013.
[42] S. R. Khan and D. J. Kok, "Modulators of urinary stone formation," *Frontiers in Bioscience*, vol. 9, no. 1-3, pp. 1450–1482, 2004.
[43] A. E. Krambeck, S. E. Handa, A. P. Evan, and J. E. Lingeman, "Brushite stone disease as a consequence of lithotripsy?," *Urological Research*, vol. 38, no. 4, pp. 293–299, 2010.
[44] A. E. Krambeck, S. E. Handa, A. P. Evan, and J. E. Lingeman, "Profile of the brushite stone former," *Journal of Urology*, vol. 184, no. 4, pp. 1367–1371, 2010.
[45] M. Straub and R. E. Hautmann, "Developments in stone prevention," *Current Opinion in Urology*, vol. 15, no. 2, pp. 119–126, 2005.
[46] S. H. Obligado and D. S. Goldfarb, "The association of nephrolithiasis with hypertension and obesity: a review," *American Journal of Hypertension*, vol. 21, no. 3, pp. 257–264, 2008.
[47] V. Butterweck and S. R. Khan, "Herbal medicines in the management of urolithiasis: alternative or complementary," *Planta Medica*, vol. 75, no. 10, pp. 1095–1103, 2009.
[48] S. Joshi, B. T. Saylor, W. Wang, A. B. Peck, and S. R. Khan, "Apocynin treatment reverses hyperoxaluria induced changes in NADPH oxidase system expression in rat kidneys: a transcriptional study," *PLoS One*, vol. 7, article e47738, 2012.
[49] I. P. Heilberg and N. Schor, "Renal stone disease: causes, evaluation and medical treatment," *Arquivos Brasileiros de Endocrinologia & Metabologia*, vol. 50, no. 4, pp. 823–831, 2006.
[50] S. Kumar, D. Sigmon, T. Miller et al., "A new model of nephrolithiasis involving tubular dysfunction injury," *Journal of Urology*, vol. 146, no. 5, pp. 1384–1389, 1991.
[51] S. R. Khan, P. N. Shevock, and R. L. Hackett, "Acute hyperoxaluria, renal injury and calcium-oxalate urolithiasis," *Journal of Urology*, vol. 147, no. 1, pp. 226–230, 1992.
[52] G. Gambaro, A. Fabris, D. Puliatta, and A. Lupo, "Lithiasis in cystic kidney disease and malformations of the urinary tract," *Urological Research*, vol. 34, no. 2, pp. 102–107, 2006.
[53] K. Mikami, K. Akakura, K. Takei et al., "Association of absence of intestinal oxalate degrading bacteria with urinary calcium oxalate stone formation," *International Journal of Urology*, vol. 10, no. 6, pp. 293–296, 2003.
[54] C. Kwak, H. K. Kim, E. C. Kim, M. S. Choi, and H. H. Kim, "Urinary oxalate levels and the enteric bacterium *Oxalobacter formigenes* in patients with calcium oxalate urolithiasis," *European Urology*, vol. 44, no. 4, pp. 475–481, 2003.
[55] M. S. Parmar, "Kidney stones," *British Medical Journal*, vol. 328, no. 7453, pp. 1420–1424, 2004.
[56] K. K. Malhotra, "Medical aspects of renal stones: review," *Journal of Indian Academy of Clinical Medicine*, vol. 9, no. 4, pp. 282–286, 2008.
[57] D. J. Kok, S. E. Papapoulos, and O. L. Bijvoet, "Crystal agglomeration is a major element in calcium oxalate urinary stone formation," *Kidney International*, vol. 37, no. 1, pp. 51–56, 1990.
[58] P. Cunningham, H. Noble, A.-K. Al-Modhefer, and I. Walsh, "Kidney stones: pathophysiology, diagnosis and management," *British Journal of Nursing*, vol. 25, no. 20, pp. 1112–1116, 2016.
[59] S. Ahmed, M. M. Hasan, and Z. M. Alam, "*In vitro* urolithiasis models: an evaluation of prophylactic management against kidney stones," *Journal of Pharmacognosy and Phytochemistry*, vol. 5, no. 3, pp. 28–35, 2016.
[60] E. O. Kajander and N. Ciftcioglu, "Nanobacteria: an alternative mechanism for pathogenic intra-and extracellular calcification and stone formation," *Proceedings of the National Academy of Sciences*, vol. 95, pp. 8274–8279, 1998.
[61] H. Xu, A. L. Zisman, F. L. Coe, and E. M. Worcester, "Kidney stones: an update on current pharmacological management and future directions," *Expert Opinion on Pharmacotherapy*, vol. 14, no. 4, pp. 435–447, 2013.
[62] V. N. Ratkalkar and J. G. Kleinman, "Mechanisms of stone formation," *Clinical Reviews in Bone and Mineral Metabolism*, vol. 9, no. 3-4, pp. 187–197, 2011.
[63] S. R. Khan, F. Atmani, P. Glenton, Z.-C. Hou, D. R. Talham, and M. Khurshid, "Lipids and membranes in the organic matrix of urinary calcific crystals and stones," *Calcified Tissue International*, vol. 59, pp. 357–365, 1996.
[64] M. S. Schepers, B. G. Vander, J. C. Romijn, F. H. Schröoderand, and C. F. Verkoelen, "Urinary crystallization inhibitors do not prevent crystal binding," *Journal of Urology*, vol. 167, no. 4, pp. 1844–1847, 2002.
[65] S. R. Khan, "Renal tubular damage/dysfunction: key to the formation of kidney stones," *Urological Research*, vol. 34, no. 2, pp. 86–91, 2006.
[66] M. Tsujihata, "Mechanism of calcium oxalate renal stone formation and renal tubular cell injury," *International Journal of Urology*, vol. 15, no. 2, pp. 115–120, 2008.
[67] C. F. Verkoelen, B. G. vander Boom, and J. C. Romijn, "Identification of hyaluronan as a crystal-binding molecule at the surface of migrating and proliferating MDCK cells," *Kidney Inernational*, vol. 58, no. 3, pp. 1045–1054, 2000.
[68] M. T. Moryama, C. Domiki, K. Miyazawa, T. Tanaka, and K. Suzuki, "Effects of oxalate exposure on Madin-Darby canine kidney cells in culture: renal prothrombin fragment-1 mRNA expression," *Urological Research*, vol. 33, no. 6, pp. 470–475, 2005.

[69] S. R. Khan, P. A. Glenton, R. Backov, and D. R. Talham, "Presence of lipids in urine, crystals and stones: Implications for the formation of kidney stones," *Kidney International*, vol. 62, no. 6, pp. 2062–2072, 2002.

[70] M. E. Barros, N. Schor, and M. A. Biom, "Effects of an aqueous extract from *Phyllanthus niruri* on calcium oxalate crystallization," *Urological Research*, vol. 30, pp. 374–379, 2003.

[71] Y. I. Rabinovich, M. Esayanur, S. Daosukho, K. J. Byer, H. E. El-Shall, and S. R. Khan, "Adhesion force between calcium oxalate monohydrate crystal and kidney epithelial cells and possible relevance for kidney stone formation," *Journal of Colloid and Interface Science*, vol. 300, no. 1, pp. 131–140, 2006.

[72] J. C. Lieske, H. Swift, T. Martin, B. Patterson, and F. G. Toback, "Renal epithelial cells rapidly bind and internalize calcium oxalate monohydrate crystals," *Proceedings of the National Academy of Sciences*, vol. 91, no. 15, pp. 6987–6991, 1994.

[73] B. Hess, "Tamm-Horsfall glycoprotein-inhibitor or promoter of calcium oxalate monohydrate crystallization processes?," *Urological Research*, vol. 20, no. 1, pp. 83–86, 1992.

[74] P. Viswanathan, J. D. Rimer, A. M. Kolbach, M. D. Ward, J. G. Kleinman, and J. A. Wesson, "Calcium oxalate monohydrate aggregation induced by aggregation of desialylated Tamm-Horsfall protein," *Urological Research*, vol. 39, no. 4, pp. 269–282, 2011.

[75] M. Carvalho, R. A. Mulinari, and Y. Nakagawa, "Role of Tamm-Horsfall protein and uromodulin in calcium oxalate crystallization," *Brazilian Journal of Medical and Biological Research*, vol. 35, no. 10, pp. 1165–1172, 2002.

[76] L. Mo, H. Y. Huang, X. H. Zhu, E. Shapiro, D. L. Hasty, and X.-R. Wu, "Tamm-Horsfall protein is a critical renal defense factor protecting against calcium oxalate crystal formation," *Kidney International*, vol. 66, no. 3, pp. 1159–1166, 2004.

[77] S. R. Khan, "Reactive oxygen species, inflammation and calcium oxalate nephrolithiasis," *Translational Andrology and Urology*, vol. 3, pp. 256–276, 2014.

[78] N. Singhto, K. Sintiprungrat, S. Sinchaikul, S.-T. Chen, and V. Thongboonkerd, "Proteome changes in human monocytes upon interaction with calcium oxalate monohydrate crystals," *Journal of Proteome Research*, vol. 9, no. 8, pp. 3980–3988, 2010.

[79] M. Asselman, A. Verhulst, M. E. De Broe, and C. F. Verkoelen, "Calcium oxalate crystal adherence to hyaluronan-, osteopontin-, and CD44-expressing injured/regenerating tubular epithelial cells in rat kidneys," *Journal of the American Society of Nephrology*, vol. 14, no. 12, pp. 3155–3166, 2003.

[80] S. Yamaguchi, J. H. Wiessner, A. T. Hasegawa, L. Y. Hung, G. S. Mandel, and N. S. Mandel, "Study of a rat model for calcium oxalate crystal formation without severe renal damage in selected conditions," *International Journal of Urology*, vol. 12, pp. 290–298, 2005.

[81] M. Hirose, T. Yasui, A. Okada et al., "Renal tubular epithelial cell injury and oxidative stress induce calcium oxalate crystal formation in mouse kidney," *International Journal of Urology*, vol. 17, pp. 83–92, 2010.

[82] Q. Xi, J. Ouyang, J. Pu, J. Hou, and S. Wang, "High concentration of calcium stimulates calcium oxalate crystal attachment to rat tubular epithelial NRK cells through osteopontin," *Urology*, vol. 86, no. 4, pp. 844.e1–844e5, 2015.

[83] S. Khan and S. Thamilselvan, "Nephrolithiasis: a consequence of renal epithelial cell exposure to oxalate and calcium oxalate crystals," *Molecular Urology*, vol. 4, pp. 305–312, 1999.

[84] S. R Khan, "Crystal induced inflammation of the kidneys results from human studies, animal models and tissue culture studies," *Journal of Clinical and Experimental Nephrology*, vol. 8, no. 2, pp. 75–88, 2004.

[85] R. Hackett, P. Shevock, and S. Khan, "Madin-Darby canine kidney cells are injured by exposure to oxalate and to calcium oxalate crystals," *Urological Research*, vol. 22, no. 4, pp. 197–203, 1994.

[86] J. M. Fasano and S. R. Khan, "Intra-tubular crystallization of calcium oxalate in the presence of membrane vesicles: an *in vitro* study," *Kidney International*, vol. 59, pp. 169–178, 2001.

[87] T. Rashed, M. Menon, and S. Thamilselvan, "Molecular mechanism of oxalate-induced free radical production and glutathione redox imbalance in renal epithelial cells: effect of antioxidants," *American Journal of Nephrology*, vol. 24, no. 5, pp. 557–568, 2004.

[88] L. S. Chaturvedi, S. Koul, A. Sekhon, A. Bhandari, M. Menon, and H. K. Koul, "Oxalate selectively activates p38 mitogen-activated protein kinase and C-Jun N-terminal kinase signal transduction pathways in renal epithelial cells," *Journal of Biological Chemistry*, vol. 277, no. 15, pp. 13321–13330, 2002.

[89] P. Peerapen and V. Thongboonkerd, "P38 MAPK mediates calcium oxalate crystal-induced tight junction disruption in distal renal tubular epithelial cells," *Scientific Reports*, vol. 3, no. 1, p. 1041, 2013.

[90] S. Koul, L. Khandrika, T. J. Pshak et al., "Oxalate upregulates expression of IL-2Rβ and activates IL-2R signaling in HK-2 cells, a line of human renal epithelial cells," *American Journal of Renal Physiology*, vol. 306, pp. 1039–1046, 2014.

[91] N. Hsieh, C. H. Shih, and H. Y. Chen, "Effects of Tamm-Horsfall protein on the protection of MCDK cells from oxalate induced free radical injury," *Urological Research*, vol. 31, pp. 10–16, 2003.

[92] J. A. Sayer, "The Genetics of nephrolithiasis," *Nephron Experimental Nephrology*, vol. 110, no. 2, pp. 37–43, 2008.

[93] S. R. Khan and B. K. Canales, "Genetic basis of renal cellular dysfunction and the formation of kidney stones," *Urological Research*, vol. 37, no. 4, pp. 169–180, 2009.

[94] N. Abrol and N. S. Kekre, "Revisiting Randall's plaque," *African Journal of Urology*, vol. 20, no. 4, pp. 174–179, 2014.

[95] A. P. Evan, J. E. Lingeman, F. L. Coe et al., "Randall's plaque of patients with nephrolithiasis begins in basement membranes of thin loops of Henle," *European Journal of Clinical Investigation*, vol. 111, no. 5, pp. 607–616, 2003.

[96] A. Evan, J. Lingeman, F. Coe, and E. Worcester, ""Randall's plaque: pathogenesis and role in calcium oxalate nephrolithiasis," *Kidney International*, vol. 69, no. 8, pp. 1313–1318, 2006.

[97] M. Daudon, D. Bazin, and E. Letavernier, "Randall's plaque as the origin of calcium oxalate kidney stones," *Journal of Urology*, vol. 43, pp. 5–11, 2015.

[98] C. H. Dawson and C. R. V. Thomson, "Kidney stone disease: pathophysiology, investigation and medical treatment," *Journal of Clinical Medicine*, vol. 12, no. 5, pp. 467–471, 2012.

[99] J. W. Yuen, M. D. I. Gohel, N. W. Poon, D. K. Y. Shum, P.-C. Tam, and D. W. T. Au, "The initial and subsequent inflammatory events during calcium oxalate lithiasis," *Clinica Chimica Acta*, vol. 411, pp. 1018–1026, 2010.

[100] D. J. Kok and S. R. Khan, "Calcium oxalate nephrolithiasis, a free or fixed particle disease," *Kidney International*, vol. 46, no. 3, pp. 847–854, 1994.

[101] V. Centeno, G. D. de Barboza, and A. Marchionatti, "Molecular mechanisms triggered by low-calcium diets," *Nutrition Research Reviews*, vol. 22, no. 2, pp. 163–174, 2009.

[102] B. Cakıroğlu, E. Eyyupoğlu, A. I. Hazar, B. S. Uyanik, and B. Nuhoğlu, "Metabolic assessment of recurrent and first renal calcium oxalate stone formers," *Archivio Italiano di Urologia e Andrologia*, vol. 88, pp. 101–105, 2016.
[103] S. R. Marengo and A. M. Romani, "Oxalate in renal stone disease: the terminal metabolite that just won't go away," *Nature Clinical Practice Nephrology*, vol. 4, no. 7, pp. 368–377, 2008.
[104] L. samal, A. K. Pattanaik, C. Mishra, B. Maharana, and L. Baithalu, "Nutritional strategies' to prevent urolithiasis in animals," *Veterinary World*, vol. 4, no. 3, pp. 142–144, 2011.
[105] S. Park and M. S. Pearle, "Pathophysiology and management of calcium stones," *Urologic Clinics of North America*, vol. 34, no. 3, pp. 323–334, 2007.
[106] NIH, *Kidney Disease*, NIH, Bethesda, Maryland, USA, 2005, http://kidney.niddk.nih.gov/kudis'eases/pubs/stonesadults/index.htm.
[107] H. G. Tiselius, "Stone incidence and prevention," *Journal of Clinical Urology*, vol. 26, pp. 452–462, 2000.
[108] L. Frassetto and I. Kohlstadt, "Treatment and prevention of kidney stones: an update," *American Family Physician*, vol. 84, no. 11, pp. 1234–1242, 2011.

4

Urinary Bladder Cancer in Egypt: Are There Gender Differences in Its Histopathological Presentation?

Fiorina Kyritsi,[1] Christopher A. Loffredo,[1] Yun-Ling Zheng,[1] George Philips,[1] and Sania Amr[2,3]

[1]*Lombardi Comprehensive Cancer Center, Georgetown University, Washington, DC, USA*
[2]*University of Maryland School of Medicine, Baltimore, MD, USA*
[3]*Marlene and Stewart Greenebaum Comprehensive Cancer Center, University of Maryland, Baltimore, MD, USA*

Correspondence should be addressed to Sania Amr; samr@som.umaryland.edu

Academic Editor: Mohammad H. Ather

We investigated gender differences in the histopathologic presentation of bladder cancer cases in Egypt, where both urothelial cell carcinoma (UC) and squamous cell carcinoma (SCC) types are highly prevalent. We used logistic regression to estimate the unadjusted (OR) and adjusted odds ratio (AOR) and 95% confidence interval (CI) of the associations between gender and different histopathologic and sociodemographic parameters of 2,186 confirmed cases of primary bladder cancer (1,775 males and 411 females; 784 SCC and 1,402 UC). There were no statistically significant gender differences in tumor grade, stage, mucosal ulcer, or inflammatory cystitis, regardless of the cancer type, but men were less likely than women to have undergone cystectomy with pelvic lymphadenectomy. Having *Schistosoma haematobium* (*SH*) ova in the bladder tissue was significantly associated with male gender in the fully adjusted model of either SCC (AOR (95% CI) = 2.12 (1.15–3.89)) or UC cases (3.78 (1.89–7.55)). Compared to females, male cases were significantly older at time of diagnosis and smokers. In Egypt, regardless of the type of bladder cancer (SCC or UC), male more than female cases had evidence of *SH* infection, but not other histopathologic differences, in bladder tissue specimens.

1. Introduction

Worldwide, the incidence and prevalence of urinary bladder cancer are higher in men than in women [1], whereas several studies, reviewed by Fajkovic et al., have shown worse outcomes after radical cystectomy in the latter than in the former [2]. Indeed, to predict recurrence of bladder cancer after surgery, the International Bladder Cancer Nomogram Consortium (IBCNC) developed a tool that includes, among other variables, sex, cancer histological type, and characteristics, as prognostic factors [3]. However, Welty et al. developed a nomogram to predict survival after cystectomy for urothelial cell carcinoma, but did not include sex, because they found age and tumor stage to be considerably stronger risk factors than sex in predicting patient survival [4].

Previous studies of the mechanisms underlying the variance in prognosis between men and women following bladder cancer diagnosis led researchers to suggest differences in exposures to carcinogens, hormones, and/or cellular and physiologic differences [5]. Known risk factors for bladder cancer include tobacco smoke, occupational exposure to aromatic amines and polycyclic aromatic hydrocarbons, and chronic urinary tract infections with *Schistosoma haematobium* (*SH*) [6–9].

The gender difference in this malignancy's incidence was at one time attributed to higher exposure to tobacco and occupational carcinogens in men than in women [10]. However, these risk factors failed to account fully for the gender disparity [11]. Other investigators focused on sex hormones and reproductive factors in searching for an explanation for the elevated bladder cancer risk among men. Both animal models [12, 13] and epidemiological studies showed evidence supporting the postulate that estrogens [14–18] and antiandrogens [19] are protective against this malignancy, particularly the urothelial type. Indeed, there are two main histological types of urinary bladder cancer, urothelial cell (UC) and squamous cell carcinoma (SCC). The latter, prevalent in areas endemic for *SH* infection, is rare (5%) in Europe and the United States, where the former is the predominant type (90%) on which most of the studies were conducted.

In their quest for understanding the gender disparity in bladder cancer incidence and outcomes after treatment, investigators focused on the clinical presentation, diagnosis, and histopathological characteristics of the bladder tumors [20, 21]. Delayed referral and diagnosis in women resulted in more advanced stage of the tumor and hence the negative outcomes following cystectomy [22, 23]. Some investigators reported high-grade and aggressive type of tumor as the reason for worse outcomes in women [24], but not others [25]. Not only were the results of these studies conflicting, and thus not conclusive, but also they involved predominantly the UC type of bladder cancer.

In Egypt, where bladder cancer is the second most common malignancy among men and 30% of the cases are SCC type, we investigated the gender differences for environmental bladder cancer risk factors separately for each of the histological types [26, 27]. In the present study, we describe the histopathological presentation of the two main types (UC and SCC) and their gender differences.

2. Materials and Methods

The present investigation used data collected on primary urinary bladder cancer in Egypt for the parent study, a multicenter case-control type that was conducted between 2006 and 2014. It was approved by the institutional review boards of the three collaborating cancer centers in Egypt: the University of Maryland in Baltimore MD, Georgetown University in Washington DC, and the National Scientific and Research Ethical Committee at the Egyptian Ministry of Health and Population.

2.1. Study Population. Bladder cancer cases were recruited from the National Cancer Institute in Cairo, the Minia Oncology Center in Minia, and the South Egypt Cancer Institute in Assiut. Participants had to be (i) adults between the ages of 19–80 years, (ii) self-identified as physically able to participate in an interview, and (iii) diagnosed with presumed urinary bladder cancer within 12 months. Individuals who had a prior history of other malignancies were excluded from the study [18, 26–28].

2.2. Questionnaire. After explaining the study and obtaining informed consent, trained interviewers administered a structured questionnaire to consented participants and collected information about sociodemographic characteristics and occupational and medical histories including the history of schistosomiasis. History of smoking and/or being exposed to secondhand smoke was documented.

2.3. Case Ascertainment. The study pathologists reviewed the pathology reports, the available surgical or biopsy specimen slides, and/or the referred slides for each urinary bladder cancer case. They first classified cases as (1) papillary transitional cell carcinoma (TCC), (2) invasive TCC, (3) squamous cell carcinoma (SCC), (4) adenocarcinoma, or (5) others, including undifferentiated carcinomas. Cases of carcinoma that had metastasized to the urinary bladder were excluded from the study. The cases of TCC were classified based on the malignancy presentation as papillary or flat and whether it is confined to the transitional epithelium or invading the other layers of the bladder wall. All TCC cases were grouped and labeled as urothelial cell carcinoma (UC). The numbers of adenocarcinomas and other malignancies were so small, and thus not included in the present study.

2.4. Histopathological Characteristic Variables. Depending on the type of specimen examined, the pathologist noted the tumor grade (from 1 to 3), the stage (from p0 to pIVb), and the presence of *SH* ova. In addition, the pathologist examined the nonneoplastic bladder tissue, whenever available, for signs of inflammatory cystitis and/or mucosal ulcer.

2.5. Variables of Interest. Gender (male, female) was the main variable of interest with the reference group being female for statistical comparisons. Smoking was categorized as none (if they had smoked less than 100 cigarettes in their lifetime and had never smoked a waterpipe), waterpipe only, cigarettes only, and both (waterpipe and cigarettes). Smoking was also dichotomized as ever versus never to include in some of the analyses. The number of pack-years of cigarettes smoked by smokers and former smokers was calculated and added in any analysis that included the smoking variable. Participants, who reported ever-been told of a diagnosis of schistosomiasis by their doctors, were classified as having positive history of the disease. Secondhand smoke exposure was categorized as none or exposure either at home, outside the home, or at work. Education was categorized as none versus some (as a large number of the cases were uneducated). Similarly, the majority was married, and hence, marital status was either yes or no; the latter included never married, divorced, widowed, or separated. Residence location was categorized as north (Cairo, Giza, and northward) versus south of Cairo and urban versus rural. We grouped age in categories for descriptive analysis and dichotomized it (≤ 55 years versus >55 years) for the multivariable analysis.

2.6. Statistical Analysis. We used, respectively, Student's t-test and χ^2 tests to compare continuous and categorical variables between males and females, separately for UC and SCC. Significance level was set at $p \leq 0.05$. We used logistic regression to estimate unadjusted (OR) and adjusted odds ratio (AOR) and 95% confidence interval (CI). We used SAS software 9.4 (SAS Institute Inc., NC) for all analyses.

3. Results

From July 2006 through July 2014, 4,049 patients presumed to have bladder cancer were asked to participate in the study. Of those patients, 3,427 were eligible and 2,891 (84%) agreed

TABLE 1: Sociodemographic characteristics of bladder cancer cases (squamous cell carcinoma (SCC) and urothelial cell carcinoma (UC)) in Egyptian men and women.

Variable	Males		Females		*p value
	SCC (N = 574)	UC (N = 1201)	SCC (N = 210)	UC (N = 201)	
Age ± SD (years)	57.2 ± 10.3	61.2 ± 10.3	53.4 ± 10.8	59.2 ± 11.1	SCC < 0.0001; UC 0.01
Age group (years)					
≤45	64 (11.1)	89 (7.4)	49 (23.4)	24 (11.9)	
>45–≤55	182 (31.7)	259 (21.6)	83 (39.5)	46 (22.9)	SCC < 0.0001
>55–≤65	206 (35.9)	421 (35.0)	53 (25.2)	73 (36.3)	UC 0.06
>65	122 (21.3)	432 (36.0)	25 (11.9)	58 (28.9)	
Marital status					
Not married	11 (1.9)	11 (0.9)	7 (3.3)	1 (0.5)	SCC 0.2
Married	563 (98.1)	1190 (99.1)	203 (96.7)	200 (99.5)	UC 0.5
Education					
None	458 (79.8)	804 (67.0)	193 (91.9)	177 (88.1)	SCC < 0.0001
Some	116 (20.2)	395 (33.0)	17 (8.1)	24 (11.9)	UC < 0.0001
Residence					
North	36 (6.3)	176 (14.7)	27 (12.9)	28 (13.9)	SCC 0.002
South	538 (93.7)	1025 (85.3)	183 (87.1)	173 (86.1)	UC 0.6
Urban	52 (9.1)	217 (18.1)	21 (10.0)	35 (17.4)	SCC 0.6
Rural	522 (90.9)	984 (81.9)	189 (90)	166 (82.6)	UC 0.8
Smoking					
None	99 (17.3)	144 (12.0)	203 (96.6)	196 (97.5)	
Waterpipe	80 (13.9)	121 (10.1)	4 (2.0)	2 (1.0)	SCC < 0.0001
Cigarette	322 (56.1)	761 (63.3)	3 (1.4)	3 (1.5)	UC < 0.0001
Both	73 (12.7)	175 (14.6)	0	0	
Schistosomiasis					
No	211 (36.8)	469 (39.0)	148 (70.5)	145 (72.1)	SCC < 0.0001
Yes	320 (55.7)	670 (55.8)	44 (20.9)	41 (20.4)	UC < 0.0001
Unknown	43 (7.5)	62 (5.2)	18 (8.6)	15 (7.5)	
Secondhand smoke					
No	46 (8.0)	92 (7.7)	5 (3.5)	3 (2.5)	SCC 0.06
Yes	527 (92.0)	1106 (92.3)	139 (96.5)	119 (97.5)	UC 0.03

*Comparison of p value between males and females was done using Student's t-test and χ^2 for continuous and categorical variables, respectively. For some variables, the sum does not add up to the total because of missing information.

to participate. The pathologists completed a review of 2,523 cases and confirmed 2,325 to be primary bladder cancer. There were 1,402 UC (60.3%), 784 SCC (33.7%), 77 adenocarcinomas (3.3%), and 62 (2.7%) cases of other types of primary bladder cancer.

Table 1 shows the sociodemographic characteristics of the SCC and UC cases separately and by gender. The mean age at diagnosis of bladder cancer was higher for men than that for women (57.2 years versus 53.4 years, p value < 0.0001; 61.2 years versus 59.2 years, p value 0.01) for SCC and UC, respectively. Very few women smoked or had some education. The majority of participants were married. Whether the cases were SCC or UC, more men (55%) than women (20%) reported having a history of schistosomiasis.

Table 2 shows the histopathological characteristics of SCC and UC separately by gender.

The men-to-women ratios were 2.7 and 5.9 for SCC and UC, respectively. Among the SCC cases, we found a significant difference (p = 0.01) between men and women in the prevalence of cystectomy; pelvic lymphadenectomy was used among women but not men for both types of malignancies. The distribution of UC types (papillary and invasive) among men and women was similar, with the majority (77.8% and 78.8%, resp.) being invasive. In both men and women, the tumor grade was predominantly 2 for SCC (62% and 70% of the cases) and 3 for UC (49%). There were no significant differences between men and women in the distribution of their tumor stages; however, more SCC (~87% of the cases for both genders) than UC (59% and 57% of the men and women cases, resp.) were stage II and above.

The presence of *SH* ova in the tumor specimen was significantly more prevalent among men (73% and 59% for SCC and UC, resp.) than among women (53% and 42% for SCC and UC, resp.) (p < 0.0001). This pattern was consistent with the self-reported history of schistosomiasis, but with a greater magnitude.

Based on the pathological stage (stage II and above), muscle invasion was noted in ~87% of SCC cases but only in 57–59% of UC cases, with no significant gender difference. There was no gender difference for either inflammatory cystitis and/or ulcer in the nonneoplastic bladder tissue specimen examined, although both signs were highly prevalent in both types of carcinoma (Table 2).

Considering the small number of subjects with grade 1, we combined it with grade 2 and compared them to grade 3 in the subsequent analysis. Table 3 shows the results of the unadjusted associations between male gender and different relevant variables, as well as the results of the multivariable

TABLE 2: Histopathological characteristics of bladder cancer cases (squamous cell carcinoma (SCC) and urothelial cell carcinoma (UC)) in Egyptian men and women.

Variable	Males		Females		p value[1]
	SCC (N = 574)	UC (N = 1201)	SCC (N = 210)	UC (N = 201)	
Referred slide	28 (4.9)	66 (5.5)	9 (4.3)	14 (7.0)	
Biopsy	292 (51.1)	786 (65.9)	83 (40.4)	140 (69.6)	UC 0.4
Cystectomy	251 (44.0)	340 (28.5)	114 (54.8)	47 (23.4)	SCC 0.01
Radical	223 (95.3)	268 (94.0)	49 (51.1)	21 (52.5)	
Simple	7 (3.0)	7 (2.5)	1 (1.0)	0	
Partial	4 (1.7)	9 (3.2)	7 (7.3)	0	SCC < 0.0001
Pelvic excision[2]	0	0	39 (40.6)	19 (47.5)	UC < 0.0001
Grade					
1	84 (15.0)	55 (4.8)	31 (15.2)	7 (3.7)	SCC 0.07
2	353 (62.9)	527 (46.2)	143 (70.1)	89 (47.1)	UC 0.8
3	124 (22.1)	558 (49.0)	30 (14.7)	93 (49.2)	
Stage					
0	0	38 (6.7)	1 (0.8)	6 (7.6)	
I	41 (12.8)	195 (34.3)	15 (11.6)	28 (35.4)	
IIa	22 (6.9)	19 (3.3)	8 (6.2)	4 (5.0)	SCC 0.6
b	82 (25.7)	72 (12.6)	29 (22.5)	10 (12.7)	UC 0.6
IIIa	33 (10.3)	54 (9.5)	12 (9.3)	4 (5.0)	
b	115 (36.0)	144 (25.3)	54 (41.8)	22 (27.8)	
IVa	26 (8.1)	44 (7.7)	10 (7.7)	5 (6.3)	
b	0	3 (0.5)	0	0	
Presence of *SH*[3] ova					
No	129 (26.8)	355 (40.7)	73 (46.5)	72 (58.1)	SCC < 0.0001
Yes	353 (73.2)	518 (59.3)	84 (53.5)	52 (41.9)	UC < 0.0001
Cystitis					
No	11 (6.7)	9 (2.8)	3 (4.7)	0	SCC 0.5
Yes	152 (93.3)	315 (97.2)	61 (95.3)	55 (100)	UC 0.2
Ulceration					
No	14 (11.2)	8 (3.3)	7 (15.6)	2 (2.7)	SCC 0.4
Yes	111 (88.8)	232 (96.7)	38 (84.4)	36 (97.3)	UC 0.8

[1]Comparison of p value between males and females was done using χ^2; [2]pelvic lymphadenectomy; [3]*Schistosoma haematobium*.

logistic regression analyses, for SCC and UC cases, separately. We included in the final model variables that were significantly associated with male gender. Among the SCC cases, having high-grade tumor (grade 3) was significantly associated with male gender (OR (95% CI) = 1.64 (1.06–2.54)), but the association became statistically nonsignificant (0.82 (0.38–1.794)) after adjustment for other significant variables. On the other hand, having *SH* ova in the bladder tissue specimen (2.12 (1.15–3.89)), older age (2.40 (1.32–4.36)), smoking (24.89 (8.58–72.21)), and residing in the south (3.31 (1.14–9.69)) remained significantly associated with male gender in the adjusted model (Table 3).

Among the UC cases, neither tumor grade nor residence in the south, but having *SH* ova in the bladder tissue (3.78 (1.89–7.55)), smoking (40.55 (9.13–180.12)), and older age (3.44 (1.73–6.83)) were associated with male gender; the associations were similar to those noted among the SCC cases (Table 3).

4. Discussion

We found male, more than female, cases of bladder cancer to have evidence of *SH* infection in their bladder tissue specimen, regardless of the type of cancer. These findings support our previous studies demonstrating that the self-reported history of *SH* infection is a risk factor, not only for SCC but also for the UC cancer type [26, 28]. Indeed, more men (55%) than women (20%) reported a history of schistosomiasis, and the pathologists reported more men (73% and 59% for SCC and UC, resp.) than women (53% and 42% for SCC and UC, resp.) to have *SH* ova in their bladder tissue specimens. The higher prevalence of *SH* infection in males, as compared to female cancer cases, can be explained by the fact that the majority of men worked in farming and thus were at risk for *SH* infection because of exposures to infested waters, while the majority of women did not work outside the house [28].

We found no gender differences in the grade and the stages of either SCC or UC; however, the male-to-female ratio was higher for UC (5.9) than for SCC (2.7). In addition, most men in this study were smokers, while few women reported smoking. It is probable that the addition of *SH* infection to smoking, which is a well-established risk factor for UC, contributed to the male-to-female ratio being higher for UC than for SCC, among bladder cancer cases in Egypt.

Bladder cancer is one of the few malignancies where women have high cancer-specific mortality [22]. One of the reasons suggested was gender differences in stage distribution [23]; the latter being worse in female than in male patients [24]. We found men and women to have similar

Table 3: Unadjusted and adjusted (multivariable regression model) associations between male gender and different variables among squamous and urothelial cell carcinoma cases in Egypt.

Variable	Squamous cell carcinoma (SCC)		Urothelial cell carcinoma (UC)	
	OR (95% CI)[1]	AOR (95% CI)[2]	OR (95% CI)[1]	AOR (95% CI)[3]
Tumor grade				
1 + 2	Ref.	Ref.	Ref.	
3	1.64 (1.06–2.54)	0.82 (0.38–1.79)	0.99 (0.72–1.34)	
Presence of *SH*[4] ova				
No	Ref.	Ref.	Ref.	Ref.
Yes	2.38 (1.64–3.45)	2.12 (1.15–3.89)	2.02 (1.38–2.96)	3.78 (1.89–7.55)
Age				
≤55 years	Ref.	Ref.	Ref.	Ref.
>55 years	2.25 (1.63–3.12)	2.40 (1.32–4.36)	1.31 (0.95–1.79)	3.44 (1.73–6.83)
Smoking				
Never	Ref.	Ref.	Ref.	Ref.
Ever	43.99 (16.97–114.05)	24.89 (8.58–72.21)	106.00 (30.28–371.10)	40.55 (9.13–180.12)
Residence				
North	Ref.	Ref.	Ref.	
South	2.20 (1.30–3.73)	3.31 (1.14–9.69)	0.94 (0.61–1.45)	

[1]Unadjusted odds ratio (95% confidence interval); [2]adjusted odds ratios (95% confidence interval) in the multivariable model that included the variables listed in the left column in addition to education and secondhand smoke; [3]adjusted odds ratios (95% confidence interval) in the multivariable model that included the variables in the left column (except residence and tumor grade), education, and secondhand smoke; [4]*Schistosoma haematobium*; whenever smoking was assessed, pack-year for ever-smokers was included in the model.

distribution of their tumor stages, whether it was UC or SCC (Table 2). High-grade tumor and thus aggressive malignancy were also suggested to occur among women more than men. We found that grade 3 SCC, but not UC, was associated with male, not female, gender; however, the association became nonsignificant after adjustment for other known risk factors (Table 3). A prior study of UC reported no gender differences in the histopathological characteristics of the tumor [25]. And more recently, Welty et al. developed a new nomogram to predict UC survival following surgery, based on the tumor characteristics, and did not include sex as a prognostic factor [4]. Our study is the first to investigate gender differences in the grade or the stage of the SCC type.

Investigators found that muscle-invasive cases occurred more frequently in men than in women, and those men were younger than the women at diagnosis [21]. In our study, we found no gender differences in the prevalence of muscle invasion: although muscle invasion was more prevalent in the SCC (~87%) than in the UC (57–59%) cases, women cases were diagnosed with bladder cancer at a significantly younger age than men, particularly with the SCC type. A Turkish study found 75% of the bladder cancer cases to be nonmuscle invasive [29].

We found that women, more commonly than men, underwent cystectomy with pelvic lymphadenectomy. This is consistent with a diagnosis made at advanced stages of the disease. However, in our study, women cases who underwent radical cystectomy were comparable to those who underwent pelvic lymphadenectomy, with respect to the grade and stage of the malignancy. Possible explanations include the existence of comorbidities leading to pelvic lymphadenectomy or differences in surgical practices between clinicians. Indeed, comparing the three referral cancer centers, Cairo NCI, Minia, and Assiut, we found that, among all women who underwent cystectomy, pelvic lymphadenectomy represented 30%, 67%, and 43% of the cases, respectively.

The search for factors associated with gender differences in bladder cancer incidence has prompted several investigators to assess the role of sex steroids. In animal studies, androgen receptor knockout (AR-KO) male mice developed fewer bladder tumors, and females without AR developed no tumors [13, 14]. Additionally, there is evidence that the presence of female hormones can inhibit bladder carcinogenesis or delay the disease progression [15], and the use of antiandrogens appears to delay the development of bladder cancer in men [19]; all of these lines of evidence support a theory that female hormones are protective against bladder cancer. Some investigators and we [16, 18] found estrogen to be protective but others did not [17]. Further studies are needed to assess the contribution of sex steroids to the gender disparity of bladder cancer in Egypt.

Our study has some weaknesses. Some of the information collected was self-reported and thus subject to bias. Despite the large sample size, very few women reported ever-smoking tobacco, and therefore, the risk estimates may not be precise. Nonetheless, our study has several strengths, such as a large sample size that included both UC and SCC cases and a large number of women with SCC, which allowed us to examine for gender-specific differences in histopathological presentation of this type of malignancy. It is a multicenter study, which recruited cases from several areas in Egypt, and it has a high participation rate (84%). Finally yet importantly, two pathologists used a standardized form to report the histopathological characteristics and ascertain the type of the tumors.

5. Conclusion

We found evidence for bladder tissue infection with *SH* to be significantly more prevalent in male than in female cases of bladder cancer, regardless of the type of cancer (SCC or UC); but there are no significant gender differences in other histopathological characteristics of either UC or SCC in Egypt. More studies are needed to elucidate the mechanism(s) underlying gender difference in bladder cancer.

Acknowledgments

The authors thank Sameera Ezzat, Tamer El Hifnawy, and Doa'a Salah who supervised the recruitment of subjects for this study. Iman Gouda, Iman Loay, and Bhaskar Kallakury performed the expert pathology review of the cases. Data management services were provided by Nabiel N. Mikhail. This study was supported by a grant from the National Cancer Institute, National Institutes of Health (R01-CA115618 to Christopher A. Loffredo).

References

[1] S. Antoni, J. Ferlay, I. Soerjomataram, A. Znaor, A. Jemal, and F. Bray, "Bladder cancer incidence and mortality: a global overview and recent trends," *European Urology*, vol. 71, no. 1, pp. 96–108, 2017.

[2] H. Fajkovic, J. A. Halpern, E. K. Cha et al., "Impact of gender on bladder cancer incidence, staging, and prognosis," *World Journal of Urology*, vol. 29, no. 4, pp. 457–463, 2011.

[3] International Bladder Cancer Nomogram Consortium, B. H. Bochner, M. W. Kattan, and K. C. Vora, "Postoperative nomogram predicting risk of recurrence after radical cystectomy for bladder cancer," *Journal of Clinical Oncology*, vol. 24, no. 24, pp. 3967–3972, 2006.

[4] C. J. Welty, T. H. Sanford, J. L. Wright et al., "The Cancer of the Bladder Risk Assessment (COBRA) score: estimating mortality after radical cystectomy," *Cancer*, vol. 123, no. 23, pp. 4574–4582, 2017.

[5] S. F. Shariat, R. L. Favaretto, A. Gupta et al., "Gender differences in radical nephroureterectomy for upper tract urothelial carcinoma," *World Journal of Urology*, vol. 29, no. 4, pp. 481–486, 2011.

[6] IARC Working Group on the Evaluation of Carcinogenic Risks to Humans, *Tobacco Smoke and Involuntary Smoking*, Vol. 83, IARC Monographs on the Evaluation of Carcinogenic Risk to Humans, Lyon, France, 2004.

[7] IARC Working Group on the Evaluation of Carcinogenic Risks to Humans, *Schistosomes, Liver Flukes and* Helicobacter pylori, Vol. 61, IARC Monographs on the Evaluation of Carcinogenic Risks to Humans, Lyon, France, 1994.

[8] D. T. Silverman, S. S. Devesa, L. E. Moore, and N. Rothman, "Bladder cancer," in *Cancer Epidemiology and Prevention*, D. Schottenfeld and J. F. J. Fraumeni, Eds., pp. 1101–1127, Oxford University Press, New York, NY, USA, 3rd edition, 2006.

[9] A. H. Al-Zalabani, K. F. Stewart, A. Wesselius, A. M. Schols, and M. P. Zeegers, "Modifiable risk factors for the prevention of bladder cancer: a systematic review of meta-analyses," *European Journal of Epidemiology*, vol. 31, no. 9, pp. 811–851, 2016.

[10] M. Burger, J. W. Catto, G. Dalbagni et al., "Epidemiology and risk factors of urothelial bladder cancer," *European Urology*, vol. 63, no. 2, pp. 234–241, 2013.

[11] M. Hemelt, H. Yamamoto, K. K. Cheng, and M. Zeegers, "The effect of smoking on the male excess of bladder cancer: a meta-analysis and geographical analyses," *International Journal of Cancer*, vol. 124, no. 2, pp. 412–419, 2009.

[12] H. Miyamoto, Z. Yang, Y. T. Chen et al., "Promotion of bladder cancer development and progression by androgen receptor signals," *Journal of the National Cancer Institute*, vol. 99, no. 7, pp. 558–568, 2007.

[13] J. W. Hsu, I. Hsu, D. Xu et al., "Decreased tumorigenesis and mortality from bladder cancer in mice lacking urothelial androgen receptor," *The American Journal of Pathology*, vol. 182, no. 5, pp. 1811–1820, 2013.

[14] S. E. Daugherty, J. V. Lacey Jr., R. M. Pfeiffer, Y. Park, R. N. Hoover, and D. T. Silverman, "Reproductive factors and menopausal hormone therapy and bladder cancer risk in the NIH-AARP Diet and Health Study," *International Journal of Cancer*, vol. 133, no. 2, pp. 462–472, 2013.

[15] M. McGrath, D. S. Michaud, and I. De Vivo, "Hormonal and reproductive factors and the risk of bladder cancer in women," *American Journal of Epidemiology*, vol. 163, no. 3, pp. 236–244, 2006.

[16] M. M. Cantwell, J. V. Lacey Jr., C. Schairer, A. Schatzkin, and D. S. Michaud, "Reproductive factors, exogenous hormone use and bladder cancer risk in a prospective study," *International Journal of Cancer*, vol. 119, no. 10, pp. 2398–2401, 2006.

[17] A. E. Prizment, K. E. Anderson, B. L. Harlow, and A. R. Folsom, "Reproductive risk factors for incident bladder cancer: Iowa Women's Health Study," *International Journal of Cancer*, vol. 120, no. 5, pp. 1093–1098, 2007.

[18] B. J. Wolpert, S. Amr, S. Ezzat et al., "Estrogen exposure and bladder cancer risk in Egyptian women," *Maturitas*, vol. 67, no. 4, pp. 353–357, 2010.

[19] E. E. Morales, S. Grill, R. S. Svateka et al., "Finasteride reduces risk of bladder cancer in a large prospective screening study," *European Urology*, vol. 69, no. 3, pp. 407–410, 2016.

[20] P. Gupta, M. Jain, R. Kapoor, K. Muruganandham, A. Srivastava, and A. Mandhani, "Impact of age and gender on the clinicopathological characteristics of bladder cancer," *Indian Journal of Urology*, vol. 25, no. 2, p. 207, 2009.

[21] M. Horstmann, R. Witthuhn, M. Falk, and A. Stenzl, "Gender-specific differences in bladder cancer: a retrospective analysis," *Gender Medicine*, vol. 5, no. 4, pp. 385–394, 2008.

[22] E. Scosyrev, K. Noyes, C. Feng, and E. Messing, "Sex and racial differences in bladder cancer presentation and mortality in the US," *Cancer*, vol. 115, no. 1, pp. 68–74, 2009.

[23] K. Mallin, K. A. David, P. R. Carroll, M. I. Milowsky, and D. M. Nanus, "Transitional cell carcinoma of the bladder: racial and gender disparities in survival (1993 to 2002), stage and grade (1993 to 2007)," *The Journal of Urology*, vol. 185, no. 5, pp. 1631–1636, 2011.

[24] N. A. Mungan, L. Kiemeney, J. van Dijck, H. J. van der Poel, and J. A. Witjes, "Gender differences in stage distribution of bladder cancer," *Urology*, vol. 55, no. 3, pp. 368–371, 2000.

[25] W. Otto, M. May, H. M. Fritsche et al., "Analysis of sex differences in cancer-specific survival and perioperative mortality following radical cystectomy: results of a large German multicenter study of nearly 2500 patients with urothelial carcinoma of the bladder," *Gender Medicine*, vol. 9, no. 6, pp. 481–489, 2012.

[26] Y. L. Zheng, S. Amr, D. A. Saleh et al., "Urinary bladder cancer risk factors in Egypt: a multicenter case-control study," *Cancer Epidemiology Biomarkers & Prevention*, vol. 21, no. 3, pp. 537–546, 2012.

[27] S. Amr, C. A. Loffredo, K. M. McClain, B. Kallakury, and Y. L. Zheng, "Adenocarcinoma of the urinary bladder in Egypt: potential risk factors," *World Journal of Nephrology and Urology*, vol. 4, no. 3, pp. 227–231, 2015.
[28] S. Amr, R. Dawson, D. Saleh et al., "Agricultural workers and urinary bladder cancer risk in Egypt," *Archives of Environmental & Occupational Health*, vol. 69, pp. 3–10, 2014.
[29] A. M. Kamat, M. Bağcıoğlu, and E. Huri, "What is new in non-muscle-invasive bladder cancer in 2016?," *Turkish Journal of Urology*, vol. 43, no. 1, pp. 9–13, 2017.

5

Efficacy of Tamsulosin plus Tadalafil versus Tamsulosin as Medical Expulsive Therapy for Lower Ureteric Stones

Diwas Gnyawali, Manish Man Pradhan, Prem Raj Sigdel, Purushottam Parajuli, Sampanna Chudal, Sujeet Poudyal, Suman Chapagain, Bhoj Raj Luitel, Pawan Raj Chalise, Uttam Sharma, and Prem Raj Gyawali

Department of Urology and Kidney Transplant Surgery, Tribhuvan University Teaching Hospital, Institute of Medicine, Maharajgung, Kathmandu 44600, Nepal

Correspondence should be addressed to Diwas Gnyawali; diwasgnyawali@gmail.com

Academic Editor: Mohammad H. Ather

Introduction. Urolithiasis is one of the common disorder with which about 1/5th is found in the ureter, of which 2/3rd is seen in the lower ureter. Medical expulsive therapy is one of the routine modalities of treatment which uses various drugs acting on the ureter smooth muscle by different mechanism. We aim to compare the efficacy of combination vs. single drug. *Methods.* This randomized controlled trial was done in 176 consecutive patients over a period of six months (March 2019 to August 2019) in Department of Urology and Kidney Transplant Surgery, Tribhuvan University Teaching. Participants were divided into two groups (Group A, tamsulosin plus tadalafil, and Group B, tamsulosin) from computer-generated random numbers. Therapy was continued for a maximum of 3 weeks. Stone expulsion rate, time to stone expulsion, analgesic use, number of colic and emergency room visits for pain, early intervention, and adverse effects of drugs were recorded. *Results.* Among 176 patients who were enrolled in study, 7 were lost to follow-up, and 5 people required immediate intervention. There was a significant higher stone passage rate in group A than group B (64 vs. 50; $P = 0.025$) and shorter expulsion time (1.66 vs. 2.32 weeks $P = 0.001$) and less number of emergency room visits and colic episodes. No significant side effects were noted during study. *Conclusion.* Tamsulosin plus Tadalafil is more effective than tamsulosin with early passage of stone and decreased number of colic episodes and emergency visits without significant side effects for lower ureteric calculi of 5 mm to 10 mm.

1. Introduction

Urolithiasis is one of the most common disorders of the urinary tract with life-time prevalence of up to 15% with men affected three times more than women [1, 2]. Improved quality of life may also have increased its prevalence. A significant proportion, about 1/5th of urinary tract stones, is found in the ureter, of which 2/3rd is seen in the distal ureter [3]. Initially, a colicky pain of various grades presents with ureteric stone. This is one of the most common problems that compel a patient to an emergency room [4].

Today, medical expulsive therapy (MET) has become the most used modality of a treatment for urolithiasis. During this treatment, the ureter smooth muscle is treated via various drugs by different mechanisms. Blocking alpha-(α-) 1 adrenergic receptors, especially in the distal third decreases basal smooth muscle contraction and causes propulsive antegrade peristalsis helping stone expulsion [2, 5, 6]. By increasing the intraureteral pressure gradient around the stone, alpha-1 adrenergic receptor antagonists eject distal ureteral stones [7]. Tamsulosin has continuously shown a proven role in increasing the stone expulsion rate and decreasing expulsion time [7]. Significant pathological changes can occur when ureteric stones are impacted. This can cause inflammatory reaction with mucosal edema which could further worsen the ureteric obstruction, increasing the risk of impaction and retention [8]. However, selective alpha-1 blockers, such as tamsulosin and silodosin, have been the treatment of choice, with proven efficacy in multiple clinical trials [8–10].

Recently, a newer PDE5 inhibitor, tadalafil, has shown action on nitric oxide-cyclic guanosine monophosphate-signaling pathway of smooth muscles, resulting in increased levels of cyclic guanosine monophosphate, causing ureteric relaxation [2, 11–13]. Due to its smooth muscle relaxation mechanism, tadalafil has received US Food and Drug Administration approval to treat many urinary tract diseases. Therefore, the combination of tamsulosin and tadalafil drugs is aimed to facilitate stone passage by better ureteric relaxation and reducing intramural ureter pressure. Though there have been few similar studies using various combinations, comparing the efficacy of tamsulosin and tadalafil vs. tamsulosin are very few, and these studies have taken longer duration of treatment (4 to 6 weeks) [5, 14] which might have affected the outcome. Meta-analysis [15] which also recommends further research has taken consideration of only one drug PDE5 inhibitor or alpha blocker in most of its studies inclusion. So, with this study, we aim to find out if the combination therapy is better than tamsulosin alone.

2. Materials and Methods

The study was conducted in the Department of Urology and Kidney Transplant surgery at Tribhuvan University Teaching Hospital, over a period of 6 months (from 1st March 2019 to 31st August 2019). All patients with lower ureteric stone from 5 mm to 10 mm in size, diagnosed by CT Scan, Ultrasound (USG) abdomen/pelvis or X-ray KUB, were only included in the study. CT scan was not done in all patients due to financial reason. Patients with the presence of multiple ureteric stones, radiolucent stones, urinary tract infection, pregnancy, and pediatric population; patients with a history of ureteral surgery or previous endoscopic procedures; patients having ischemic heart disease, congestive cardiac failure, or complicated hypertension; patients requiring emergency intervention; and patients with raised creatinine were not included in the study.

Previously performed other studies [5, 13, 16] were taken as a reference for $P1$ and $P2$ values for sample size, and it was calculated by the following formula and K value from (Table 1); a power of 80% and a level of significance of 95% was used for the test. With 10% drop out rate, the sample size was calculated as 176. The formula is

$$N = K\frac{p_1(1-p_1)+p_2(1-p_2)}{(p_1-p_2)^2}, \tag{1}$$

where N = sample size, p_1 = successful passage in the tamsulosin and tadalafil group, and p_2 = successful passage in the tamsulosin group.

Written informed consent was taken from all participants. Study methodology and protocol were approved from the Institutional Review Board of Institute of Medicine, Tribhuvan University (reference no. 359(6-11) E2/075/76). This trial was registered retrospectively in the University Hospital Medical Information Network (UMIN) (registration no UMIN000038125).

Table 1: K value for sample size calculation

		Power			
		50% $\beta=0.5$	80% $\beta=0.2$	90% $\beta=0.1$	95% $\beta=0.05$
α	0.10	2.7	6.2	8.6	10.8
	0.05	3.8	7.9	10.5	13.0
	0.02	5.4	10.0	13.0	15.8
	0.01	6.6	11.7	14.9	17.8

Detailed history and clinical examination and routine urine examination and/or urine culture, serum creatinine, digital X-ray KUB and/or USG abdomen and pelvis, and/or CT-KUB were carried out in all patients. The stone size was determined using largest dimension.

Patients were randomized and divided into two equal groups of 88 based on a computer-generated random number table (Figure 1). Patients in Group A were prescribed tamsulosin of 0.4 mg and tadalafil of 10 mg once a day, whereas those in group B were prescribed tamsulosin of 0.4 mg. Both groups received diclofenac of 50 mg three times a day, hyoscine butylbromide of 10 mg three times a day for one day followed by as per need basis, and proton pump inhibitor (Pantoprazole 40 mg) once a day. Drugs were continued until stone expulsion.

In both groups, drugs were continued until stone expulsion or for a period of 3 weeks. There was no strong evidence that, the longer duration of drugs user will increase the expulsion rate and deleterious effect of obstruction on kidney function will be minimized. Patients were instructed to take plenty of fluids and filter their urine by using a net. All patients were evaluated by physical examination, serum creatinine, and the same imaging modality by which lower ureteric stones were conformed previously in those who either could not present the stone or presented the stone that did not match the original size and shape. In case of doubt, CT KUB was done despite previous imaging modality to conform stone expulsion. Expulsion of the ureteric calculi, total dose of analgesic used, number of colic episodes and emergency room visits, and side effect of drugs were recorded. Semirigid ureteroscopy was done to those who did not pass stones after 3 weeks of follow-up for stone removal. Unpaired Student's t-test and the χ^2-test were used for the analysis of the variables and categorical data. Differences were considered significant at a P value less than 0.05.

3. Results

Out of 190 patients, 176 met the inclusion criteria who were randomly assigned into 2 groups. Three patients from Group A and four patients from Group B lost their follow-up for various reasons. Four patients from both groups required early intervention, whereas the remaining patients completed the study. There were no statistically significant differences in patients' age, gender, and stone size (Table 2).

The stone expulsion rate was 79.0% in Group A and 62.5% in Group B; Group A showed a higher stone expulsion rate than Group B (P value = 0.025). The mean time for

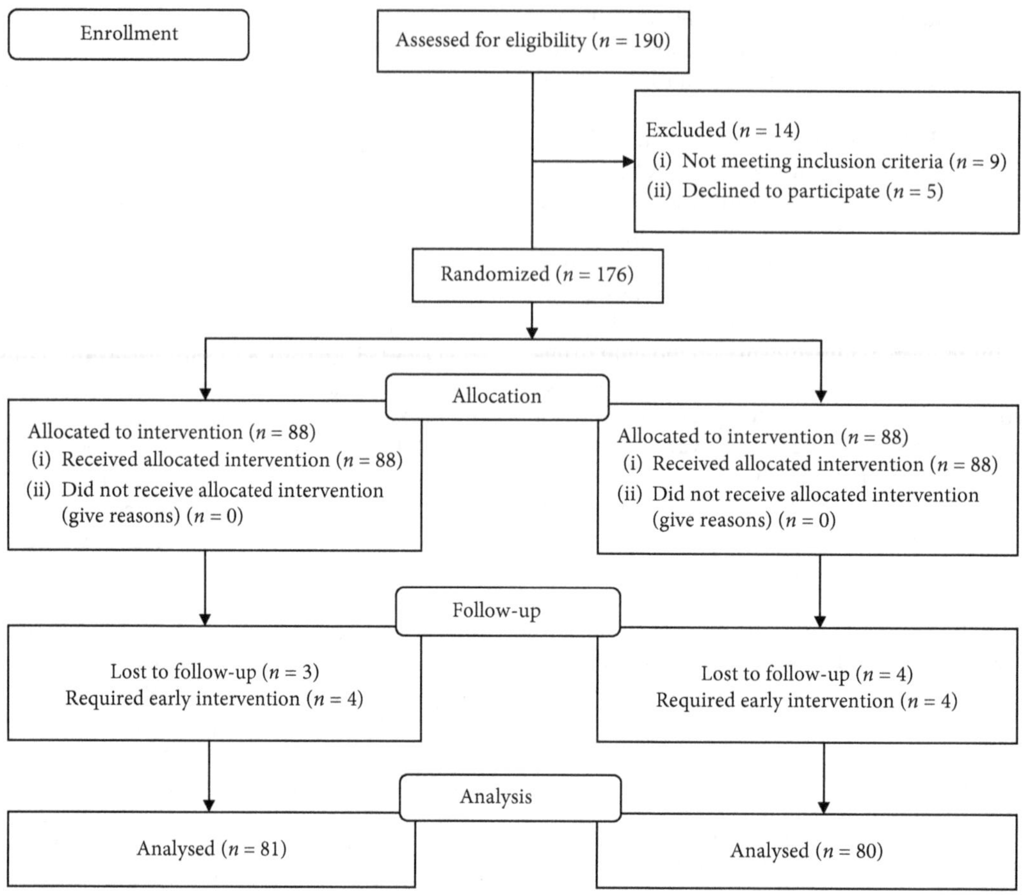

Figure 1: Patient flow diagram.

stone expulsion in Group A was 1.66 vs. 2.32 weeks in Group B (P value = 0.001). Out of 161 patients, stones were not expelled in 47 patients (17 and 30 patients in groups A and B, respectively) at the end of 3rd week of therapy. These patients underwent semirigid ureteroscopic stone removal with laser lithotripsy. While comparing Group A (2.02), the patients had significantly less episodes of colicky pain than Group B (2.32) (P value = 0.001) with significantly less number of emergency room visits.

Table 2: Demographic and results.

Parameter	Group A	Group B	P value
Mean age (years)	33.75 ± 10.01	32.85 ± 10.36	0.575
No. of patients (male/female)	58/23	50/30	0.243
Mean stone size (mm)	7.43 ± 1.23	7.34 ± 1.13	0.618
Expulsion rate (%)	64/81	50/80	0.025
Mean expulsion time (weeks)	1.66 ± 0.87	2.32 ± 0.76	0.001
Mean analgesic use (mg)	403 ± 131	526 ± 86	0.001
Mean no. of colic episodes	2.02 ± 0.80	2.34 ± 0.67	0.008
Mean no. of emergency visits	1.48 ± 0.61	1.70 ± 0.60	0.024

Statistical significance was analyzed by Student's t-test and χ^2-test. Values are presented as mean ± standard deviation. Group A: tamsulosin and tadalafil. Group B: tamsulosin.

Additionally, the mean requirement of analgesia (diclofenac) was significantly less in Group A (403) than in Group B (526) (Table 2).

Drug-related adverse effects such as headache, dizziness, postural hypotension, backache, and running nose were comparable between two groups (Table 3). Out of 58 males from Group A, 31 of them (55%) developed mild degree of penile tumescence lasting for 20–30 minutes, but none of them developed priapism.

4. Discussion

Urolithiasis is common urological disease. Among all urinary tract stones, about 1/5th are ureteral stones, of which 2/3rd are found in the lower third [17]. In last two decades, the development and improvisation of new, minimally invasive

Table 3: Side effects.

Variable	Group A	Group B	P value
Headache	10	8	0.62
Dizziness	9	7	0.47
Postural hypotension	4	3	0.81
Backache	11	7	0.41
Runny nose	2	1	0.91
Abnormal ejaculation	5	6	0.78

Statistical significance was analyzed by the χ^2-test. Group A: tamsulosin and tadalafil. Group B: tamsulosin.

procedures (extracorporeal shock wave lithotripsy and ureteroscopy) for ureteral stones has considerably changed the management of ureteral stones [18, 19]. But on the contrary, these methods are not only risky and inconvenient but also very expensive. This can affect the quality of life of a patient as patient daily activities can be reduced [20]. Hence, there has been paradigm shift in the treatment of distal ureteric stone with a primary focus on MET. According to the available literature, spontaneous passage of distal ureteric stone using a conservative approach for stones of 5–10 mm is less likely [21], with a mean expulsion time of >10 days [20].

Factors influencing the spontaneous expulsion of stones, such as stone location, stone size, stone number, stone structure, ureteral spasm, mucosal edema or inflammation, and ureteral anatomy. Therefore, the use of medical therapy is justifiable to reduce edema, reduce spasm, and relax the smooth muscles for stone expulsion [21]. MET has recently emerged as an alternative strategy for the initial management of selected patients with distal ureteral stones [19, 20].

Since Sigala et al., described that the most common adrenoceptors found in the ureter are α-1D and α-1A [22], several studies have been carried out to determine the effect of a combined α-1A and α-1D selective antagonist, tamsulosin, which showed an improved expulsion rate of medium sized (3–10 mm) stones. We also observed an expulsion rate of 62.5% with tamsulosin, which is better than historical controls used in earlier studies of 30–43% [16, 23, 24].

Tadalafil, PDE-5 inhibitors, act via the nitric oxide/cGMP-signaling pathway, which results in increased levels of cGMP, leading to ureteric smooth muscle relaxation, which helps in stone passage [25, 26]. Tadalafil was used as it is more selective compared with sildenafil for PDE5 with long duration of action (~36 h, and a half-life of 17.5 h) and its activity unaffected by meals [12] and combination of tamsulosin and tadalafil was found to be safe [27, 28] by Kloner et al. Bechara et al. showed effectiveness of combination when they used for LUTS [29].

While comparing the efficacy of drugs in our study, we found Group A (tamsulosin plus tadalafil) patients had higher expulsion rate than Group B (tamsulosin) 79.01% vs. 62.50% (P value 0.025), respectively. Stone passage rate in tamsulosin plus tadalafil was comparable with Jayant et al. of 83% [5] but was less than Rahman et al. of 90% [8] which may be they have used silodusin and tadalafil as combination.

Tamsulosin and tadalafil when used in combination facilitates stone passage and also decreases the stone passage duration 11.66 days which is shorter than 14.9 days of Jayant et al. [5] and comparable to 12 days of Rahman et al. [8].

In the present study, the mean analgesic requirement in group A was significantly less with respect to group B (403 mg vs. 531 mg ($P = 0.001$)), this better pain control was also reflected by the lesser number of colic episodes and emergency room visits in group A. The abovementioned effects may be due to decrease in frequency and amplitude of phasic contractions that accompany ureteric obstruction; that is, an improved antispasmodic effect of tamsulosin and tadalafil [14].

There was no significant difference in side effects. These were mild and well tolerated by the study population who were relatively younger in age and lack of any comorbidity. Similar result was shown on various other studies. There was no significant difference in side effects between two groups and side effects were comparable with other studies [5, 8, 13, 14].

5. Conclusion

With this study, we can conclude that combination of tamsulosin and tadalafil is more efficacious than tamsulosin alone when used in lower ureteric stones of 5 mm to 10 mm with significant low-dose analgesic requirement, less number of colic episodes, and few number of emergency room visits without extra side effects.

Additional Points

CT KUB was not done in all cases as a diagnostic modality due to financial reasons, and follow-up was up to three weeks as if we increase follow-up, then there may be more drop out cases and also patients in our region already presented late to hospital.

Acknowledgments

The authors thank all patients, collogues, and hospital radiology and laboratory staffs for their help in conducting this research. This research was conducted as a part of employment of authors on Institute of Medicine, Tribhuvan University Teaching Hospital.

References

[1] D.-U. Tchey, Y. S. Ha, W. T. Kim, S. J. Yun, S. C. Lee, and W. J. Kim, "Expectant management of ureter stones: outcome and clinical factors of spontaneous passage in a single institution's experience," *Korean Journal of Urology*, vol. 52, no. 12, pp. 847–851, 2011.

[2] S. Puvvada, P. Mylarappa, K. Aggarwal, A. Patil, P. Joshi, and R. Desigowda, "Comparative efficacy of tadalafil versus tamsulosin as the medical expulsive therapy in lower ureteric stone: a prospective randomized trial," *Central European Journal of Urology*, vol. 69, no. 69, pp. 178–182, 2016.

[3] A.-f. Abdel-maguid Ahmed and A.-y. S. Al-Sayed, "Tamsulosin versus alfuzosin in the treatment of patients with distal ureteral stones: prospective, randomized, comparative study," *Korean Journal of Urology*, vol. 51, no. 3, pp. 193–197, 2010.

[4] J. M. Hollingsworth, M. A. M. Rogers, S. R. Kaufman et al., "Medical therapy to facilitate urinary stone passage: a meta-analysis," *The Lancet*, vol. 368, no. 9542, pp. 1171–1179, 2006.
[5] K. Jayant, R. Agrawal, and S. Agrawal, "Tamsulosin versus tamsulosin plus tadalafil as medical expulsive therapy for lower ureteric stones: a randomized controlled trial," *International Journal of Urology*, vol. 21, no. 10, pp. 1012–1015, 2014.
[6] F. Porpiglia, D. Vaccino, M. Billia et al., "Corticosteroids and tamsulosin in the medical expulsive therapy for symptomatic distal ureter stones: single drug or association?" *European Urology*, vol. 50, no. 2, pp. 339–344, 2006.
[7] C.-J. Wang, S.-W. Huang, and C.-H. Chang, "Efficacy of an alpha1 blocker in expulsive therapy of lower ureteral stones," *Journal of Endourology*, vol. 22, no. 1, pp. 41–46, 2008.
[8] M. J. Rahman, M. S. Faridi, N. Mibang, and R. S. Singh, "Comparing tamsulosin, silodosin versus silodosin plus tadalafil as medical expulsive therapy for lower ureteric stones: a randomised trial," *Arab Journal of Urology*, vol. 16, no. 2, pp. 245–249, 2018.
[9] K. Sridharan and G. Sivaramakrishnan, "Efficacy and safety of alpha blockers in medical expulsive therapy for ureteral stones: a mixed treatment network meta-analysis and trial sequential analysis of randomized controlled clinical trials," *Expert Review of Clinical Pharmacology*, vol. 11, no. 3, pp. 291–307, 2018.
[10] M. D. Jayawardene, B. Balagobi, A. L. A. M. C. Ambegoda et al., "Outcome of uncomplicated ureteric calculi managed with medical expulsive therapy in the outpatient clinic of a urology unit in Sri Lanka," *BMC Research Notes*, vol. 10, no. 1, p. 636, 2017.
[11] C. Gratzke, S. Ückert, O. Reich et al., "PDE5 inhibitors," *Der Urologe*, vol. 46, no. 9, pp. 1219–1223, 2007.
[12] C. Gratzke, S. Ückert, G. Kedia et al., "In vitro effects of PDE5 inhibitors sildenafil, vardenafil and tadalafil on isolated human ureteral smooth muscle: a basic research approach," *Urological Research*, vol. 35, no. 1, pp. 49–54, 2007.
[13] H. B. Kc, A. Shrestha, G. B. Acharya, R. B. Basnet, A. K. Shah, and P. M. Shrestha, "Tamsulosin versus tadalafil as a medical expulsive therapy for distal ureteral stones: a prospective randomized study," *Investigative and Clinical Urology*, vol. 57, no. 5, pp. 351–356, 2016.
[14] S. Kumar, K. Jayant, S. Agrawal, and S. K. Singh, "Comparative efficacy of tamsulosin versus tamsulosin with tadalafil in combination with prednisolone for the medical expulsive therapy of lower ureteric stones: a randomized trial," *Korean Journal of Urology*, vol. 55, no. 3, pp. 196–200, 2014.
[15] C. E. Montes Cardona and H. A. García-Perdomo, "Efficacy of phosphodiesterase type 5 inhibitors for the treatment of distal ureteral calculi: a systematic review and meta-analysis," *Investigative and Clinical Urology*, vol. 58, no. 2, pp. 82–89, 2017.
[16] M. P. S. Pradhan, S. Chapagain, B. R. Luitel, P. R. Chalise et al., "Efficacy of tamsulosin in expulsion of lower ureteric stone upto 10 mm," *Journal of Urology and Research*, vol. 4, no. 2, p. 1085, 2017.
[17] W. A. Hübner, P. Irby, and M. L. Stoller, "Natural history and current concepts for the treatment of small ureteral calculi," *European Urology*, vol. 24, no. 2, pp. 172–176, 1993.
[18] M. Dellabella, G. Milanese, and G. Muzzonigro, "Efficacy of tamsulosin in the medical management of juxtavesical ureteral stones," *Journal of Urology*, vol. 170, no. 6, pp. 2202–2205, 2003.
[19] J. W. Segura, G. M. Preminger, D. G. Assimos et al., "Ureteral stones clinical guidelines panel summary report on the management of ureteral calculi," *Journal of Urology*, vol. 158, no. 5, pp. 1915–1921, 1997.
[20] K. Bensalah, M. Pearle, and Y. Lotan, "Cost-effectiveness of medical expulsive therapy using alpha-blockers for the treatment of distal ureteral stones," *European Urology*, vol. 53, no. 2, pp. 411–419, 2008.
[21] C. Seitz, E. Liatsikos, F. Porpiglia, H.-G. Tiselius, and U. Zwergel, "Medical therapy to facilitate the passage of stones: what is the evidence?," *European Urology*, vol. 56, no. 3, pp. 455–471, 2009.
[22] S. Sigala, M. Dellabella, G. Milanese et al., "Evidence for the presence of alpha1 adrenoceptor subtypes in the human ureter," *Neurourology and Urodynamics*, vol. 24, no. 2, pp. 142–148, 2005.
[23] F. Porpiglia, G. Ghignone, C. Fiori, D. Fontana, and R. M. Scarpa, "Nifedipine versus tamsulosin for the management of lower ureteral stones," *Journal of Urology*, vol. 172, no. 2, pp. 568–571, 2004.
[24] J. K. Parsons, L. A. Hergan, K. Sakamoto, and C. Lakin, "Efficacy of alpha-blockers for the treatment of ureteral stones," *Journal of Urology*, vol. 177, no. 3, pp. 983–987, 2007.
[25] Y. Bai, Y. Yang, X. Wang, Y. Tang, P. Han, and J. Wang, "Tadalafil facilitates the distal ureteral stone expulsion: a meta-analysis," *Journal of Endourology*, vol. 31, no. 6, pp. 557–563, 2017.
[26] A. A. Shokeir, M. A. Tharwat, A. E. Abolazm, and A. Harraz, "Sildenafil citrate as a medical expulsive therapy for distal ureteric stones: a randomised double-blind placebo-controlled study," *Arab Journal of Urology*, vol. 14, no. 1, pp. 1–6, 2016.
[27] R. A. Kloner, G. Jackson, J. T. Emmick et al., "Interaction between the phosphodiesterase 5 inhibitor, tadalafil and 2 alpha-blockers, doxazosin and tamsulosin in healthy normotensive men," *Journal of Urology*, vol. 172, no. 5, pp. 1935–1940, 2004.
[28] R. A. Kloner, "Cardiovascular effects of the 3 phosphodiesterase-5 inhibitors approved for the treatment of erectile dysfunction," *Circulation*, vol. 110, no. 19, pp. 3149–3155, 2004.
[29] A. Bechara, S. Romano, A. Casabé et al., "Comparative efficacy assessment of tamsulosin vs. tamsulosin plus tadalafil in the treatment of LUTS/BPH. Pilot study," *The Journal of Sexual Medicine*, vol. 5, no. 9, pp. 2170–2178, 2008.

6

Efficacy of Neoadjuvant Targeted Therapy in Treatment of Patients with Localised Clear-Cell Renal Cell Carcinoma

O. A. Voylenko,[1] O. E. Stakhovsky,[1] I. V. Vitruk,[1] O. A. Kononenko,[2] M. V. Pikul,[3] S. L. Semko,[3] and E. O. Stakhovsky[4]

[1]*Senior Researcher of Department of Plastic and Reconstructive Oncological Urology, National Cancer Institute, 33/43 Lomonosova Str., Kyiv 03022, Ukraine*

[2]*Researcher of Department of Plastic and Reconstructive Oncological Urology, National Cancer Institute, 33/43 Lomonosova Str., Kyiv 03022, Ukraine*

[3]*Urologist of Department of Plastic and Reconstructive Oncological Urology, National Cancer Institute, 33/43 Lomonosova Str., Kyiv 03022, Ukraine*

[4]*Head of Department of Plastic and Reconstructive Oncological Urology, National Cancer Institute, 33/43 Lomonosova Str., Kyiv 03022, Ukraine*

Correspondence should be addressed to O. A. Voylenko; voilenko@rambler.ru and M. V. Pikul; urogenetics@gmail.com

Academic Editor: Muhammad Shahid

Aim. This study aimed to evaluate the efficacy of neoadjuvant targeted therapy (TT) in patients with localised clear-cell renal cell carcinoma (RCC). *Materials and Methods.* A special randomised trial was planned and conducted by the Research Department of Plastic and Reconstructive Oncology in the National Cancer Institute of Ukraine for testing the clinical efficacy of neoadjuvant TT in the treatment of clear-cell localised RCC, and the primary endpoint was tumour response evaluation after TT. The secondary endpoints included evaluation of dependence between the use of neoadjuvant TT and the probability of partial nephrectomy and the correlation between tumour size, stage, remaining functioning parenchyma volume, and response to systemic therapy. *Results.* Overall, 118 patients met the inclusion criteria and were randomly assigned to receive combined treatment or surgery alone. The percentage of tumour regression ranged from 0% to 60%, and the median was (95% confidence interval) 20.5 ± 14.3 (16.8–24.3%). Most of the patients had a slightly positive response to TT (3%–29% decrease in tumour size); $n = 44$ (76.9%) cases. Partial response by the Response Evaluation Criteria in Solid Tumours, version 1.1, was observed in 14 (24.1%) patients and reached a maximum of 60% regression. Tumour reduction in the neoadjuvant TT group allowed kidney preservation in 53 (91.4%) patients. In the control group, the number of organ-sparing procedures was significantly lower ($n = 20$, 33.3%). The statistical difference was relevant ($x^2 = 42.1$; $p < 0.001$). *Conclusion.* The positive results of neoadjuvant TT obtained in our study indicate the clinical validity of combined treatment in patients with localised RCC.

1. Introduction

Partial nephrectomy is considered to be the surgery of choice in the treatment of localised renal cell carcinoma (RCC) [1, 2], and its oncological and functional efficacy have been proven in numerous clinical trials. However, the indications for this organ-sparing surgery have not been clearly determined.

Radical nephrectomy is commonly used in clinical practice in cases of renal hilum tumours or large tumours (>4 cm) and significantly impairs patient survival due to a decrease in filtration rate and quality of life [3–6]. In such cases, tumour size reduction can prompt kidney preservation, resulting in significant preferences for the patient. This goal can be achieved using neoadjuvant targeted therapy (TT).

According to modern literature analysis, neoadjuvant TT in localised RCC can be used only in elective clinical cases. The current data suggest performing it only during imperative indications (single kidney tumour, bilateral kidney tumours, pathology in the opposite kidney, significantly affecting its function) [7–12], and there are no randomised trials concerning the use of TT for the treatment of localised RCC.

2. Patients and Methods

2.1. Study Design. A special randomised trial was planned and conducted by the Research Department of Plastic and Reconstructive Oncology at the National Cancer Institute of Ukraine, testing the clinical efficacy of neoadjuvant TT in the treatment of clear-cell localised RCC. The eligibility of participating surgeons included sufficient surgical experience of >100 partial/radical nephrectomies per surgeon annually. The study was approved by the Institutional Review Board and local ethics committee, which was conducted as per with the Declaration of Helsinki and the Good Clinical Practice guidelines. The study flowchart is shown in Figure 1.

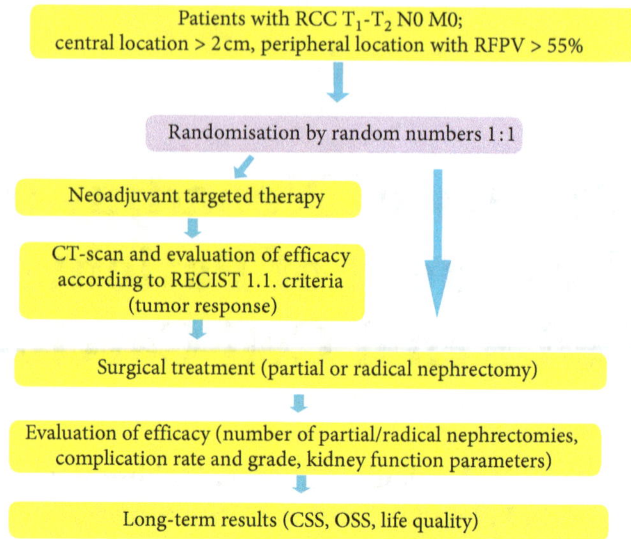

FIGURE 1: Efficacy of neoadjuvant targeted therapy in treatment of patients with localised clear-cell renal cell carcinoma study flowchart.

2.2. Patients. The inclusion criteria were clinically and histologically confirmed localised clear-cell RCC (ccRCC) (T1-T2 N0 M0) with intermediate indications for both radical and partial nephrectomy:

(1) Lesion larger than 20 mm located in the renal hilum
(2) Peripheral or polar RCC extending to kidney sinus
(3) Remaining functioning parenchyma volume (RFPV) over 55%

Patients with chronic kidney disease, expected estimated glomerular filtration rate (eGFR) > 30 mL/min after surgery, coexisting malignant disease, and a history of any other systemic therapy were excluded. It was mandatory to exclude tumour extension and metastatic disease before patient enrolment. A special informed consent form was obtained from the study team and signed along with the National Health Care system form during the investigation. Tumour biopsy to confirm ccRCC was performed routinely, not less than 2 weeks before randomisation.

2.3. Randomisation and Treatment. Patients were randomly assigned in a 1 : 1 ratio to receive either a combination of neoadjuvant TT with surgery (main group) or surgery alone (control group). Randomisation was performed using a random number generation method at the randomisation centre of the National Cancer Institute.

TT in the main group was performed according to the standard schedule with drugs provided by the National Health Care System: pazopanib 800 mg daily orally for two cycles (one cycle equals 4 weeks of intake) or sunitinib 50 mg daily for two cycles (one cycle equals 4 weeks of intake/2 weeks washout interval). Patients were informed by the investigators about the side effects and oncological efficacy of both drugs before signing the informed consent form and choosing precise medication. In cases of AE greater than level 2, dose reduction was planned, with interruption in patients who might have had life-threatening conditions. Patient safety was the primary goal of the study.

Surgical treatment of the main group was planned to start from 2 weeks after neoadjuvant TT cessation or termination for complete excretion of the target drug from the body for better tissue regeneration after surgical treatment. Patients in the control group underwent surgery for 14 days after randomisation. Preference was given for partial nephrectomy in both the groups. The surgical strategy was discussed on a multidisciplinary board. The main indication for kidney preservation was an RFPV over 55%.

Treatment efficacy was evaluated based on imaging methods (computed tomography (CT) and magnetic resonance imaging), which were used in the initial examination and in all control examinations. The primary tumour was evaluated using the Response Evaluation Criteria in Solid Tumours, version 1.1 (RECIST) [13]. In the main group, kidney lesions were assessed as target lesions following response evaluation after two cycles of TT according to imaging data.

2.4. Follow-Up. According to the standard of care, the patients did not receive any adjuvant therapy. Follow-up examinations, including CT, were performed every 6 months up to 2 years postoperatively. Thereafter, it was performed once a year.

2.5. Outcomes. The primary endpoint was tumour response evaluation after TT. The secondary endpoints included evaluation of dependence between the use of neoadjuvant TT and the probability of partial nephrectomy and correlation between tumour size, RFPV, and response to systemic therapy. Recurrence-free survival, cancer-specific survival, and overall survival were not reached at the period of data cutoff.

2.6. Statistical Analysis. The results were statistically analysed using SPSS (version 24.0) software. The distribution of continuous data in the group was estimated using the Kolmogorov–Smirnov criterion. Descriptive statistics included calculating the median with a standard deviation or median of 25–75 percentiles. Quantitative comparisons between groups were conducted using the Mann–Whitney criterion and qualitative comparisons using the Pearson test. A total statistical estimation of regression was performed using the analysis of variance (ANOVA) test. Type I errors less than 5% ($p < 0.05$) were considered to be statistically significant differences.

3. Results

3.1. Patients and Treatment. Patients were enrolled between January 2017 and October 2018. Overall, 118 patients met the inclusion criteria and were randomly assigned to receive combined treatment or surgery alone. TT was performed in 58 (49%) patients, whereas surgery alone was performed in 60 (51%) patients.

Information on baseline patient characteristics, tumour stage and size, kidney function, and concomitant pathology are summarised in Table 1. As shown in Table 1, no statistical difference between baseline characteristics was found between the groups at randomisation.

It should be noted that about half of the patients ($n = 57$; 48%) had concomitant pathology in other organs and systems, which affected kidney function both in the preoperative and postoperative periods. The most frequent complications were hypertension in 47 (39.8%) patients, obesity in 41 (34.7%), contralateral kidney cysts in 14 (11.9%), urinary stone disease in 11 (9.3%), diabetes in five (4.2%), contralateral kidney hypoplasia in two (1.7%), and a history of myocardial infarction in three (2.5%) patients.

3.2. Clinical Outcome. According to the primary endpoint, we estimated the percentage of tumour regression in 58 patients in the neoadjuvant TT group. The degree of tumour regression in each case is shown in Figure 2. The results showed that tumour size in the prevalence of cases decreased after neoadjuvant TT. Thus, the percentage of the tumour regression ranged from 0% to 60% and the median was (95% confidence interval (CI)) 20.5 ± 14.3 (16.8–24.3%). Patients who underwent neoadjuvant TT had no evidence of disease progression. No response to targeted therapy (0% regression) was observed in eight (13.8%) cases. Thus, most of the patients had a slight positive response to TT (3%–29% of tumour size decrease); $n = 44$ (76.9%) cases. A partial response was observed in 14 patients (24.1%) and reached a maximum of 60% regression. No complete response events were observed in the study cohort. After two blocks of neoadjuvant TT in patients with localised RCC, the mean kidney tumour size reduction was 12.3 mm from ($M \pm SD$ (95% CI)) 60.8 ± 19.7 (55.7–66) to 48.5 ± 16.4 (44.2–52.8) mm (*t*-test; $p < 0.001$), which could have influenced surgical tumour complexity.

We performed a comparative analysis of RFPV before and after neoadjuvant TT in patients with localised RCC. The use of neoadjuvant TT in patients with localised RCC (Mann–Whitney *U* test; $p < 0.001$) increased the median (Me) RFPV by 21% from (Me [25%; 75%]) 62 (57; 77) mm to 83 (70; 90) mm. (Additional information is provided in Supplementary Materials.)

The distribution of partial and radical nephrectomies in the study groups is shown in Table 2. Provided with the same baseline clinical and nephrometric parameters in groups of comparison before treatment, tumour reduction seen in the neoadjuvant TT group allowed kidney preservation in 53 cases (91.4%). In the control group, the number of organ-sparing procedures was significantly lower, accounting for only 20 (33.3%). The statistical difference was relevant ($x^2 = 42.1$; $p < 0.001$).

The correlation between tumour size before and after neoadjuvant TT using Pearson correlation analysis revealed a relevant direct correlation ($r = 0.77613$; $p < 0.001$) of the tumour size before neoadjuvant treatment on the expected outcome. (Additional information is provided in Supplementary Materials.)

Furthermore, we analysed the dependence between the objective response level and the size of the primary lesion. The data indicated that there was no direct correlation between the tumour objective response level and tumour size. Thus, for a 113 mm tumour, the objective response rate was 43%, while another large tumour (93 mm) did not respond to neoadjuvant TT at all (0% regression). Similar differences in objective responses were observed in small tumours. (Additional information is provided in Supplementary Materials.)

The evaluation was also performed in terms of comparing the T-stage and regression. Total statistical estimation performed using the ANOVA test revealed no influence of stage on tumour regression. However, the effect $\eta^2 = 0.01$, with an impact power of 0.1, was not significant ($p = 0.72$). Post hoc analysis using the Newman–Keuls test showed no significant difference between all subgroups of the study. Thus, between T1a and T1b, the confidence indicator was $p = 0.8$ (between groups T1b and T2; $p = 0.6$). Therefore, we have not confirmed the theory of greater efficacy of TT in patients with primary small RCC [14].

3.3. Adverse Events and Complication Rates. Adverse events (AEs) and complication rates are being evaluated by another part of the presented clinical trial and will be further presented. There were no cases of TT interruption, with most patients suffering from AE not higher than Gr 1 during the treatment period. There were no severe surgical complications in either group according to the Clavien–Dindo scoring system that required repeated intervention during the 90-day postoperative period.

4. Discussion

The results of a randomised prospective study evaluating the efficacy of neoadjuvant TT in the treatment of patients with localised RCC showed promising results.

Table 1: Baseline patients characteristics, tumour stage and size, kidney function, and concomitant pathology, $n = 118$.

Indicator	Statistical units	Main group, $n = 58$ (%)	Control group, $n = 60$ (%)	Statistical evaluation
Age, years	M ± SD (95% CI)	55.3 ± 10.3 (52.6–58)	54.5 ± 12 (51.4–57.6)	Mann–Whitney *U* test; $p = 0.8$
Sex	Male, *n* (%)	39 (67.2)	34 (56.7)	$x^2 = 1.39$
	Female, *n* (%)	19 (32.7)	26 (43.3)	$p = 0.24$
T	1a, *n* (%)	7 (12.1)	5 (8.3)	$x^2 = 7.3$; $p = 0.63$
	1b, *n* (%)	3 5 (60.3)	31 (51.7)	
	2a, *n* (%)	1 2 (20.7)	22 (36.7)	
	2b, *n* (%)	4 (6.9)	2 (3.3)	
ECOG	Me [25%; 75%]	1 [0, 1]	1 [0, 1]	Mann–Whitney *U* test; $p = 0.63$
Body mass index	Me [25%; 75%]	28.6 [25.3; 33.2]	28, 4 [26.9; 30.4]	Mann–Whitney *U* test; $p = 0.64$
Haemoglobin	Me [25%; 75%]	130, 5 [115; 141]	135 [118; 149]	Mann–Whitney *U* test; $p = 0.2$
Kidney tumour size, mm	M ± SD (95% CI)	60.7 ± 19.8 (55.5–66)	62.5 ± 16.7 (58.2–66.9)	Mann–Whitney *U* test; $p = 0.56$
Total glomerular	M ± SD (95% CI)	88.6 ± 26.1(76.7–100.5)	90.5 ± 22.5 (80.5–100.5)	Mann–Whitney *U* test; $p = 0.83$
Blood creatinine (μmol/L)	M ± SD (95% CI)	94.5 ± 2 (89.3–99.7)	90 ± 2.4 (83.7–96.5)	Mann–Whitney *U* test; $p = 0.17$
CKD	*n* (%)	4 (6, 9)	3 (5)	$x^2 = 0.19$; $p = 0.66$
Concomitant pathology	*n* (%)	29 (50)	28 (46.7)	$x^2 = 0.13$; $p = 0.71$

SD, standard deviation; CKD, chronic kidney disease; ECOG, East Cooperation Oncology Group status.

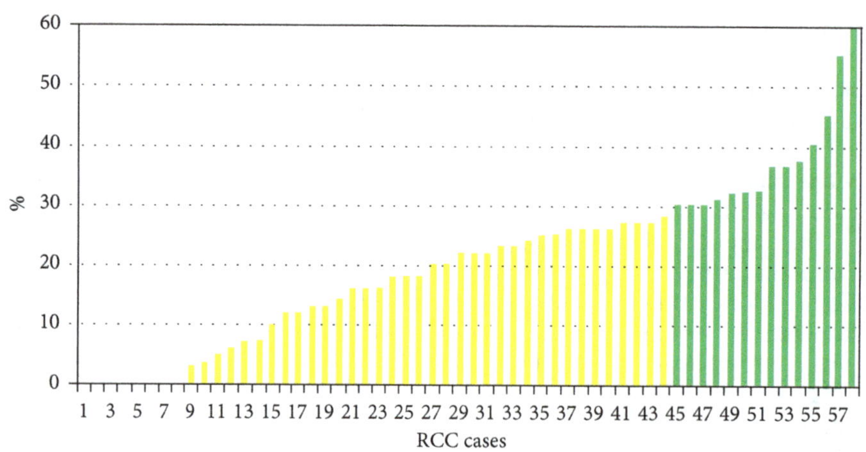

Figure 2: Percentage of regression of localised RCC after 2 cycles of neoadjuvant TT according to the results of spiral CT with bolus contrast enhancement, $n = 58$. Stable disease according to RECIST 1.1 (up to 30% regression) is shown as yellow, and partial regression according to RECIST 1.1 (30% regression to 100%), green. RCC, renal cell carcinoma; CT, computed tomography; TT, targeted therapy; RECIST, Response Evaluation Criteria in Solid Tumours.

Table 2: Distribution of surgical interventions in groups, $n = 118$.

Type of surgical treatment	Main group (neoadjuvant targeted therapy) $n = 58$	Control group (neoadjuvant targeted therapy) $n = 60$	Statistical evaluation
Partial nephrectomy, *n* (%)	53 (91.4)	20 (33.3)	$x^2 = 42.1$; $p < 0.001$
Radical nephrectomy, *n* (%)	5 (8.6)	40 (66.7)	

Data from clinical trials indicate a connection between chronic kidney disease and cardiovascular risks. Conservative treatment allows preservation of additional functioning nephrons with reference rates of oncologic survival compared to nephrectomy. Currently, indications for conservative surgical treatment beyond the standard T1a stage are expanding. Particular attention is given to bilateral kidney lesions, single kidney tumours, and RCC with simultaneous opposite kidney pathology, which significantly diminishes its function, while nephrectomy may result in dialysis for such patients. This could induce a problem due to the insufficient number of dialysis beds and their high costs [15]. In these cases, TT aims to reduce the RCC size and increase the likelihood of partial nephrectomy. This appears to be quite attractive from the perspective of RFPV preservation [16, 17].

The principle of neoadjuvant TT in RCC is based on the concept of increasing procedural safety and improving locoregional control [18]. A potential advantage of this approach is its cytoreductive effect and the movement of patients from radical treatment to nephron-sparing surgery.

The efficacy of this option was evaluated using sunitinib, sorafenib, pazopanib, and axitinib [19].

The positive effect of neoadjuvant TT was first described by Thomas et al. [12]. The study included 19 patients with advanced RCC ineligible for initial nephrectomy and who were indicated to be treated with sunitinib. Partial response of the primary tumour was observed in 16% ($n = 3$) of patients, stable disease in 37% ($n = 7$), and progression in 47% ($n = 9$). A reduction in tumour size was observed in 8/19 (42%) patients, with an average of 24% reduction, which allowed nephrectomy in four cases.

The role of neoadjuvant TT is even more significant in increasing the likelihood of conservative treatment for RCC. Silberstein et al. demonstrated TT efficacy in a group of 14 tumours (12 patients) with imperative indications, who showed an average reduction in RCC size of 21.1%. In all cases, a partial nephrectomy with a negative surgical margin was performed. No patients required further haemodialysis [8]. These results confirmed the feasibility of using this strategy in highly selective patients to increase the likelihood of organ-sparing surgery.

Another study by Rini et al. showed the feasibility of pazopanib (800 mg) in optimising parenchyma preservation within high-complexity tumours. A common criterion was that the expected eGFR would be less than 30 mL/min/1.73 m^2 in the case of nephrectomy. In total, 25 patients were enrolled in the study, 71% of whom showed a decrease in the lesion complexity and 92% showed a decrease in the tumour volume after TT. Kidney preservation was eventually performed in 80% (20/25) of cases with an increased probability of parenchyma preservation from 107 to 173 cm^3 ($p = 0.0015$) [10]. Other similar studies by Karam et al. and Lane et al. showed downsizing of primary tumours up to 28.3% and 32%, respectively. A reliable high level of patients responded to axitinib and sunitinib, which eventually allowed conservative surgery [11, 20]. The limitations of these studies were their small cohorts, group heterogeneity, and the absence of randomisation.

The results of the study evaluating the efficacy of neoadjuvant TT in the treatment of localised ccRCC have shown promising results. The high sensitivity of localised RCC to neoadjuvant TT with an objective response of 91% prompted the search for surgical strategy optimisation. A hidden benefit is an increase in the possibility of conservative treatment for complex kidney tumours. This might also lead to a reduction in the incidence of chronic kidney disease in this group and induce life expectancy and quality.

This approach facilitates the selection of surgical tactics for anatomically complex kidney tumours. The neoadjuvant treatment in oncology aims to reduce side effects and improve the tolerability of the selected therapy. This could be explained by the presence of two functioning kidneys, which significantly increased the body's detoxification capabilities.

Our analysis of the correlation between the kidney tumour size before and after neoadjuvant TT using the Pearson method revealed a reliable direct correlation ($r = 0.77613$; $p < 0.001$). We could predict the expected tumour volume after neoadjuvant TT based on the initial tumour size according to tomography (refer to Supplementary Materials). This could help predict possible localised RCC regression and shift tactics to conservative surgical treatment. In contrast, we could conclude on its feasibility (in case of unfavourable results) and prevent unnecessary systemic toxicity.

The dependence of the correlation between the RCC size and regression degree under the influence of neoadjuvant TT was described by Kroon et al. [14]. The authors found a direct correlative dependence based on the treatment of 78 patients with metastatic RCC with different drugs of the group of tyrosine kinase inhibitors. They concluded that the smaller the primary RCC size, the greater the likelihood and more effective the tumour regression. However, the results we obtained did not reveal the dependence of the level of objective tumour response to neoadjuvant TT on the size of the lesion. This could be explained by biological differences within RCC, which could not be evaluated by size.

Considering the above mentioned, it should be noted that neoadjuvant TT in localised ccRCC is a promising method aimed at improving functional outcomes of treatment, thus decreasing the level of patients with further disability. Additionally, the implementation of the technique aims to facilitate the choice of surgical tactics for anatomically complex kidney tumours.

The ongoing study on neoadjuvant TT in localised RCC is aimed at increasing the understanding of anatomical and functional changes in the kidneys affected by TT, evaluation of its efficacy, determination of its indications, prediction of the course of treatment stages, and the choice of surgery type.

5. Conclusion

Neoadjuvant TT in patients with surgically complex localised RCC resulted in clinical tumour regression, which provided a higher rate of conservative surgical treatment compared to similar patients without TT.

The positive results of neoadjuvant TT obtained in our study indicate the clinical validity of further investigating preoperative systemic therapy in localised ccRCC.

Ethical Approval

Research involving human participants and/or animals and all procedures performed in studies involving human participants were as per the ethical standards of the Institutional and/or National Research Committee and with the 1964 Helsinki Declaration and its later amendments or comparable ethical standards. The study was approved by the Bioethics Committee of the National Cancer Institute of Ukraine.

Consent

The informed consent form was obtained from the study team and signed along with the National Health Care system form during the investigation. This form was approved by the local ethics committee.

Authors' Contributions

OA Voylenko contributed to protocol/project development, data collection or management, and manuscript writing/editing. OE Stakhovskiy, YV Vitruk, and OA Kononenko contributed to data collection or management. MV Pikul contributed to protocol/project development and manuscript writing/editing. SL Semko performed data analysis. EO Stakhovskiy contributed to protocol/project development and manuscript writing/editing.

Acknowledgments

The authors thank the Institutional Review Board and Local Ethics Committee for their expertise and conceptual help with the study design. The authors also thank the Scientific Committee of the National Health Care System for providing support and follow-up of the study results. The authors thank Editage (http://www.editage.com) for English language editing.

Supplementary Materials

Additional Figure 3: comparative assessment of the mean size of localised RCC before and after neoadjuvant TT based on spiral CT data, $n = 58$. Additional Figure 4: correlation of localised RCC size before and after neoadjuvant TT using Pearson correlation analysis. Additional Figure 5: dependence of the localised RCC regression level on the size of the primary tumour in the kidney, $n = 58$. Additional Table 3: RFPV before and after neoadjuvant TT in the main group according to the bolus contrast enhancement spiral CT results, $n = 58$. Additional Table 4: evaluation of objective response according to RECIST 1.1 in localised RCC after neoadjuvant targeted therapy based on spiral CT data, $n = 58$. Additional Table 5: dependence of regression level and tumour stage after neoadjuvant targeted therapy, $n = 58$ (*Supplementary Materials*)

References

[1] NCCN Guidelines Version 2.2019, "Kidney cancer," 2019, https://www.nccn.org/professionals/physician_gls/pdf/kidney.pdf.

[2] European Association of Urology, "EAU guidelines on renal cell carcinoma 2018 ISBN/EAN: 978-94-92671-01-1," 2018, https://uroweb.org/guideline/renal-cell-carcinoma.

[3] D. H. Smith, M. L. Thorp, J. H. Gurwitz et al., "Chronic kidney disease and outcomes in heart failure with preserved versus reduced ejection fraction," *Circulation: Cardiovascular Quality and Outcomes*, vol. 6, no. 3, pp. 333–342, 2013.

[4] A. S. Go, G. M. Chertow, D. Fan, C. E. McCulloch, and C.-Y. Hsu, "Chronic kidney disease and the risks of death, cardiovascular events, and hospitalization," *New England Journal of Medicine*, vol. 351, no. 13, pp. 1296–1305, 2004.

[5] C. A. Herzog, R. W. Asinger, A. K. Berger et al., "Cardiovascular disease in chronic kidney disease. A clinical update from Kidney Disease: improving Global Outcomes (KDIGO)," *Kidney International*, vol. 80, no. 6, pp. 572–586, 2011.

[6] W. C. Huang, A. S. Levey, A. M. Serio et al., "Chronic kidney disease after nephrectomy in patients with renal cortical tumours: a retrospective cohort study," *The Lancet Oncology*, vol. 7, no. 9, pp. 735–740, 2006.

[7] T. Powles, I. Kayani, C. Blank et al., "The safety and efficacy of sunitinib before planned nephrectomy in metastatic clear cell renal cancer," *Annals of Oncology*, vol. 22, no. 5, pp. 1041–1047, 2011.

[8] J. L. Silberstein, F. Millard, R. Mehrazin et al., "Feasibility and efficacy of neoadjuvant sunitinib before nephron-sparing surgery," *BJU International*, vol. 106, no. 9, pp. 1270–1276, 2010.

[9] N. J. Hellenthal, W. Underwood, R. Penetrante et al., "Prospective clinical trial of preoperative sunitinib in patients with renal cell carcinoma," *Journal of Urology*, vol. 184, no. 3, pp. 859–864, 2010.

[10] B. I. Rini, E. R. Plimack, T. Takagi et al., "A phase II study of pazopanib in patients with localized renal cell carcinoma to optimize preservation of renal parenchyma," *Journal of Urology*, vol. 194, no. 2, pp. 297–303, 2015.

[11] B. R. Lane, I. H. Derweesh, H. L. Kim et al., "Presurgical sunitinib reduces tumor size and may facilitate partial nephrectomy in patients with renal cell carcinoma," *Urologic Oncology: Seminars and Original Investigations*, vol. 33, no. 3, pp. e15–112, 2015.

[12] A. A. Thomas, B. I. Rini, B. R. Lane et al., "Response of the primary tumor to neoadjuvant sunitinib in patients with advanced renal cell carcinoma," *Journal of Urology*, vol. 181, no. 2, pp. 518–523, 2009.

[13] E. A. Eisenhauer, P. Therasse, J. Bogaerts et al., "New response evaluation criteria in solid tumours: revised RECIST guideline (version 1.1)," *European Journal of Cancer*, vol. 45, no. 2, pp. 228–247, 2009.

[14] B. K. Kroon, R. de Bruijn, W. Prevoo, S. Horenblas, T. Powles, and A. Bex, "Probability of downsizing primary tumors of renal cell carcinoma by targeted therapies is related to size at presentation," *Urology*, vol. 81, no. 1, pp. 111–115, 2013.

[15] B. Shuch, W. M. Linehan, and G. Bratslavsky, "Repeat partial nephrectomy," *Current Opinion in Urology*, vol. 21, no. 5, pp. 368–375, 2011.

[16] E. O. Stakhovskiy, O. A. Voylenko, Y. V. Vitruk, and O. E. Stakhovskiy, "Application of nephrometry for choice of the treatment tactics in patients, suffering nephrocellular cance," *Klin Khir*, vol. 3, pp. 55–60, 2015.

[17] O. Voylenko, I. Vitruk, O. Stakhovskyi et al., "UNCI nephrometry and remaining functional parenchyma as a new tool indicator for partial nephrectomy in RCC," in *Proceedings of the 29th Annual EAU Congress*, Stockholm, Sweden, April 2014.

[18] A. Bindayi, Z. A. Hamilton, M. L. McDonald et al., "Neoadjuvant therapy for localized and locally advanced renal cell carcinoma," *Urologic Oncology: Seminars and Original Investigations*, vol. 36, no. 1, pp. 31–37, 2018.

[19] T. E. Hutson, G. R. Thoreson, R. A. Figlin, and B. I. Rini, "The evolution of systemic therapy in metastatic renal cell carcinoma," *American Society of Clinical Oncology Educational Book*, vol. 36, pp. 113–117, 2016.

[20] J. A. Karam, C. E. Devine, D. L. Urbauer et al., "Phase 2 trial of neoadjuvant axitinib in patients with locally advanced nonmetastatic clear cell renal cell carcinoma," *European Urology*, vol. 66, no. 5, pp. 874–880, 2014.

7

The Use of Modified Templates in Early and Advanced Stage Nonseminomatous Germ Cell Tumor

Timothy A. Masterson and Clint Cary

Department of Urology, Indiana University School of Medicine, Indianapolis, IN 46202, USA

Correspondence should be addressed to Timothy A. Masterson; tamaster@iupui.edu

Academic Editor: Jason M. Hafron

The surgical management of both early and advanced stage germ cell tumors of the testis remains a complex process of surgical decision making to maximize oncologic control while minimizing morbidity. Over the past 5 decades, the evolution of the surgical template for retroperitoneal lymphadenectomy (RPLND) has resulted in important modifications to achieve these goals. In this review, we will characterize the historical motivating factors that led to the modified template, outline patient and clinical factors in selecting these approaches in both early and advanced stage disease, and briefly discuss future horizons for their implementation.

1. Introduction

Few topics generate more discussion and consideration than the extent and laterality of the surgical template when managing the retroperitoneum (RP) in germ cell tumor (GCT) patients. The implications of limiting the surgical template inappropriately leave patients at risk for RP relapses. Conversely, extending the template beyond necessary boundaries increases the risk of surgical complications and long-term side effects. Several modifications have been incorporated that allow for an optimization between functional and oncologic outcomes. Understanding the historical rationale for these alterations and the clinical scenarios in which implementation of a limited dissection can be safely integrated is imperative. For the purposes of this review, our goal is to highlight the motivating factors and clinical experience that led to changes in the surgical boundaries for retroperitoneal lymph node dissection (RPLND).

2. Historical Perspectives and Rationale for Template Modifications

Prior to effective chemotherapy for metastatic GCT, wide surgical resection of retroperitoneal (RP) disease was necessary to provide patients their only chance for durable, cancer-free survival. Additionally, cross-sectional imaging was unavailable and staging of disease limited. Accordingly, the burden of disease in this era was great; therefore, suprahilar and bilateral retroperitoneal dissections were routinely performed. With the development of curative, platinum-based chemotherapy regimens [1] along with the introduction of cross-sectional imaging of the abdomen with computed tomography [2] and discovery of serum tumor markers (STM) [3], the management of testicular cancer patients shifted. Surgery was associated with significant morbidity, with the loss of ejaculatory function representing the most pressing issue for young men and their fertility, occurring in roughly 90% of patients undergoing bilateral template dissections. Surveillance protocols were implemented for patients without detectable metastatic disease (CSI) to avoid this morbidity, utilizing chemotherapy in those that relapsed or failed observation. Limitations of surveillance protocols included the inaccuracies of clinical staging in roughly 30% of patients [4] and the greater burden of surveillance imaging and salvage treatments at the time of relapse.

Several surgical advancements improved our understanding of nodal dissemination of disease to the RP and neural pathways that impacted ejaculatory function were discovered, setting the stage for surgical modifications and refinement. Preceded by cadaveric and lymphangiographic

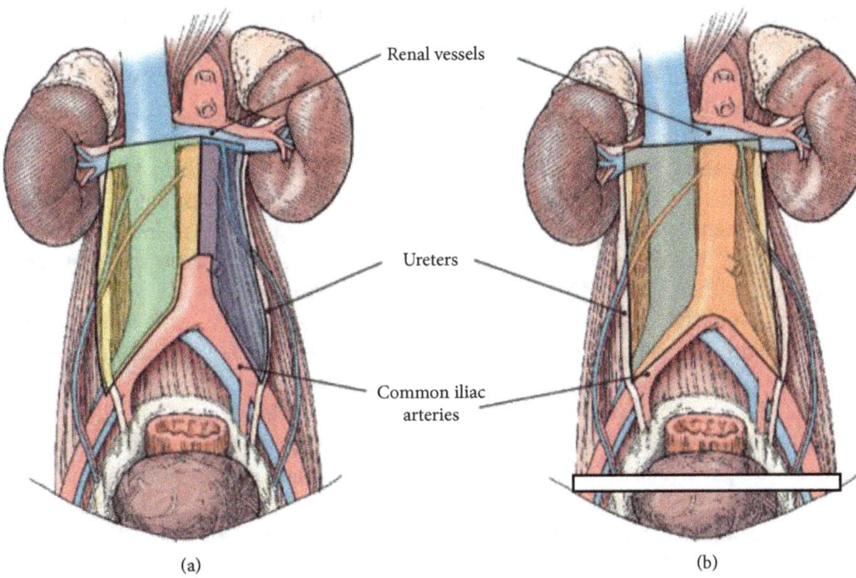

Figure 1: Template boundaries for left and right modified RPLND (a) and bilateral template rPLND (b).

studies elucidating the primary and secondary lymphatic drainage of the testicle [5–10], Ray et al. presented their nearly 30-year experience with bilateral, infrahilar RPLND in 283 patients [11]. Among the 122 patients with resectable metastatic disease, they characterized distinct patterns of spread based upon the laterality of the testicular primary. The authors noted the absence of crossover relative to the primary landing zones among patients with solitary metastases of the right or left testes. In 1982, Donohue et al. reported their findings among 104 patients with node-positive disease who were not previously treated with chemotherapy and underwent routine full bilateral dissections, including the suprahilar regions [12]. This study confirmed the predictable patterns of disease spread as reported by Ray et al. and provided pathologic rationale for the safe omission of suprahilar, interiliac, and contralateral RP dissections in low-volume disease. These modifications resulted in a reduction in the risk of postoperative chylous ascites, renovascular injury, pancreatic complications, and improved preservation of antegrade ejaculation.

Weissbach and Boedefeld reported on a prospective, multi-institutional trial of 214 consecutive patients undergoing a bilateral dissection for clinical stage II disease [13]. The goals of this study were to determine the localization and distribution of solitary and multiple lymph node metastases. These authors again confirmed the uncommon occurrence of contralateral disease relative to the aorta in the setting of early stage tumors, defined as solitary metastases measuring 5 cm or less. More importantly, when a limited template was compared prospectively by this same group among patients with CSI disease, no differences were seen regarding relapse rates or perioperative complications, while preservation of ejaculatory function was noted in 74% undergoing a modified dissection as compared to 34% subjected to a radical (bilateral) dissection [14].

Despite data from several published series, incorporation of these template modifications into clinical guidelines has remained controversial. Patient selection remains key for maximizing the cancer control and limiting the morbidity. In the primary setting, the risk of contralateral spread increases with increasing tumor burden. For patients with residual disease after chemotherapy, locations of disease both pre- and postchemotherapy, IGCCCG risk classification, along with tumor size have been suggested as criteria to consider when selecting patients for template modifications. Included in Figure 1 are the current templates utilized at our institution for right and left modified boundaries (A), in addition to bilateral template surgery (B). The following sections report on the current data and guidelines.

3. Outcomes in Early Stage NSGCT

Several institutions have assessed oncologic and functional outcomes with modifications in the surgical template over time. While significant variability exists among groups as to the type of modifications made to the template, outcomes regarding RP relapse rate, and recovery of ejaculatory function are uniformly reported. In one of the earliest studies out of Italy, Pizzocaro et al. reported on 61 CSI patients, of which 10 experienced relapse in the absence of adjuvant therapy. None of these occurred in the RP and 87% reported preservation of antegrade ejaculation with template modification alone [15]. Similar findings were seen in a cohort of 85 CSI patients from Brigham & Women's Hospital in Boston, again with no RP recurrences identified and 94% recovering antegrade ejaculation [16]. Donohue et al. from Indiana published their experience with unilateral template modifications, this time with ipsilateral nerve-sparing [17]. In this series of 75 patients published in 1990, 73 of which were CSI and 2 patients had low-volume CSIIa disease.

One RP recurrence was reported and later salvaged. When assessing survival outcomes across all studies, cancer specific and overall survival approaches 100%.

Proponents of bilateral, infrahilar dissections with unilateral or bilateral nerve-sparing have suggested that limited templates subject patients to higher rates of unresected disease in the RP, leaving them at greater risk for late relapse, higher burdens of chemotherapy, and potentially a greater risk of death. Eggener et al. reported upon 191 cases of pathologic node-positive cases undergoing primary RPLND for early stage NSGCT [18]. Comparing published templates to the distribution of disease mapped within their cohort, they estimate that 3% to 23% of patients with unilaterally modified dissections would have nodal disease outside of the field of surgery. A couple points are worth further discussion in this study. Interestingly, there were 136 patients with clinical stage IIA disease; however, only 80 (58%) were found to have pathologic disease. Further, there were 20 patients with elevated tumor markers at the time of RPLND. In the only prospective trial comparing outcomes between surgical approaches, no difference in oncologic outcomes was identified, and a twofold increase in functional outcomes was reported with the unilateral template (Weissbach). To date, no randomized trials have compared template modifications to full bilateral dissections for difference in cancer control, 90-day morbidity, and long-term functional outcomes regarding ejaculatory function. Additionally, the Eggener study omits any consideration for intraoperative findings that may influence the judgment of the surgeon to expand the dissection. Nevertheless, improving upon the oncologic and functional outcomes reported among these open series when template modifications are performed at high-volume centers with therapeutic intent would be difficult to accomplish.

4. Postchemotherapy RPLND Template Outcomes

Early experience in using full bilateral templates following cisplatin-based chemotherapy was reported by Donohue et al. in 1982 [19]. Given the uncertainties of frozen section pathologic evaluation in the postchemotherapy setting and bulky disease with what is now considered suboptimal chemotherapy, the authors supported the use of complete bilateral RPLND. Since that time, several centers have investigated the oncologic safety of modified unilateral templates in appropriately selected individuals in contemporary series. In 2007, Beck et al. evaluated 100 patients who underwent a modified dissection with a median follow-up of 31.9 months [20]. Patient selection criteria were: nonseminomatous GCT's with normal serum tumors markers after cisplatin-based chemotherapy and tumors limited to the primary landing zone both before and after chemotherapy. There were 4 recurrences during follow-up, all of which were outside the boundaries of a full bilateral template. This study was recently updated with 10-year follow-up data with an additional 3 patients demonstrating a recurrence [21]. Again, no recurrences were within the bounds of a full bilateral template with the majority of recurrences being in the chest. An additional series of 102 patients from the Austrian group also evaluated the safety of template surgery in the post-chemotherapy setting [22]. The inclusion criteria in this series were normal serum tumor markers after first-line cisplatin-based chemotherapy with stage II disease. All patients underwent template surgery based on the location of the primary tumor. There was 1 recurrence in the RP within the boundary of a full bilateral template for a recurrence rate of 0.9% at a median follow-up of 8.5 years. The majority (73%) of these patients demonstrated a complete response to chemotherapy with residual masses <1 cm. Heidenreich et al. described the German experience in 98 patients who underwent a modified template RPLND [23]. The inclusion criteria in this series were similar to the prior studies and also limited the residual mass to ≤5 cm in diameter. One patient developed a RP recurrence in this series for a 1% recurrence rate at 3 years of follow-up. These studies in combination demonstrate a risk of RP recurrence of 0.6% in approximately 300 patients.

Others have published on the pathologic findings of disease outside the boundary of a modified template. For example, Carver et al. published the results of 269 patients who had a full bilateral template performed and described the pathologic findings outside the bounds of a modified template [24]. They demonstrate that extra-template disease was present in 7% to 32% depending on the boundaries used for template dissections. However, the inclusion criteria in this study were quite different than other published reports. In the Carver et al. study, unselected patients with bulky disease, significant receipt of salvage chemotherapy regimens, elevated STMs at the time of surgery, and positive pre-operative imaging outside the modified template boundaries were included. These factors limit the relevance of this study in determining the utility of template surgery in the post-chemotherapy setting.

5. Functional Outcomes with Template Modifications

Historical comparisons for bilateral RPLND are associated with loss of seminal emission and ejaculation in the majority of patients. With the incorporation of unilateral templates, preservation of antegrade ejaculation was attributable to the exclusion of any dissection or disruption of the contralateral efferent, postganglionic sympathetic nerve fibers as they course to the hypogastric plexus. Donohue reported ejaculatory rates of 90% with modified, unilateral templates without any compromise in oncologic efficacy [4]. Similar rates of preservation were reported from the Italian group among 61 CSI patients [15]. In the only prospective trial assessing functional and oncologic outcomes among patients undergoing either a unilateral template compared to the standard bilateral template, the modified template was associated with a twofold improvement in ejaculatory rates without any greater risk of in field relapse [14]. With further modifications to include ipsilateral nerve-sparing within the surgical template, rates of ejaculatory preservation were improved. Jewett et al. demonstrated feasibility in a series of 30 patients, with 18 of 20 patients in whom successful nerve-sparing was accomplished ultimately recovering function [25]. The Indiana group published their experience combining unilateral template modifications with ipsilateral nerve-sparing in 1990. In this cohort of 75 early-staged patients, 100% were able to achieve successful antegrade ejaculation [17]. In a more contemporary series of 135 men undergoing nerve-sparing primary RPLND at Indiana, 134 achieve normal function, and nearly 75% were able to conceive [26].

While data exist describing the safety of template surgery in the postchemotherapy setting from an oncologic standpoint, functional data also support an improved ejaculatory status in modified template surgery. In the Indiana series with 10-year follow-up data, antegrade ejaculation occurred in 97.7% of patients, who were contacted [21]. Additionally, Heidenreich et al. evaluated the likelihood of being able to perform nerve-sparing surgery and found that 74.5% versus 55.5% of patients could undergo preservation of the postganglionic sympathetic nerve fibers in modified template versus bilateral template surgery, respectively [23]. Furthermore, antegrade ejaculation occurred in 85% of modified template resections versus 25% of full bilateral resections in their series, ($p < 0.001$). Additional clinical outcomes are also improved with a modified template dissection in the appropriately selected patient, such as shorter operative times, less blood loss, less transfusions, and fewer postoperative complications [23].

6. Future Directions

The majority of the current data supports the oncologic safety of modified template surgery in strictly defined cohorts. Efforts to determine the safety in other patient populations such as poor-risk disease and late relapse offer areas of potential study. These studies would require meticulous design to ensure patient safety. For example, patients with a late relapse 10 years following their primary tumor with a small solitary recurrence in the ipsilateral landing zone could be reasonable to apply modified template principles. The assumption here would be that the disease has declared itself to the ipsilateral landing zone of the primary tumor and there has been a 10-year lag time to monitor the contralateral side with no recurrence.

Data surrounding the use of minimally invasive surgery and template dissection is limited particularly in the postchemotherapy setting, but this should and will be held to the same standards of the open approach. Oncologic outcomes regarding the therapeutic value of template surgery in laparoscopic and robot-assisted primary RPLND are significantly lacking due to small numbers of patients, even smaller numbers with true pathologic disease, and the majority of patients with pathologic stage II disease receiving adjuvant chemotherapy. While some early reports of nerve-sparing success in the robotic settings are promising in the primary RPLND setting [27], this is not consistent across studies with some series demonstrating lower antegrade ejaculation rates with the robotic approach [28, 29]. Others have shown inferior ejaculatory rates in clinical stage I patients with the laparoscopic technique compared to robotic techniques [30]. Ejaculatory outcomes in the postchemotherapy setting with minimally invasive techniques are unclear. Overall, the high bar of 99% ejaculatory success [26] and subsequent fertility in open primary RPLND using modified templates cannot be compromised by incorporating a robotic approach.

7. Conclusions

With more than 35 years of experience, several studies have confirmed the safety of modified templates for RPLND both in the primary and postchemotherapy setting. Benefits include limiting the morbidity of surgery, without compromising the therapeutic impact among appropriately selected patients. Expansion of its use within other patient populations warrants exploration but must be integrated in a thoughtful manner to ensure patient outcomes are not compromised.

References

[1] L. H. Einhorn and J. Donohue, "Cis-diamminedichloroplatinum, vinblastine, and bleomycin combination chemotherapy in disseminated testicular cancer," *Annals of Internal Medicine*, vol. 87, no. 3, pp. 293–298, 1977.

[2] J. E. Husband, A. Barrett, and M. J. Peckham, "Evaluation of computed tomography in the management of testicular teratoma," *British Journal of Urology*, vol. 53, no. 2, pp. 179–183, 1981.

[3] W. E. Barzell and W. F. Whitmore, "Clinical significance of biologic markers: Memorial Hospital experience," *Seminars in Oncology*, vol. 6, no. 1, pp. 48–52, 1979.

[4] J. P. Donohue, J. A. Thornhill, R. S. Foster et al., "Retroperitoneal lymphadenectomy for clinical stage A testis cancer (1965 to 1989): modifications of technique and impact on ejaculation," *Journal of Urology*, vol. 149, no. 2, pp. 237–243, 1993.

[5] B. Cuneo, "Note sure les lymphatiques du testicle," *Bulletin Society of Anatomic*, vol. 76, pp. 107–110, 1901.

[6] L. K. Jamieson and J. F. Dobson, "The lymphatics of the testicle," *The Lancet*, vol. 175, no. 4512, pp. 493–495, 1910.

[7] H. Most, "Uber maligue hoden ges chwulste und ihre metastasen," *Archiv für Pathologische Anatomie und Physiologie und für Klinische Medicin*, vol. 154, no. 1, pp. 138–177, 1898.

[8] H. Rouviere, "Lymphatiques de l'Homme," *Mason et Cie*, 1932.

[9] S. Chiappa, C. Uslenghi, G. Galli, G. Ravasi, and G. Bonadonna, "Lymphangiography and endolymphatic radiotherapy in testicular tumours," *British Journal of Radiology*, vol. 39, no. 463, pp. 498–512, 1966.

[10] S. Chiappa, C. Uslenghi, G. Bonadonna, P. Marano, and G. Ravasi, "Combined testicular and foot lymphangiography in testicular carcinomas," *Surgery, Gynecology & Obstetrics*, vol. 123, pp. 10–14, 1966.

[11] B. Ray, S. I. Hajdu, and W. F. Whitmore, "Distribution of retroperitoneal lymph node metastases in testicular germinal tumors," *Cancer*, vol. 33, no. 2, pp. 340–348, 1974.

[12] J. P. Donohue, J. M. Zachary, and B. R. Maynard, "Distribution of nodal metastases in nonseminomatous testis cancer," *Journal of Urology*, vol. 128, no. 2, pp. 315–320, 1982.

[13] L. Weissbach and E. A. Boedefeld, "Localization of solitary and multiple metastases in stage II nonseminomatous testis

tumor as basis for a modified staging lymph node dissection in stage I," *Journal of Urology*, vol. 138, no. 1, pp. 77–82, 1987.

[14] L. Weissbach, E. A. Boedefeld, and B. Horstmann-Dubral, "Surgical treatment of stage-I non-seminomatous germ cell testis tumor. Final results of a prospective multicenter trial 1982-1987. Testicular Tumor Study Group," *European Urology*, vol. 17, no. 2, pp. 97–106, 1990.

[15] G. Pizzocaro, R. Salvioni, and F. Zanoni, "Unilateral lymphadenectomy in intraoperative stage I nonseminomatous germinal testis cancer," *Journal of Urology*, vol. 134, no. 3, pp. 485–489, 1985.

[16] J. P. Richie, "Clinical stage 1 testicular cancer: the role of modified retroperitoneal lymphadenectomy," *Journal of Urology*, vol. 144, no. 5, pp. 1160–1163, 1990.

[17] J. P. Donohue, R. S. Foster, R. G. Rowland, R. Bihrle, J. Jones, and G. Geier, "Nerve-sparing retroperitoneal lymphadenectomy with preservation of ejaculation," *Journal of Urology*, vol. 144, no. 2, pp. 287–291, 1990.

[18] S. E. Eggener, B. S. Carver, D. S. Sharp et al., "Incidence of disease outside modified retroperitoneal lymph node dissection templates in clinical stage I or IIA nonseminomatous germ cell testicular cancer," *Journal of Urology*, vol. 177, no. 3, pp. 937–942, 2007.

[19] J. P. Donohue, L. M. Roth, J. M. Zachary, R.G. Rowland, L. H. Einhorn, and S. G. Williams, "Cytoreductive surgery for metastatic testis cancer: tissue analysis of retroperitoneal masses after chemotherapy," *Journal of Urology*, vol. 127, no. 6, pp. 1111–1114, 1982.

[20] S. D. W. Beck, R. S. Foster, R. Bihrle, J. P. Donohue, and L. H. Einhorn, "Is full bilateral retroperitoneal lymph node dissection always necessary for postchemotherapy residual tumor?," *Cancer*, vol. 110, no. 6, pp. 1235–1240, 2007.

[21] J. S. Cho, H. Z. Kaimakliotis, C. Cary, T. A. Masterson, S. Beck, and R. Foster, "Modified retroperitoneal lymph node dissection for post-chemotherapy residual tumour: a long-term update," *BJU International*, vol. 120, no. 1, pp. 104–108, 2017.

[22] H. Steiner, R. Peschel, and G. Bartsch, "Retroperitoneal lymph node dissection after chemotherapy for germ cell tumours: is a full bilateral template always necessary?," *BJU International*, vol. 102, no. 3, pp. 310–314, 2008.

[23] A. Heidenreich, D. Pfister, R. Witthuhn, D. Thüer, and P. Albers, "Postchemotherapy retroperitoneal lymph node dissection in advanced testicular cancer: radical or modified template resection," *European Urology*, vol. 55, no. 1, pp. 217–226, 2009.

[24] B. S. Carver, B. Shayegan, S. Eggener et al., "Incidence of metastatic nonseminomatous germ cell tumor outside the boundaries of a modified postchemotherapy retroperitoneal lymph node dissection," *Journal of Clinical Oncology*, vol. 25, no. 28, pp. 4365–4369, 2007.

[25] M. A. Jewett, Y. S. Kong, S. D. Goldberg et al., "Retroperitoneal lymphadenectomy for testis tumor with nerve sparing for ejaculation," *Journal of Urology*, vol. 139, no. 6, pp. 1220–1224, 1988.

[26] S. D. W. Beck, A. L. Bey, R. Bihrle, and R. S. Foster, "Ejaculatory status and fertility rates after primary retroperitoneal lymph node dissection," *Journal of Urology*, vol. 184, no. 5, pp. 2078–2080, 2010.

[27] S. M. Pearce, S. Golan, M. A. Gorin et al., "Safety and early oncologic effectiveness of primary robotic retroperitoneal lymph node dissection for nonseminomatous germ cell testicular cancer," *European Urology*, vol. 71, no. 3, pp. 476–482, 2017.

[28] S. Stepanian, M. Patel, and J. Porter, "Robot-assisted laparoscopic retroperitoneal lymph node dissection for testicular cancer: evolution of the technique," *European Urology*, vol. 70, no. 4, pp. 661–667, 2016.

[29] S. M. Cheney, P. E. Andrews, B. C. Leibovich, and E. P. Castle, "Robot-assisted retroperitoneal lymph node dissection: technique and initial case series of 18 patients," *BJU International*, vol. 115, no. 1, pp. 114–120, 2015.

[30] K. T. Harris, M. A. Gorin, M. W. Ball, P. M. Pierorazio, and M. E. Allaf, "A comparative analysis of robotic vs laparoscopic retroperitoneal lymph node dissection for testicular cancer," *BJU International*, vol. 116, no. 6, pp. 920–923, 2015.

8

Toxicities Associated with Cisplatin-Based Chemotherapy and Radiotherapy in Long-Term Testicular Cancer Survivors

Chunkit Fung,[1] Paul Dinh Jr.,[2] Shirin Ardeshir-Rouhani-Fard,[2] Kerry Schaffer,[1] Sophie D. Fossa,[3] and Lois B. Travis[2]

[1]*James P. Wilmot Cancer Institute, University of Rochester Medical Center, Rochester, NY, USA*
[2]*Melvin and Bren Simon Cancer Center, Indiana University, Indianapolis, IN, USA*
[3]*Department of Oncology, Oslo University Hospital, Radium Hospital, Oslo, Norway*

Correspondence should be addressed to Chunkit Fung; chunkit_fung@urmc.rochester.edu

Academic Editor: Aditya Bagrodia

Testicular cancer has become the paradigm of adult-onset cancer survivorship, due to the young age at diagnosis and 10-year relative survival of 95%. This clinical review presents the current status of various treatment-related complications experienced by long-term testicular cancer survivors (TCS) free of disease for 5 or more years after primary treatment. Cardiovascular disease and second malignant neoplasms represent the most common potentially life-threatening late effects. Other long-term adverse outcomes include neuro- and ototoxicity, pulmonary complications, nephrotoxicity, hypogonadism, infertility, and avascular necrosis. Future research efforts should focus on delineation of the genetic underpinning of these long-term toxicities to understand their biologic basis and etiopathogenetic pathways, with the goal of developing targeted prevention and intervention strategies to optimize risk-based care and minimize chronic morbidities. In the interim, health care providers should advise TCS to adhere to national guidelines for the management of cardiovascular disease risk factors, as well as to adopt behaviors consistent with a healthy lifestyle, including smoking cessation, a balanced diet, and a moderate to vigorous intensity exercise program. TCS should also follow national guidelines for cancer screening as currently applied to the general population.

1. Introduction

Testicular cancer (TC) is the most common cancer, affecting young men aged 18–39 years [1]. Due to effective cisplatin-based chemotherapy introduced in the 1970s [2], TC is highly curable with a 10-year relative survival approaching 95% [3, 4]. However, treatment-related complications, including cardiovascular disease (CVD), second malignant neoplasms (SMN), neuro- and ototoxicity, pulmonary complications, nephrotoxicity, hypogonadism, infertility, avascular necrosis, cognitive impairment, anxiety/depression, and chronic cancer-related fatigue, accompany these remarkable successes [5–7]. These adverse outcomes of TC and its therapy have emerged as important issues for this young cohort of survivors. In this review article, we will focus on toxicities due to cisplatin-based chemotherapy and radiotherapy experienced by long-term survivors of TC, which are defined as individuals who are disease-free 5 years or more after primary treatment [8]. Due to sparse data, the risks of long-term toxicities after single-dose carboplatin for stage I seminoma or one to two cycles of bleomycin, etoposide, and cisplatin (BEP) for stage I nonseminoma will not be reviewed.

2. Cardiovascular Disease and Raynaud Phenomenon

A few hypotheses have been proposed to explain the pathophysiology of CVD in TC survivors (TCS), including the direct vascular damage hypothesis, the indirect hypothesis, and more recently the multiple-hit hypothesis [9, 10]. The direct vascular damage hypothesis proposes that cisplatin-based chemotherapy causes direct damage to the vascular endothelium [9]. In vitro exposure of endothelial cells to cisplatin or bleomycin causes cytokine release and cytotoxicity [11, 12]. Von Willebrand factor, an inflammatory marker released by endothelial cells in response to vascular damage, increases in TC patients during chemotherapy [13]. Other markers of inflammation and endothelial dysfunction are also evident after cisplatin-based chemotherapy, including fibrinogen, tissue-type plasminogen activator, and high-sensitivity C-reactive protein [14, 15]. Microalbuminuria is present in an increased number of TC patients treated with cisplatin-based chemotherapy [14, 16], which is a clinical manifestation of systemic vascular dysfunction that independently predicts for vascular events, including stroke and myocardial infarction (MI) [17]. In one study, microalbuminuria persisted in 22% of TCS treated with cisplatin-based chemotherapy after a median follow-up of 14 years [16].

A prior investigation [15] showed that the carotid intimal medial thickness of TC patients, which correlates with increased risk of cerebrovascular accidents and MI [18], significantly increased during a 3.5-month course of cisplatin-based chemotherapy. This rate of increase was significantly higher than the annual change observed in carotid intimal medial thickness in the general population. Acute alterations in diastolic heart function were reported in a study [19] of 14 TC patients three months after initiation of 3 to 4 cycles of chemotherapy with BEP; these included significant decreases in the left ventricular end-diastolic and stroke volumes. Other suggested mechanisms of direct vascular damage include cisplatin-induced vasospasm due to hypomagnesemia [20–23] and increased formation of procoagulant endothelial microparticles released by endothelial cells, triggering thrombin generation and hypercoagulability [24, 25].

Raynaud phenomenon is another clinical manifestation of vascular damage and is estimated to be present in approximately 25% to 61% of TCS [26–30]. The onset of symptoms from Raynaud phenomenon generally begins within 4 to 12 months of chemotherapy, with 25% experiencing these symptoms up to 20 years [14]. Bleomycin is strongly associated with the development of Raynaud phenomenon. In a randomized study [31] of 395 patients with good-risk metastatic nonseminoma, 8% of patients randomized to BEP developed Raynaud phenomenon compared to none undergoing etoposide and cisplatin (EP). Vinblastine and cisplatin are other chemotherapeutic agents that may contribute to this toxicity [28–30, 32].

The indirect hypothesis postulates that cisplatin-based chemotherapy increases the prevalence of CVD risk factors in TCS, resulting in increased CVD events [9]. Multiple studies [14, 16, 30, 33–40] have reported increased frequency of hyperlipidemia, hypertension, diabetes, insulin resistance, and metabolic syndrome among TC patients after treatment with chemotherapy compared to surgery-only comparison groups or controls derived from the general population (Table 1). Although several studies [36, 38, 41] showed that metabolic syndrome and its individual components are associated with testosterone deficiency and hypogonadism, most TCS with CVD risk factors have normal testosterone levels [33]. Decreased testosterone levels may cause endothelial dysfunction, impair vascular smooth muscle reactivity, increase intima and media thickness of vessels, and increase synthesis of proinflammatory cytokines [42–44]. In an investigation by Haugnes et al. [33], relationships with both hypogonadism and cumulative dose of cisplatin and metabolic syndrome were evaluated among 1135 Norwegian TCS. Compared to the surgery group, TCS who received a cumulative dose of cisplatin >850 mg had a significant 2.8-fold increased odds of metabolic syndrome, with both total serum testosterone and smoking history (≥20 pack-years) being independent predictive factors in multiple regression models.

A multiple-hit hypothesis that encompasses both the direct and indirect hypotheses has recently been proposed to explain the elevated risk of CVD among TCS [10, 45]. This model hypothesizes that multiple factors interact synergistically to increase the risks of CVD among TCS, including orchiectomy-derived subclinical hypogonadism, chemotherapy-induced vascular injury, chemotherapy-related disturbance of metabolic homeostasis, and other TC treatment-related toxicities [10].

The relative risk of CVD among TCS treated with chemotherapy is 1.4- to 7.1-fold significantly higher compared to the general population or to those managed with surveillance only [16, 34, 35, 46, 47]. A British study [35] of 390 TCS treated with chemotherapy between 1982 and 1992 at a median follow-up of 9.7 years showed a 7% incidence of angina, MI or sudden cardiac death, with an elevated age-adjusted relative risk (RR) of 2.6 (95% confidence interval (CI) 1.2–5.8) when compared with TC patients treated with surgery alone. In a retrospective study [46] of a nationwide cohort of 2707 5-year TCS in the Netherlands (1965–1995) after a median follow-up of 17.6 years, cisplatin-based chemotherapy (cisplatin, vinblastine, bleomycin (PVB) or BEP) increased the risk of CVD by 1.7-fold (95% CI 1.1–2.5) when compared with age and sex-matched data in the general Dutch population.

To determine CVD risk after modern-era cisplatin-based chemotherapy in TC patients, Haugnes et al. [34] evaluated the prevalence of cardiovascular risk factors and long-term incidence of CVD among 990 5-year TC survivors (median follow-up: 19 years). All cytotoxic treatment groups (radiation only, chemotherapy only, and combined radiation/chemotherapy) had significantly increased prevalence of usage of antihypertensive medications compared with age-matched male controls in the general population. The odds of diabetes were higher in the radiation (odds ratio (OR) 2.3; 95% CI 1.5–3.7) and radiation/chemotherapy groups (OR 3.9; 95% CI 1.4–10.9) compared to controls [34]. Using age-adjusted Cox regression analyses, increased risks of atherosclerotic disease were reported in the radiation only (hazard ratio (HR) 2.3; 95% CI 1.04–5.3), chemotherapy only (HR 2.6; 95% CI 1.1–5.9), and combined radiation/chemotherapy cohorts (HR 4.8; 95% CI 1.6–14.4) compared to those managed with surgery only [34]. Treatment with BEP alone increased the risk of coronary artery disease by 5.7-fold (95% CI 1.9–17.1) compared with surgery only, while the risk for MI increased by 3.1-fold (95% CI 1.2–7.7) compared with age-matched male controls [34].

Using age-adjusted Cox regression analyses, increased risks of atherosclerotic disease were reported after radiation only (HR 2.3; 95% CI 1.04–5.3), chemotherapy only (HR 2.6;

TABLE 1: Prevalence of cardiovascular disease risk factors in chemotherapy-treated patients in select studies since 2000.

						Prevalence of cardiovascular risk factors versus Controls[b] (%)				
Author (year)	*N*[a]	Treatment dates	Median length of follow-up (range)	Median age at follow-up (range)	Control group (*N*)	HTN (definition)	Increased lipids[c] (definition)	DM (definition)	Obesity (definition)	Metabolic syndrome (definition)
Meinardi et al. (2000) [16]	62	Before 1987	14 y (10–20 y)	42 y (30–50 y)	Stage I TC (40)	39 versus 13 (SBP > 150 mmHg, DBP > 95 mmHg)	79 versus 53 (TC ≥ 201 mg/dL)	NA	21 versus 28[d] (BMI > 27.8)	NA
Strumberg et al. (2002) [30]	32	1977–1981	15 y (13–17 y)	40 y (30–59 y)	None	25 versus NA (DBP > 95 mmHg)	81 versus NA (TC ≥ 200 mg/dL)	NA	48 versus NA (BMI ≥ 25)	NA
Huddart et al. (2003) [35]	390	1982–1992	10 y (0–20 y)	41 y (23–72 y)	Stage I TC (242)	13 versus 9[d] (antihypertension medication)	1 versus 2[d] (lipid-lowering medication)	NA	NA	NA
Nuver et al. (2004) [14]	90	1988–1999	7 y (NA)	37 y (20–65 y)	Stage I TC (44) and healthy patients (47)	22 versus 23 versus 11[d] (SBP ≥ 135 mmHg, DBP ≥ 85 mmHg)	71 versus 59 versus 45[e] (LDL > 131 mg/dL)	NA	22 versus 27 versus 11[e] (BMI ≥ 30)	NA
Nuver et al. (2005) [36]	86	1988–1999	7 y (3–13 y)	37 y (20–65 y)	Stage I TC (44) and healthy patients (47)	NA	NA	NA	NA	26 versus 36 versus 9[e] (≥3 factors per NCEP definition [163])
Sagstuen et al. (2005) [37]	500	1980–1994	11 y (4–22 y)	44 y (23–75 y)	Surgery-only[f] (242)[g]	50 versus 39 (SBP ≥ 140 mmHg or DBP ≥ 90 mmHg or antihypertension medication)	NA	NA	18 versus 13[h] (BMI ≥ 30)	NA
Haugnes et al. (2007) [33]	464	1980–1994	11 y (5–22 y)	43 y (15–52 y)	Surgery-only[f] (225) and healthy population (1150)	45 versus 34 versus 50[i] (SBP ≥ 140 mmHg or DBP ≥ 90 mmHg or antihypertension medication)	68 versus 67 versus 84[d] (TC ≥ 201 mg/dL)	3 versus 2 versus 3[d] (by patient self-report)	18 versus 13 versus 21[d] (BMI ≥ 30)	9 versus 7 versus 15[h] (≥3 factors per NCEP definition [163])
Haugnes et al. (2010) [34]	364	1980–1994	19 y (13–28 y)	49 y (31–69 y)	Surgery-only[f] (206) and healthy population (990)	26 versus 12 versus 13 (antihypertension medication)	14 versus 14 versus 9[e] (lipid-lowering medication)	5 versus 4 versus 4[d] (by patient self-report or fasting glucose ≥ 198 mg/dL)	17 versus 19 versus 23[d] (BMI ≥ 30)	NA

Table 1: Continued.

Author (year)	N[a]	Treatment dates	Median length of follow-up (range)	Median age at follow-up (range)	Control group (N)	Prevalence of cardiovascular risk factors versus Controls[b] (%)				
						HTN (definition)	Increased lipids[c] (definition)	DM (definition)	Obesity (definition)	Metabolic syndrome (definition)
Willemse et al. (2013) [38]	194[j]	1977–2008	7.8 y (0.1–30 y)	39.6 y (18–70 y)	Surgery-only (57) and healthy population (360)	29 versus 14 versus 22.5[k] (per NCEP definition [163])	NA	NA	29 versus 18 versus 19[k] (per NCEP definition [163])	16 versus 9 versus 8[k] (per NCEP definition [163])
de Haas et al. (2013) [39]	173	1977–2004	5 y (3–20 y)	37 y (19–59 y)	Healthy population (1085)	59 versus NA (SBP ≥ 130 mmHg or DBP ≥ 85 mmHg or antihypertension medication) (AHA/NHLBI definition)	44 versus NA (HDL <1.03 mmol/l or lipid-lowering medication) (AHA/NHLBI definition)	14 versus NA (fasting glucose ≥5.6 mmol/l or medication) (AHA/NHLBI definition)	17 versus NA (waist circumference ≥ 102 cm) (AHA/NHLBI definition)	25 versus NA (≥3 factors per AHA/NHLBI definition)
Fung et al. (2017) [40]	952	1979–2015	4.3 y (1.0–29.9)	37 y (19–68 y)	NHANES matched controls (952)	16.8 versus 19.4[d] ever diagnosed with high blood pressure and current use of antihypertension medication	10.5 versus NA[l] current use of cholesterol lowering medication	3.1 versus NA[l] diabetes requiring insulin or diabetes requiring medication	31.3 versus 35.4[k] BMI ≥ 30	NA

*Adapted with permission from Feldman et al. [9] (Table 2). AHA: American Heart Association; BMI: body mass index; DBP: diastolic blood pressure; DM: diabetes mellitus; NHLBI: National Heart, Lung, and Blood Institute; NHANES: National Health and Nutrition Examination Survey; TC: testicular cancer; HTN: hypertension; LDL: low-density lipoprotein; NA: not available; NCEP: National Cholesterol Education Program; SBP: systolic blood pressure; TC: total cholesterol. (a) N varies slightly for individual factors due to missing data in papers for some variables. (b) Definitions of individual factors vary by study. Comparisons of chemotherapy group to controls significant unless otherwise stated; percentages vary slightly due to missing data for individual factors. (c) Cholesterol and fasting glucose values in definitions were converted from mml/L to mg/dL, where necessary for uniformity. (d) Not significant. (e) Significant versus healthy population controls but not versus surgery patients. (f) Includes both orchiectomy and primary retroperitoneal lymph node dissection patients. (g) A healthy population control group was also included in this study, but prevalence rates of cardiovascular risk factors were not reported for this control group, and therefore these data are not included in the table. (h) Significant only for patients who received >850 mg of cisplatin. (i) Significant versus surgery patients but not versus healthy controls. (j) 20 patients received carboplatin and 174 patients received combination chemotherapy. (k) Significant for patients who received combination chemotherapy compared to healthy population. (l) Significance versus controls not tested.

95% CI 1.1–5.9), and combined radiation/chemotherapy (HR 4.8; 95% CI 1.6–14.4) compared with surgery only (P-trend = 0.02) [34]. In particular, treatment with BEP alone increased CAD risk by 5.7-fold (95% CI 1.9–17.1) compared with surgery only and increased MI risk by 3.1-fold (95% CI 1.2–7.7) compared with age-matched male controls [34].

Several studies [48–50] have examined the extent to which increased CVD mortality might result from TC treatment. In an international population-based study [48] of 38,907 TCS (1943–2002) at a median follow-up of 10 years, a 1.6-fold (95% CI 1.3–2.0) increased risk of mortality from all circulatory diseases was reported for those treated with chemotherapy after 1975. Another population-based study [49] using the SEER program (1973–2008) found that patients with either mediastinal or nonmediastinal extragonadal GCT had significantly increased 4.5-fold and 2.8-fold risks of CVD mortality, respectively, compared to patients with primary testicular GCT. The increased number of cycles of primary chemotherapy and additional salvage chemotherapy typically required to treat extragonadal TC were hypothesized to contribute to this higher risk, although detailed chemotherapy data were not available [49]. Recently, Fung et al. [50] reported a significant 5.3-fold increase in CVD mortality during the first year after chemotherapy in a population-based study of 15,006 TCS managed initially with either chemotherapy or surgery alone without radiotherapy during 1980–2010. In contrast, excess CVD mortality was not observed more than one year after chemotherapy, likely due to advances in cardiovascular disease management, as reflected in the 31% decline in US cardiovascular death rates from 2000 to 2010 [51]. In multivariable analyses, increased CVD mortality after chemotherapy was confined to the first year after TC diagnosis (HR 4.86; 95% CI, 1.25–32); distant disease ($P < 0.05$) and older age at diagnosis ($P < 0.01$) were independent risk factors [50].

Currently, there are no established evidence-based CVD screening recommendations developed specifically for TCS. In November 2013, the American College of Cardiology and the American Heart Association released guidelines for the assessment of cardiovascular disease risk, the management of elevated cholesterol and increased body weight, and lifestyle modifications to reduce CVD risk in adults in the general population [52]. Health care professionals should monitor and modify cardiovascular risk factors of TCS by referring to these guidelines [52] and by leveraging TC diagnosis as a teachable moment to promote lifestyle changes, including smoking cessation, optimal nutrition, and a non-sedentary lifestyle [7, 53].

3. Second Malignant Neoplasms

Syndromic, cancer treatment, and shared etiologic exposures are the major causative factors of SMN [54]. Figure 1 shows the influence of lifestyle factors, genetic susceptibility, environmental exposures, host effects, and a combination of influences, including gene-environment interactions in the development of SMN. Age at exposure and attained age are modifiers for the risks of selected SMN [55].

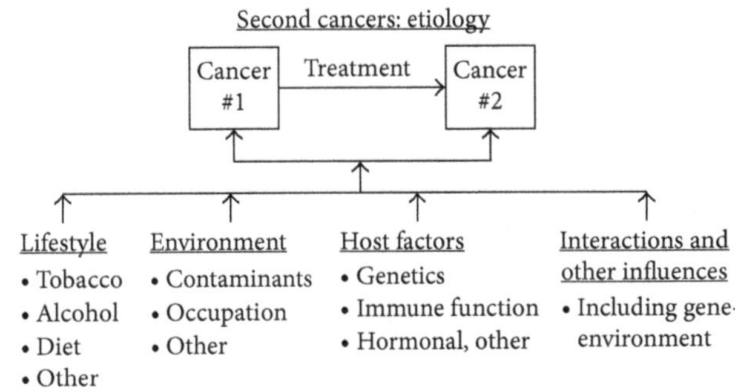

Figure 1: Risk factors for second primary cancer (refer to text). Many influences some of which are diagrammed here may contribute to the development of multiple primary cancers, including interactions between exposures. *Adapted with permission from Travis [169].

After receiving radiotherapy for TC treatment, TCS have significantly increased risks of leukemia [56] and solid cancers [46, 55, 57–59] (Table 2). An international population-based study of 18,567 TCS reported a significantly 3-fold increased risk of leukemia after abdominal and pelvic radiotherapy with a mean dose of 10.9 Gy to active bone marrow [56]. The median latency for leukemia was 5.0 years with a quarter of survivors developing leukemia more than one decade later (maximum latency: 17.3 years) [56]. After radiation treatment, long-term TCS also have significantly 1.4 to 1.9-fold increased risks of second solid cancers compared to the general population (Table 2) [46, 55, 57]. An international population-based investigation of 10-year TCS reported that the RR of SMN at sites included in typical infradiaphragmatic radiotherapy fields were significantly larger than risks at unexposed sites (RR 2.7 versus 1.6; $P < 0.05$), which remained elevated for more than 35 years. In another study [46], infradiaphragmatic radiotherapy administered at doses 40–50 Gray (Gy) compared with 26–35 Gy increased the HR for SMN from 2.3 to 3.2, respectively, when using a surgery-only group as control. Two recent studies of 5-year TCS reported a 5.9-fold increased risk of stomach cancer (95% CI 1.7–20.7) [58] and a 2.9-fold increased risk of pancreatic cancer (95% CI 1.0–7.8) after radiotherapy [59]. The risks of stomach and pancreatic cancers increased with higher radiation doses to stomach [58] and pancreas [59], respectively (P trend < 0.001), and risks remained elevated for ≥20 years after exposure ($P < 0.01$) [58, 59]. Several other studies of TCS [46, 60, 61] similarly reported significant associations between radiotherapy and SMN risks.

Cisplatin and etoposide are integral chemotherapeutic agents used in standard chemotherapy regimens to treat TC [62]. Both cisplatin and etoposide are associated with significantly elevated risks of secondary leukemia [56, 63–65]. An international nested case-control study [56] among TCS estimated a 3.2-fold risk of leukemia after cumulative cisplatin dose of 650 mg, although the excess risk was small with only 16 excess cases among 10,000 TC patients after 15 years of follow-up. The same study also reported a significant dose-response relationship between cumulative dose of cisplatin and leukemia risk after adjustment for radiation dose

Table 2: Relative risks of second malignant neoplasms (SMN) in testicular cancer survivors.

	No. of patients	Calendar years of testicular cancer diagnosis	Duration of follow-up (years)	Treatment	Obs.	RR	(95% CI)
Study populations[a]							
All SMNs							
Norwegian radium hospital [66]	2006	1952–1990	Mean = 12.5	Any	153[b]	1.7	1.4–1.9
				RT	130	1.6	1.3–1.9
				CT	4	1.3	0.4–3.4
				RT + CT	15	3.5	2.0–5.8
Fourteen population-based tumor registries in Europe and North America [55]	40,576	1943–2001	Mean = 11.3	Any	1694	1.9	1.8–2.1
				RT	892	2.0	1.9–2.2
				CT	35	1.8	1.3–2.5
				RT + CT	25	2.9	1.9–4.2
Thirteen International Cancer Registries [164]	29,511	1943–2000	Median = 8.3	Any	1811[c]	1.7	1.6–1.7
Netherlands testicular cancer survivor cohort [46]	2707	1965–1995	Median = 17.6	Any	270[d]	1.7	1.5–1.9
				RT	199	1.7	1.5–2.0
				CT	23	1.4	0.9–2.1
				RT + CT	29	3.0	2.0–4.4
				SDRT	N/A	2.6[g]	1.7–4.0
				SDRT + MRT	N/A	3.6[g]	2.1–6.0
				PVB/BEP	N/A	2.1[g]	1.4–3.1
				SDRT (26–35 Gy)	N/A	2.3[g]	1.5–3.6
				SDRT (40–50 Gy)	N/A	3.2[g]	2.1–5.1
Swedish family cancer database [165]	5533	1980–2006	N/A	Any	274[e]	2.0	1.8–2.2
Second solid cancers							
Sixteen population-based registries within the SEER program [67]	12,691	1980–2008	Median = 7.0	Initial surgery only	99	0.9	0.8–1.1
				Initial CT (no RT)	111[f]	1.4	1.2–1.7
Therapy-associated leukemia							
Nested case-control study of leukemia in 8 population-based tumor registries in Europe and North America [56]	18,567	1970–1993	N/A	No RT/CT	4	1.0	—
				RT	22	3.1	0.7–2.2
				CT	8	5.0	1.1–40
				RT + CT	2	5.1	0.5–28

*Adapted with permission from Fung et al. *J Natl Compr Canc Netw 2012; 10:545-56* (Table 2). RR: relative risk; CI: confidence interval; Obs.: observed number of cases; RT: any radiation treatment; CT: chemotherapy; IDRT: infradiaphragmatic radiation; SDRT: supradiaphragmatic radiation; MRT: mediastinal radiation; PVB: cisplatin, vinblastine, bleomycin; BEP: bleomycin, etoposide, cisplatin; N/A: not available (data not provided). (a) There was overlap in the cancer registries included in the cohort studies by Richiardi et al. [164] and Travis et al. [55], with the following countries contributing patients to both studies: Denmark, Finland, Norway, and Sweden; (b) six cases of leukemia were observed with a RR of 1.9 (95% CI: 0.7–4.1); (c) thirty-eight cases of myeloid leukemia were observed with a RR of 3.6 (95% CI: 2.6–5.0); thirteen cases of lymphoid leukemia were observed with a RR of 1.0 (95% CI: 0.5–1.7); twenty-three cases of other types of leukemia were observed with a RR of 3.5 (95% CI: 2.2–5.2); (d) six cases of leukemia were observed with a RR of 1.6 (95% CI: 0.6–3.5); (e) hazard ratios are shown, with the referent group consisting of patients treated with surgery alone (HR = 1.0). Twelve cases of leukemia were observed with a RR of 3.8 (95% CI: 2.0–6.7); (f) significantly increased risks occurred for cancers of the kidney (SIR = 3.4; 95% CI 1.8–5.7; $n = 13$); thyroid (SIR = 4.4; 95% CI: 2.2–7.9; $n = 11$); and soft tissue (SIR = 7.5; 95% CI: 3.6–13.8; $n = 10$).

(P trend = 0.001) [56]. The 5-year cumulative incidence of leukemia is approximately 0.5% after a cumulative etoposide dose of <2000 mg/m^2 and 2.0% after a cumulative etoposide dose of ≥2000 mg/m^2 [65].

Most prior studies of second solid cancer focused on TCS treated before modern cisplatin-based chemotherapy became widely adopted prior to early 1980s (Table 2) [10, 13, 22, 23]. Whereas an international series of more than 40,000 TCS showed a 1.8-fold (95% CI 1.3–2.5) significantly increased risk of second solid cancers among a subgroup of 10-year TCS who received initial chemotherapy during 1943–2001, three smaller epidemiologic studies [10, 39, 57] (ranging from 346 to 710 patients) found no significantly elevated risk of SMN after chemotherapy [27, 46, 66], though they may have inadequate statistical power. To evaluate the risks of second solid cancer among TCS treated in the modern era of cisplatin-based chemotherapy during 1980 to 2008, a recent large population-based investigation by Fung et al. [67] of more than 12,000 TCS reported a 1.4-fold significantly increased risk of solid cancers after initial treatment with chemotherapy compared to those who underwent initial surgery alone. Significantly increased three- to seven-fold risks of cancers of the kidney (standardized incidence ratio (SIR) 3.4), thyroid (SIR 4.4), and soft tissue (SIR 7.5) were also observed. After chemotherapy, elevated risks of solid cancer were reported in most follow-up periods with a median latency of 12.5 years, including at more than 20 years after treatment (SIR 1.54; 95% CI 0.96–2.3). However, detailed information on cytotoxic drug name and dose were not available [67].

TCS should follow national guidelines for cancer screening as applied to the general population, given their increased risks of SMN [53]. Earlier or additional cancer screening may be clinically indicated in TCS deemed at high risk due to prior treatment history and/or health habits [53]. In addition, health care providers should advise TCS of the modest 15-year cumulative risk (1.9%) of metachronous contralateral testicular cancer [68].

4. Neurotoxicity

Approximately 20 to 40% of long-term TCS experience symptoms of peripheral neuropathy after cisplatin-based chemotherapy [28, 29, 69]. Common clinical manifestations of peripheral neuropathy include numbness, tingling, and a decrease in vibratory sense in distal extremities [70]. The cumulative dose of cisplatin administered affects the incidence of peripheral neuropathy. At a median of 11 years after TC treatment, 46% of TCS in a population-based long-term Norwegian survey self-reported paresthesia after ≥5 cycles of cisplatin-based chemotherapy compared to 28% after 1 to 4 cycles of chemotherapy or 10% after orchiectomy alone [28]. Compared to TCS who did not receive chemotherapy, those who underwent 1 to 4 cycles and ≥5 cycles of cisplatin-based chemotherapy had higher risks of symptomatic paresthesia of the hands (OR 2.0, 95% CI 1.5–2.7; OR 3.9, 95% CI 2.1–7.3, resp.) and feet (OR 2.2, 95% CI 1.7–3.0; OR 3.1, 95% CI 1.7–5.7, resp.) [28]. In the same study [28], radiotherapy was significantly associated with symptomatic paresthesias of the feet (OR 1.5), but retroperitoneal lymph node dissection (RPLND) was not an independent risk factor. Increasing levels of residual serum platinum are also directly associated with severity of neurotoxicity after adjusting for initial cisplatin dose [71]. Sprauten et al. reported [71] that the total score for the Scale for Chemotherapy Induced Neuropathy (SCIN) had a significant four-to five-fold association with the highest residual serum platinum quartile in cisplatin-treated TC patients.

Oldenburg et al. [72] investigated the impact of germline single nucleotide polymorphisms (SNPs) of glutathione S-transferase (*GST*) *P*1, *M*1, and *T*1 on self-reported paresthesia among long-term TCS. The *GSTP1-GG* genotype conferred a significantly lower risk of developing paresthesia in the fingers (OR = 0.46, 95% CI 0.22–0.96) and toes (OR = 0.42, 95% CI 0.20–0.88) than the *GSTP1-AA* and *GSTP1-AG* genotypes. Recently, a genome-wide analysis of cisplatin-induced peripheral neuropathy in survivors of adult-onset cancer reported that genetically determined expression level of *RPRD1B* was associated with cisplatin-induced peripheral neuropathy [73]. Defects in *RPRD1B* expression or knockdown cause a deficiency in DNA repair mechanisms known to be critical in repairing cisplatin-induced lesions [74] and result in increased sensitivity to cisplatin in a breast cancer cell line, MDA-123 [75].

No therapeutic agents are currently recommended for the prevention of peripheral neuropathy due to the paucity of high-quality, consistent evidence. For management of drug-induced peripheral neuropathy, the ASCO Clinical Practice Guideline [76] recommends treatment with duloxetine as potentially the most effective drug. Health care providers may also offer tricyclic antidepressants (i.e., nortriptyline), gabapentin, and a compounded topical gel containing baclofen, amitriptyline HCL, and ketamine based on clinical benefits observed for other neuropathic pain conditions [76].

5. Ototoxicity

Cisplatin selectively damages the outer hair cells of the cochlea [77], causing tinnitus and hearing loss that predominantly affect high frequencies [77–79] similar to age-related presbycusis. After a median follow-up of 58 months, Bokemeyer et al. [78] found that 20% of TCS (median age: 31 years) reported symptomatic ototoxicity (59% tinnitus, 18% hearing loss, 23% both) after cisplatin-based chemotherapy. For TCS who received >400 mg/m^2 of cumulative cisplatin dose, 50% self-reported tinnitus and hearing loss compared to 20% of those treated with ≤400 mg/m^2 [78]. Older age, higher cumulative cisplatin dose, a history of noise exposure, hypertension, and impaired baseline renal function and hearing are each independently associated with more severe ototoxicity [78–80]. A recent comprehensive audiometric analysis of 488 North American TCS [79] reported that almost one in five (18%) had severe to profound hearing loss as defined by the American Speech-Language-Hearing Association criteria (median follow-up: 4.25 years after completion of cisplatin-based chemotherapy). Tinnitus (40% patients) was significantly correlated with reduced hearing at each frequency ($P < 0.001$). The same study [79] also found that increasing cumulative cisplatin dose was significantly related to hearing loss at 4, 6, 8, 10, and 12 kHz (P trend for each <0.05). For each 100 mg/m [2] increase in cumulative cisplatin dose, a 3.2 dB impairment in age-adjusted overall hearing threshold (4–12 kHz; $P < 0.001$) resulted. However, cisplatin dose did not affect noise-induced hearing damage (10% patients) ($P = 0.59$) [79].

A few reports have identified significant associations of germline genetic polymorphisms of various genes with platinum-related ototoxicity, including megalin [81], *GSTP1* [72, 82], *GSTM3* [72, 82], *COMT* [83], *TPMT* [83], and *WFS1* [84]. Both alleles of *105Val-GSTP1* protected against cisplatin-induced ototoxicity in cisplatin-treated TCS, whereas *GSTM1* positivity was detrimental for hearing ability [82]. Functional polymorphisms of the glutathione S-transferases (*GSTs*) genes likely cause differential expression of the cisplatin-detoxifying enzymes, consequently rendering TCS suspcetible to varying degrees of cisplatin-induced hearing impairment. A recent genome-wide association study [85] of 511 TC patients of European genetic ancestry reported that one SNP, rs62283056, in the first intron of *WFS1* (wolframin ER transmembrane glycoprotein) was significantly associated with cisplatin-associated ototoxicity ($P = 1.4 \times 10^{-8}$), with higher cisplatin doses exacerbating hearing loss in TC patients with the risk allele. In the general population, *WSF1* mutations causes the Mendelian disorders DFNA6 (deafness, autosomal dominant 6) and the recessive Wolfram syndrome (with hearing loss) [86, 87].

There are no effective pharmacologic agents available to prevent or treat cisplatin-induced ototoxicity. TCS should use ear protection to minimize noise exposure and additional hearing loss. Since the peak concentration of cisplatin may be directly associated with the severity of ototoxicity [28, 88], where indicated, the 5-day BEP regimen seems preferable to a 3-day regimen [7].

6. Pulmonary Toxicity

The incidence of fatal bleomycin-induced pulmonary toxicity is approximately 1–3% [89, 90]. Corticosteroids remain the mainstay of treatment of bleomycin-induced pneumonitis, although there are no data from prospective randomized trials to support this approach [91]. Health care providers should withhold bleomycin at the earliest signs or symptoms of bleomycin-induced pulmonary toxicities during chemotherapy. Since age of more than 40 years [89] and increased tobacco use [92] are both significantly associated with pulmonary toxicity during bleomycin treatment, a careful assessment of patient history (i.e., age, smoking status, and preexisting lung disease) are important to consider prior to the administration of any bleomycin-containing regimen [93]. Avoiding perioperative overhydration is important to minimize the risk of perioperative lung complications, but perioperative oxygen restriction in patients a few months after administration of bleomycin is not necessary [94, 95].

Bleomycin hydrolase is an enzyme encoded by the *BLMH* gene, which inactivates bleomycin [96]. A Dutch investigation of 340 TC patients treated with bleomycin-containing chemotherapy between 1977 and 2003 reported that the genetic polymorphism of 1450A > G was not associated with bleomycin-induced pneumonitis or changes in pulmonary function tests [97].

A large Norwegian study [92] of 1049 long-term TCS treated during 1980 to 1994 (median follow-up: 11.2 years) reported that 8% of survivors had restrictive lung disease as defined by predicted FVC <80% and a value of ≥70% for forced expiratory volume (FEV) 1/forced vital capacity (FVC). In multivariate analyses adjusting for bleomycin, etoposide, and vinblastine doses, higher cumulative cisplatin dose ($P = 0.007$) and older age ($P = 0.008$) were both significantly related to restrictive lung disease [92]. Compared with men treated with surgery only, patients who received large cumulative doses of cisplatin (>850 mg) as well as combined chemotherapy and pulmonary surgery were at significantly increased risk of demonstrating decreased spirometry variables, including age-adjusted FVC, FEV1, FVC% predicted, and FEV1% predicted [92]. A population-based study of TCS reported to North American and European cancer registries found that patients treated with chemotherapy (with or without radiotherapy) in 1975 or later had a 1.6-fold higher risk of mortality (95% CI 1.25–2.01) (median follow-up: 10 years) due to respiratory diseases compared to the general population. The extent to which bleomycin-induced lung toxicity may have contributed to these excesses is not known.

7. Nephrotoxicity

Cisplatin damages the proximal and distal renal tubular epithelium and the renal collecting duct system, as well as the glomeruli at higher doses [98, 99]. Two long-term studies [100, 101] reported persistently decreased renal function in TCS for years after completion of treatment compared with baseline assessments. A Norwegian study [100] of 85 TC patients more than 10 years after treatment showed that renal function among TCS who received radiotherapy alone decreased by 8%, whereas survivors who had cisplatin-based chemotherapy had reductions of 14%. Cumulative cisplatin dose and age at treatment were both directly associated with long-term impairment of renal function ($P < 0.05$). A Danish investigation [101] of 34 TCS who received systemic chemotherapy with PVB (median dose of cisplatin: 583 mg/m^2) reported that the glomerular filtration rate (GFR) decreased by a median of 18% during treatment. At a median follow-up of 65 months (range, 43 to 97 months), 38% of survivors had persistent renal dysfunction. Research in the general population has demonstrated a relationship between decreased GFR and the presence of microalbuminuria, leading to increased risks of CVD and all-cause mortality [102, 103]. Among long-term TCS, treatment-related nephrotoxicity may contribute to the reported increases in incident CVD events, including hypertension and MI [34, 35, 47]. To limit the severity of acute- and long-term renal damage, health care providers should administer hydration [104] and avoid nephrotoxic drugs [7] during cisplatin-based chemotherapy.

8. Hypogonadism

Orchiectomy, testicular dysgenesis syndrome, postorchiectomy chemotherapy or radiotherapy, and aging are the predominant causes of hypogonadism and premature hormonal aging in long-term TCS [105]. A Norwegian investigation [105] reported that 307 TCS treated between 1980 and 1994 had significantly increased risks of low testosterone as well as high-luteinizing hormone (LH) and follicle-stimulating hormone (FSH) levels after radiotherapy or chemotherapy at long-term follow-up. The degree of hypogonadism was directly related to the intensity of TC treatment [105–110]. A recent meta-analysis reported that both standard cisplatin-based chemotherapy (OR: 1.8) and infradiaphragmatic radiotherapy (OR: 1.6) significantly increased the risk of hypogonadism among TCS, as defined by total testosterone levels less than reference levels or use of testosterone replacement therapy, when compared to orchiectomy alone [110]. Hypogonadism may lead to reduced sexual functioning and well-being, fertility problems, muscle weakness, osteoporosis, loss of energy, and depression [111–117]. Further, hypogonadism is directly associated with the metabolic syndrome and CVD [29, 30, 32]. A recent multi-institutional cross-sectional study [118] reported that over one-third of North American TCS had hypogonadism at a median age of 38 years; in addition, hypogonadism was associated with increased CVD risk factors (i.e., dyslipidemia, hypertension, and diabetes), erectile dysfunction, and medication use for anxiety/depression ($P < 0.05$). Health care providers should regularly assess TCS for symptoms of hypogonadism and check hormonal status as clinically indicated. Clinical symptoms of hypogonadism should guide treatment decisions with testosterone replacement therapy [7]. Referral to endocrinologists for evaluation and management of difficult cases should also be considered.

9. Infertility

The association of infertility and TC is well established. Approximately 50% of patients with newly diagnosed TC have decreased sperm counts (<20 million/mL), low sperm motility indices (<40), and a high percentage of abnormal sperm cells (>80%) prior to initiation of any radiation or chemotherapy [119]. In a multicenter prospective study of 2318 TC patients in Germany and Austria [120], TC patients had significantly reduced spermatogenesis in their contralateral testicles confirmed histologically when compared to healthy subjects. The overall conception and paternity rates among long-term TCS with known intention to conceive a child after treatment completion range from 49% to 88% in several investigations (range of median follow-up: 7 to 12 years) [109, 121–123].

Radiotherapy can adversely affect reproductive function of TCS in the short-term [124, 125], since spermatogonia are the most sensitive germ cells to radiation treatment [126]. In the SWOG-8711 clinical trial of 207 patients with seminoma [124], sperm concentration reached a nadir 4 to 6 months after completion of radiotherapy, but returned to pretreatment level by 10 to 24 months after end of treatment. Similarly, Gandini et al. [127] reported that the sperm counts of TC patients reached a nadir at 6 months after radiation treatment, but 94% of patients recovered sperm counts by 2 years after end of radiotherapy. Higher dose of radiation is directly associated with longer recovery time for sperm concentration, and the use of testicular shielding devices significantly improves recovery of spermatogenesis [124]. A recent investigation of 1191 Norwegian TCS (median follow-up: 11 years) confirmed that radiotherapy had no significant long-term effects on sperm counts when compared to the surgery-only cohort [125].

In a retrospective study [128] of 178 TC patients treated with cisplatin-based chemotherapy in England, 64%, 24%, and 15% of patients who were normospermic, oligospermic and azoospermic, respectively, in the prechemotherapy period recovered normal spermatogenesis at least one year after chemotherapy completion. Prechemotherapy normospermia (HR 6.0), use of carboplatin versus cisplatin (HR 4.4), and noninclusion of a vinca alkaloid (HR 5.3) in chemotherapy regimen were significantly associated with normal recovery of sperm counts [128]. Cumulative dose of cisplatin-based chemotherapy is directly associated with infertility risk [112, 123, 125, 128]. In a multicenter investigation [123] of 316 Norwegian TCS (median follow-up: 12 years), 100%, 83%, and 76% of survivors self-reported achieving posttreatment paternity after 2, 3, and 4 cycles of standard cisplatin-based chemotherapy, respectively ($P = 0.022$). However, sperm counts were not significantly related to number of cycles of chemotherapy in a limited cohort of patients for whom the results of semen analysis were available ($N = 71$) [123]. After a median follow-up of 10.6 years, another study [112] showed that TCS treated with high-dose chemotherapy (>850 mg cumulative cisplatin dose) had the lowest 15-year actuarial posttreatment paternity rate (48%) compared to 92% in the surveillance group and 60% in those treated with low-dose chemotherapy (≤850 mg cumulative cisplatin) ($P < 0.001$). Similarly, a recent investigation [125] reported that sperm counts and serum level of inhibin B were significantly lower in TCS treated with >850 mg cumulative cisplatin dose compared to those who had either surgery only or ≤850 mg cumulative cisplatin, whereas the serum FSH was significantly higher.

Among patients with stage II or III nonseminomatous germ cell tumor who have had a serologic complete response but have persistent enlarged retroperitoneal lymph nodes after cisplatin-based chemotherapy, RPLND is a standard treatment. To potentially avoid toxicities associated with cisplatin-based chemotherapy, RPLND is another treatment option for low-volume stage II nonseminomatous germ cell tumor with normal β-hCG and AFP levels after orchiectomy [62]. Injury to the retroperitoneal postganglionic sympathetic nerves during RPLND may result in retrograde ejaculation [126], leading to inability to conceive without use of cryopreserved sperm. The rate of retrograde ejaculation ranges from 1 to 9% after primary RPLND [129–131], 11% to 29% after nerve-sparing postchemotherapy RPLND [130, 132–134], and 75% after full bilateral postchemotherapy RPLND [135].

Health care providers should address the possibility of infertility and discuss fertility preservation options with TC patients as detailed by the American Society of Clinical Oncology Clinical Practice Guideline for fertility preservation for patients with cancer [136]. If clinically indicated, referral to appropriate reproductive specialists should be considered [136]. Sperm cryopreservation is a standard fertility preservation practice [136] that may be offered to interested TC patients undergoing treatment.

10. Avascular Necrosis

Avascular necrosis commonly affects the femoral head, often bilaterally [137], with an incidence of approximately 1-2% in long-term TCS treated with cisplatin-based chemotherapy [137, 138]. The etiology for avascular necrosis is multifactorial [7] but likely to be partially attributable to corticosteroids used as antiemetics during TC treatment [137–140]. Bleomycin and vinblastine have also been hypothesized as causative agents in a case of avascular necrosis in one TCS who did not receive corticosteroids during chemotherapy [141]. Health care providers should review with TC patients who receive high-dose corticosteroids the potential risk of avascular necrosis. For any long-term TCS who develops early symptoms suggestive of avascular necrosis, including decreased hip motion and/or limp, prompt evaluation with plain radiograph or MRI is critical [7].

11. Cognitive Impairment

The underlying mechanisms of chemotherapy-related cognitive impairment have not been elucidated. Several neuroimaging studies of breast cancer survivors have reported that white matter activation patterns involved in cognitive functioning are altered after chemotherapy [142–144], likely due to neurotoxic effects [145]. A study [146] of 66 TC patients suggested that cortisol levels prior to chemotherapy may be a predictor of later cognitive complaints. The prevalence of cognitive impairment in men with newly diagnosed TC before receipt of any chemotherapy ranges from 46% to 58% and is significantly higher than expected in the healthy normal population ($P < 0.01$) [146, 147]. A prospective clinical trial [88] of 666 patients with metastatic TC in Europe showed that cognitive function decreased at 3 months after chemotherapy, though not at the level of clinical relevance but recovered to baseline values at 2 years for most patients, with 19% still having worsened cognitive function at that time. However, the association of cisplatin-based chemotherapy with cognitive impairment in TCS remains unclear. Whereas three studies [148–150] of TCS ($N = 70$–112; median follow-up: 1–3 years) reported no significant differences in performance on cognitive tests between TC treatment groups (i.e., surgery only versus chemotherapy), two investigations [151, 152] reported increased risks of cognitive impairment after chemotherapy. Among 1173 TCS with a median follow-up of 9 years, Skoogh et al. [151] reported a 2-fold increased risk (95% CI 1.3–3.1) of long-term compromised speech in survivors who completed five or more cycles of cisplatin-based chemotherapy compared to those who received no chemotherapy. Similarly, a single institutional prospective study [152] of TC patients after orchiectomy who either received adjuvant chemotherapy ($N = 55$) or no additional treatment ($N = 14$) reported that chemotherapy was significantly associated with cognitive decline with a dose-response relationship observed at 12 months (surveillance group: 0%; 2-3 cycles of chemotherapy: 52%; and 4–7 cycles of chemotherapy: 67%). Although the extent to which cisplatin-based chemotherapy may have negative effects on long-term cognitive function in TCS is unclear, cognitive complaints among long-term survivors are common and independent of treatment modality [88, 148–151]. These subjective complaints may reflect the effects of anxiety and depression, which are prevalent in TCS [148]. The first step in managing cognitive complaints may include managing specific stressors by implementing effective coping strategies.

12. Anxiety/Depression

A Norwegian study [153] reported a significantly higher prevalence of a Hospital Anxiety and Depression Scale-(HADS-) defined anxiety disorder among TCS (mean follow-up time: 11.3 years) compared to age-adjusted men from the general population (19.2% versus 13.5%, $P < 0.001$). Young age, peripheral neuropathy, economic difficulties, excess alcohol use, sexual concerns, and prior treatment for mental illness were significantly associated with HADS-defined anxiety disorder [153]. A recent investigation [154] showed that the prevalence of clinically significant anxiety among TCS (mean: 11.6 years after diagnosis) in Germany was 6.1%. Anxiety was significantly associated with younger age at diagnosis and shorter time since diagnosis in multivariate analyses. Prior studies [153–156] reported that the prevalence of depression among TCS ranges from 7.9% to 20%, but the extent to which TCS may experience significantly more depressive orders compared to the general population is uncertain. Feeling helpless/hopeless [156], lower social support [156], a higher number of physical symptoms [154], and having children [154] were reported to be significantly associated with higher levels of depression.

13. Fatigue

Chronic fatigue, defined as symptoms with a duration of ≥6 months, is a common and distressing cancer-related adverse effect [157]. The prevalence of chronic cancer-related fatigue among Norwegian TCS was significantly higher compared to age-matched men in the general population (17.1% versus 9.7%) [158]. A recent longitudinal investigation [159] of 812 TCS treated between 1980 and 1994 in Norway reported that the prevalence of chronic fatigue increased from 15% at survey I (1998–2002) to 27% at survey II (2007-2008) ($P < 0.001$). Several factors were significantly associated with chronic fatigue in this study: [159] high level of neuropathy, Raynaud-like phenomena, testosterone level in the lowest quartile, low level of physical activity, as well as higher levels of anxiety and depression. Health care professionals should consider exercise and psychological interventions for early prevention and treatment of chronic fatigue among TCS. A recent meta-analysis of cancer survivors [160] reported that exercise and psychological interventions are effective for reducing cancer-related fatigue during and after cancer treatment and significantly more effective than available pharmaceutical options.

14. Adverse Health Outcomes

To develop risk-stratified, evidence-based follow-up recommendations for TCS, characterization of long-term adverse health outcomes (AHOs) is critical. A recent multi-institutional investigation [40] of 952 North American TCS examined the type and prevalence of AHOs after chemotherapy with four cycles of EP (EPX4) or three or four cycles of BEP (BEPX3/BEPX4) (Table 3). At a median age of 37 years, more than one-third of survivors reported three or more AHOs with similar prevalence and type after EPX4 and BEPX3, except for Raynaud phenomenon (11.6% versus 21.4%; $P < 0.01$), peripheral neuropathy (29.2% versus 21.4%; $P = 0.02$), and obesity (25.5% versus 33.0%; $P = 0.04$). The type and prevalence of AHOs after BEPX4 were largely similar to EPX4 and BEPX3. Increasing age at clinical evaluation, current tobacco use, and nonmarried status were associated with increased numbers of AHOs, whereas weekly vigorous

TABLE 3: Numbers and types of self-reported adverse health outcomes among 952 cisplatin-treated germ cell tumor survivors in North America*.

Adverse health outcomes (AHOs)	Total patients (N = 952) N (%)	Treatment regimen EP (4 cycles) (N = 294) N (%)	BEP (3 cycles) (N = 364) N (%)	BEP (4 cycles) (N = 170) N (%)
Total number of AHOs				
Median (range)	2 (0–11)	2 (0–9)	2 (0–11)	2 (0–10)
0	194 (20.4)	64 (21.8)	83 (22.8)	25 (14.7)
1	209 (21.9)	68 (23.1)	71 (19.5)	42 (24.7)
2	191 (20.1)	61 (20.8)	82 (22.5)	27 (15.9)
3	143 (15.0)	48 (16.3)	48 (13.2)	25 (14.7)
4	96 (10.1)	28 (9.5)	38 (10.4)	18 (10.6)
5 or more	119 (12.5)	25 (8.5)	42 (11.5)	33 (19.4)
Type of AHOs†				
Yes	353 (37.1)	104 (35.4)	130 (35.7)	65 (38.2)
No‡	599 (62.9)	190 (64.6)	234 (64.3)	105 (61.8)
Hearing impairment§				
Yes	300 (31.5)	95 (32.3)	109 (30.0)	56 (33.0)
No	652 (68.5)	199 (67.7)	255 (70.0)	114 (67.0)
Peripheral neuropathy‖				
Yes	257 (27.0)	86 (29.2)	78 (21.4)	54 (31.8)
No	695 (73.0)	208 (70.8)	286 (78.6)	116 (68.2)
Peripheral neuropathy plus tinnitus and/or hearing issue				
Yes	156 (16.4)	49 (16.7)	48 (13.2)	31 (18.2)
No	796 (83.6)	245 (83.3)	316 (86.8)	139 (81.8)
Hypertension and on prescription medication				
Yes	110 (11.6)	35 (11.9)	45 (12.4)	15 (8.8)
No¶	842 (88.4)	259 (88.1)	319 (87.6)	155 (91.2)
Hypercholesterolemia and on prescription medication				
Yes	100 (10.5)	32 (10.9)	31 (8.5)	20 (11.8)
No**	852 (89.5)	262 (89.1)	333 (91.5)	150 (88.2)
Cardiovascular disease††				
Yes	14 (1.5)	4 (1.4)	4 (1.1)	2 (1.2)
No‡‡	938 (98.5)	290 (98.6)	360 (98.9)	168 (98.8)
Raynaud phenomenon				
Yes	178 (18.7)	34 (11.6)	78 (21.4)	49 (28.8)
No§§	774 (81.3)	260 (88.4)	286 (78.6)	121 (71.2)
Peripheral vascular disease				
Yes	29 (3.0)	5 (1.7)	8 (2.2)	10 (5.9)
No‖‖	923 (97.0)	289 (98.3)	356 (97.8)	160 (94.1)
Thromboembolic disease¶¶				
Yes	5 (0.5)	0	0	4 (2.4)
No	947 (99.5)	294 (100)	364 (100)	166 (97.6)
Renal disease				
Yes	25 (2.6)	7 (2.4)	6 (1.6)	7 (4.1)
No***	927 (97.4)	287 (97.6)	358 (98.4)	163 (95.9)
Diabetes and on prescription medication†††				
Yes	30 (3.1)	9 (3.1)	10 (2.7)	3 (1.8)
No	922 (96.9)	285 (96.9)	354 (97.3)	167 (98.2)
Benign thyroid disease				
Yes	23 (2.4)	6 (2.0)	9 (2.5)	5 (2.9)

Table 3: Continued.

Adverse health outcomes (AHOs)	Total patients (N = 952) N (%)	Treatment regimen EP (4 cycles) (N = 294) N (%)	BEP (3 cycles) (N = 364) N (%)	BEP (4 cycles) (N = 170) N (%)
No‡‡‡	929 (97.6)	288 (98.0)	355 (97.5)	165 (97.1)
Problems with balance/vertigo/dizziness§§§				
Yes	89 (9.3)	26 (8.8)	37 (10.2)	16 (9.4)
No	863 (90.7)	268 (91.2)	327 (89.8)	154 (90.6)
Hypogonadism with testosterone therapy‖‖‖				
Yes	93 (9.9)	25 (8.6)	37 (10.3)	16 (9.5)
No	851 (90.1)	267 (91.4)	323 (89.7)	152 (90.5)
Erectile dysfunction				
Yes	115 (12.1)	28 (9.5)	39 (10.7)	34 (20.0)
No¶¶¶	837 (87.9)	266 (90.5)	325 (89.3)	136 (80.0)
*Psychotropic prescription medication for anxiety and/or depression*****				
Yes	99 (10.4)	34 (11.6)	27 (7.4)	20 (11.8)
No	853 (89.6)	260 (88.4)	337 (92.6)	150 (88.2)

*Adapted with permission from Fung et al. [40] (Table 3). BEP: bleomycin, etoposide, cisplatin; CAD: coronary artery disease; EP: etoposide, cisplatin; MI: myocardial infarction. †P values are derived from the chi-square test comparing the proportions of AHOs reported by TCS in the EPX4 and BEPX3 treatment groups. Except for Raynaud phenomenon ($P < 0.01$) and peripheral neuropathy ($P = 0.02$), the P values for all other AHOs were >0.05; category includes 3 participants for whom this outcome was not stated; among all 952 participants, 270 (28.4%) reported problems hearing words, sounds, or language in crowds, 13 (1.4%) required hearing aid, and 2 (0.2%) had complete deafness (questions derived from the hearing handicap inventory by Ventry and Weinstein) [166]; 109 (11.4%) had "quite a bit" or "very much" difficulty hearing and 75 (7.9%) had "quite a bit" or "very much" reduced hearing (EORTC-CIPN20 and SCIN) ([167, 168]). Category includes 48 participants for whom this outcome was not stated; among all 952 participants, the number of patients reporting "quite a bit" or "very much" to the following questions are as follows: 123 (12.9%) tingling fingers or hands, 167 (17.5%) tingling toes or feet, 121 (12.7%) numbness in fingers or hands, 161 (16.9%) numbness in toes or feet, 34 (3.6%) shooting/burning pain in fingers or hands, 70 (7.4%) shooting/burning pain in toes or feet (EORTC-CIPN20) [167]; 134 (14.1%) pain and tingling in toes or feet, and 86 (9.0%) pain and tingling in hands or fingers (SCIN) [168]. Category includes 16 participants for whom this outcome was not stated; category includes 11 participants for whom this outcome was not stated; ** category includes 3 participants for whom this outcome was not stated; ††includes coronary artery disease, heart failure, and cerebrovascular disease (categories not mutually exclusive, and each category was counted as one AHO). Among all participants, 7 (0.7%) reported coronary artery disease (3 occurrences for coronary artery disease, 5 occurrences of angioplasty or stent, and 5 occurrences of heart attack or myocardial infarction); 1 patient reported heart failure; and 10 (1.0%) reported cerebrovascular disease (6 occurrences of transient ischemic attacks, 4 occurrences of stroke, and 1 occurrence of carotid artery surgery); ‡‡category includes 21 participants for whom this outcome was not stated; §§category includes 12 participants for whom this outcome was not stated; ‖‖category includes 19 participants for whom this outcome was not stated; ¶¶deep vein thrombosis (DVT) and pulmonary embolism (PE) developed simultaneously in 3 participants and was counted as one thromboembolic event for each. The remaining 2 participants reported DVT only. Category includes 19 participants for whom this outcome was not stated; ***category includes 26 participants for whom this outcome was not stated; †††among all participants, 13 (1.4%) and 22 (2.3%) reported use of insulin and oral antiglycemic agents, respectively (categories not mutually exclusive). Category includes 15 participants for whom this outcome was not stated; ‡‡‡category includes 19 participants for whom this outcome was not stated; §§§of the 89 patients, 47 reported persistent dizziness or vertigo and 63 reported symptoms of dizziness when standing up (categories not mutually exclusive). Category includes 40 participants for whom this outcome was not stated; ‖‖‖eight participants who underwent bilateral orchiectomy were excluded from this category; ¶¶¶category include 7 participants for whom this outcome was not stated; ****participants could report more than one psychotropic medication. Psychotropic medications used by the 99 participants include aripirazole (n=2), alprazolam ($n = 5$), amphetamine-dextroamphetamine ($n = 9$), bupropion ($n = 10$), buspirone ($n = 1$), citalopram ($n = 6$), clonazepam ($n = 8$), desvenlafaxine ($n = 1$), diazepam ($n = 1$), duloxetine ($n = 7$), escitalopram ($n = 16$), fluvoxamine ($n = 1$), fluoxetine ($n = 4$), hydroxyzine ($n = 1$), lisdexamfetamine ($n = 4$), lorazepam ($n = 6$), methylphenidate ($n = 5$), nortriptyline ($n = 2$), olanzapine ($n = 2$), paroxetine ($n = 7$), trazodone ($n = 5$), sertraline ($n = 11$), and venlafaxine ($n = 7$).

physical activity was protective ($P < 0.05$). Self-reported health was excellent/very good in approximately 60% of TCS, but this proportion decreased as number of AHOs increased ($P < 0.001$) (Figure 2).

15. Conclusions

Due to their young age at diagnosis, long-term survival, and current use of largely homogeneous therapies, TCS comprise an ideal cohort for adult-onset cancer survivorship research [161]. Moreover, these patients now comprise approximately 4% of all male cancer survivors [162]. Table 4 summarizes major research priorities for TC survivors set forth at an international consensus conference [161]. An overarching recommendation was the development of longitudinal cohort studies to evaluate the life-long burden and latency trends of medical and psychosocial morbidities by category of treatment. TC is relatively unique among cancer types in that it provides for the ready availability of a "comparison group" cured with surgery only without the confounding effects of cytotoxic treatment, with which to compare the late effects of radiotherapy and chemotherapy. Moreover, study of the surgery-only group itself is informative and presents a unique opportunity to study the long-term history of a cancer cured without cytotoxic therapy, including any inherently preprogrammed development of adverse metabolic and other outcomes. This type of proposed cohort investigation, which gathers comprehensive exposure and outcome

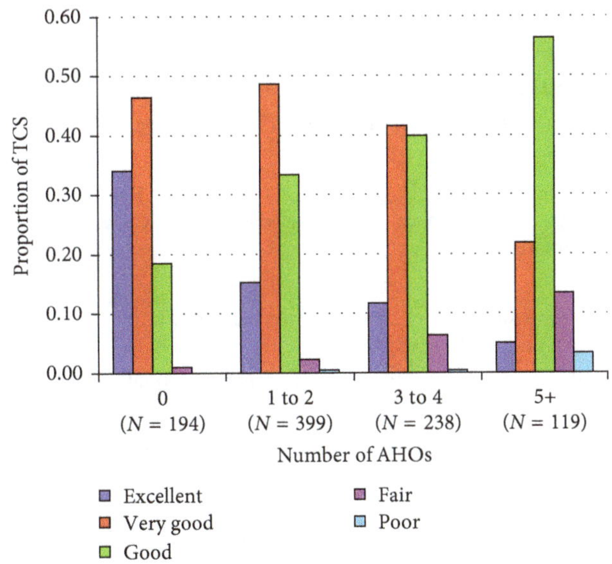

FIGURE 2: Proportion of testicular cancer survivors (TCS) with excellent, very good, good, fair, and poor self-reported health by number of adverse health outcomes (AHOs). *P* value for association of number of AHOs with self-reported health was <0.01 (Mantel 1 df chi-square test of trend). Self-reported health was not indicated by one participant with 1-2 AHOs and one participant with 3-4 AHOs. *Adapted with permission from Fung et al. [40] (Figure 1).

TABLE 4: Summary of major research recommendations: late effects of testicular cancer and its treatment.

(1) *Overarching recommendation: lifelong follow-up of all testicular cancer survivors (TCS)*
(i) Integrate observational and analytic epidemiologic studies with molecular and genetic approaches to ascertain the risk of emerging toxicities and to understand the evolution of known late effects, especially with the aging of TCS.
(ii) Evaluate the influence of race and socioeconomic status (SES) on the late effects of TC and its treatment.
(iii) Characterize long-term tissue deposition of platinum (sites and reactivity), serum levels, and correlation with late effects.
(iv) Evaluate the life-long burden of medical and psychosocial morbidity by treatment.
(v) Utilize research findings to establish evidence-based, risk-adapted, long-term follow-up care.
(2) *Specific recommendations*
(i) Second malignant neoplasms (SMN) and late relapses
(a) Determine the effect of reductions in field size and dose of radiotherapy, along with the use of carboplatin as adjuvant therapy in seminoma patients, on the risk of SMN.
(b) Examine relation between platinum-based chemotherapy and site-specific risk of solid tumors, the associated temporal patterns, and the influence of age at exposure and attained age.
(c) Compare risk of SMN in TCS managed with surgery alone to cancer incidence in the general male population.
(d) Examine delaying influence of platinum-based chemotherapy (and duration and magnitude of effect) on development of contralateral testicular cancer.
(e) Characterize the evolution of cured testicular cancer, in particular, the molecular underpinnings of late recurrences.
(ii) Cardiovascular disease (CVD)
(a) Evaluate the contributions and interactions of subclinical hypogonadism, platinum-based chemotherapy, radiotherapy, lifestyle factors (diet, tobacco use, and physical activity), body mass index, family history of CVD, race, socioeconomic status, abnormal laboratory values, and genetic modifiers.
(b) Develop comprehensive risk prediction models, considering the above variables, to stratify TCS into risk groups in order to customize follow-up strategies and develop evidence-based interventions.
(iii) Neurotoxicity
(a) Evaluate evolution of neurotoxicity across TCS lifespan, role of genetic modifiers, and extent to which symptoms impact on work ability and quality of life.
(iv) Nephrotoxicity
(a) Determine whether the natural decline in renal function associated with aging is accelerated in TCS, any influence of low-level platinum exposure, and the impact of decreased GFR on CVD and all-cause mortality.
(b) Determine the incidence of hypomagnesemia, together with the role of modifying factors and resultant medical consequences, in long-term TCS.

Table 4: Continued.

(v) Hypogonadism and decreased fertility (a) Address the incidence, course, and clinical effects of subclinical hypogonadism. (b) Evaluate effect of all levels of gonadal dysfunction in TCS on CVD, premature aging, fatigue, osteoporosis, mental health, quality of life, and sexuality. (vi) Pulmonary function (a) Examine role of platinum compounds on long-term pulmonary damage in TCS, and interactions with other influences, including bleomycin, tobacco use, and occupational risk factors. (vii) Psychosocial effects (a) Identify prevalence and predictors of depression, cancer-related anxiety, fatigue, infertility-related distress, problems with sexuality and paired relationships, and posttraumatic growth. (b) Examine the impact of different cultural backgrounds on posttreatment quality of life. (c) Evaluate TCS work ability throughout life. (d) Determine whether normal age-related declines in cognitive function are accelerated in TCS.
(3) *Interventions* (i) Conduct targeted intervention trials aimed at promoting smoking cessation, healthy dietary habits, and an increase in physical activity. (ii) Evaluate the role of information and communication technologies in promoting a healthy lifestyle among TCS. (iii) Consider randomized, pharmacologic intervention trials among TCS with biochemical parameters approaching threshold values to avoid accelerated development into treatment-requiring CVD. (iv) Determine optimal schedule of testosterone replacement therapy among TCS with clinical hypogonadism. (v) Consider screening strategies for selected SMN.
(4) *Genetic and molecular considerations* (i) Evaluate genetic risk factors (identified in the general male population) as modifiers for all late effects in TCS, in particular, CVD, SMN, neurotoxicity, nephrotoxicity, hypogonadism, and psychosocial effects. (ii) Investigate the role of genome-wide association studies, epigenetics, mitochrondrial DNA, microRNA, proteomics and related approaches in identifying genetic variants that contribute to the late effects of treatment. (iii) Develop standardized procedures for biospecimen collection to support genetic and molecular studies, as reviewed previously.
(5) *Risk prediction models* (i) Develop comprehensive risk prediction models that incorporate genetic modifiers of late sequelae.

*Adapted with permission from Travis et al. [161] (Table 2).

data, can provide the basis for identifying predictors of AHOs, either singly or jointly, for the eventual development of preventive and interventional measures. An important goal not only for TCS, but for cancer survivors in general, is the identification of genetic variants that predispose to the development of acute and long-term treatment toxicities. This elucidation of etiopathogenetic pathways provides another step towards developing targeted prevention and intervention strategies to optimize risk-based care, minimize chronic morbidities, and improve patients' quality of life.

References

[1] R. L. Siegel, K. D. Miller, and A. Jemal, "Cancer Statistics, 2017," *CA: A Cancer Journal for Clinicians*, vol. 67, no. 1, pp. 7–30, 2017.

[2] L. H. Einhorn and J. Donohue, "Cis-diamminedichloroplatinum, vinblastine, and bleomycin combination chemotherapy in disseminated testicular cancer," *Annals of Internal Medicine*, vol. 87, no. 3, pp. 293–298, 1977.

[3] N. Hanna and L. H. Einhorn, "Testicular cancer: a reflection on 50 years of discovery," *Journal of Clinical Oncology*, vol. 32, no. 28, pp. 3085–3092, 2014.

[4] A. Verdecchia, S. Francisci, H. Brenner et al., "Recent cancer survival in Europe: a 2000-02 period analysis of EUROCARE-4 data," *Lancet Oncology*, vol. 8, no. 9, pp. 784–796, 2007.

[5] L. H. Einhorn, "Testicular cancer as a model for a curable neoplasm: the Richard and Hinda Rosenthal Foundation Award Lecture," *Cancer Research*, vol. 41, no. 1, pp. 3275–3280, 1981.

[6] L. B. Travis, A. K. Ng, J. M. Allan et al., "Second malignant neoplasms and cardiovascular disease following radiotherapy," *Journal of the National Cancer Institute*, vol. 104, no. 5, pp. 357–370, 2012.

[7] H. S. Haugnes, G. J. Bosl, H. Boer et al., "Long-term and late effects of germ cell testicular cancer treatment and implications for follow-up," *Journal of Clinical Oncology*, vol. 30, no. 30, pp. 3752–3763, 2012.

[8] N. M. Aziz, "Cancer survivorship research: state of knowledge, challenges and opportunities," *Acta Oncologica*, vol. 46, no. 4, pp. 417–432, 2007.

[9] D. R. Feldman, W. L. Schaffer, and R. M. Steingart, "Late cardiovascular toxicity following chemotherapy for germ cell tumors," *Journal of the National Comprehensive Cancer Network*, vol. 10, no. 4, pp. 537–544, 2012.

[10] J. F. Christensen, M. Bandak, A. Campbell, L. W. Jones, and P. Højman, "Treatment-related cardiovascular late effects and exercise training countermeasures in testicular germ cell cancer survivorship," *Acta Oncologica*, vol. 54, no. 5, pp. 592–599, 2015.

[11] L. Y. Dirix, M. Libura, J. Libura, P. B. Vermeulen, E. A De Bruijn, and A. T. Van Oosterom, "In vitro toxicity studies with mitomycins and bleomycin on endothelial cells," *Anticancer Drugs*, vol. 8, no. 9, pp. 859–868, 1997.

[12] Y. Shi, S. Inoue, R. Shinozaki, K. Fukue, and T. Kougo, "Release of cytokines from human umbilical vein endothelial cells treated with platinum compounds in vitro," *Japanese Journal of Cancer Research*, vol. 89, no. 7, pp. 757–767, 1998.

[13] K. P. Dieckmann, W. J. Struss, and U. Budde, "Evidence for acute vascular toxicity of cisplatin-based chemotherapy in patients with germ cell tumour," *Anticancer Research*, vol. 31, no. 12, pp. 4501–4505, 2011.

[14] J. Nuver, A. J. Smit, D. T. Sleijfer et al., "Microalbuminuria, decreased fibrinolysis, and inflammation as early signs of atherosclerosis in long-term survivors of disseminated testicular cancer," *European Journal of Cancer*, vol. 40, no. 5, pp. 701–706, 2004.

[15] J. Nuver, A. J. Smit, J. van der Meer et al., "Acute chemotherapy-induced cardiovascular changes in patients with testicular cancer," *Journal of Clinical Oncology*, vol. 23, no. 36, pp. 9130–9137, 2005.

[16] M. T. Meinardi, J. A. Gietema, W. T. van der Graaf et al., "Cardiovascular morbidity in long-term survivors of metastatic testicular cancer," *Journal of Clinical Oncology*, vol. 18, no. 8, pp. 1725–1732, 2000.

[17] H. C. Gerstein, J. F. Mann, Q. Yi et al., "Albuminuria and risk of cardiovascular events, death, and heart failure in diabetic and nondiabetic individuals," *Journal of the American Medical Association*, vol. 286, no. 4, pp. 421–426, 2001.

[18] D. H. O'Leary, J. F. Polak, R. A. Kronmal et al., "Carotid-artery intima and media thickness as a risk factor for myocardial infarction and stroke in older adults. Cardiovascular Health Study Collaborative Research Group," *New England Journal of Medicine*, vol. 340, no. 1, pp. 14–22, 1999.

[19] L. D. van Schinkel, P. M. Willemse, R. W. van der Meer et al., "Chemotherapy for testicular cancer induces acute alterations in diastolic heart function," *British Journal of Cancer*, vol. 109, no. 4, pp. 891–896, 2013.

[20] D. J. Brenner and E. J. Hall, "Computed tomography–an increasing source of radiation exposure," *New England Journal of Medicine*, vol. 357, no. 22, pp. 2277–2284, 2007.

[21] R. L. Schilsky and T. Anderson, "Hypomagnesemia and renal magnesium wasting in patients receiving cisplatin," *Annals of Internal Medicine*, vol. 90, no. 6, pp. 929–931, 1979.

[22] P. D. Turlapaty and B. M. Altura, "Magnesium deficiency produces spasms of coronary arteries: relationship to etiology of sudden death ischemic heart disease," *Science*, vol. 208, no. 4440, pp. 198–200, 1980.

[23] N. J. Vogelzang, J. L. Torkelson, and B. J. Kennedy, "Hypomagnesemia, renal dysfunction, and Raynaud's phenomenon in patients treated with cisplatin, vinblastine, and bleomycin," *Cancer*, vol. 56, no. 12, pp. 2765–2770, 1985.

[24] G. I. Togna, A. R. Togna, M. Franconi, and L. Caprino, "Cisplatin triggers platelet activation," *Thrombosis Research*, vol. 99, no. 5, pp. 503–509, 2000.

[25] D. Lechner, M. Kollars, A. Gleiss, P. A. Kyrle, and A. Weltermann, "Chemotherapy-induced thrombin generation via procoagulant endothelial microparticles is independent of tissue factor activity," *Journal of Thrombosis and Haemostasis*, vol. 5, no. 12, pp. 2445–2452, 2007.

[26] D. Bissett, L. Kunkeler, L. Zwanenburg et al., "Long-term sequelae of treatment for testicular germ cell tumours," *British Journal of Cancer*, vol. 62, no. 4, pp. 655–659, 1990.

[27] C. Bokemeyer and H. J. Schmoll, "Secondary neoplasms following treatment of malignant germ cell tumors," *Journal of Clinical Oncology*, vol. 11, no. 9, pp. 1703–1709, 1993.

[28] M. Brydoy, J. Oldenburg, O. Klepp et al., "Observational study of prevalence of long-term Raynaud-like phenomena and neurological side effects in testicular cancer survivors," *Journal of the National Cancer Institute*, vol. 101, no. 24, pp. 1682–1695, 2009.

[29] J. L. Glendenning, Y. Barbachano, A. R. Norman et al., "Long-term neurologic and peripheral vascular toxicity after chemotherapy treatment of testicular cancer," *Cancer*, vol. 116, no. 10, pp. 2322–2331, 2010.

[30] D. Strumberg, S. Brugge, M. W. Korn et al., "Evaluation of long-term toxicity in patients after cisplatin-based chemotherapy for non-seminomatous testicular cancer," *Annals of Oncology*, vol. 13, no. 2, pp. 229–236, 2002.

[31] R. de Wit, G. Stoter, S. B. Kaye et al., "Importance of bleomycin in combination chemotherapy for good-prognosis testicular nonseminoma: a randomized study of the European Organization for Research and Treatment of Cancer Genitourinary Tract Cancer Cooperative Group," *Journal of Clinical Oncology*, vol. 15, no. 5, pp. 1837–1843, 1997.

[32] C. Bokemeyer, C. C. Berger, M. A. Kuczyk, and H. J. Schmoll, "Evaluation of long-term toxicity after chemotherapy for testicular cancer," *Journal of Clinical Oncology*, vol. 14, no. 11, pp. 2923–2932, 1996.

[33] H. S. Haugnes, N. Aass, S. D. Fossa et al., "Components of the metabolic syndrome in long-term survivors of testicular cancer," *Annals of Oncology*, vol. 18, no. 2, pp. 241–248, 2007.

[34] H. S. Haugnes, T. Wethal, N. Aass et al., "Cardiovascular risk factors and morbidity in long-term survivors of testicular cancer: a 20-year follow-up study," *Journal of Clinical Oncology*, vol. 28, no. 30, pp. 4649–4657, 2010.

[35] R. A. Huddart, A. Norman, M. Shahidi et al., "Cardiovascular disease as a long-term complication of treatment for testicular cancer," *Journal of Clinical Oncology*, vol. 21, no. 8, pp. 1513–1523, 2003.

[36] J. Nuver, A. J. Smit, B. H. Wolffenbuttel et al., "The metabolic syndrome and disturbances in hormone levels in long-term survivors of disseminated testicular cancer," *Journal of Clinical Oncology*, vol. 23, no. 16, pp. 3718–3725, 2005.

[37] H. Sagstuen, N. Aass, S. D. Fossa et al., "Blood pressure and body mass index in long-term survivors of testicular cancer," *Journal of Clinical Oncology*, vol. 23, no. 22, pp. 4980–4990, 2005.

[38] P. M. Willemse, J. Burggraaf, N. A. Hamdy et al., "Prevalence of the metabolic syndrome and cardiovascular disease risk in chemotherapy-treated testicular germ cell tumour survivors," *British Journal of Cancer*, vol. 109, no. 1, pp. 60–67, 2013.

[39] E. C. de Haas, R. Altena, H. M. Boezen et al., "Early development of the metabolic syndrome after chemotherapy for testicular cancer," *Annals of Oncology*, vol. 24, no. 3, pp. 749–755, 2013.

[40] C. Fung, H. D. Sesso, A. M. Williams et al., "Multi-institutional assessment of adverse health outcomes among north American testicular cancer survivors after modern cisplatin-based chemotherapy," *Journal of Clinical Oncology*, vol. 35, no. 11, pp. 1211–1222, 2017.

[41] C. Bogefors, S. Isaksson, J. Bobjer et al., "Hypogonadism in testicular cancer patients is associated with risk factors of cardiovascular disease and the metabolic syndrome," *Andrology*, vol. 5, no. 4, pp. 711–717, 2017.

[42] A. M. Traish, F. Saad, R. J. Feeley, and A. Guay, "The dark side of testosterone deficiency: III. Cardiovascular disease," *Journal of Andrology*, vol. 30, no. 5, pp. 477–494, 2009.

[43] A. M. Traish, F. Saad, and A. Guay, "The dark side of testosterone deficiency: II. Type 2 diabetes and insulin resistance," *Journal of Andrology*, vol. 30, no. 5, pp. 23–32, 2009.

[44] A. M. Traish, A. Guay, R. Feeley, and F. Saad, "The dark side of testosterone deficiency: I. Metabolic syndrome and erectile dysfunction," *Journal of Andrology*, vol. 30, no. 5, pp. 10–22, 2009.

[45] L. W. Jones, M. J. Haykowsky, J. J. Swartz, P. S. Douglas, and J. R. Mackey, "Early breast cancer therapy and cardiovascular injury," *Journal of the American College of Cardiology*, vol. 50, no. 15, pp. 1435–1441, 2007.

[46] A. W. van den Belt-Dusebout, R. de Wit, J. A. Gietema et al., "Treatment-specific risks of second malignancies and cardiovascular disease in 5-year survivors of testicular cancer," *Journal of Clinical Oncology*, vol. 25, no. 28, pp. 4370–4378, 2007.

[47] A. W. van den Belt-Dusebout, J. Nuver, R. de Wit et al., "Long-term risk of cardiovascular disease in 5-year survivors of testicular cancer," *Journal of Clinical Oncology*, vol. 24, no. 3, pp. 467–475, 2006.

[48] S. D. Fossa, E. Gilbert, G. M. Dores et al., "Noncancer causes of death in survivors of testicular cancer," *Journal of the National Cancer Institute*, vol. 99, no. 7, pp. 533–544, 2007.

[49] S. R. Alanee, D. R. Feldman, P. Russo et al., "Long-term mortality in patients with germ cell tumors: effect of primary cancer site on cause of death," *Urologic Oncology*, vol. 32, no. 1, pp. 26.e9–26.e15, 2014.

[50] C. Fung, S. D. Fossa, M. T. Milano et al., "Cardiovascular disease mortality after chemotherapy or surgery for testicular nonseminoma: a population-based study," *Journal of Clinical Oncology*, vol. 33, no. 28, pp. 3105–3115, 2015.

[51] A. S. Go, D. Mozaffarian, V. L. Roger et al., "Heart disease and stroke statistics–2014 update: a report from the American Heart Association," *Circulation*, vol. 129, no. 3, pp. e28–e292, 2014.

[52] D. C. Goff Jr., D. M. Lloyd-Jones, G. Bennett et al., "2013 ACC/AHA guideline on the assessment of cardiovascular risk: a report of the American College of Cardiology/ American Heart Association Task Force on Practice Guidelines," *Circulation*, vol. 129, no. 2, pp. S49–S73, 2013.

[53] M. E. Wood, V. Vogel, A. Ng, L. Foxhall, P. Goodwin, and L. B. Travis, "Second malignant neoplasms: assessment and strategies for risk reduction," *Journal of Clinical Oncology*, vol. 30, no. 30, pp. 3734–3745, 2012.

[54] L. B. Travis, C. S. Rabkin, L. M. Brown et al., "Cancer survivorship-genetic susceptibility and second primary cancers: research strategies and recommendations," *Journal of the National Cancer Institute*, vol. 98, no. 1, pp. 15–25, 2006.

[55] L. B. Travis, S. D. Fossa, S. J. Schonfeld et al., "Second cancers among 40,576 testicular cancer patients: focus on long-term survivors," *Journal of the National Cancer Institute*, vol. 97, no. 18, pp. 1354–1365, 2005.

[56] L. B. Travis, M. Andersson, M. Gospodarowicz et al., "Treatment-associated leukemia following testicular cancer," *Journal of the National Cancer Institute*, vol. 92, no. 14, pp. 1165–1171, 2000.

[57] L. B. Travis, R. E. Curtis, H. Storm et al., "Risk of second malignant neoplasms among long-term survivors of testicular cancer," *Journal of the National Cancer Institute*, vol. 89, no. 19, pp. 1429–1439, 1997.

[58] M. Hauptmann, S. D. Fossa, M. Stovall et al., "Increased stomach cancer risk following radiotherapy for testicular cancer," *British Journal of Cancer*, vol. 112, no. 1, pp. 44–51, 2015.

[59] M. Hauptmann, T. Borge Johannesen, E. S. Gilbert et al., "Increased pancreatic cancer risk following radiotherapy for testicular cancer," *British Journal of Cancer*, vol. 115, no. 7, pp. 901–908, 2016.

[60] A. W. van den Belt-Dusebout, B. M. Aleman, G. Besseling et al., "Roles of radiation dose and chemotherapy in the etiology of stomach cancer as a second malignancy," *International Journal of Radiation Oncology, Biology, Physics*, vol. 75, no. 5, pp. 1420–1429, 2009.

[61] J. M. Bachaud, F. Berthier, M. Soulie et al., "Second non-germ cell malignancies in patients treated for stage I-II testicular seminoma," *Radiotherapy and Oncology*, vol. 50, no. 2, pp. 191–197, 1999.

[62] N. H. Hanna and L. H. Einhorn, "Testicular cancer–discoveries and updates," *New England Journal of Medicine*, vol. 371, no. 21, pp. 2005–2016, 2014.

[63] D. F. Bajorin, M. F. Sarosdy, D. G. Pfister et al., "Randomized trial of etoposide and cisplatin versus etoposide and carboplatin in patients with good-risk germ cell tumors: a multiinstitutional study," *Journal of Clinical Oncology*, vol. 11, no. 4, pp. 598–606, 1993.

[64] C. Kollmannsberger, J. Beyer, J. P. Droz et al., "Secondary leukemia following high cumulative doses of etoposide in patients treated for advanced germ cell tumors," *Journal of Clinical Oncology*, vol. 16, no. 10, pp. 3386–3391, 1998.

[65] C. Kollmannsberger, J. T. Hartmann, L. Kanz et al., "Therapy-related malignancies following treatment of germ cell cancer," *International Journal of Cancer*, vol. 83, no. 6, pp. 860–863, 1999.

[66] E. H. Wanderas, S. D. Fossa, and S. Tretli, "Risk of subsequent non-germ cell cancer after treatment of germ cell cancer in 2006 Norwegian male patients," *European Journal of Cancer*, vol. 33, no. 2, pp. 253–262, 1997.

[67] C. Fung, S. D. Fossa, M. T. Milano, J. Oldenburg, and L. B. Travis, "Solid tumors after chemotherapy or surgery for testicular nonseminoma: a population-based study," *Journal of Clinical Oncology*, vol. 31, no. 30, pp. 3807–3814, 2013.

[68] S. D. Fossa, J. Chen, S. J. Schonfeld et al., "Risk of contralateral testicular cancer: a population-based study of 29,515 U.S. men," *Journal of the National Cancer Institute*, vol. 97, no. 14, pp. 1056–1066, 2005.

[69] P. B. Rossen, A. F. Pedersen, R. Zachariae, and H. von der Maase, "Health-related quality of life in long-term survivors of testicular cancer," *Journal of Clinical Oncology*, vol. 27, no. 35, pp. 5993–5999, 2009.

[70] S. D. Williams, R. Birch, L. H. Einhorn, L. Irwin, F. A. Greco, and P. J. Loehrer, "Treatment of disseminated germ-cell tumors with cisplatin, bleomycin, and either vinblastine or etoposide," *New England Journal of Medicine*, vol. 316, no. 23, pp. 1435–1440, 1987.

[71] M. Sprauten, T. H. Darrah, D. R. Peterson et al., "Impact of long-term serum platinum concentrations on neuro- and ototoxicity in Cisplatin-treated survivors of testicular cancer," *Journal of Clinical Oncology*, vol. 30, no. 3, pp. 300–307, 2012.

[72] J. Oldenburg, S. M. Kraggerud, M. Brydoy, M. Cvancarova, R. A. Lothe, and S. D. Fossa, "Association between long-term neuro-toxicities in testicular cancer survivors and polymorphisms in glutathione-s-transferase-P1 and -M1, a retrospective cross sectional study," *Journal of Translational Medicine*, vol. 5, no. 1, p. 70, 2007.

[73] M. E. Dolan, O. El Charif, H. E. Wheeler et al., "Clinical and genome-wide analysis of cisplatin-induced peripheral neuropathy in survivors of adult-onset cancer," *Clinical Cancer Research*, vol. 23, no. 19, pp. 5757–5768, 2017.

[74] A. Sawant, A. Kothandapani, A. Zhitkovich, R. W. Sobol, and S. M. Patrick, "Role of mismatch repair proteins in the processing of cisplatin interstrand cross-links," *DNA Repair*, vol. 35, pp. 126–136, 2015.

[75] J. C. Morales, P. Richard, A. Rommel et al., "Kub5-Hera, the human Rtt103 homolog, plays dual functional roles in transcription termination and DNA repair," *Nucleic Acids Research*, vol. 42, no. 8, pp. 4996–5006, 2014.

[76] D. L. Hershman, C. Lacchetti, R. H. Dworkin et al., "Prevention and management of chemotherapy-induced peripheral neuropathy in survivors of adult cancers: American Society of Clinical Oncology clinical practice guideline," *Journal of Clinical Oncology*, vol. 32, no. 18, pp. 1941–1967, 2014.

[77] C. A. Bauer and T. J. Brozoski, "Cochlear structure and function after round window application of ototoxins," *Hearing Research*, vol. 201, no. 1-2, pp. 121–131, 2005.

[78] C. Bokemeyer, C. C. Berger, J. T. Hartmann et al., "Analysis of risk factors for cisplatin-induced ototoxicity in patients with testicular cancer," *British Journal of Cancer*, vol. 77, no. 8, pp. 1355–1362, 1998.

[79] R. D. Frisina, H. E. Wheeler, S. D. Fossa et al., "Comprehensive audiometric analysis of hearing impairment and tinnitus after cisplatin-based chemotherapy in survivors of adult-onset cancer," *Journal of Clinical Oncology*, vol. 34, no. 23, pp. 2712–2720, 2016.

[80] L. P. Rybak, "Mechanisms of cisplatin ototoxicity and progress in otoprotection," *Current Opinion in Otolaryngology & Head and Neck Surgery*, vol. 15, no. 5, pp. 364–369, 2007.

[81] L. Riedemann, C. Lanvers, D. Deuster et al., "Megalin genetic polymorphisms and individual sensitivity to the ototoxic effect of cisplatin," *Pharmacogenomics Journal*, vol. 8, no. 1, pp. 23–28, 2008.

[82] J. Oldenburg, S. M. Kraggerud, M. Cvancarova, R. A. Lothe, and S. D. Fossa, "Cisplatin-induced long-term hearing impairment is associated with specific glutathione s-transferase genotypes in testicular cancer survivors," *Journal of Clinical Oncology*, vol. 25, no. 6, pp. 708–714, 2007.

[83] C. J. Ross, H. Katzov-Eckert, M. P. Dube et al., "Genetic variants in TPMT and COMT are associated with hearing loss in children receiving cisplatin chemotherapy," *Nature Genetics*, vol. 41, no. 12, pp. 1345–1349, 2009.

[84] H. E. Wheeler, E. R. Gamazon, R. D. Frisina et al., "Variants in WFS1 and other Mendelian deafness genes are associated with cisplatin-associated ototoxicity," *Clinical Cancer Research*, vol. 23, no. 13, pp. 3325–3333, 2016.

[85] H. E. Wheeler, R. D. Frisina, E. R. Gamazon et al., "Genome-wide association study (GWAS) of cisplatin-related hearing loss in testicular cancer survivors (TCS) to reveal associated variant in wolfram syndrome 1 (WFS1) gene," *Journal of Clinical Oncology*, vol. 34, no. 15, p. 10015, 2016.

[86] K. Cryns, T. A. Sivakumaran, J. M. Van den Ouweland et al., "Mutational spectrum of the WFS1 gene in Wolfram syndrome, nonsyndromic hearing impairment, diabetes mellitus, and psychiatric disease," *Human Mutation*, vol. 22, no. 4, pp. 275–287, 2003.

[87] H. Inoue, Y. Tanizawa, J. Wasson et al., "A gene encoding a transmembrane protein is mutated in patients with diabetes mellitus and optic atrophy (wolfram syndrome)," *Nature Genetics*, vol. 20, no. 2, pp. 143–148, 1998.

[88] S. D. Fossa, R. de Wit, J. T. Roberts et al., "Quality of life in good prognosis patients with metastatic germ cell cancer: a prospective study of the European Organization for Research and Treatment of Cancer Genitourinary Group/ Medical Research Council Testicular Cancer Study Group (30941/TE20)," *Journal of Clinical Oncology*, vol. 21, no. 6, pp. 1107–1118, 2003.

[89] J. M. O'Sullivan, R. A. Huddart, A. R. Norman, J. Nicholls, D. P. Dearnaley, and A. Horwich, "Predicting the risk of bleomycin lung toxicity in patients with germ-cell tumours," *Annals of Oncology*, vol. 14, no. 1, pp. 91–96, 2003.

[90] A. B. Simpson, J. Paul, J. Graham, and S. B. Kaye, "Fatal bleomycin pulmonary toxicity in the west of Scotland 1991-95: a review of patients with germ cell tumours," *British Journal of Cancer*, vol. 78, no. 8, pp. 1061–1066, 1998.

[91] S. Sleijfer, "Bleomycin-induced pneumonitis," *Chest*, vol. 120, no. 2, pp. 617–624, 2001.

[92] H. S. Haugnes, N. Aass, S. D. Fossa et al., "Pulmonary function in long-term survivors of testicular cancer," *Journal of Clinical Oncology*, vol. 27, no. 17, pp. 2779–2786, 2009.

[93] H. S. Haugnes, J. Oldenburg, and R. M. Bremnes, "Pulmonary and cardiovascular toxicity in long-term testicular cancer survivors," *Urologic Oncology*, vol. 33, no. 9, pp. 399–406, 2015.

[94] S. M. Donat and D. A. Levy, "Bleomycin associated pulmonary toxicity: is perioperative oxygen restriction necessary?," *Journal of Urology*, vol. 160, no. 4, pp. 1347–1352, 1998.

[95] R. de Wit, S. Sleijfer, S. B. Kaye et al., "Bleomycin and scuba diving: where is the harm?," *Lancet Oncology*, vol. 8, no. 11, pp. 954-955, 2007.

[96] A. A. Ferrando, A. M. Pendas, E. Llano, G. Velasco, R. Lidereau, and C. López-Otín, "Gene characterization, promoter analysis, and chromosomal localization of human bleomycin hydrolase," *Journal of Biological Chemistry*, vol. 272, no. 52, pp. 33298–33304, 1997.

[97] J. Nuver, M. F. Lutke Holzik, M. van Zweeden et al., "Genetic variation in the bleomycin hydrolase gene and bleomycin-induced pulmonary toxicity in germ cell cancer patients," *Pharmacogenetics and Genomics*, vol. 15, no. 6, pp. 399–405, 2005.

[98] A. E. Vickers, K. Rose, R. Fisher, M. Saulnier, P. Sahota, and P. Bentley, "Kidney slices of human and rat to characterize cisplatin-induced injury on cellular pathways and morphology," *Toxicologic Pathology*, vol. 32, no. 5, pp. 577–590, 2004.

[99] H. Tanaka, E. Ishikawa, S. Teshima, and E. Shimizu, "Histopathological study of human cisplatin nephropathy," *Toxicologic Pathology*, vol. 14, no. 2, pp. 247–257, 1986.

[100] S. D. Fossa, N. Aass, M. Winderen, O. P. Börmer, and D. R. Olsen, "Long-term renal function after treatment for malignant germ-cell tumours," *Annals of Oncology*, vol. 13, no. 2, pp. 222–228, 2002.

[101] S. W. Hansen, S. Groth, G. Daugaard, N. Rossing, and M. Rørth, "Long-term effects on renal function and blood pressure of treatment with cisplatin, vinblastine, and bleomycin in patients with germ cell cancer," *Journal of Clinical Oncology*, vol. 6, no. 11, pp. 1728–1731, 1988.

[102] J. M. Peacock, T. Ohira, W. Post, N. Sotoodehnia, W. Rosamond, and A. R. Folsom, "Serum magnesium and risk of sudden cardiac death in the Atherosclerosis Risk in Communities (ARIC) Study," *American Heart Journal*, vol. 160, no. 3, pp. 464–470, 2010.

[103] B. C. Astor, S. I. Hallan, E. R. Miller III, E. Yeung, and J. Coresh, "Glomerular filtration rate, albuminuria, and risk of cardiovascular and all-cause mortality in the US population," *American Journal of Epidemiology*, vol. 167, no. 10, pp. 1226–1234, 2008.

[104] J. T. Hartmann, C. Kollmannsberger, L. Kanz, and C. Bokemeyer, "Platinum organ toxicity and possible prevention in patients with testicular cancer," *International Journal of Cancer*, vol. 83, no. 6, pp. 866–869, 1999.

[105] M. Sprauten, M. Brydoy, H. S. Haugnes et al., "Longitudinal serum testosterone, luteinizing hormone, and follicle-stimulating hormone levels in a population-based sample of long-term testicular cancer survivors," *Journal of Clinical Oncology*, vol. 32, no. 6, pp. 571–578, 2014.

[106] J. Eberhard, O. Stahl, M. Cwikiel et al., "Risk factors for post-treatment hypogonadism in testicular cancer patients," *European Journal of Endocrinology*, vol. 158, no. 4, pp. 561–570, 2008.

[107] C. Nord, T. Bjoro, D. Ellingsen et al., "Gonadal hormones in long-term survivors 10 years after treatment for unilateral testicular cancer," *European Urology*, vol. 44, no. 3, pp. 322–328, 2003.

[108] M. Brydoy, S. D. Fossa, O. Dahl, and T. Bjøro, "Gonadal dysfunction and fertility problems in cancer survivors," *Acta Oncologica*, vol. 46, no. 4, pp. 480–489, 2007.

[109] R. A. Huddart, A. Norman, C. Moynihan et al., "Fertility, gonadal and sexual function in survivors of testicular cancer," *British Journal of Cancer*, vol. 93, no. 2, pp. 200–207, 2005.

[110] M. Bandak, N. Jorgensen, A. Juul et al., "Testosterone deficiency in testicular cancer survivors - a systematic review and meta-analysis," *Andrology*, vol. 4, no. 3, pp. 382–388, 2016.

[111] J. Eberhard, O. Stahl, G. Cohn-Cedermark et al., "Sexual function in men treated for testicular cancer," *Journal of Sexual Medicine*, vol. 6, no. 7, pp. 1979–1989, 2009.

[112] M. Brydoy, S. D. Fossa, O. Klepp et al., "Paternity following treatment for testicular cancer," *Journal of the National Cancer Institute*, vol. 97, no. 21, pp. 1580–1588, 2005.

[113] A. A. Dahl, R. Bremnes, O. Dahl, O. Klepp, E. Wist, and S. D. Fosså, "Is the sexual function compromised in long-term testicular cancer survivors?," *European Urology*, vol. 52, no. 5, pp. 1438–1447, 2007.

[114] J. Hintikka, L. Niskanen, H. Koivumaa-Honkanen et al., "Hypogonadism, decreased sexual desire, and long-term depression in middle-aged men," *Journal of Sexual Medicine*, vol. 6, no. 7, pp. 2049–2057, 2009.

[115] S. Bhasin, G. R. Cunningham, F. J. Hayes et al., "Testosterone therapy in men with androgen deficiency syndromes: an Endocrine Society clinical practice guideline," *Journal of Clinical Endocrinology & Metabolism*, vol. 95, no. 6, pp. 2536–2559, 2010.

[116] M. Ondrusova, D. Ondrus, L. Dusek, and B. Spanikova, "Damage of hormonal function and bone metabolism in long-term survivors of testicular cancer," *Neoplasma*, vol. 56, no. 6, pp. 473–479, 2009.

[117] V. Rochira, A. Balestrieri, B. Madeo, L. Zirilli, A. R. Granata, and C. Carani, "Osteoporosis and male age-related hypogonadism: role of sex steroids on bone (patho)physiology," *European Journal of Endocrinology*, vol. 154, no. 2, pp. 175–185, 2006.

[118] M. Abu Zaid, A. G. Menendez, O. E. Charif et al., "Adverse health outcomes in relationship to hypogonadism (HG) after platinum-based chemotherapy: a multicenter study of North American testicular cancer survivors (TCS)," *Journal of Clinical Oncology*, vol. 35, no. 18, 2017.

[119] S. D. Fossa, T. Abyholm, and A. Aakvaag, "Spermatogenesis and hormonal status after orchiectomy for cancer and before supplementary treatment," *European Urology*, vol. 10, no. 3, pp. 173–177, 1984.

[120] K. P. Dieckmann, J. Linke, U. Pichlmeier, M. Kulejewski, and V. Loy, "Spermatogenesis in the contralateral testis of patients with testicular germ cell cancer: histological evaluation of testicular biopsies and a comparison with healthy males," *BJU International*, vol. 99, no. 5, pp. 1079–1085, 2007.

[121] E. Huyghe, T. Matsuda, M. Daudin et al., "Fertility after testicular cancer treatments: results of a large multicenter study," *Cancer*, vol. 100, no. 4, pp. 732–737, 2004.

[122] J. R. Spermon, L. A. Kiemeney, E. J. Meuleman, L. Ramos, A. M. M. Wetzels, and J. A. Witjes, "Fertility in men with testicular germ cell tumors," *Fertility and Sterility*, vol. 79, pp. 1543–1549, 2003.

[123] M. Brydoy, S. D. Fossa, O. Klepp et al., "Paternity and testicular function among testicular cancer survivors treated with two to four cycles of cisplatin-based chemotherapy," *European Urology*, vol. 58, no. 1, pp. 134–140, 2010.

[124] W. Gordon Jr., K. Siegmund, T. H. Stanisic et al., "A study of reproductive function in patients with seminoma treated with radiotherapy and orchidectomy: (SWOG-8711). Southwest Oncology Group," *International Journal of Radiation Oncology Biology Physics*, vol. 38, no. 1, pp. 83–94, 1997.

[125] M. Brydoy, S. D. Fossa, O. Klepp et al., "Sperm counts and endocrinological markers of spermatogenesis in long-term survivors of testicular cancer," *British Journal of Cancer*, vol. 107, no. 11, pp. 1833–1839, 2012.

[126] K. A. Ostrowski and T. J. Walsh, "Infertility with testicular cancer," *Urologic Clinics of North America*, vol. 42, no. 3, pp. 409–420, 2015.

[127] L. Gandini, P. Sgro, F. Lombardo et al., "Effect of chemo- or radiotherapy on sperm parameters of testicular cancer patients," *Human Reproduction*, vol. 21, no. 11, pp. 2882–2889, 2006.

[128] H. Lampe, A. Horwich, A. Norman et al., "Fertility after chemotherapy for testicular germ cell cancers," *Journal of Clinical Oncology*, vol. 15, no. 1, pp. 239–245, 1997.

[129] S. D. Beck, A. L. Bey, R. Bihrle et al., "Ejaculatory status and fertility rates after primary retroperitoneal lymph node dissection," *Journal of Urology*, vol. 184, no. 5, pp. 2078–2080, 2010.

[130] V. S. Subramanian, C. T. Nguyen, A. J. Stephenson et al., "Complications of open primary and post-chemotherapy retroperitoneal lymph node dissection for testicular cancer," *Urologic Oncology*, vol. 28, no. 5, pp. 504–509, 2010.

[131] A. Heidenreich, P. Albers, M. Hartmann et al., "Complications of primary nerve sparing retroperitoneal lymph node dissection for clinical stage I nonseminomatous germ cell tumors of the testis: experience of the German Testicular Cancer Study Group," *Journal of Urology*, vol. 169, no. 5, pp. 1710–1714, 2003.

[132] K. D. Jacobsen, S. Ous, H. Waehre et al., "Ejaculation in testicular cancer patients after post-chemotherapy retroperitoneal lymph node dissection," *British Journal of Cancer*, vol. 80, no. 1-2, pp. 249–255, 1999.

[133] J. A. Pettus, B. S. Carver, T. Masterson, J. Stasi, and J. Sheinfeld, "Preservation of ejaculation in patients

undergoing nerve-sparing postchemotherapy retroperitoneal lymph node dissection for metastatic testicular cancer," *Urology*, vol. 73, no. 2, pp. 328–331, 2009.

[134] C. L. Coogan, M. J. Hejase, G. R. Wahle et al., "Nerve sparing post-chemotherapy retroperitoneal lymph node dissection for advanced testicular cancer," *Journal of Urology*, vol. 156, no. 5, pp. 1656–1658, 1996.

[135] A. Heidenreich, D. Pfister, R. Witthuhn, D. Thüer, and P. Albers, "Postchemotherapy retroperitoneal lymph node dissection in advanced testicular cancer: radical or modified template resection," *European Urology*, vol. 55, no. 1, pp. 217–224, 2009.

[136] A. W. Loren, P. B. Mangu, L. N. Beck et al., "Fertility preservation for patients with cancer: American Society of Clinical Oncology clinical practice guideline update," *Journal of Clinical Oncology*, vol. 31, no. 19, pp. 2500–2510, 2013.

[137] E. W. Winquist, G. S. Bauman, and J. Balogh, "Nontraumatic osteonecrosis after chemotherapy for testicular cancer: a systematic review," *American Journal of Clinical Oncology*, vol. 24, no. 6, pp. 603–606, 2001.

[138] A. M. Cook, A. S. Dzik-Jurasz, A. R. Padhani, A. Norman, and R. A. Huddart, "The prevalence of avascular necrosis in patients treated with chemotherapy for testicular tumours," *British Journal of Cancer*, vol. 85, no. 11, pp. 1624–1626, 2001.

[139] R. Kaila and R. L. Wolman, "Groin pain in athletes: a consequence of femoral head avascular necrosis after testicular cancer chemotherapy," *Clinical Journal of Sport Medicine*, vol. 16, no. 2, pp. 175-176, 2006.

[140] F. van den Berkmortel, R. de Wit, J. de Rooy, and P. DeMulder, "Osteonecrosis in patients with testicular tumours treated with chemotherapy," *Netherlands Journal of Medicine*, vol. 62, no. 1, pp. 23–27, 2004.

[141] P. G. Harper, C. Trask, and R. L. Souhami, "Avascular necrosis of bone caused by combination chemotherapy without corticosteroids," *British Medical Journal*, vol. 288, no. 6413, pp. 267-268, 1984.

[142] M. B. de Ruiter, L. Reneman, W. Boogerd et al., "Cerebral hyporesponsiveness and cognitive impairment 10 years after chemotherapy for breast cancer," *Human Brain Mapping*, vol. 32, no. 8, pp. 1206–1219, 2011.

[143] S. R. Kesler, F. C. Bennett, M. L. Mahaffey, and D. Spiegel, "Regional brain activation during verbal declarative memory in metastatic breast cancer," *Clinical Cancer Research*, vol. 15, no. 21, pp. 6665–6673, 2009.

[144] D. H. Silverman, C. J. Dy, S. A. Castellon et al., "Altered frontocortical, cerebellar, and basal ganglia activity in adjuvant-treated breast cancer survivors 5–10 years after chemotherapy," *Breast Cancer Research and Treatment*, vol. 103, no. 3, pp. 303–311, 2007.

[145] B. Weiss, "Chemobrain: a translational challenge for neurotoxicology," *Neurotoxicology*, vol. 29, no. 5, pp. 891–898, 2008.

[146] A. Amidi, L. M. Wu, M. Agerbaek et al., "Cognitive impairment and potential biological and psychological correlates of neuropsychological performance in recently orchiectomized testicular cancer patients," *Psycho-Oncology*, vol. 24, no. 9, pp. 1174–1180, 2015.

[147] J. S. Wefel, D. J. Vidrine, T. L. Veramonti et al., "Cognitive impairment in men with testicular cancer prior to adjuvant therapy," *Cancer*, vol. 117, no. 1, pp. 190–196, 2011.

[148] S. B. Schagen, W. Boogerd, M. J. Muller et al., "Cognitive complaints and cognitive impairment following BEP chemotherapy in patients with testicular cancer," *Acta Oncologica*, vol. 47, no. 1, pp. 63–70, 2008.

[149] A. D. Pedersen, P. Rossen, M. Y. Mehlsen et al., "Long-term cognitive function following chemotherapy in patients with testicular cancer," *Journal of the International Neuropsychological Society*, vol. 15, no. 2, pp. 296–301, 2009.

[150] T. Skaali, S. D. Fossa, S. Andersson et al., "Self-reported cognitive problems in testicular cancer patients: relation to neuropsychological performance, fatigue, and psychological distress," *Journal of Psychosomatic Research*, vol. 70, no. 5, pp. 403–410, 2011.

[151] J. Skoogh, G. Steineck, U. Stierner et al., "Testicular-cancer survivors experience compromised language following chemotherapy: findings in a Swedish population-based study 3-26 years after treatment," *Acta Oncologica*, vol. 51, no. 2, pp. 185–197, 2012.

[152] J. S. Wefel, D. J. Vidrine, S. K. Marani et al., "A prospective study of cognitive function in men with non-seminomatous germ cell tumors," *Psycho-Oncology*, vol. 23, no. 6, pp. 626–633, 2014.

[153] A. A. Dahl, C. F. Haaland, A. Mykletun et al., "Study of anxiety disorder and depression in long-term survivors of testicular cancer," *Journal of Clinical Oncology*, vol. 23, no. 10, pp. 2389–2395, 2005.

[154] S. Vehling, A. Mehnert, M. Hartmann, C. Oing, C. Bokemeyer, and K. Oechsle, "Anxiety and depression in long-term testicular germ cell tumor survivors," *General Hospital Psychiatry*, vol. 38, pp. 21–25, 2016.

[155] E. H. Shinn, K. Basen-Engquist, B. Thornton, P. E. Spiess, and L. Pisters, "Health behaviors and depressive symptoms in testicular cancer survivors," *Urology*, vol. 69, no. 4, pp. 748–753, 2007.

[156] A. B. Smith, P. Butow, I. Olver et al., "The prevalence, severity, and correlates of psychological distress and impaired health-related quality of life following treatment for testicular cancer: a survivorship study," *Journal of Cancer Survivorship*, vol. 10, no. 2, pp. 223–233, 2016.

[157] J. E. Bower, "Cancer-related fatigue–mechanisms, risk factors, and treatments," *Nature Reviews Clinical Oncology*, vol. 11, no. 10, pp. 597–609, 2014.

[158] I. J. Orre, S. D. Fossa, R. Murison et al., "Chronic cancer-related fatigue in long-term survivors of testicular cancer," *Journal of Psychosomatic Research*, vol. 64, no. 4, pp. 363–371, 2008.

[159] M. Sprauten, H. S. Haugnes, M. Brydoy et al., "Chronic fatigue in 812 testicular cancer survivors during long-term follow-up: increasing prevalence and risk factors," *Annals of Oncology*, vol. 26, no. 10, pp. 2133–2140, 2015.

[160] K. M. Mustian, C. M. Alfano, C. Heckler et al., "Comparison of pharmaceutical, psychological, and exercise treatments for cancer-related fatigue: a meta-analysis," *JAMA Oncology*, vol. 3, no. 7, pp. 961–968, 2017.

[161] L. B. Travis, C. Beard, J. M. Allan et al., "Testicular cancer survivorship: research strategies and recommendations," *Journal of the National Cancer Institute*, vol. 102, no. 15, pp. 1114–1130, 2010.

[162] K. D. Miller, R. L. Siegel, C. C. Lin et al., "Cancer treatment and survivorship statistics, 2016," *CA: A Cancer Journal for Clinicians*, vol. 66, no. 4, pp. 271–289, 2016.

[163] Expert Panel on Detection, Evaluation, and Treatment of High Blood Cholesterol in Adults, "Executive summary of the third report of the national cholesterol education program (NCEP) expert panel on detection, evaluation, and treatment of high blood cholesterol in adults (adult treatment panel III)," *Journal of the American Medical Association*, vol. 285, no. 19, pp. 2486–2497, 2001.

[164] L. Richiardi, G. Scelo, P. Boffetta et al., "Second malignancies among survivors of germ-cell testicular cancer: a pooled analysis between 13 cancer registries," *International Journal of Cancer*, vol. 120, no. 3, pp. 623–631, 2007.

[165] K. Hemminki, H. Liu, and J. Sundquist, "Second cancers after testicular cancer diagnosed after 1980 in Sweden," *Annals of Oncology*, vol. 21, no. 7, pp. 1546–1551, 2010.

[166] I. M. Ventry and B. E. Weinstein, "The hearing handicap inventory for the elderly: a new tool," *Ear and Hearing*, vol. 3, no. 3, pp. 128–134, 1982.

[167] European Organisation for Research and Treatment of Cancer, *First EORTC Cancer Survivorship Summit*, Vol. 12, European Journal of Cancer Supplements, Brussels, Belgium, June 2014.

[168] J. Oldenburg, S. D. Fossa, and A. A. Dahl, "Scale for chemotherapy-induced long-term neurotoxicity (SCIN): psychometrics, validation, and findings in a large sample of testicular cancer survivors," *Quality of Life Research*, vol. 15, no. 5, pp. 791–800, 2006.

[169] L. B. Travis, "Therapy-associated solid tumors," *Acta Oncologica*, vol. 41, no. 4, pp. 323–333, 2002.

9

A Vaginal Inlay for Reduction of Stress Urinary Incontinence: Outcome of a Randomized Clinical Trial and Four User Acceptance Studies

Aino Fianu Jonasson,[1] **Karin Bryder**,[2] **and Elisabeth Sthengel**[2]

[1]*Division of Obstetrics and Gynaecology, Karolinska University Hospital, Huddinge, 141 86, Stockholm, Sweden*
[2]*Invent Medic Sweden AB, Medicon Village, 223 81, Lund, Sweden*

Correspondence should be addressed to Aino Fianu Jonasson; aino.fianu.jonasson@ki.se

Academic Editor: Muhammad Shahid

A multicenter, randomized, controlled clinical trial and four postmarket user acceptance investigations were carried out to document the safety, performance, and user acceptance of Efemia Bladder Support, a novel vaginal inlay for the temporary reduction of stress urinary incontinence (SUI). The clinical investigation enrolled 97 women diagnosed with SUI, randomized 3 : 1 to either treatment or standard care (control). The primary endpoint was reduction of urine leakage, measured as change in pad weight baseline week compared with treatment week. Secondary endpoints were treatment success, calculated as the percentage of subjects with >70% reduction in pad weight, reduction in incontinence episodes, and quality of life (QoL). 75 women (77%) completed the clinical investigation. No serious adverse events occurred. The treatment group reached a 55% ($p < 0.001$) mean reduction of total leakage compared to the control arm. A subanalysis, involving only leakage during provocation testing (coughing and jumping), showed a 67% ($p < 0.001$) mean reduction of leakage. No significant effect on QoL could be observed. 51% of the women answered "yes" to the question if they would use the device to reduce SUI. The user acceptance of the device was further investigated in four postmarket studies, using an improved device design with a slimmer centerpiece and a thinner handle, while keeping the effect achieving parts of the device unchanged. An average of 74% of the 102 participants in the postmarket studies reported that they were likely to continue using Efemia. The highest user satisfaction was seen in the two studies evaluating the use of Efemia during exercise, where 83% and 88% of the women were likely to continue using Efemia. It can be concluded that Efemia is a safe, well-tolerated, and effective alternative for reducing SUI, both in everyday life and during physical exercise.

1. Introduction

Urinary incontinence (UI) in women is a distressing condition that restricts quality of life and interferes with daily activities. In a review of reported UI prevalence in studies, Milsom et al. found that most studies reported a prevalence of female UI in the range of 25 to 45%. Stress urinary incontinence accounted for approximately half of the UI cases and the prevalence increases with increasing age [1]. However, SUI occurs also in younger, physically active women. According to Abrams et al., it is clear that high impact exercise leads to stress UI, with a dose-dependent deleterious effect, while low-impact sports might be protective [2]. In a review of 36 publications addressing the associations between physical activity and SUI, Chisholm et al. found evidence for increased rates of SUI among women who are physically active [3]. In a study quantifying SUI in 104 young female athletes, 52% of the participants self-reported SUI according to the ICQ_UI_SF score [4]. These results show the importance of not only evaluating device performance on the target group of elderly women clinically diagnosed with SUI but also including younger, active women that experience urine leakage during exercise, but not necessarily define themselves as being incontinent.

There are several treatment options for SUI available. In clinical practice, it is the convention that nonsurgical therapies are tried first because they usually carry the least risk of harm. Containment devices (absorbent pads, urinary catheters, and intravaginal devices) play an important role, especially for individuals who prefer to avoid the risks of interventional treatments, or in whom active treatment is impossible for any reason. [5]. Insertion of a synthetic sling to give support to the midurethra is currently the first in line recommended surgical approach [5, 6]. However, as more women are treated, concerns of the safety of the surgery have been raised. In a data analysis of incontinence surgery registered in The Swedish National Registry for Gynecologic Surgery (GynOP), presented at the ICS 2019 conference, S. Zacharias et al. reported that, out of 4,160 Swedish women that went through incontinence surgery during 2017, 681 women (16%) responded that they either had a complication, were worse off in their incontinence than before, or were unhappy with the results. The most common problems were urinating problems, pain, infection, and rupture/erosion of the tape in the vagina [7]. It is clear from this data that there is a need for effective nonsurgical alternatives for treatment or alleviation of SUI.

In a review of studies on the use of vaginal pessaries for the management of SUI, Ghadeer et al. concluded that they are an effective alternative to surgery if they are fit properly [8]. Several models of vaginal inserts designed to give support to the urethra or bladder neck to temporarily reduce urine leakage have been evaluated in clinical studies. Examples are Uresta [9], Diveen [10], Contrelle [11], Impressa [12], and Contiform [13]. Due to differences in vaginal anatomy and personal preferences, it cannot be expected that one design will suit all women. The introduction of Efemia gives women a new choice of device, with a handle for easy self-positioning, ensuring correct placement at the midurethra.

The aim of the present clinical investigation and postmarket studies was to evaluate the safety, efficacy, and usabillity of Efemia.

2. Materials and Methods

2.1. Investigational Device. Efemia Bladder Support is intended to temporarily reduce SUI in women by supporting the midurethra through the vaginal wall. It is reusable and can be used continuously up to 16 hours a day or on occasion when urine leakage is expected. It is made from medical grade silicone rubber and is available with three support ring diameters: 30 mm, 35 mm, and 40 mm. A first design was used during the clinical investigation TVS1000. After the clinical investigation, the device design was improved with a slimmer centerpiece and a thinner handle, while keeping the effect achieving parts of the original trial device unchanged. The revised device was used in the postmarket studies TVS2000, TVS3000, TVS4000, and TVS5000. Figure 1 shows the two device designs. The two rings (A) support the midurethra through the vaginal wall, thereby preventing involuntary urine leakage upon abdominal pressure. The midsection (B) positions the device correctly at the urethral knee. The handle (C) holds the device in place and is placed against the vaginal introitus. The handle is also used as an aid at insertion and removal of the device.

2.2. Study Design of the Clinical Investigation TVS1000

2.2.1. Study Title. The study title is an Open Randomized Controlled Multicenter Clinical Investigation with an Intravaginal Device for Stress Urinary Incontinence in Comparison to Using Standard of Care.

2.2.2. Study Population. All study participants were diagnosed with stress urinary incontinence, had normal voiding, were above 18 years, and leaked at least 10 g per 24 hours. Women with dominated urgency or neurogenic incontinence, hysterectomized, with a pronounced prolapse, pregnant, with a vaginal infection, or with a history of not being able to use tampons were excluded from the study.

2.2.3. Randomization. Subjects fulfilling the exclusion and inclusion criteria were randomly assigned at a 3 : 1 ratio to either the TVS treatment group or the standard-of-care (SoC) group at visit 2, using block design. Each site was provided with closed envelopes with consecutive numbering. Those assessing the outcomes were blinded to treatment allocation until the database was validated and locked.

2.2.4. Primary Endpoint. Absolute reduction in pad weight from the run-in week (week 1) compared with the final week (week 3). The weight of the pad is defined as the mean weight over the entire week of measurement.

2.2.5. Secondary Endpoints

Overall success rate, defined as at least 70% reduction in pad weight from run-in to the final week (week 3)

Reduction of SUI episodes

Reduced incontinence impact on QoL, measured using the validated patient reported outcome questionnaires EQ-5D-5 L, IIQ-7, and UDI-6

2.2.6. Study Size and Statistical Analysis. The aim was to enroll 96 female study subjects. A study size of 96 patients was calculated using a standard deviation of 9 g, a power of 90%, a significance level of 5%, and a 20% dropout rate. A mean leakage reduction of 13 g was assumed for the active group and 5 g for the control group (MIREDIF = 8 g). The full analysis set, defined as randomized subjects with at least one test measurement after randomization (FAS), was used for safety primary and secondary efficacy endpoints. A subanalysis, involving only leakage during provocation testing, was also planned. Center and treatment were used as covariates in the analysis of the primary variable. Hypothesis was tested using a two-sided Student's *t*-test with a 5% significance level. No adjustments for multiplicity were performed. Outliers were not excluded. Data from prematurely withdrawn subjects was included in the analysis as far as possible. No imputation of missing data was performed.

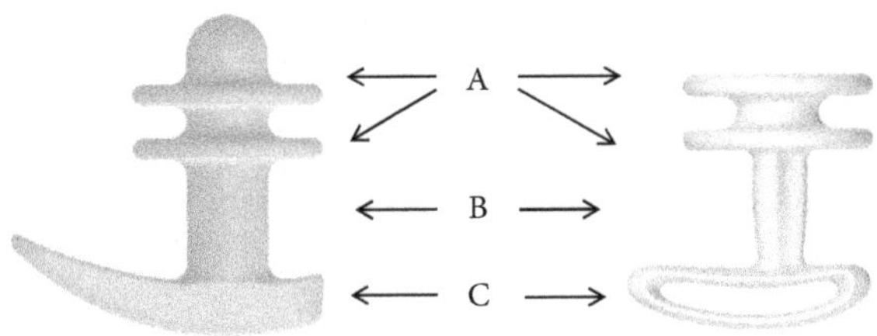

FIGURE 1: Investigational device, size 30 mm. Left: the design used in the clinical investigation; right: the design used in the postmarket studies. A = support rings, B = midsection, and C = handle.

2.2.7. Study Procedures. The clinical investigation was conducted at four clinics with Aino Fianu Jonasson, Dr, Md, PhD, urogynecology specialist at Karolinska University Hospital, as coordinating investigator. Participants were recruited via advertisements in newspapers and on Facebook. At the screening visit, a medical and surgical history, a physical examination (including gynecological examination), and a confirmation of the diagnosis of SUI were performed, followed by a confirmation of the inclusion/exclusion criteria. SUI was diagnosed by pad testing and measurement of residual urine after filling the bladder with 300 ml saline and provoking urine leakage by coughing, jumping, and rinsing hands in cold running water. A positive cough/jump test indicates stress incontinence while a positive rinsing test indicates urge incontinence. Calibrated scales were distributed to the participants for weighing pads. Baseline data was collected during the first week. During week 2, the women in the TVS group selected the device size and practiced how to use the device prior to the start of treatment at week 3. The control group continued with conventional treatment, i.e., using pads during weeks 2 and 3. For women who were menstruating, the study was interrupted, due to the fact that menstruation could affect the weight of the pads and consequently the study data. Specific instructions for re-entering the study were given to the subjects prior to start. The women used a diary to record their incontinent episodes, pad weight, physical activities, and general observations during the first three weeks of the study. They also performed a daily provocation test by coughing 10 times and jumping in place (or sit and stand if unable to jump) 20 times with a full bladder. At the weekly visits to the clinic, the women were asked QoL questions (IIQ-7, UDI-6, and EQ-5D-DL) and were asked to rate their experience of the device. After completing week 3, women in the control group were offered to use the device for two weeks. If they chose to do so, they switched over to a SoC-TVS group and went to a 5th visit to the clinic to answer questions regarding their experience. Both the TVS and the control group had a follow-up telephone call after 8 weeks.

2.2.8. Safety Monitoring. Subjects were carefully monitored for the occurrence of adverse events (AE) during the investigation period from randomization to the completion of follow-up. The clinical investigators collected AE information using nonleading questions. Events directly observed or spontaneously volunteered by subjects were also recorded.

2.2.9. Ethical Considerations. The investigation was conducted in compliance with the ethical principles of the latest revision of the Declaration of Helsinki as well as ISO 14155 : 2011. The study was reviewed and permission granted by Ethical Committee and Competent Authority prior to start (EC registration #2016/1899/31/1, CA registration#: CIV-16-10–017304). Clincaltrial.gov identifier: NCT03186651.

2.3. Study Design of Postmarket Studies: TVS2000, TVS3000, TVS4000, and TVS5000. The four postmarket studies were designed as observational user satisfaction studies. The identity of the participants was not revealed to the sponsor (Invent Medic Sweden AB). The subject recruitment, informed consent, subject ID-log, and distribution of questionnaires and study products were handled by independent study administrators at the Ladulaas Clinic (TVS2000), Aller Media (TVS3000), Tilling Träning (TVS4000), and the Urotherapy Clinic at Skelleftea Hospital (TVS5000). Participants received a free package containing the three sizes of Efemia. Participants recruited from the Aller Media test panel collected loyalty points that could be used for purchase in the Aller Media webshop. No other compensation or rewards were given for participation.

2.3.1. Sample Size. The sample size calculation in the TVS2000 and TVS3000 study was based on the standard deviations for the average IIQ-7 score in the TVS1000 study. A study size of 25 subjects is required to detect a significant difference of at least 25% with a power of 80% and a significance level of 5%, expecting a standard deviation of 32%.

The sample sizes of the TVS4000 and TVS5000 studies were not based on power calculations, since the primary endpoint was user satisfaction and they do not contain any hypothesis evaluations. It was estimated that a sample size of 20 women would represent a sufficient basis for evaluating user satisfaction during exercise.

2.3.2. Study Objectives. The first two studies, TVS2000 and TVS3000, had the objective to investigate the effect on quality of life (measured as reduction in IIQ-7 score) and user satisfaction when using Efemia in everyday life. The participants answered the IIQ-7 questionnaire before using Efemia and after 4 weeks of usage. The other two studies had the objective to evaluate user satisfaction when using Efemia during physical exercise. Table 1 shows a comparison of the design of the four studies.

2.3.3. Ethical Considerations. The studies were designed and performed by adhering to the ICC/ESOMAR international code of marketing and social research [14]. In addition, ethical approval was obtained for the TVS2000 study

TABLE 1: Comparison of study design of the four postmarket surveillance studies.

Parameter	Study: TVS2000	TVS3000	TVS4000	TVS5000
Recruitment	Previous participants in TVS1000	Through the Aller Media test panel	Visitors at the gym Tilling Träning	Urotherapist at Skellefteå Hospital
Study size	34	40	19	9
Treatment length	4 weeks	4 weeks	6 weeks	6 weeks
Target group	Women clinically diagnosed with SUI	Women self-diagnosed with SUI	Women with urine leakage during weightlifting	Women with urine leakage during cross-fit training
Study objectives	Change in the IIQ-7 score after 4 w device usage	Change in the IIQ-7 score after 4 w device usage	User satisfaction when using Efemia during weight training	User satisfaction when using Efemia during cross-fit training

because it included participants from the previous clinical investigation TVS1000 (EC ref: EPN Lund, Dnr: 2018/959).

3. Results and Discussion

3.1. Results of TVS1000 Clinical Investigation. A total of 191 women at four clinical sites were screened for eligibility. Of these, 97 women met all the inclusion and none of the exclusion criteria and were thereafter randomized.

The most common screening failure was <10 g urine leakage during 24 h ($n = 25$), followed by prolapse reaching hymen when coughing ($n = 12$). Recruitment started in Feb 2017 and the study was completed in Jan 2018. The women were randomized 3 : 1 to either use the device or standard care (SoC).

The groups had similar baseline demographics and clinical characteristics, and the mean age was 54.7 years. The mean leakage weight at the controlled provocation test during the screening visit was 53.5 g. The baseline characteristics and demographics are shown in Table 2.

20 subjects in the TVS group and 2 subjects in the control group discontinued the investigation. A chart of participant flow and reasons for discontinuation is shown in Figure 2.

3.2. Primary Outcome. The absolute reduction in mean pad weight from baseline (week 1) compared with the final week (week 3) was 18.2 g. The estimated treatment effect compared with the control group for total leakage was 12.4 g (55%) with a p value of 0.0005 in favour for the TVS group.

The absolute reduction in pad weight during provocation testing was 28.2 g (67%, $p < 0.0001$). Analysis of covariance for the variables: treatment group, site, age, weight, and residual volume showed no association between the covariate and the primary outcome measure. The outcome is summarised in Table 3.

3.3. Secondary Outcome. Overall success rate, defined as at least 70% reduction in pad weight from the run-in week to the final week (week 3): 42% of the subjects in the TVS arm and 4% of the subjects in the control arm had more than 70% reduction in pad weight with a p value = 0.0008 in favour for the TVS group.

The number of SUI episodes at week 3 compared to baseline was reduced with a median of 28% ($n = 52$, max-min, -95-150%) for the TVS group and 0% ($n = 23$, max-min, -46-557%) for the control group with a p value = 0.0019 in favour for the TVS group.

Incontinence Impact Questionnaire (IIQ-7): IIQ-7 score was reduced with 10% for the TVS group and 12% for the control group. There was no statistical difference between the TVS group and the control group (p = 0.414).

Urogenital Distress Inventory (UDI-6): UDI-6 score was reduced with 12% for the TVS group and 18% for the control group. No statistical difference between TVS group and control group was observed (p = 0.1971).

3.4. Safety. A total of 92 women were exposed to the device for two weeks during the investigation. No device-related serious adverse effects occurred. 32 of the 92 subjects using the device reported device-related adverse effects (45 episodes). The most frequent adverse device effect was discomfort (30), followed by bleeding (4), vaginal discharge (4), contusion (4), itching (2), and candidiasis (1). All adverse effects were resolved when TVS use was reduced, except for the single incident of candidiasis that needed medical intervention.

3.5. Usability. The usability analysis included all 72 women that had been exposed to the device at any time during the investigation and answered the usability questions. 85% of the women rated the device as easy or very easy to insert or remove. 51% answered "yes" to the question if they would use the device to reduce SUI, and 75% of them would recommend the device to a friend. 58% found the device to be comfortable (acceptable or perfectly acceptable), 13% were neutral, and 29% found it to be unacceptable.

4. Results of Postmarket Surveillance Studies: TVS2000, TVS3000, TVS4000, and TVS5000

A total of 102 women were enrolled in the four user satisfaction studies. 79 women used Efemia in their daily lives or during exercise and are included in the analysis. All studies were performed during 2019. A chart of participant flow in the four studies is shown in Figure 3.

TABLE 2: Demographics.

Variable	Treatment arm		
	TVS Mean (SD)	SoC Mean (SD)	Total Mean (SD)
Number of women	73	24	97
Age (years)	54.8 (10.8)	54.6 (9.38)	54.7 (10.4)
Weight (kg)	78.6 (15.8)	78.2 (17.7)	78.5 (16.2)
Height (cm)	166 (6.22)	167 (6.55)	166 (6.28)
Residual urine (ml)	27.1 (23.9)	29.1 (21.6)	27.6 (23.3)
Urine leakage, controlled provocation test (g)	56.6 (63.3)	43.9 (49.9)	53.5 (60.3)

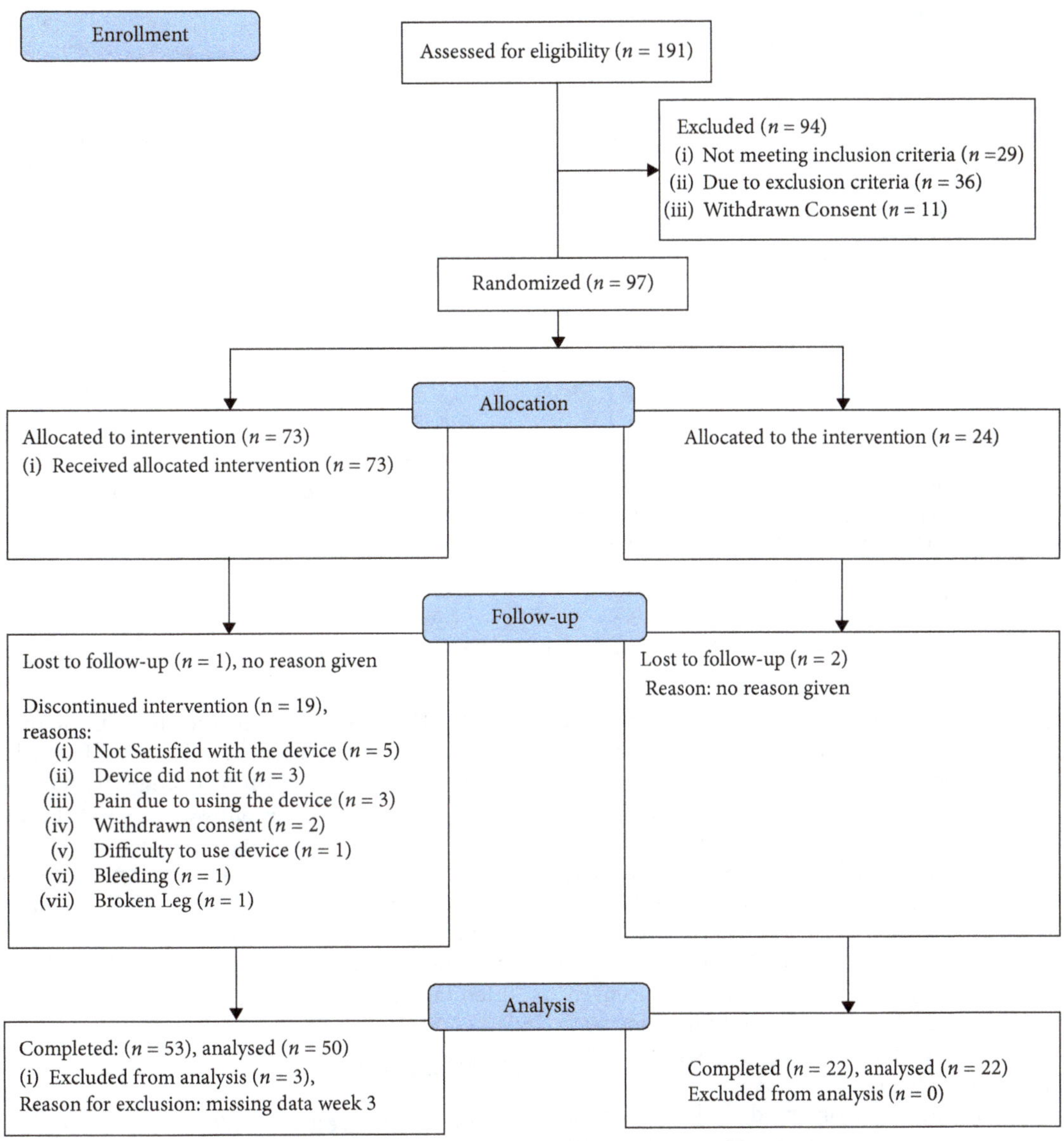

FIGURE 2: TVS1000 participant flow.

TABLE 3: Efemia effect on mean urine leakage (average daily pad weight), analysed on the full analysis set.

Variable	SoC ($n = 22$)			TVS ($n = 50$)			Treatment effect
	Week 1	Week 3	Change (g)	Week 1	Week 3	Change (g)	TVS-SoC
Mean total leakage (g)	27.1	22.5	−5.2	27.3	10.5	−18.2	55%
(SD, p value)	(33.2)	(20.8)	(34.4)	(33.6)	(21.9)	(35.5)	p = 0.0005
Mean provoked leakage	32.4	31.2	−1.2	38.2	10.0	−28.2	67%
(SD, p value)	(33.0)	(29.2)	(9.5)	(42.6)	(22.1)	(30.0)	$p < 0.0001$

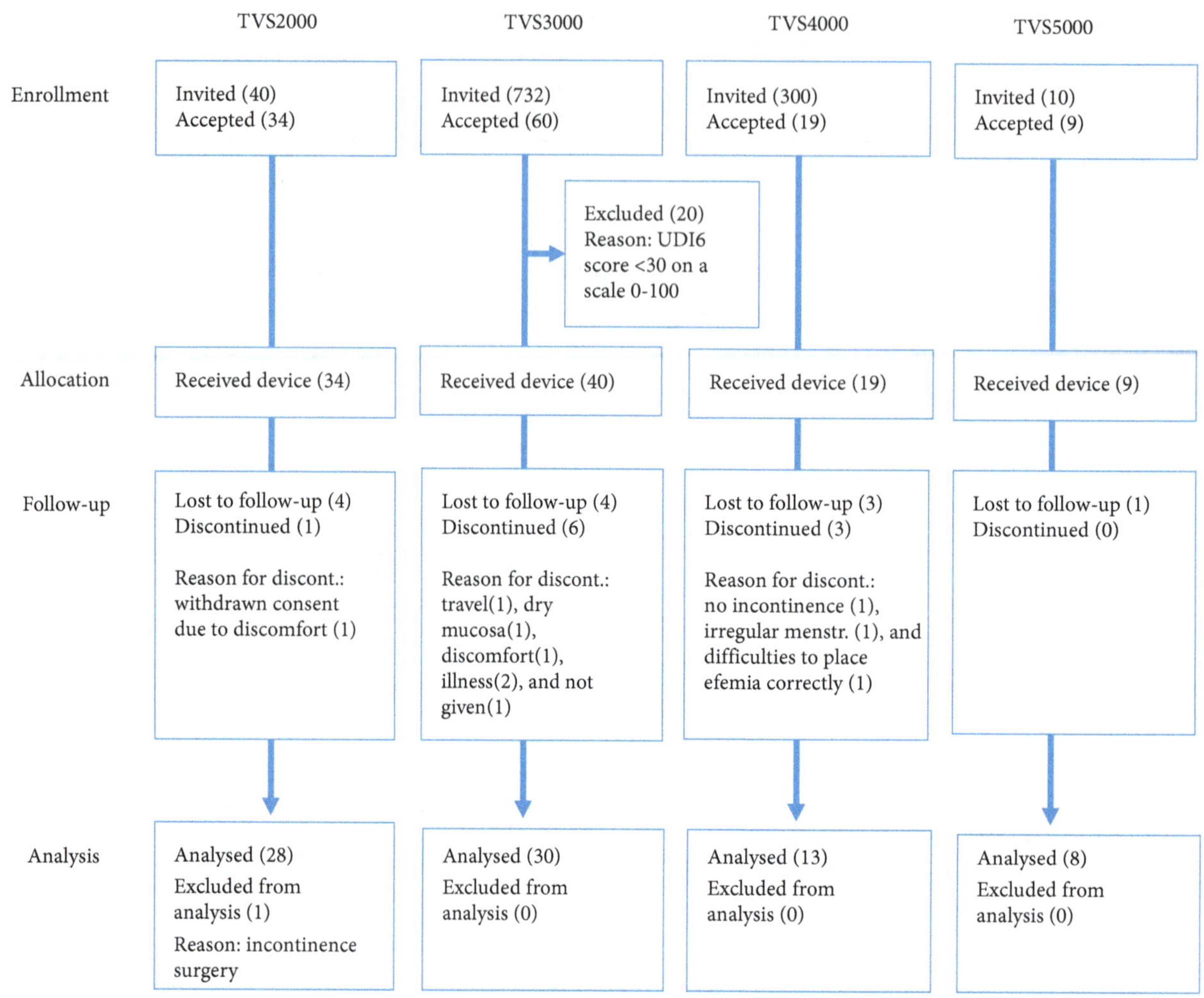

Figure 3: Participant flow, postmarket surveillance studies.

User satisfaction was measured as likelihood to continue to use Efemia and to recommend Efemia to a friend. The women were asked to grade their answers 0–10, where 0 = " not at all likely" and 10 = " extremely likely." A grading of 6 or above was regarded as a positive answer. The frequency of women likely to recommend Efemia to a friend in the TVS2000, TVS3000, TVS4000, and TVS5000 studies was 82%, 62%, 92%, and, 100%, respectively. The frequency of women likely to continue using Efemia in the TVS2000, TVS3000, TVS4000, and TVS5000 studies was 68%, 55%, 83%, and 88%, respectively. The median gradings of the likelihood to continue using or to recommend Efemia to a friend, for each study separately and pooled, are shown in Figure 4.

The impact of incontinence on the daily life was measured in TVS2000 and TVS3000 using the validated Incontinence Impact Questionnaire IIQ-7, where the women were asked to grade the impact of their incontinence in 7 areas of everyday life before and after having tried Efemia for 4 weeks. A grading of 0–3 was used, where 0 = not at all, 1 = slightly, 2 = moderately, and 3 = greatly. There was a significant improvement in IIQ-7 scores with a 27% mean decrease in TVS2000 ($p = 0.0015$) and a 29% mean decrease in TVS3000 ($p = 0.012$).

In the TVS3000 study, the effect of Efemia on quality of life was also measured by asking if Efemia had facilitated daily life. A comparison of change in IIQ-7 score with facilitation of daily life showed no significant correlation, while there was a strong positive correlation between facilitation of everyday life and willingness to continue to use or recommend the device with a R^2 of 0.499 and 0.587, respectively. Graphs plotting facilitation of everyday life with change in the IIQ-7 score or likelihood to recommend Efemia are shown in Figure 5.

5. Discussion

The clinical investigation TVS1000 confirmed that Efemia Bladder Support is safe and achieves its primary performance objective to reduce involuntary urine leakage with a 55% ($p < 0.0001$) mean reduction of leakage compared to the control group. The subanalysis of leakage during the daily provocation tests showed a 67% ($p < 0.0001$) mean reduction of leakage.

The secondary endpoints for the study were also met. 42% of the subjects in the TVS arm had >70% reduction in pad weight and the number of SUI episodes was reduced by 28%.

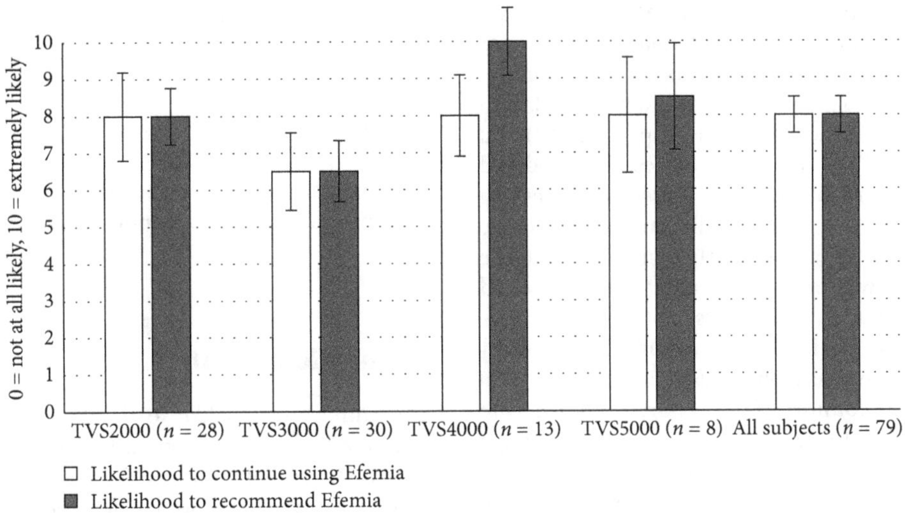

FIGURE 4: Median gradings of the questions: on a scale of 0–10, how likely are you to continue using Efemia or to recommend Efemia to a friend? Error bars = 95% CI.

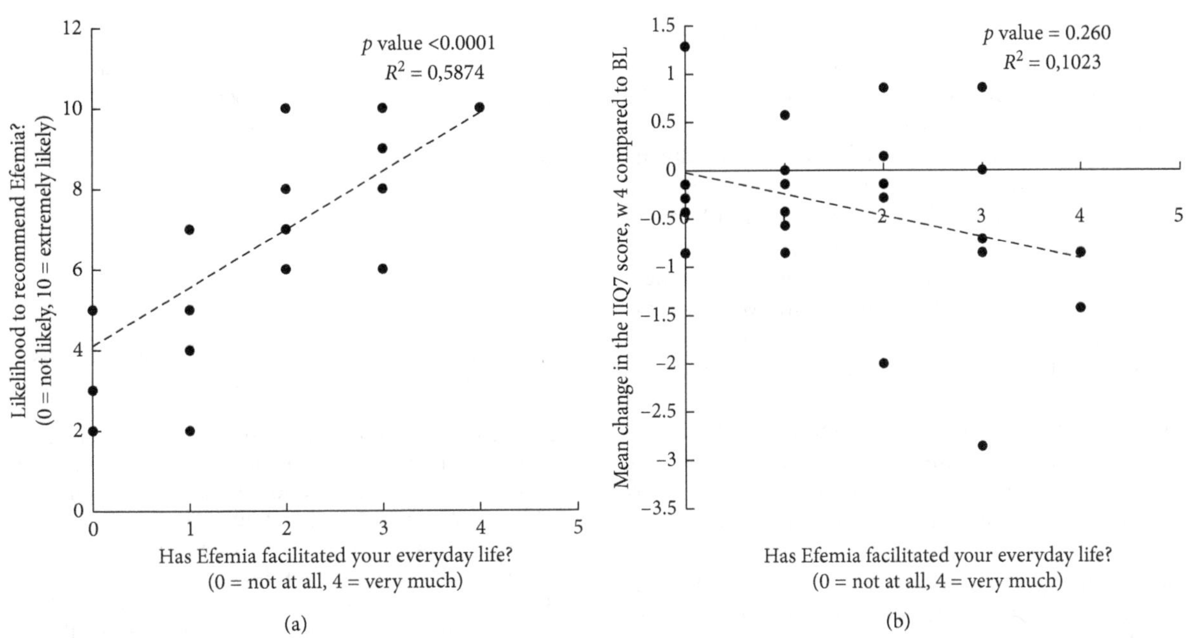

FIGURE 5: Likelihood to recommend (graph (a)) and mean change in the IIQ-7 score (graph (b)), plotted against facilitation of everyday life, TVS3000 ($n = 30$).

The quality of life endpoints in TVS1000 were not met. No clinically significant decrease in the IIQ-7 score, compared to controls, could be detected after 2-week use of the device, while there was a modest but significant decrease of the IIQ-7 score in the two user satisfaction studies TVS2000 and TVS3000, with 27% and 29% reduction, respectively. The published validation of the Swedish form of the IIQ-7 questionnaire reported a strong-to-moderate correlation with treatment satisfaction and reduction of the IIQ-7 score [15]. It was therefore surprising to note that there was no significant correlation between any of the treatment satisfaction variables (willingness to continue using or recommending Efemia), and reduction of IIQ-7 scores in the present investigations. In fact, 6 of the 8 women in the TVS3000 study and 5 of the 7 women in the TVS2000 study, with an increase or no change in the IIQ-7 score after treatment, reported that they were likely to continue using Efemia. It is difficult to understand why anyone will want to continue to use Efemia if it has no effect or even worsens the impact of incontinence on their daily life, as measured with IIQ-7. An explanation might be that women with mild SUI cannot relate to the IIQ-7 questions because most of them are likely to use protective pads in situations where they expect to leak. Therefore, their incontinence has very little impact on their ability to perform daily activities. As one of the women comments, "I think the IIQ-7 questions are wrongly designed. Incontinence is unpleasant but it does not affect my ability to do things." The inadequacy of IIQ-7 for quantifying the objective severity of SUI is confirmed in the publication by Franco et al. where they found no correlation between reduction in urine leakage (1-hour pad weight) and change in IIQ-7 score [16]. In future studies, the validated ICQ-SF questionnaire might be better suited for assessing incontinence impact on the quality of life in relation to the use of Efemia. However, it can be clearly concluded that the treatment satisfaction was high and that Efemia facilitated the daily lives of the study participants.

No serious adverse device effects occurred. The most commonly reported adverse device effect in the TVS1000 investigation was discomfort (30 reports). Since the TVS1000 investigation, there has been a design change resulting in a lighter and more appealing product. It is therefore interesting to compare the device comfort in the TVS1000 investigation where the old design was used with the TVS2000 study in which the current design was used. In the TVS1000 investigation, 33% of the women considered the device to be uncomfortable while discomfort was experienced by only 7% of the women in the TVS2000 study, where the current device design was used.

The postmarket studies, using the current version of the device, showed a high user satisfaction. This was particularly noteworthy in the two studies where Efemia was used during exercise, where >80% of the women were likely to continue to use Efemia and >90% were likely to recommend Efemia to a friend. However, it is important to note that the evaluation of Efemia during exercise is based on a total of 21 women, using Efemia during cross-fit training and weightlifting. Studies, involving other sports and more women, would therefore be useful for evaluating the use of Efemia by physically active women.

For women diagnosed with SUI, Efemia can be an effective and safe alternative, either temporarily, while waiting for surgery, or to be able to avoid surgery altogether. Furthermore, since Efemia is available "over-the-counter," it might improve the daily lives of active women experiencing urine leakage during physical exercise, who might not see themselves as generally incontinent and therefore do not seek medical help. A weakness of the TVS3000 investigation is that the device usage was surprisingly low, such that most of the responders had used Efemia only a few times during the 4-week trial period. The reason for this is not clear. It could be either that the participants had very mild incontinence and only experienced urine leakage a few times during the 4-week trial period or that they were not fully dedicated to the study, but rather participated to collect loyalty points from Aller Media.

6. Conclusion

It can be concluded that Efemia is a safe, well-tolerated, and effective alternative for reducing SUI, both in everyday life and during physical exercise. It is clear from the studies that even though most women found Efemia comfortable, it does not suit all. Further studies, evaluating comfort and user satisfaction on a larger group of women, over a longer time, could be useful as a guidance in further device development.

Disclosure

The primary author and coordinating investigator, Aino Fianu Jonasson, takes responsibility for the integrity of the data.

Acknowledgments

The authors would like to thank the principal investigators, Katarina Berndtsson-Blom at Ladulaas Clinical Investigations, Margareta Hellgren at PCT, Skaraborg, and Johan Ellbin Andersson at PTC, Gothia, for their excellent work in the clinical conduct of the TVS1000 clinical investigation, Fredrik Hansson at CTC for the statistical analysis, and Christina Schönborg at Devicia AB for monitoring and coordination. The authors would also like to thank Kristina Agriwill at Aller Media, Sara Tilling at Tilling Träning AB, and Jenny Norrgren at Skellefteå Hospital for recruitment and coordination of the user acceptance studies TVS3000, TVS4000, and TVS5000, respectively. This research was funded by Invent Medic, a medical technology company at Medicon Village in Lund, Sweden.

References

[1] I. Milsom Gyhagen and M. Gyhagen, "The prevalence of urinary incontinence," *Climacteric*, vol. 22, no. 3, pp. 217–222, 2018.

[2] P. Abrams, L. Cardozo, A. Wagg, and A. Wein, *Incontinence*, 6th international consultation on incontinence, ICI-ICS. International Continence Society, Bristol, UK, 6th edition, 2016.

[3] L. Chisholm, S. Delpe, T. Priest, and W. S. Reynolds, "Physical activity and stress incontinence in women," *Current Bladder Dysfunction Reports*, vol. 14, no. 3, pp. 174–179, 2019.

[4] K. M. dos Santos, T. Da Roza, S. C. Tonon da Luz et al., "Quantification of urinary loss in nulliparous athletes during 1 hour of sports training," *PM&R*, vol. 11, no. 5, pp. 495–502, 2019.

[5] F. C. Burkhard, *EAU Guidelines on Urinary Incontinence in Adults*, European Association of Urology, Arnhem, Netherlands, 2018.

[6] C. R. Chapple, "Contemporary surgical management of stress urinary incontinence," *Current Opinion in Urology*, vol. 30, no. 2, p. 271, 2020.

[7] E. Uuustal and S. Zacharias, "Complications one year after mid urethal slings in Sweden, the womens descriptions classified," in *Proceedings of the ICS 2019 Gothenburg Conference*, Gothenburg, Sweden, September 2019.

[8] G. Al-Shaikh, S. Syed, S. Osman, A. Bogis, and A. Al-Badr, "Pessary use in stress urinary incontinence: a review of advantages, complications, patient satisfaction, and quality of life," *International Journal of Women's Health*, vol. 10, pp. 195–201, 2018.

[9] S. A. Farell, S. Baydock, B. Amir, and C. Fanning, "Effectiveness of a new self-positioning pessary for the management

of urinary incontinence in women," *Gynecology & Obstetrics*, vol. 196474.e1 pages, 2007.

[10] J.-N. Cornu, S. Mouly, S. Mouly et al., "75NC007 device for noninvasive stress urinary incontinence management in women: a randomized controlled trial," *International Urogynecology Journal*, vol. 23, no. 12, pp. 1727–1734, 2012.

[11] H. Thyssen, J. Bidmead, G. Lose, K. Møller Bek, P. Dwyer, and L. Cardozo, "A new intravaginal device for stress incontinence in women," *BJU International*, vol. 88, no. 9, pp. 889–892, 2001.

[12] E. Ziv, S. L. Stanton, and A. Joseph, "Efficacy and safety of a novel disposable intravaginal device for treating stress urinary incontinence," *Gynecology & Obstetrics*, vol. 198, no. 5, pp. 594.e1–594.e7, 2008.

[13] W. A. Allen, H. Leek, A. Izurieta, and K. H. Moore, "Update: the "Contiform" intravaginal device in four sizes for the treatment of stress incontinence," *International Urogynecology Journal*, vol. 19, no. 6, pp. 757–761, 2008.

[14] International Chamber of Commerce, Opinion and Social Research and Data Analytics, *ICC/ESOMAR International Code on Market*, Opinion and Social Research and Data Analytics, International Chamber of Commerce, Paris, France, 2016.

[15] K. Franzén, J.-E. Johansson, J. Karlsson, and K. Nilsson, "Validation of the Swedish version of the incontinence impact questionnaire and the urogenital distress inventory," *Acta Obstetricia et Gynecologica Scandinavica*, vol. 92, no. 5, pp. 555–561, 2013.

[16] A. V. M. Franco, F. Lee, and M. M. Fynes, "Is there an alternative to pad tests? Correlation of subjective variables of severity of urinary loss to the 1-h pad test in women with stress urinary incontinence," *BJU International*, vol. 102, no. 5, pp. 586–590, 2008.

10

Outcomes from the Introduction of a Combined Urology Outpatient Clinic

Clíodhna Browne, Catherine M. Dowling, Patrick O'Malley, Nadeem Nusrat, Kilian Walsh, Syed Jaffry, Eamonn Rogers, Garrett C. Durkan, and Frank T. D'Arcy

Department of Urology, University College Hospital Galway, Newcastle Road, Galway, Ireland

Correspondence should be addressed to Clíodhna Browne; cliodhnabrowne@rcsi.ie

Academic Editor: Fabio Campodonico

Background. A combined urology clinic staffed by four consultants and four non-consultant hospital doctors (NCHDs) was introduced in our institution in October 2015. This clinic is supported by a pre-clinic radiology meeting and a synchronous urology clinical nurse specialist (CNS) clinic with protected uroflow/trial of void slots. Herein, we report on the outcomes of this clinic in comparison with the standard format of urology outpatient review. *Methods.* We carried out a retrospective review of clinic attendances from May to July 2016. We recorded the number of new and return attendances, which team members had reviewed the patient and patient outcomes. We also calculated the waiting times for new patients to be reviewed in the outpatient clinic. *Results.* The combined urology clinic reviewed an average of 12 new and 46 return patients per clinic. The standard urology clinic reviewed an average of 8 new and 23 return patients per clinic. 54% of patients were seen by a consultant in the combined urology clinic, and 20% of patients were seen by a consultant in the standard urology clinic. The rate of patient discharge for new patients was 14.8% in the combined clinic compared to 5.9% in the standard clinic. Overall patient outcomes are outlined in the table. The waiting time for review of new patients in the combined clinic was reduced by 39% from 144 days to 89 days over a one-year period. *Conclusions.* The introduction of a combined urology outpatient clinic with the support of pre-clinic radiology meeting and synchronous urology CNS clinic facilitates patient discharge.

1. Introduction

Urology is a speciality with a large volume of outpatient work. Hospital outpatient services make up a significant proportion of urologists' working hours. Manpower and workforce crisis issues have a significant impact on outpatient services in our hospitals. The British Association of Urological Surgeons (BAUS) has produced guidelines that suggest ideal clinic numbers and outline the proportion of the working week that should be dedicated to outpatient clinics. In many urology departments, these numbers are not adhered to, due to long outpatient waiting lists and unfilled consultant posts. It has been suggested that a comprehensive combined "one-stop" clinic review, incorporating imaging and endoscopy, would facilitate discharge of patients after one clinic visit.

A combined urology clinic staffed by four consultant urologists with different subspecialist interests was introduced in our institution in October 2015. A total of eight doctors staff the combined clinic, four consultant urologists and four non-consultant hospital doctors (NCHDs). Every second week, there were three consultants and three NCHDs in attendance. In comparison with the standard clinic, the combined clinic staffing structure is such that although an equivalent number of patients per doctor are seen in both clinics, there are more consultants present in the combined clinic compared to the standard clinic. The intention of the increased consultant to patient ratio compared to the standard clinic is to facilitate early senior decision-making and fast-track the patient journey through the outpatient system.

Clinic lists are reviewed by the consultant in advance. Patients attending for follow-up of normal results are often contacted by phone and letter as a virtual clinic review, negating the need for them to travel to the clinic. The combined clinic is supported by a pre-clinic radiology meeting in the style of a standard multidisciplinary team meeting, where patient's imaging is reviewed by a consultant radiologist in the presence of the clinic team. This meeting lasts one hour and happens immediately before the clinic. Individual cases are discussed to plan surgical approaches or patient follow-up as required. A synchronous urology clinical nurse specialist (CNS) clinic with protected slots for uroflow measurements and trials of voiding runs in tandem with the combined urology clinic. Herein, we aim to report on the outcomes of the combined clinic in comparison with the standard format of the urology outpatient clinic that was traditionally employed in this institution.

2. Methods and Materials

We carried out a retrospective review of clinic attendances from a representative time period after pilot introduction of the combined clinic (May to July 2016). We recorded the number of new and return attendances, which team members had reviewed the patient and patient outcomes. We also calculated the waiting times for new patients to be reviewed in the outpatient clinic. These outcomes were compared to the clinic attendances at the standard urology clinic over the same time period.

3. Results

3.1. Referral Sources. A total of 757 patients attended the combined urology clinic over the study period. There were 183 new patients and 574 return patients seen in the combined clinic. A total of 372 patients attended the standard urology clinic over the study period. There were 118 new patients and 254 return patients in this group. The combined urology clinic reviewed an average of 12 new and 46 return patients per clinic. The standard urology clinic reviewed an average of 8 new and 23 return patients per clinic. The staffing structure of the clinics as outlined above means that the combined clinic reviewed an average of 17 patients per whole-time equivalent consultant compared to an average of 31 patients per whole-time equivalent consultant in the standard clinic.

The sources of new patient referrals to the combined urology clinic were 51% from general practitioners, 21% from other hospitals, 12% from other consultants in our hospital, 7% from inpatient consultations, 5% from the emergency department, and 4% from previous clinic non-attendances (Figure 1). The sources of new patient referrals to the standard urology clinic were 63% from general practitioners, 16% from other hospitals, 11% from other consultants in our hospital, 4% from the emergency department, 4% from previous clinic non-attendances, and 2% from inpatient consultations (Figure 2).

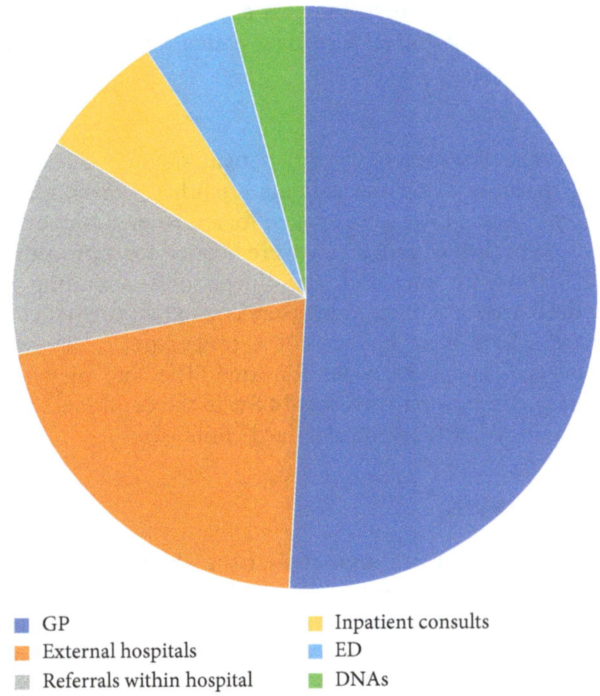

Figure 1: Standard urology clinic referrals.

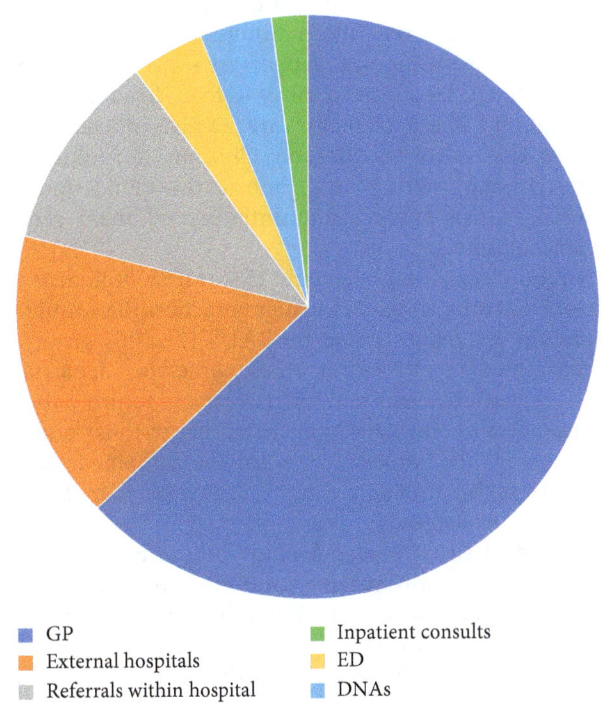

Figure 2: Combined urology clinic referrals.

3.2. Waiting Times. The median waiting time for new patients to be seen in the combined clinic was 53 days. The median waiting time for new patients to be seen in the standard urology clinic was 98 days. The mean waiting time for new patients was reduced by 38% during the first year of the combined urology clinic.

3.3. Patient Reviews. Fifty-four percent of patients were seen by a consultant in the combined urology clinic, and 20% of patients were seen by a consultant in the standard urology clinic. A consultant reviewed 56% of the new patients in the combined clinic and 21% of new patients in the standard urology clinic.

3.4. Patient Outcomes. Overall patient outcomes are outlined in Table 1. Of the patients attending the combined urology clinic, 51.8% were booked for a further clinic review, 21.1% were discharged, 26.8% were booked for a procedure, and 0.3% were admitted. Of the patients attending the standard urology clinic, 55.4% were booked for further clinic review, 34.1% were booked for a procedure, 10.2% were discharged, and 0.3% were admitted. The rate of patient discharge for new patients was 14.8% in the combined clinic compared to 5.9% in the standard clinic.

Table 1: Outcomes of clinic review.

Patient outcome	Combined clinic (%)	Standard clinic (%)
Discharged	21.1	10.2
Procedure booked	26.8	34.1
Admitted	0.3	0.3
Further clinic review	51.8	55.4

4. Discussion

Manpower and workforce crisis issues have a significant impact on outpatient services in Irish hospitals. The British Association of Urological Surgeons (BAUS) guidelines suggest ideal clinic numbers of eleven new patients and fifteen return patients per consultant per outpatient clinic [1]. In total, combined new and review patients should be limited at 12 patients per consultant per clinic. BAUS recommends allocating twenty minutes per consultation for new patients and two to fifteen minutes per consultation for review patients. Complex patients referred for specialist opinion should be allocated thirty to forty-five minutes per consultation. These numbers are rarely adhered to in practice due to restrictions on clinician time and prohibitively long waiting lists. Indeed, the clinic numbers reported in this study significantly exceed these recommended numbers.

Gilmore et al. found that only 25% of Irish urologists and 21% of UK urologists had outpatient practices that would fall within the guidelines issues by BAUS [2]. This group reported a median of two outpatient clinics per department per week, with thirteen new and twenty-six return patients. The numbers in our institution are similar to those outlined in this study. The numbers attending the combined urology clinic are higher, but this clinic is staffed by four different consultant urologists.

The ideal situation for urology outpatient services is full access to comprehensive combined "one-stop" clinic review that incorporates imaging and endoscopy. Some centres have implemented a similar strategy in the form of rapid access haematuria clinics with access to laboratory blood tests, upper tract imaging, and flexible cystoscopy. Traditionally, several clinic visits were required to diagnose one issue. Coull et al. reported on the implementation of a "one-stop" diagnostic clinic for urology patients [3]. They report an impressive 42% discharge rate back to GP care during the pilot period of this clinic. While neither clinic in this study has reached such discharge rates, the discharge rate in the combined clinic is double that of the standard clinic. This is likely as a result of the increased number of senior decision-makers in attendance at the clinic and the access to adjuncts such as the pre-clinic radiology meeting and CNS clinic. Availability of same-day imaging and endoscopy in our combined clinic would likely further improve outpatient efficiency.

Combined clinics have been reported in the literature in a variety of different complimentary specialities, including ophthalmology, renal disease, diabetes, cardiovascular disease, orthopaedics, and rheumatology. Patient outcomes have been favourable in these studies, with reductions in the number of clinic visits required for individual patients [4–7]. These approaches have also proven to be cost effective. Weber et al. reported on a group of patients with multiple related medical issues (kidney disease, cardiovascular disease, and diabetes) who attended a combined clinic with all the relevant speciality doctors, rather than individual speciality clinics [8]. Hospitalisation, dialysis, and mortality rates were no different between patients in the combined group and patients attending the individual clinics. However, differences in the cost of clinic visits were $86,400 per year in favour of the combined clinic.

The most significant difference in the results from our clinic was the rate of patients discharged versus those booked for further investigations or procedures. This can most likely be explained by a number of factors unique to the combined clinic. The pre-clinic X-ray conference enables a comprehensive review of imaging with a consultant radiologist in a formal multidisciplinary team setting. This informs the discussion with the patient and assists with decision-making, e.g., regarding follow-up of renal cysts or in planning operative approach in complex stone disease. The better consultant to patient ratio facilitates senior decision-making in a timely fashion, reducing the number of patients being sent for unnecessary investigations and increasing patient discharge rates. The combined clinic is staffed by four consultants with different subspecialist interests. This enables cross-referral between consultants, further facilitating senior decision-making and negating the need for return outpatient visits to see the appropriate surgeon.

5. Conclusions

The introduction to our department of a combined urology outpatient clinic with the support of pre-clinic radiology meeting and synchronous urology CNS clinic has facilitated patient discharge and enabled prompt senior decision-making for our outpatients. The presence of a senior decision-maker results in more consultant-led care and facilitates patient discharge. The introduction of same-day imaging and endoscopy would likely further improve outpatient clinic efficiency.

Ethical Approval

This research follows the principles of the Declaration of Helsinki.

References

[1] BAUS, *A guide to Job Planning for Consultant Urologists*, British Association of Urological Surgeons, London, UK, 2016, http://www.baus.org.uk.

[2] P. E. Gilmore, D. C. Shackley, N. W. Clarke, C. D. Betts, and K. J. O'Flynn, "National review of urology outpatient practice in the UK," *Postgraduate Medical Journal*, vol. 81, no. 951, pp. 55–57, 2005.

[3] N. Coull, G. Rottenberg, S. Rankin et al., "Assessing the feasibility of a one-stop approach to diagnosis for urological patients," *Annals of the Royal College of Surgeons of England*, vol. 91, no. 4, pp. 305–309, 2009.

[4] R. C. Han, J. M. Jefferis, J. P. Taylor, N. K. Archibald, and M. P. Clarke, "A novel, multidisciplinary clinic for complex visual problems in older people," *Eye*, vol. 26, no. 12, pp. 1536–1541, 2012.

[5] M. Patel, I. R. Shilliday, and G. A. McKay, "A combined diabetes renal clinic improves risk factor management and progression of renal disease in a district general hospital," *Journal of Evaluation in Clinical Practice*, vol. 15, no. 5, pp. 832–835, 2009.

[6] R. J. Newman, J. Belch, I. G. Kelly, and R. D. Sturrock, "Are combined orthopaedic and rheumatology clinics worth while?," *BMJ*, vol. 294, no. 6584, pp. 1392-1393, 1987.

[7] M. K. Jayapaul, R. Messersmith, D. N. Bennett-Jones, P. A. Mead, and D. M. Large, "The joint diabetic-renal clinic in clinical practice: 10 years of data from a district general hospital," *QJM*, vol. 99, no. 3, pp. 153–160, 2006.

[8] C. Weber, M. Beaulieu, O. Djurdjev et al., "Towards rational approaches of health care utilization in complex patients: an exploratory randomized trial comparing a novel combined clinic to multiple specialty clinics in patients with renal disease-cardiovascular disease-diabetes," *Nephrology Dialysis Transplantation*, vol. 27, no. 3, pp. 104–110, 2012.

11

Evaluation of the Extent of Primary Buccal Mucosal Graft Contracture in Augmentation Urethroplasty for Stricture Urethra: A Prospective Observational Study at a Tertiary Healthcare Centre

A. BhalaguruIyyan,[1] P. Puvai Murugan,[1] Chandranaath C. Alakhananda,[2] and B. M. Zeeshan Hameed[3]

[1]*Department of Urology, PSG Institute of Medical Sciences and Research, Coimbatore, Tamil Nadu, India*
[2]*Department of Surgery, PSG Institute of Medical Sciences and Research, Coimbatore, Tamil Nadu, India*
[3]*Department of Urology, Kasturba Medical College Manipal, Manipal Academy of Higher Education, Manipal, Karnataka, India*

Correspondence should be addressed to P. Puvai Murugan; puovai@gmail.com

Academic Editor: Kostis Gyftopoulos

Introduction. Buccal mucosal graft (BMG) urethroplasty is considered as gold standard in the treatment of urethral stricture disease. The successful outcome after BMG urethroplasty varies between 66 and 99%. One of the possible causes for failure is BMG contracture. Primary BMG contracture rate is poorly understood and unreported. The present study aimed to evaluate the extent of contracture of buccal mucosa immediately after harvesting. *Materials and Methods.* This was a prospective observational study conducted in the Department of Urology at our institute between January 2016 and December 2019. All patients with urethral stricture disease undergoing BMG urethroplasty for the first time were enrolled in the study after obtaining informed consent. Demographic and patient clinical profile was noted. Based on the intraoperative urethral stricture size, the preharvest graft was marked on the buccal mucosa and the size was calculated. Postharvest unstretched size of the graft was measured immediately after graft removal from the oral cavity. Alteration in BMG size was analysed using paired *t*-test. *Results.* Forty-four patients were included in the study. Mean age of the patient was 53.6 years. Mean stricture length was 7.45 cm (range 4–12 cm). Mean pre- and postharvest BMG size was 8.3×1.5 cm and 7.6×1.3 cm, respectively. There was a 8.4% decrease in length and 9.5% decrease in width of the buccal mucosal graft. *Conclusion.* Primary buccal mucosal graft contracture is around 8.4% in length and 9.5% in width. It would be better to mark wider than necessary while harvesting buccal mucosa so that tension-free anastomosis is performed.

1. Introduction

Buccal mucosal graft (BMG) urethroplasty is considered as the treatment of choice for long segment anterior urethral stricture disease [1]. Easy availability, exposure to moisture, and quick regeneration in the donor area make buccal mucosa a near ideal substitute for the urethra [2]. Still, successful outcomes after BMG urethroplasty are highly variable and range between 66 and 99% [3–6].

The failure of BMG urethroplasty has been attributed to various reasons such as progression of primary disease and loss of vascularity due to over mobilisation of urethra, recurrent infections, and possible contracture of graft.

Graft contracture can be primary or secondary. Primary graft contracture happens immediately after harvest from the donor site is a well-described phenomenon in skin grafts [7]. It can be overcome by increasing the area of the graft from the donor site. However, there is lack of knowledge regarding the extent of primary BMG shrinkage. Hence, in this study, we explored objectively the extent of primary contracture of BMG and its clinical implications in this procedure.

2. Materials and Methods

A prospective observational study was conducted in the Department of Urology at a tertiary institute from January 2016 to December 2019 after obtaining the institute's ethical committee approval (project no. 20/128). Patients planned for augmentation urethroplasty using BMG were included in the study, after obtaining consent. Patients' demographic and clinical findings were noted. All cases were operated by a team of three urologists alternating between the buccal graft harvesting and the urethroplasty (BIA, PMP, and ACC). Stricture characteristics were recorded. A thorough oral cavity examination was performed. Patients who had undergone previous oral surgeries or radiation were excluded from the study.

2.1. The Procedure-Harvesting of Buccal Mucosal Graft. BMG urethroplasty was performed under general anaesthesia with nasal intubation. After intubation, the patient was in lithotomy position, preliminary urethro-cystoscopy was done using 6/7.5 Fr semirigid ureteroscope, and findings were noted. Through a midline perineal incision, the urethra was identified, isolated, and stricture segment was laid open. The stricture length was measured using a measuring ruler.

BMG harvesting was done in rose position with a sandbag under the shoulder blade and neck extended. Dingman retractor was used to retract the jaws apart. The graft that needs to be harvested was outlined with a marker pen for one centimeter more than the measurement of stricture (Figures 1(a) and 1(b)), taking care to exclude the opening of Stensen's duct. 10 ml solution of 2% lignocaine diluted with adrenaline (1 : 80,000) was injected to achieve hydrodissection. Using a scalpel, the margins of the graft were defined over the pen markings. Holding sutures were taken at the ends of the graft, for better grip. Metzenbaum curved scissor was used to dissect buccal mucosa from underlying buccinator muscle, and the graft was harvested. The donor site haemostasis was secured, was packed with adrenaline-saline soaked gauze pack, and left to heal with secondary intention. The harvested graft was then placed in a kidney tray, and the unstretched length and width of the grafts were measured (Figures 1(c) and 1(d)). The measurement was double-checked by different members of the surgical team to minimise measurement errors. Defattening of the graft was done. The oral gauze pack was removed after 4 hours, and the patient was advised to take fluid diet for 48 hours followed by bland semisolids till they could tolerate normal diet. The oral buccal mucosal wound was inspected every 12 hours for bleeding, wound infection, or restriction of mouth opening till the hospital stay.

2.2. Statistical Analysis. Pre- and postharvest size of BMG was compared using a paired t-test. Descriptive data were presented in the form of mean, range, percentage, and standard deviation. Statistical analysis was completed using SPSS software, version 21.0 (IBM Corp, NY, USA). Statistical significance was kept below 0.05. The confidence interval was set at 95%.

3. Results

Forty four patients who fulfilled the inclusion and exclusion criteria were included in this study. Demographic data are presented in Table 1.

Forty patients (91%) underwent dorsolateral onlay (Kulkarni technique) [8], and 4 (9%) underwent ventral onlay BMG urethroplasty. The mucosal graft was taken from one cheek in 59%, whereas from both cheeks in 41%. The mean operative time for unilateral buccal mucosal graft harvesting was 23 minutes, and for bilateral harvesting, it was 41 minutes. Table 2 lists the pre- and postharvest measurement of the graft.

Mean preharvest and postharvest BMG length was 8.3 and 7.6 cm, respectively (Figure 2) which showed a statistically significant decrease (8.4%, $p < 0.001$) in length. Mean pre- and postharvest BMG width was 1.5 and 1.3 cm, respectively (Figure 2) which also showed a statistically significant decrease (9.5%, $p < 0.001$) in width.

In patients aged more than 55 years, the mean pre- and postharvest BMG dimensions were 8.9×1.5 and 8.2×1.3 cm, respectively. While in patients aged less than 55 years, the mean pre- and postharvest BMG dimensions were 8.1×1.5 and 7.5×1.3 cm, respectively. However, the differences in the contracture between the age groups were not statistically significant (Table 3). Tobacco usage was found in 59% of patients. The mean pre- and postharvest BMG dimensions were $8.3 \times 1.5$and 7.6×1.3 cm, respectively in tobacco users. The mean pre- and postharvest BMG dimensions were 8.4×1.4 and 7.7×1.3 cm in those not using tobacco. However, the differences in the contracture between both the groups were statistically insignificant (Table 3).

The complications in the donor site are listed in Table 4.

4. Discussion

Outcome-related variables in augmentation urethroplasty can be listed as surgical technique, graft quality, stricture characteristics, and patient-related factors. Nontransection of urethra during urethroplasty had better results than transecting urethroplasty [9]. Kulkarni et al. [8] reported that dorsolateral mobilisation of the urethra and preservation of unilateral urethral vascularity is associated with better outcomes of augmentation urethroplasty. Breyer et al. [10] reported that length, site of stricture, and previous surgeries are independent predictors of stricture in multivariate analysis.

Type of graft and graft contracture are other outcome-related variables in augmentation urethroplasty. Skin, bladder, and intestinal and oral mucosa (buccal, lingual, and labial) grafts are the preferred sites of donors for the reconstruction of the urethra [11]. The properties of buccal mucosa such as the absence of hair follicle, highly vascular lamina propria promoting early in growth, wet environment compatibility [12], and ease of harvest with a concealed donor site scar makes it a near ideal substitute for urethra.

The incidence of graft contracture in BMG urethroplasty varies from 3 to 22.5% in various studies [13–18]. Oral mucosal grafts are also used in the ocular reconstructive

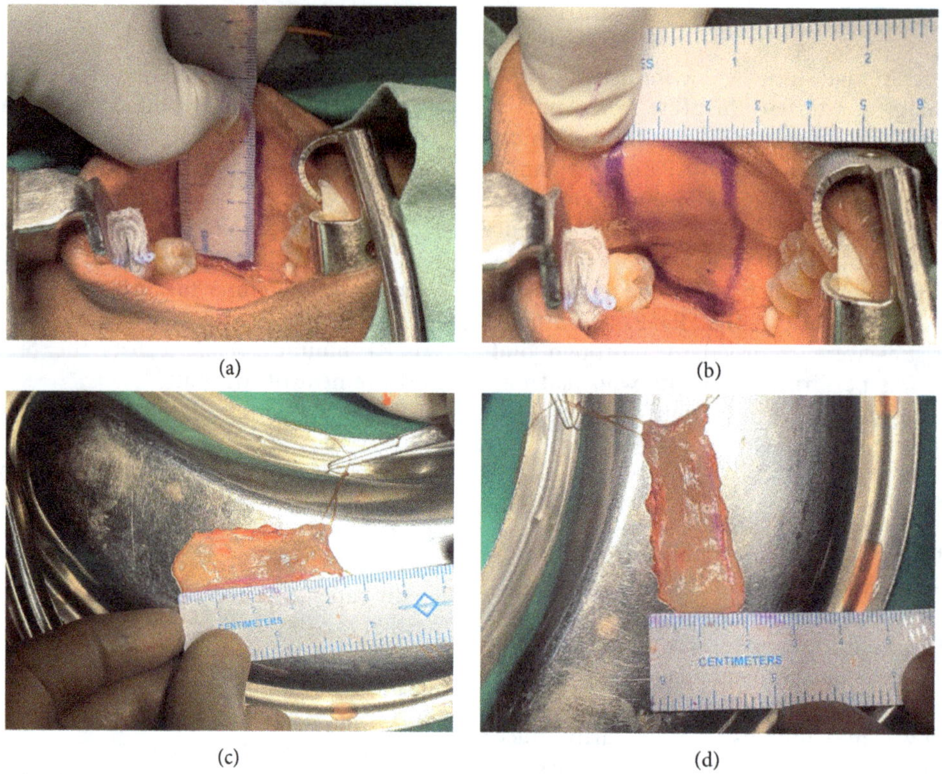

FIGURE 1: The marking and measurement of the preharvest buccal mucosal graft (a, b) and postharvest measurements of length and breadth (c, d).

TABLE 1: Demographic data.

Parameters	Total ($N = 44$)
Age (years)	53.6 (28–74)*
Length of the stricture (cm)	7.45 (3–12)*
Tobacco users, n (%)	26 (59.09)

*Data expressed as mean and range in brackets.

TABLE 2: Pre- and postharvest measurement of the graft.

Buccal mucosal graft	Preharvest	Postharvest	Shrinkage in %
Length in cm (mean (±SD))	8.33 (±2.41)	7.64 (±2.34)	8.43 (±2.56)
Breadth in cm (mean (±SD))	1.46 (±0.13)	1.32 (±0.11)	9.51 (±3.69)

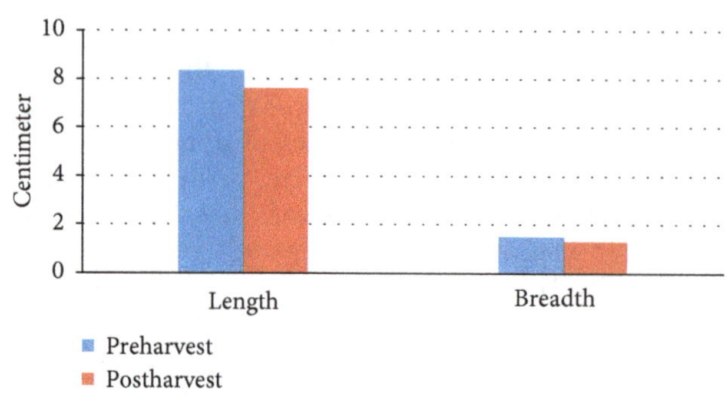

FIGURE 2: Preharvest vs. postharvest measurements.

surgeries [19]. Graft contracture has been noticed in these ocular reconstructive surgeries [19]. It has been reported that graft contracture is less when harvested from hard palate [19].

Graft contracture leads to suboptimal results in BMG urethroplasty. Primary graft contracture, if not accounted for, can lead to overstretching of the graft. This graft overstretching can widen the urethral lumen initially, but in long term, the graft can shrink rapidly, especially after the removal of the catheter. Prior knowledge of the extent of primary graft contracture can give an estimate of extra size of the graft needed. To some extent, primary graft contracture can be dealt by meshing, spreading, and suture fixation of the graft. However, this can be challenging if the size of the urethral defect is large. Surprisingly, no study has focused on this issue in BMG urethroplasty. In our study, we found 8.4% decrease in length and 9.5% decrease in the width of the BMG. As we took one centimeter extrasize graft, tension-free anastomosis was possible. Loss of elastic recoil is the reason for primary graft contracture [20]. The extent of primary skin graft contracture ranges from 9 to 22% [20, 21]. Age is postulated to affect the extent of primary graft contracture in skin grafts [21]. But in our study, age did not influence primary graft contracture of BMG significantly. Smoking and oral tobacco usage is known to cause various intraoral pathologies such as smoker's palate, smoker's melanosis, oral submucosal fibrosis, leukoplakia, leukoedema, and oral cancers [22]. However, the extent of BMG contracture did not vary significantly between tobacco users and nontobacco users. Patel et al. reported that there was not

Table 3: Comparison of factors associated with the contracture of buccal mucosal graft.

Factors	% contracture in length	% contracture in width
Age <55 years ($n = 32$)	8.54	10.10
Age >55 years ($n = 12$)	8.27	8.94
p value	0.63	0.38
Smokers/tobacco users ($n = 26$)	8.52	9.60
Nonsmokers/nontobacco users ($n = 18$)	8.24	9.11
p value	0.63	0.66

Table 4: Postoperative donor site complication.

Donor site complications	Total ($n = 44$)
Immediate complications n (%)	
Oral cavity bleeding	2 (4.54)
Pain	38 (86.37)
Facial swelling	28 (63.64)
Restriction of mouth opening	30 (68.18)
Oral numbness	25 (56.82)
Persistent (>4 weeks) complications n (%)	
Restriction of mouth opening	1 (2.27)
Oral numbness	4 (9.09)

much long-term difference in the restriction of mouth opening after BMG harvest in smokers and nonsmokers [23].

Larger size graft creates larger raw area in the donor site. It leads to inability to close the donor site. Muruganandham et al. [24] reported no changes in long-term graft site morbidity when the graft site is left open or closed. Wood et al. [25] reported no significant difference in obtaining a repeat graft from the buccal mucosal donor site, whether it was closed or left open in the previous harvest. In fact, the severity of pain in the immediate postoperative period is less when the graft site is left open. Immediate postoperative pain (86.4%) is the commonest complication following BMG harvest in our study. Akyüz et al. [26] reported the similar incidence of facial pain (85.7%), while Muruganandam et al. [24] reported to be 83%. The pain and swelling resolves with short duration anti-inflammatory therapy.

Previous studies have reported oral cavity bleeding after BMG harvest in 5–21% [2, 24, 27]. The incidence of persistent oral cavity bleeding is 4.5% in our study. Patel et al. [23] showed that, after achieving complete haemostasis, the buccal mucosal graft site could be left open without suturing to heal by secondary intention and without any significant complications.

Persistent oral numbness (9.1%) and restricted mouth opening (2.3%) are the common long-term sequelae following BMG harvest in our study. Behura et al. [22] in their study noted that the restriction of mouth opening was transient and resolved with time. Castagnetti et al. [27] reported that these complications are not related to the size of graft but are a consequence of dissection of buccinator muscle. They further reported that these complications can be minimised by infiltrating diluted local anaesthesia or saline, aiding hydrodissection of the graft followed by surgical dissection.

Salivatory problems such as excessive salivation or decreased salivation have been reported following BMG harvest [24, 27]. These problems are attributed to parotid/Stensen's duct opening and minor salivary glands injury and are usually transient [27]. None of our patients reported any long-term salivatory problems. Moreover, our patients could tolerate their regular diet within 72 hours, when compared to prior studies [27].

The relatively small sample size was one of the limitations of this study. We did not measure the thickness of the graft and hence could not relate the bearing of graft thickness with the shrinkage rate. Since all the donor sites were left open for healing, we could not compare the morbidity with the donor sites which could have been sutured.

5. Conclusion

Primary graft contracture in buccal mucosa is around 8.4% in length and 9.5% in width. It would be better to mark wider than necessary while harvesting buccal mucosa to obtain a tension-free and successful BMG urethroplasty. Donor site morbidity is reasonable if it is left open and allowed to heal by secondary intention.

References

[1] S. Bhargava and C. R. Chapple, "Buccal mucosal urethroplasty: is it the new gold standard?" *BJU International*, vol. 93, no. 9, pp. 1191–1193, 2004.

[2] M. R. Markiewicz, J. L. DeSantis, J. E. Margarone, M. A. Pogrel, and S. K. Chuang, "Morbidity associated with oral mucosa harvest for urological reconstruction: an overview," *Journal of Oral and Maxillofacial Surgery*, vol. 66, pp. 739–744, 2008.

[3] S. P. Elliott, M. J. Metro, and J. W. McAninch, "Long-term followup of the ventrally placed buccal mucosa onlay graft in bulbar urethral reconstruction," *Journal of Urology*, vol. 169, no. 5, pp. 1754–1757, 2003.

[4] T. Heinke, E. W. Gerharz, R. Bonfig, and H. Riedmiller, "Ventral onlay urethroplasty using buccal mucosa for complex stricture repair," *Urology*, vol. 61, no. 5, pp. 1004–1007, 2003.

[5] C. J. Kane, G. J. Tarman, D. J. Summerton et al., "Multi-institutional experience with buccal mucosa onlay urethroplasty for bulbar urethral reconstruction," *The Journal of Urology*, vol. 167, pp. 1314–1317, 2002.

[6] D. S. Kellner, J. A. Fracchia, and N. A. Armenakas, "Ventral onlay buccal mucosal grafts for anterior urethral strictures: long-term followup," *Journal of Urology*, vol. 171, no. 2, pp. 726–729, 2004.

[7] G. Patino, M. Y. Zheng, B. N. Breyer, and A. J. Cohen, "Skin grafting applications in urology," *Reviews in Urology*, vol. 21, no. 1, pp. 8–14, 2019.

[8] S. Kulkarni, G. Barbagli, S. Sansalone, and M. Lazzeri, "One-sided anterior urethroplasty: a new dorsal onlay graft technique," *BJU International*, vol. 104, no. 8, pp. 1150–1155, 2009.

[9] S. Ivaz, S. Bugeja, A. Frost, D. Andrich, and A. R. Mundy, "The nontransecting approach to bulbar urethroplasty," *Urologic Clinics of North America*, vol. 44, no. 1, pp. 57–66, 2017.

[10] B. N. Breyer, J. W. McAninch, J. M. Whitson et al., "Multivariate analysis of risk factors for long-term urethroplasty outcome," *The Journal of Urology*, vol. 183, no. 2, pp. 613–617, 2010.

[11] M. E. Levy and S. P. Elliott, "Graft use in bulbar urethroplasty," *Urologic Clinics of North America*, vol. 44, no. 1, pp. 39–47, 2017.

[12] D. Filipas, M. Fisch, J. Fichtner et al., "The histology and immunohistochemistry of free buccal mucosa and full-skin grafts after exposure to urine," *BJU International*, vol. 84, no. 1, pp. 108–111, 1999.

[13] K. N. Haxhirexha, M. Castagnetti, W. Rigamonti, and G. A. Manzoni, "Two-stage repair in hypospadias," *Indian Journal of Urology*, vol. 24, pp. 226–232, 2008.

[14] M. Spilotros, N. Sihra, S. Malde et al., "Buccal mucosal graft urethroplasty in men-risk factors for recurrence and complications: a third referral centre experience in anterior urethroplasty using buccal mucosal graft," *Translational Andrology and Urology*, vol. 6, no. 3, pp. 510–516, 2017.

[15] M. Selim, S. Salem, E. Elsherif, A. Badawy, M. Elshazely, and M. Gawish, "Outcome of staged buccal mucosal graft for repair of long segment anterior urethral stricture," *BMC Urology*, vol. 19, no. 1, p. 38, 2019.

[16] H. A. Aldaqadossi, H. Shaker, H. Youssof, Y. Kotb, and M. Eladawy, "Outcomes of staged lingual mucosal graft urethroplasty for redo hypospadias repair," *Journal of Pediatric Urology*, vol. 15, no. 5, pp. 519.el–519.e7, 2019.

[17] F. Campos-Juanatey, S. Bugeja, M. Dragova et al., "Single-stage tubular urethral reconstruction using oral grafts is an alternative to classical staged approach for selected penile urethral strictures," *Asian Journal of Andrology*, vol. 22, no. 2, pp. 134–139, 2020.

[18] A. Sakr, E. Elkady, M. Abdalla et al., "Lingual mucosal graft two-stage Bracka technique for redo hypospadias repair," *Arab Journal of Urology*, vol. 15, no. 3, pp. 236–241, 2017.

[19] C. Mai and E. Bertelmann, "Oral mucosal grafts: old technique in new light," *Ophthalmic Research*, vol. 50, no. 2, pp. 91–98, 2013.

[20] A. B. Berezovsky, V. A. Pagkalos, E. Silberstein, Y. Shoham, L. Rosenberg, and Y. Krieger, "Primary contraction of skin grafts: a porcine preliminary study," *Plastic and Aesthetic Research*, vol. 2, pp. 22–26, 2015.

[21] C. A. Harrison and S. MacNeil, "The mechanism of skin graft contraction: an update on current research and potential future therapies," *Burns*, vol. 34, no. 2, pp. 153–163, 2008.

[22] S. S. Behura, M. K. Masthan, and A. B. Narayanasamy, "Oral mucosal lesions associated with smokers and chewers—a case-control study in Chennai population," *Journal of Clinical and Diagnostic Research: JCDR*, vol. 9, no. 7, pp. ZC17–ZC22, 2015.

[23] K. Patel, J. Kalathia, and V. Krishnamoorthy, "Objective assessment of mouth opening after buccal mucosal graft urethroplasty: a prospective study," *Urology Annals*, vol. 12, pp. 259–265, 2020.

[24] K. Muruganandam, D. Dubey, A. K. Gulia et al., "Closure versus nonclosure of buccal mucosal graft harvest site: a prospective randomized study on post operative morbidity," *Indian Journal of Urology*, vol. 25, pp. 72–75, 2009.

[25] D. N. Wood, S. E. Allen, D. E. Andrich, T. J. Greenwell, and A. R. Mundy, "The morbidity of buccal mucosal graft harvest for urethroplasty and the effect of nonclosure of the graft harvest site on postoperative pain," *Journal of Urology*, vol. 172, no. 2, pp. 580–583, 2004.

[26] M. Akyüz, M. Gunes, O. Koca, Z. Sertkaya, H. Kanberoglu, and M. I. Karaman, "Evaluation of intraoral complications of buccal mucosa graft in augmentation urethroplasty," *Türk Üroloji Dergisi/Turkish Journal of Urology*, vol. 40, no. 3, pp. 156–160, 2014.

[27] M. Castagnetti, V. Ghirardo, A. Capizzi, M. Andretta, and W. Rigamonti, "Donor site outcome after oral mucosa harvest for urethroplasty in children and adults," *Journal of Urology*, vol. 180, no. 6, pp. 2624–2628, 2008.

12

Risk Factors of Ureteral Stenosis in Kidney Transplant Recipients: A Retrospective Study in National Referral Hospital in Indonesia

Gampo A. Irdam, Bobby Sutojo, and Putu A. R. Raharja

Department of Urology, Faculty of Medicine Universitas Indonesia, Cipto Mangunkusumo Hospital, Jakarta 10430, Indonesia051

Correspondence should be addressed to Gampo A. Irdam; gampoai@gmail.com

Academic Editor: Paddy Dewan

Ureteral stenosis is one of the most common urological complications following kidney transplantations. It is occurred in 2–10% of patients and poses a significant problem to the patients as it may lead to permanent damage to renal damage. Identification of risk factors is important to prevent the incidence of ureteral stenosis. Thus, we aim to determine the risk factors of ureteral stenosis in the Indonesian population. This is a retrospective analysis of 487 kidney transplant patients performed in Cipto Mangunkusumo Hospital between 2014 and 2018. We collected and compared donor and recipient demography data in recipients who developed ureteral stenosis and recipients who did not develop ureteral stenosis. Ureteral stenosis was defined as the presence of hydronephrosis from ultrasound and increased number of serum creatinine. The overall incidence of ureteral stenosis post-kidney transplantation in our center is 6.6% (32 from 487 patients) from January 2014 until June 2018. We found that older donor and recipient age more frequent in developing ureteral stenosis post-kidney transplantation ($p < 0.001$). We also found that donors with number of arteries more than 2 ($p < 0.001$) and prolonged warm ischemic time ($p < 0.05$) are more frequently to develop ureteral stenosis post-kidney transplantation. There is no association between type II diabetes mellitus and hypertension with ureteral stenosis in this study. Donor age, recipient age, donor number of arteries more than 2, and prolonged warm ischemia time are associated with ureteral stenosis after kidney transplantation.

1. Introduction

End-stage renal disease (ESRD) is a worldwide public health problem with increasing prevalence each year. Based on the Medicare-funded program, there was an increase from approximately 10,000 cases in 1973 to 703,243 in 2015 in the United States [1]. In 2014, the Indonesian Renal Registry showed the annual ESRD incidence of 35,000 patients and prevalence of 120,000 patients [2]. There are some renal replacement therapy modalities for ESRD including hemodialysis, peritoneal dialysis, and kidney transplantation [1, 2]. Kidney transplantation has been considered as the best treatment for ESRD which provides not only better long-term survival but also a better quality of life than other types of renal replacement therapy [3, 4]. Acute graft rejection once becomes a major concern in kidney transplantation [5–7], but advances in the management of graft rejection have led to decreased number of graft failures and improvement of patient survival rates [5, 6]. Reduced number of graft failures apparently is followed by an increase in posttransplant urological complications [7]. The most common urological complication following kidney transplantation is ureteral stenosis [5], which occurred in 2–10% of patients receiving kidney transplantation [4]. Ureteral stenosis poses significant problems to patients with kidney transplantation as it may lead to permanent damage to the renal allograft [6].

Almost 70% of ureteral obstructions following kidney transplantation were observed within 3 months [8]. Ischemia is probably the main reason, but it is difficult to demonstrate this directly. Some authors reported donor age as the risk factor for stenosis [9], while some other authors denied this finding [10]. The number of allograft arteries is the other risk factor. Some authors even reported cases of ureteral stenosis caused by CMV infection [8]. However, no studies have been conducted in Indonesian population to identify the risk factors of ureteral stenosis after kidney transplantation. Thus, we aim to determine the risk factors of allograft ureteral stenosis following kidney transplantation in Indonesian population.

2. Methods

This is a retrospective cohort study of 487 renal transplants performed in Cipto Mangunkusumo Hospital (National Referral Hospital in Indonesia) between January 2014 and June 2018. The surgical transplantation technique was quite homogeneous during the entire study. We included all the patients that underwent kidney transplantation between the study time. Diagnosis of ureteral stenosis is defined as the presence of hydronephrosis (dilated renal calyces and pelvis) from ultrasound and increased number of serum creatinine and decreased urine output (<100 mL/day) [10]. These findings were then confirmed using antegrade or retrograde pyelography. All other causes of graft function impairment, i.e., acute rejection, hematoma, lymphocele, and urine collections, were ruled out. All patients were stented.

Transplantation procedure was done by the technique of anastomosis of the renal vein followed by renal artery anastomosis. We performed end-to-side anastomosis between the graft renal vein and the recipient's external iliac vein by extraperitoneal approach. The arterial anastomosis was done by end-to-side anastomosis to the external iliac artery. Extravesical ureteroneocystostomy was done by Lich–Gregoir technique. Vascular reconstruction in multiple renal arteries was done by side-to-side anastomosis on small vessels with end-to-side anastomosis of the smaller artery to the main artery, side-to-side anastomosis of similar-sized arteries, and anastomosis to the recipient internal, external, or common iliac and hypogastric arteries [11].

We collected the demographic data, intraoperative parameters, and postoperative parameters from both donor and recipient. Data were presented using tables. We then compared the demographic, intraoperative, and postoperative data with the occurrence of ureteral stenosis with statistical analysis using Statistical Package for the Social Sciences (SPSS) version 23. The data were compared, and the p value was measured to define the clinical significance. The data were presented in frequency and mean or median (mean if the data's distribution is normal and median if the distribution is abnormal). Continuous variables were compared using independent t-test if the data were normally distributed or Mann–Whitney test if the data were not normally distributed. Categorical variables were compared with chi-square test. p value less than 0.05 was considered statistically significant.

3. Results

The overall incidence of ureteral stenosis post-kidney transplantation in our center is 6.6% (32 from 487 patients) from January 2014 until June 2018. In this study, the median age of the donor is 31 (18–50) years; meanwhile, the median age of the recipient is 47 (8–78) years and majority of donor and recipient is male (69.6% and 73.3%, respectively). About 29.6% of the recipients had a history of diabetes mellitus and 60.8% had a history of hypertension. Only 5 recipients had neurogenic bladder condition. The demographic data of subjects are shown in Table 1.

The comparison of demographic data, intraoperative parameters, and postoperative parameters between ureteral stenosis and nonureteral stenosis groups is shown in Table 2. We found that there were significant differences in donor and recipient age in patients who develop ureteral stenosis following kidney transplantation. The older age of donor and recipient was more likely to develop ureteral stenosis postoperatively ($p < 0.001$). No difference was found in donor and recipient sex between the two groups ($p = 0.2$ and $p = 0.85$). The relationship between donor and recipient also did not play a significant role in developing ureteral stenosis after kidney transplantation ($p = 0.68$).

We found that donors with more than 2 allograft arteries were more frequently to develop ureteral stenosis post-kidney transplantation (12.5% vs. 0.9%, $p < 0.001$); meanwhile, the number of allograft veins did not play a significant role. We also found that prolonged warm ischemic time is correlated with the development of ureteral stenosis ($p = 0.038$). Recipient comorbidities (type 2 diabetes mellitus and hypertension) also did not seem to have a major role in causing ureteral stenosis postoperatively ($p = 0.55$ and $p = 0.08$, respectively). History of previous kidney transplantation also did not seem to increase the risk of ureteral stenosis ($p = 0.47$). The difference between preoperative and postoperative levels of creatinine in the two groups also did not show statistical significance ($p = 0.65$ and $p = 0.94$).

4. Discussion

In spite of recent advances in urological surgical technique, continuous improvement, and center's experience, ureteral stenosis remains the most common urological complication following kidney transplantation. We report an incidence of 6.8% (37 from 545 patients) of ureteral stenosis after kidney transplantation in our center from 2014 until 2018. This number is not much different from previously reported in the literature as Karam et al. and Fontana et al. reported incidence of ureteral stenosis in the first month after transplantation is between 2 and 7.5% [6, 7].

There are various etiologies of ureteral stenosis, as mentioned before, such as technical error and external compression (hematoma, lymphocele, abscess, kinking redundant ureter, ureteral stone, anastomotic edema, and ureteral ischemia) [12]. Ureteral ischemia is known as the most common etiology for ureteral stenosis, which accounted for 60–95% of cases of ureteral stenosis. The distal ureter is the most vulnerable part of the ureter to develop ureteral ischemia owing to its anatomical location that is the furthest part of the renal artery [5]. In our center, we also found many patients with impaired ureteral vascularization that might precipitate ureteral ischemia.

From this study, we found that donor age, recipient age, number of arteries > 2, and prolonged warm ischemia time

TABLE 1: Demographic data of the patients.

	Frequencies or mean
Donor age (years)	31 (18–50)
Recipient age (years)	47 (8–78)
Donor sex (male)	339 (69.6%)
Recipient sex (male)	357 (73.3%)
Recipient with type II diabetes mellitus	144 (29.6%)
Recipient with hypertension	396 (60.8%)
Recipient with neurogenic bladder	5 (1.03%)

TABLE 2: Comparison of demographic data, intraoperative parameters, and postoperative parameters between the ureteral stenosis group and nonureteral stenosis group.

	Ureteral stenosis ($n = 32$ patients)	Without ureteral stenosis ($n = 455$ patients)	p value
Donor age (years)	40.5 (24–50)	30 (18–50)	<0.001*
Donor sex			
Male, n (%)	18 (56.3%)	321 (70.5%)	0.13
Female, n (%)	14 (43.7%)	134 (29.5%)	
Donor-recipient relationship			0.68
Not related, n (%)	6 (18. 8%)	99 (21.8%)	
Related, n (%)	26 (81. 2%)	356 (78.2%)	
Donor site of transplant			0.83
Right, n (%)	2 (6.3%)	33 (7.3%)	
Left, n (%)	30 (93.7%)	422 (92.7%)	
Donor history of abdominal surgery	2 (6.3%)	27 (5.9%)	0.94
Donor number of veins			0.40
>1, n (%)	1 (3.1%)	6 (1.3%)	
≤1, n (%)	31 (96.9%)	449 (98.7%)	
Donor number of arteries			<0.001*
>2, n (%)	4 (12.5%)	4 (0.9%)	
≤2, n (%)	28 (87.5%)	451 (99.1%)	
Warm ischemic time (min)	2422 (1892–4473)	2295 (293–5523)	0.038*
Cold ischemic time (min)	1737 (1658–1817)	1892 (836–6480)	0.42
Time to urinate (sec)	328 (151–506)	125 (32–982)	0.93
Donor body mass index (kg/m^2)	19.9 (19–20.8)	23 (17.1–33.5)	0.62
Recipient preoperative creatinine (mg/dL)	6.1 (1–14.4)	5.35 (5.3–5.4)	0.65
Recipient postoperative creatinine (mg/dL)	1.25 (1.1–1.4)	1.1 (0.3–19)	0.94
Recipient length of prior dialysis (month)	52.5 (21–84)	10 (1–216)	0.75
Recipient resistive index	0.67 (0.61–0.73)	0.72 (0.06–0.91)	0.98
Recipient age (years)	44 (19–77)	48 (8–78)	<0.001*
Recipient sex			0.85
Male, n (%)	23 (71.9%)	334 (73.4%)	
Female, n (%)	9 (28.1%)	121 (26.6%)	
Recipient history of type II DM			0.55
Yes, n (%)	8 (25%)	136 (29.9%)	
No, n (%)	24 (75%)	319 (70.1%)	
Recipient history of HT			0.08
Yes, n (%)	24 (75%)	272 (59.8%)	
No, n (%)	8 (25%)	183 (40.2%)	
Recipient history of transplantation			0.47
Yes, n (%)	2 (6.3%)	17 (3.7%)	
No, n (%)	30 (93.7%)	438 (96.3%)	

*Significant difference.

were associated with ureteral stenosis after kidney transplantation. Arpalli et al [13] reported that advanced donor age has a higher risk for developing ureteral stenosis after kidney transplantation (Cox HR: 1.03 (1.01–1.05) $p = 0.03$). Fontana et al. also reported the same result that donor age >65 years is more likely to develop ureteral stenosis ($p = 0.001$). Advanced age donor has been established as the independent risk factor for ureteral obstruction following kidney transplantation from various literature studies. Older donors usually have vascular problems that favorably cause ureteral ischemia. Older donor kidneys are also usually more susceptible to damage from cold ischemia, and small differences can have a significant impact on organ function. It is also reported that there is a higher rate of lymphocele formation in older donor kidney transplant, possibly due to more difficult surgical resection in older patients. This is due to higher fragility of renal lymphatic vessels and more abundant perihilar fatty tissue [6, 7, 13].

Recipient donor age was also reported as an independent factor for developing ureteral stenosis. Arpalli reported that younger recipient age at donor is 3% more unlikely to develop a ureteral stenosis over 15 years (Cox HR: 0.97 (0.95–0.99) $p = 0.01$). This is due to more frequent vascular problems that can cause ureteral ischemia and due to underdiagnosed benign prostate hypertrophy (BPH) in previously anuric or oliguric patients that cause many posttransplantation complications [13].

More than two renal arteries were found to be associated with ureteral stenosis after kidney transplant in this study. Rahnemai-Azar et al. [14] also reported the same result (OR 2.48 (1.16–3.34), $p = 0.02$) that is explained by relative ischemia of the ureter due to malperfusion of accessory arteries from small anastomosis, greater turbulence, or more vulnerability of the arteries for traction injury. Multiple renal arteries, theoretically, pose a significant risk for postoperative risk after renal transplantation. Even at the beginning of the transplantation era, multiple renal arteries are considered as a contraindication. However, several techniques have been developed to reconstruct the multiple renal arteries and reported to significantly reduce vascular complications.

The clinical significance of these results can be taken for early diagnosis and prevention of ureteral stenosis after kidney transplantation in Indonesian population. Patients with high-risk profiles have to undergo several monitoring techniques to diagnose and evaluate the development of ureteral stenosis over time [15]. The modalities include ultrasonography, computed tomography scan, magnetic resonance urography, and scintigraphy. Identification of high-risk profiles can lead to more cost-efficient evaluation of patients with kidney transplantation. Also, prevention of ureteral stenosis can be taken by the placement of ureteral stent that has proven effective to prevent ureteral stenosis [16].

5. Conclusion

Donor age, recipient age, number of arteries > 2, and prolonged warm ischemia time are associated with ureteral stenosis after kidney transplantation.

References

[1] United States Renal Data System, *USRDS 2010 Annual Data Report: Atlas of Chronic Kidney Disease and End-Stage Renal Disease in the United States*, National Institute of Diabetes and Digestive and Kidney Diseases, Bethesda, MD, USA, 2010.

[2] K. L. C. Afiatin and E. Kristin, "Economic evaluation of policy options for dialysis in end-stage renal disease patients under the universal health coverage in Indonesia," *PLoS One*, vol. 12, no. 5, Article ID e0177436, 2017.

[3] L. S. Borden, V. M. Pais, and D. G. Assimos, "Repetitive ureteral stenting for management of transplant graft ureteral obstruction," *International Brazilian Journal of Urology*, vol. 32, no. 2, 2006.

[4] S. Kumar, J. H. Jeon, A. Hakim, S. Shrivastava, D. Banerjee, and U. Patel, "Long-term graft and patient survival after balloon dilation of ureteric stenosis after renal transplant: a 23-year retrospective matched cohort study," *Radiology*, vol. 281, no. 1, pp. 301–310, 2016.

[5] P. Leonardou, S. Gioldasi, and P. Pappas, "Percutaneous management of ureteral stenosis of transplanted kidney: technical and clinical aspects," *Urologia Internationalis*, vol. 87, no. 4, pp. 375–379, 2011.

[6] G. Karam, J.-F. Hetet, F. Maillet et al., "Late ureteral stenosis following renal transplantation: risk factors and impact on patient and graft survival," *American Journal of Transplantation*, vol. 6, no. 2, pp. 352–356, 2006.

[7] I. Fontana, M. Bertocchi, A. M. Rossi et al., "Late ureteral stenosis after kidney transplantation: a single-center experience," *Transplantation Proceedings*, vol. 42, no. 4, pp. 1174-1175, 2010.

[8] B. F. Schwartz, J. R. Chatham, P. Bretan, R. Goharderakhshan, and M. L. Stoller, "Treatment of refractory kidney transplant ureteral strictures using balloon cautery endoureterotomy," *Urology*, vol. 58, no. 4, pp. 536–539, 2001.

[9] J. Safa, N. Nezami, M. K. Tarzamni et al., "Post-transplant urological and vascular complications," *Saudi Journal of Kidney Disease and Transplantation*, vol. 20, pp. 867–871, 2009.

[10] J. A. Lowell, R. J. Stratta, J. J. Morton, P. C. Kolbeck, and R. J. Taylor, "Invasive cytomegalovirus infection in A renal transplant ureter after combined pancreas-kidney transplantation: an unusual cause of renal allograft dysfunction," *Journal of Urology*, vol. 152, no. 5 Part 1, pp. 1546–1548, 1994.

[11] E. C. Jeong, S. H. Hwang, and S. R. Eo, "Vascular augmentation in renal transplantation: supercharging and turbocharging," *Archives of Plastic Surgery*, vol. 44, no. 3, pp. 238–242, 2017.

[12] B. D. Duty and J. M. Barry, "Diagnosis and management of ureteral complications following renal transplantation," *Asian Journal of Urology*, vol. 2, no. 4, pp. 202–207, 2015.

[13] E. Arpali, T. Al-Qaoud, E. Martinez et al., "Impact of ureteral stricture and treatment choice on long-term graft survival in kidney transplantation," *American Journal of Transplantation*, vol. 18, no. 8, pp. 1977–1985, 2018.

[14] A. A. Rahnemai-Azar, B. F. Gilchrist, and L. K. Kayler, "Independent risk factors for early urologic complications after kidney transplantation," *Clinical Transplantation*, vol. 29, no. 5, pp. 403–408, 2015.

[15] D. Hernández, M. Rufino, S. Armas et al., "Retrospective analysis of surgical complications following cadaveric kidney transplantation in the modern transplant era," *Nephrology Dialysis Transplantation*, vol. 21, no. 10, pp. 2908–2915, 2006.

[16] R. S. Mangus and B. W. Haag, "Stented versus nonstented extravesical ureteroneocystostomy in renal transplantation: a metaanalysis," *American Journal of Transplantation*, vol. 4, no. 11, pp. 1889–1896, 2004.

13

Histoprotective Effect of Essential Oil from *Citrus aurantifolia* in Testosterone-Induced Benign Prostatic Hyperplasia Rat

Desmond O. Acheampong,[1] Isaac K. Barffour,[1] Alex Boye,[2] Ernest A. Asiamah,[1] Francis A. Armah,[1] Christian K. Adokoh,[1] Joy F. Oluyemi,[1] Benjamin Adrah,[1] Richard Opoku,[1] and Emmanuel Adakudugu[1]

[1]*Department of Biomedical Sciences, School of Allied Health Sciences, University of Cape Coast, Cape Coast, Ghana*
[2]*Department of Medical Laboratory Science, School of Allied Health Sciences, University of Cape Coast, Cape Coast, Ghana*

Correspondence should be addressed to Desmond O. Acheampong; dacheampong@ucc.edu.gh

Academic Editor: Kostis Gyftopoulos

Background. Benign prostatic hyperplasia (BPH) is a common urological disorder reported among ageing men. *Objective.* The study assessed histoprotective effect of lime essential oil (LEO) in a rat model of testosterone-induced benign prostatic hyperplasia (BPH) and evaluated its ability to reverse testosterone-mediated changes in the testis, kidney, and liver. *Materials and Methods.* Adult Sprague Dawley (aged 12 weeks, 240–390 g) male rats were intramuscularly injected with testosterone enanthate (TE) (10 mg/kg) reconstituted in olive oil for ten days to establish benign prostatic hyperplasia (serum PSA level ≥ 1.24 ng/ml) in. After confirmation of BPH (sustained serum PSA level ≥ 1.24 ng/ml), rats in all groups (LEO: 30, 100, and 300 mg/kg, *po*, $n = 6$; finasteride: 15 mg/kg, *po*, $n = 6$) except model (BPH without treatment) and sham (no BPH and no treatment) groups were treated for 21 days. At the end of treatment, rats were anesthetised and blood was collected via cardiac puncture to determine serum PSA and total antioxidant capacity (TAC) levels. The prostate gland, testis, kidney, and liver were harvested, weighed, histologically processed and stained with H&E. *Results.* LEO- and finasteride-treated groups recorded lesser mean prostatic weights relative to their model group. Baseline mean serum PSA level of LEO- and finasteride-treated groups reduced significantly ($p < 0.05$) relative to model group. Serum TAC levels were also higher in LEO- and finasteride-treated groups relative to model group. LEO-treated groups had less thickened glandular epithelium, smaller acini, fewer prostatic secretions and more fibromuscular stroma relative to model group. LEO and finasteride treatment produced improved histomorphological characteristics of testis, kidney, and liver compared to model group. *Conclusion.* By the current results, *Citrus aurantifolia* LEO may possess active agents that can be explored for translational medicine against BPH.

1. Introduction

Benign prostatic hyperplasia (BPH) is a common urological disorder reported among ageing men [1]. The disorder is a non-malignant uncontrolled proliferation of the parenchymal cells of the prostate gland, resulting in the enlargement of the prostate gland [2]. The prostate gland is a critical reproductive organ in males and consists of branched tubuloacinar glandular epithelium embedded in a fibromuscular stroma. Secretion from the gland contributes one-fifth to one-third (20–33.3%) of seminal volume, and it is necessary for sperm activation owing to the composition of its secretions including citrate and enzymes such as fibrinolysin, hyaluronidase, and acid phosphate [3]. The pathophysiology of BPH is not clearly understood; however, its etiology is attributable to inflammatory [4] and/or oxidative stress [5]. Inflammation is known to have an association with excessive cell proliferation and death as compensatory hyperplasia could occur after cell death from chronic inflammation [6]. Oxidative stress also generates unstable chemical species that cause damage to mRNA, DNA, and proteins involved in cell death and proliferation [7]. Thus, antioxidant-rich and/or anti-inflammatory drug especially those of natural product origin may prevent or delay the progression of BPH. Interestingly, essential oils from *Citrus aurantifolia* have demonstrated both anti-inflammatory and antioxidant properties.

Lime essential oil is obtained from fruit peels of the *Citrus aurantifolia*. Lime essential oils have been investigated for their medicinal properties [8–11]. Nonetheless, its effect on uncontrolled BPH is yet to be studied and explored. Lime essential oil is locally used as a sweetener in the food industry but has recently been shown to possess antimicrobial [12, 13], anti-inflammatory [13], anticancer [8] and antioxidative [14] properties attributable to its phytochemical constituents. Thus, lime essential oil may be able to ameliorate variables which are indicative of benign prostatic hyperplasia. The study investigated the protective potential of lime essential oil (LEO) on the prostate gland in Sprague Dawley male albino rats experimentally induced with BPH.

BPH is also characterized by high serum and plasma testosterone levels. Hypertestosteronemia is reported to cause damage in the kidney, testis, and possibly, other body organs [15, 16]. The study also aimed at investigating if lime essential oil could ameliorate testosterone-induced histological changes in selected organs including the prostate gland, testis, liver, and kidney.

2. Materials and Methods

2.1. Drugs and Chemicals. Testosterone was purchased from ADD Pharma (GH) LTD, Accra, Ghana. Finasteride was purchased from Cape Coast Teaching Hospital pharmacy, Abura, Cape Coast, Ghana. Chemicals used in the study included phosphomolybdenum, a reagent prepared by mixing in 1 : 1 : 1 ratio, ammonium molybdate (4 mM), sodium phosphate (28 mM), and sulphuric acid (0.6 M), and ascorbic acid (20–200 μg/mL) from the biochemistry department, University of Cape Coast, Ghana.

2.2. Preparation of Essential Oil from Citrus aurantifolia Fruits. Oil was extracted from the unripened fruit peels of *Citrus aurantifolia* by hydrodistillation using a modified Clevenger apparatus. The unripe fruits of *Citrus aurantifolia* of the family Rutaceae were collected from Amissakrom Ekroful in the Mfantseman West District of the Central Region, Ghana. The samples were examined and authenticated at the Herbarium Unit of School of Biological Sciences, University of Cape Coast, Ghana, where a voucher specimen (SBS/UCC/102) was deposited.

2.3. GC/Mass Spectrometry Analysis of the Unripe LEO Chemical Composition. The LEO was stored in a refrigerator at 4°C prior to Gas chromatography Mass Spectrometry (GC-MS) analyses using a Hewlett Packard 6890 Series, equipped with a HP Chemstation data processor, fitted with a HP-Innowax bonded phase capillary column: 30 m × 320 μm id. and 0.50 μm film thickness (Hewlett Packard, Palo Alto, USA). The Column temperature was 40°C (8 min.) to 180°C at 3°C/min., 180–230°C at 20°C/min., 230°C (20 min.); injector temperature was 250°C and a detector temperature of 250°C was used. Carrier gas was H_2 (34 kPa), and split ratio 1 : 50, volume injected was 1 μL and was diluted in hexane (1 : 10) for hydrodistillation samples and 1 μL neat for supercritical extraction samples.

The GC/MS analysis was done in a 6890/MSD5973 Hewlett gas chromatograph with a mass selective detector, equipped with HP Chemstation software and using Wiley 275 spectra data [17] with few modifications. Briefly, a fused silica capillary column HP-Innowax: 30 m × 250 μm, 0.25 μm film thickness (Hewlett Packard, Palo Alto, USA) was used. The programmed temperature for GC/MS was the same as that of the GC analysis. The interface temperature and split ratio were 280°C and 1 : 100 respectively. The carrier gas He (56 kPa), flow rate: 1.0 mL/min., ionization energy 70 eV, mass range 40–350, volume injected 0.5 μL, and solvent cut 3.5 min. were used. The characterization of individual components was based on comparison of their GC retention indices (RI) on polar columns and comparison of their mass spectra by GC/MS to those described in literature.

2.4. Induction of BPH in Rats. Thirty-six (36) healthy adult male Sprague Dawley rats aged 12-week-old and weighing 240–390 g were purchased from the Animal Breeding Unit of Noguchi Memorial Institute for Medical Research, University of Ghana, Legon, Ghana, and transported to the Animal House of the School of Biological Science, University of Cape Coast, Ghana, where the experiment was conducted. The rats were allowed two weeks to acclimatize to laboratory conditions before commencement of the experiments under ambient conditions of temperature, relative humidity, and 12 hours light/dark cycle. They were provided with a standard pellet diet (Grower Mash, Essaar, Ghana) and water *ad libitum*.

BPH was established in 30 adult male rats by injecting (IM) testosterone enanthate (10 mg/kg) reconstituted in olive oil in alternate thighs of each rat for ten days. The remaining six rats were injected (IM) with olive oil (5 ml/kg) on alternate thighs for ten days. On the 11th day, rats were anesthetised with petroleum ether, and a cardiac puncture was carried out by a trained technician to collect blood for baseline serum PSA level determination. All the rats injected with testosterone enanthate had a serum PSA ≥ 1.24 ng/ml and were randomly reassigned into five groups of six. Rats were treated with LEO (30, 100, and 300 mg/kg, *po*) and finasteride (15 mg/kg, *po*) daily for 21 days, while rats in the model group had no any treatment except access to food and water. Rats which received only olive oil injection had a serum PSA of ≤ 0.0010 ng/ml and were used as the sham group.

Group 1: testosterone-enanthate + no lime essential oil/finasteride (model) ($n = 6$).

Group 2: testosterone-enanthate + 30 mg/kg of lime essential oil ($n = 6$).

Group 3: testosterone-enanthate + 100 mg/kg of lime essential oil ($n = 6$).

Group 4: testosterone-enanthate + 300 mg/kg of lime essential oil ($n = 6$).

Group 5: testosterone-enanthate + 15 mg/kg of finasteride ($n = 6$).

Group 6: olive oil + no lime essential oil/finasteride (sham) ($n = 6$).

2.5. Anesthesia Induction and Isolation of Organs. At the end of 21-day treatment, all the rats were anesthetised using chloroform inhalation, and cardiac puncture was performed following thoracotomy to collect blood for serum PSA levels and total antioxidant capacity (TAC) determination. The rats were sacrificed, and some organs (prostate gland, liver, kidney, and testis) were carefully harvested for routine tissue processing and HE staining.

2.6. Serum PSA Measurements Using ELISA. Commercial quantitative enzyme-linked immunosorbent assay was used to determine serum PSA levels in BPH induced rats. Twenty-five microlitres (25 μL) of either serum sample or calibrators (0, 2.5, 5.0, 10, 25, and 50 ng/ml of serum matrix PSA) were placed in microtitre wells precoated with 100 μL of antibody-enzyme conjugate (HRP-labeled anti-mouse PSA), mixed to form the sandwich complex on the surface of the wells, and were incubated for 30 minutes at 20–25°C. Excess conjugate and unbound antigen were washed five times using 300 μL solution consisting of 1 : 19 dilution of Tris-Buffered saline. A 100 μL substrate-reagent mixture made up of 1.2 mM 3,3′, 5,5′- tetramethylbenzidine (TMB) and ≤6.0 mM hydrogen peroxide was then added to each well after which the total mixture was incubated at 20–25°C at 15 minutes. The reaction was halted using 100 μL of 0.5 M sulphuric acid. The absorbance of the mixture was measured using Urit 680 microplate analyser at a wavelength of 450 nm. Serum PSA concentration subsequently computed from a straight line graph plotted using absorbance (as ordinate) and respective calibrator concentration (as abscissa).

2.7. Plasma Total Antioxidant Capacity (TAC). Total antioxidant capacity of the plasma was determined using the phosphomolybdenum method as described by Prieto et al. [18]. A reagent solution was prepared by mixing in 1 : 1 : 1 ratio, ammonium molybdate (4 mM), sodium phosphate (28 mM) and sulphuric acid (0.6 M). Five hundred microlitres (500 μL) of the plasma was mixed with 3 mL of the reagent solution in separate test tubes, and the reaction mixture was subsequently incubated at 95°C for 70 minutes. The absorbance of the mixture was measured at 695 nm using a spectrophotometer against blank after cooling to room temperature. The method was repeated using various concentrations (20–200 μg/mL) of the standard, ascorbic acid. Each concentration was prepared in duplicates. A mixture containing 0.5 mL methanol and 3 mL reagent solution was used as a blank. The total antioxidant capacity (TAC) of the plasma was expressed in ascorbic acid (AscAE) equivalents.

2.8. Statistical Analysis. Data were analysed using GraphPad Prism 7.00 software (GraphPad, La Jolla, CA, USA). The data were expressed as means ± standard error of mean (SEM) of each group. Statistical significance was then determined using analysis of variance (ANOVA). Tests that showed a significant difference among groups were analysed by a multiple comparison procedure using Bonferroni's multiple comparison tests. The level of significance was set at $p < 0.05$.

2.9. Ethical Approval. Experimental animals were handled in strict compliance with the guide for the Care and Humane Use of Laboratory Animals (National Research Council, 1996) and the U. Animals (Scientific Procedures) Act, 1986, and associated guidelines, EU Directive 2010/63/EU for animal experiments.

3. Results

3.1. Chemical Composition and Characterization of LEO. The GC/MS analyses of LEO led to the identification of ten (10) phyto-constituents (Table 1). The two major isomers of germacrene, A and B, were identified (61.2%), and were followed by pinene (14%) and bornane (11%), respectively. As presented in Table 1, the remaining components were linalool dimmer (2.9%), citral (2.9%), anethole (1.5%), anisole (1.1%), 2,6-dimethylheptan-2-ol (demitol) (0.6%), and safrole (0.3%). From the GC spectrum and extracted m/z data (Table 1), the component labeled 8 with m/z 152 was identified as citral with a typical fragmentation pattern depicted in the MS spectra comparable to literature data [19]. To confirm the compounds, mechanisms of fragmentation were also computed which matched with dictionary of Natural Products online database theoretical values (http://dnp.chemnetbase.com/). According to the MS fragmentation patterns, several terpenes derivatives were identified (Table 1). Accordingly, molecules 2, 3, and 4 (supplementary data Figure S2 and Scheme S2) were identified as isomers of germacrene and dimmer of linalool, respectively. Presented in Table 1 is molecule 1 at retention time (Rt) 5.05 min. produced a precursor ion at m/z 136 [M + H] ($C_{10}H_{16}$). Mass spectrometer fragmentation of this molecule (supplementary data Figure S1 and Scheme S1) generated product ions at m/z 121, resulting from the loss of methyl (−15 Da) after a possible 1, 2 methyl rearrangement of dimethyl derivative of pinene to a more stable derivative of β-pinene (Scheme S1). Product ions at m/z 93 also correspond to the loss of propenyl group (forty-three mass units (−43 Da)) with a bass peak of 100% intensity. The molecule was recorded as β-pinene since the abundance of ion $m/z = 41$ is more than half of the base peak whilst that for the α-isomer is always less than one-quarter [20]. This molecule (m/z 136) is also distinguished from other isomers such as limonene with base peak at m/z 68 [21]. Based on the individual molecular fragmentation patterns, molecules 2–10 were positively identified and characterized similarly as presented in the supplementary data (Figure and Scheme S1–S6). Other constituents such as demitol (m/z 145), safrole (m/z 161), anethole (m/z 147), and anisole (m/z 110) were also identified with unique fragmentation patterns as reported in Table 1.

3.2. Effect of LEO on the Prostate Gland. The mean prostate gland weights for the experimental groups (Figure 1): normal, model, low dose, middle dose, high dose, and finasteride were

Table 1: Percentage composition and retention time of chemical composition of unripe lime essential oil.

Peak no.	Components	Formulae	Measured (m/z) $[M+H]^+$	Relative (%)	Retention time (min.)	Main product ions $[M+H]^+$
1	Pinene	$C_{10}H_{16}$	136	14.3	5.05	136, 121, 107, 93, 81, 79, 69, 43
2	Germacrene A	$C_{15}H_{26}$	207	49.0	6.08	206, 136, 121, 106, 93, 68, 44
3	Germacrene B	$C_{15}H_{26}$	207	12.2	6.79	206, 136, 121, 106, 93, 68, 44
4	Linalool dimer	$2(C_{10}H_{18}O)$	309	2.9	7.52	110, 94, 79, 59, 44, 40
5	Anisole	C_7H_8O	110	1.1	9.64	110, 94, 84, 79, 77, 69, 59
6	Bornane	$C_{10}H_{18}$	139	11.3	10.32	139, 136, 121, 107, 93, 81, 43
7	Anethole	$C_{10}H_{12}O$	148	1.5	11.67	147, 119, 108, 94, 69, 55
8	Citral/geranial	$C_{10}H_{16}O$	152	2.9	12.48	152, 137, 123, 109, 94, 69
9	Safrole	$C_{10}H_{10}O_2$	161	0.3	14.48	161, 136, 121, 108, 93, 77, 55
10	Demitol	$C_9H_{20}O$	145	0.6	15.04	145, 128, 114, 97, 83, 69, 57, 44

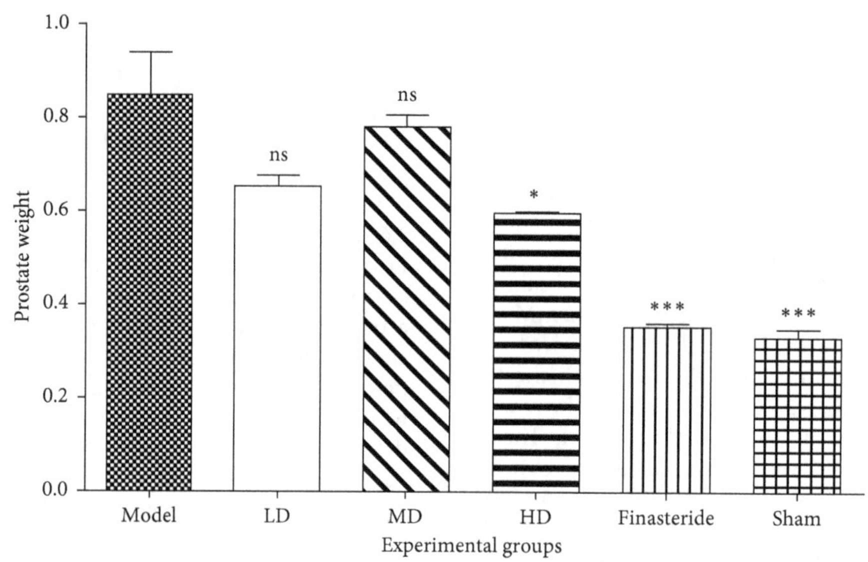

Figure 1: Mean prostate gland weights of experimental groups after 21 days of treatment. Data are presented as mean ± standard error of mean ($n = 6$) (ns = no significance, $^*p < 0.05$ and $^{***}p < 0.0001$). Compared to the disease control group (one way ANOVA followed by Bonferroni's post hoc). This figure demonstrates the change in prostate weights of various groups after treatment. When prostate weights were compared to disease (testosterone groups), there was a statistically significant decrease in prostate weights. Groups treated with 30 mg/kg·b.wt. and 100 mg/kg·b.wt. resulted in no significant reduction in prostate weight, while those treated with 300 mg/kg·b.wt. produced a significant decrease in prostate weight.

0.333 ± 0.018 g; 0.853 ± 0.091 g; 0.657 ± 0.023 g; 0.785 ± 0.026 g; 0.600 ± 0.003 g and 0.356 ± 0.008 g respectively (Supplementary Table S1). The mean prostate gland weight of testosterone-injected groups: model, LD, MD, HD, and finasteride were 155.93% ($p = 0.0001$), 97.12% ($p = 0.0246$), 135.52% ($p = 0.0008$), 80.02% ($p = 0.0803$) and 6.66% ($p = 0.9998$) greater than that of normal control group respectively (Supplementary Table S1). The mean prostate gland weights of the essential oil-treated rats were lesser than that of the model group, but the differences were not significant ($p > 0.05$). Finasteride-treated group had significantly lower mean prostate gland weight than all essential oil-treated groups ($p < 0.05$) except for the high-dose group ($p = 0.1243$) (Supplementary Table S1).

3.3. Effect of Treatments on Serum PSA Levels. The mean serum PSA levels (ng/ml) (Figure 2) of experimental groups before and after treatment were sham group (0.0010 ± 0.0002 and 0.0010 ± 0.0000), model group (1.4720 ± 0.0370 and 1.4890 ± 0.0870), LD (1.4570 ± 0.1060 and 0.1870 ± 0.1080), MD (1.6350 ± 0.2920 and 0.5020 ± 0.1550), HD (1.3450 ± 0.3960 and 0.0010 ± 0.0000), and finasteride (1.2490 ± 0.2130 and 0.0010 ± 0.0001). The mean serum PSA levels of the testosterone-injected groups were significantly greater than the normal which did not receive testosterone-injection. After twenty-one days of treatment, all the essential oil and finasteride treatment groups had their serum PSA levels significantly reduced ($p < 0.05$) except the model group. The normal group which received no testosterone injection had no significant change in the serum PSA levels.

3.4. Effect of Treatments on Prostate Gland Histology. After ten days of testosterone enanthate injection, Testosterone-injected group had thicker epithelium, larger acini, and more prostatic secretions. Sham group had thinner epithelium and fewer prostatic secretions (Figure 3). After

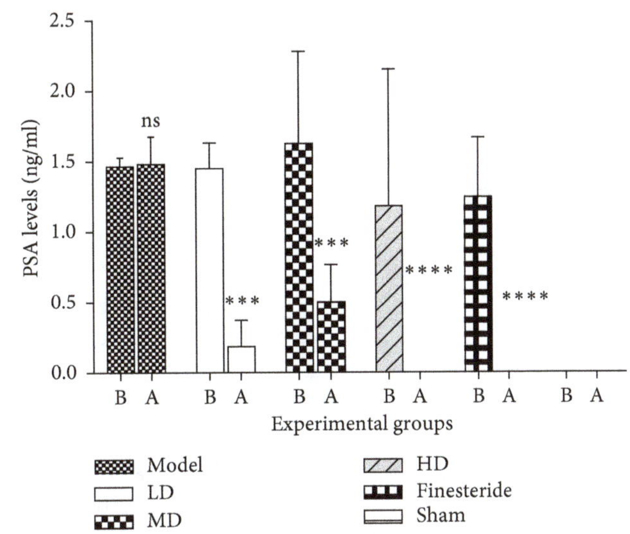

FIGURE 2: Mean serum PSA level before and after treatment for various experimental groups. Data are presented as mean ± standard error of mean ($n = 6$) (ns = no significance, $^{***}p < 0.05$ and $^{****}p < 0.0001$). B represents before treatment, and A represents after treatment. There was a decrease in the serum PSA levels of all treatment groups compared to the disease control (testosterone) group. The low-dose, mid-dose, and high-dose *Citrus aurantifolia* groups all produced a significant reduction in serum PSA levels, together with the finasteride and normal control groups. This implies that the reduction in serum PSA levels was statistically significant, upon treatment with all doses of *Citrus aurantifolia*. A greater and more significant decrease was observed in the high-dose group than the low-dose and the mid-dose groups.

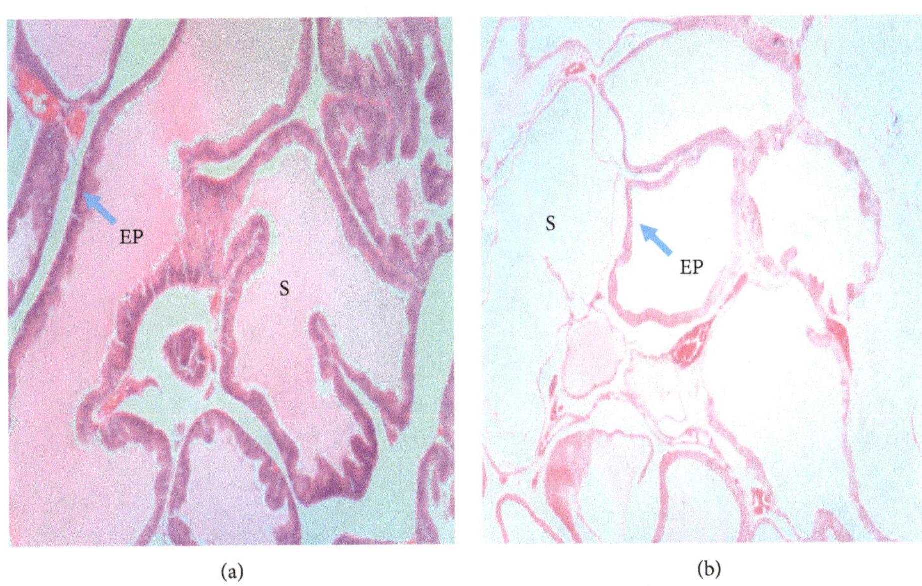

FIGURE 3: Photomicrograph of prostate glands of experimental rats after testosterone-induced benign prostatic hyperplasia: prostatic secretions (S); epithelium (EP). (a) Testosterone-injected group. (b) Sham group. The testosterone-injected group had thicker epithelium, larger acini, and more prostatic secretions. Sham group had thinner epithelium and fewer prostatic secretions.

twenty-one days of treatment, testosterone-injected rats had more prostatic secretions and thinner layers of fibromuscular stroma in between acini when compared to the normal control (Figure 4). Rats which were administered with the low dose (LD), 30 mg/kg of the lime essential oil showed no significant restoration of the tissue histoarchitecture. There were very thinner strands of fibromuscular stroma in between each acinus, and more prostatic secretory activity was observed when compared to the model group. Rats in the mid-dose group (MD), 100 mg/kg, appeared to have a thick layer of fibromuscular stroma in between the acini and also had more prostatic secretions, compared to the low-dose group. Treatment with the high dose (HD), 300 mg/kg, appeared to have a thicker layer of fibromuscular stroma in between the acini, with more prostatic secretions in the acini.

3.5. Effect of Treatments on Total Antioxidant Capacity. The mean plasma total antioxidant capacities (TAC) (AscAEq μg/ml) of the experimental groups were as follows:

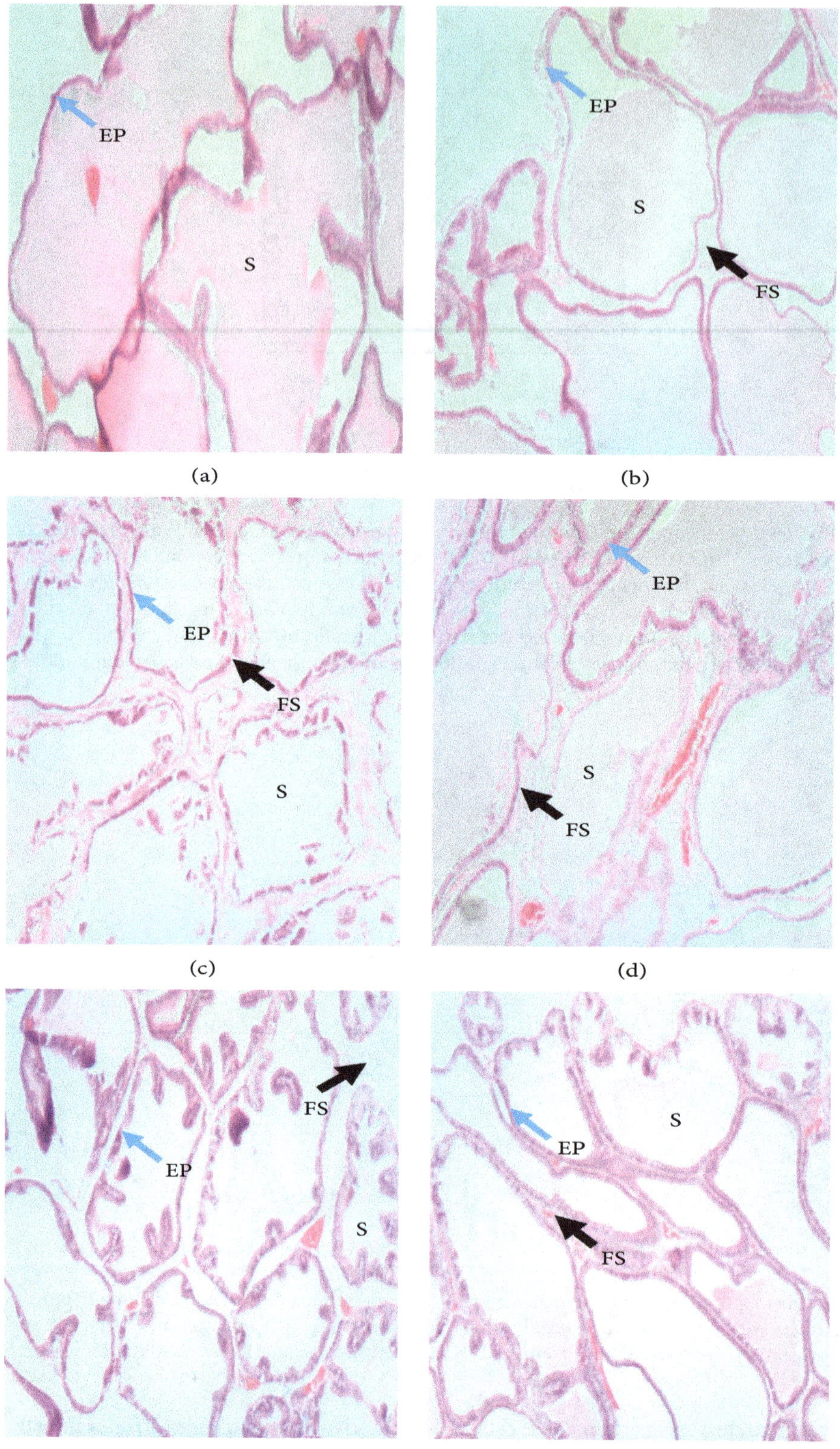

(a) (b) (c) (d) (e) (f)

FIGURE 4: Photomicrographs of prostate glands of experimental groups after 21 days of treatment: (a) model; (b) low dose of oil (30 mg/kg); (c) mid-dose of oil (100 mg/kg); (d) high dose of oil (300 mg/kg); (e) finasteride (15 mg/kg); (f) normal control. Prostatic secretions (S), epithelium (EP), and fibromuscular stroma (FS), model group had larger acini with thicker epithelium, more prostatic secretions, and thinner fibromuscular stroma. Low dose group had slightly large acini, light prostatic secretions and thin fibromuscular stroma. Mid-dose group shows smaller acini with thinner epithelium, moderate prostatic secretion, thick strand of the fibromuscular stroma. High-dose group shows small-sized acini, moderate prostatic secretions, thin epithelium and thick fibromuscular stroma. Finasteride group had almost absent prostatic secretions and a very few amount of fibromuscular stroma, sham group had small-sized acini, little or no prostatic secretion, together with few strands of the fibromuscular stroma.

model (453.3 ± 42.1), low dose (685.5 ± 35.61), middle dose (783.2 ± 73.14), high dose (901.6 ± 0.7782), finasteride (909.4 ± 20.44) and sham (1015 ± 168.2). The essential oil-treated groups recorded a dose-dependent increase in mean plasma TAC. One-way ANOVA test showed the mean plasma TAC of the high dose-treated, finasteride-treated and sham groups was significantly greater than the model group ($p < 0.05$) (Figure 5).

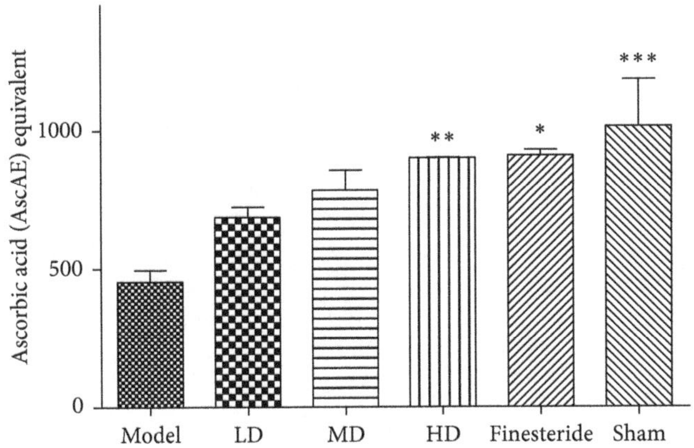

Figure 5: Mean plasma TAC among various treatment groups (*$p < 0.05$ and **$p < 0.01$). Data are presented as mean ± standard error of mean. One-way ANOVA test showed a p value >0.05.

3.6. Effect of Treatments on Testicular Histology. When compared with sham group, seminiferous tubules of rats from the model group were shrunken with the germinal epithelium appearing less compact or eroded off and as an eosinophilic secretion in the intertubular space (Figure 6). Sperm cells were mostly absent in the centre of the tubules. Tubules with sperms present had an eosinophilic pithing. Also, most cells forming the germinal epithelium of their seminiferous tubules and those of the tubulointerstitium had pyknotic nuclei. The finasteride-treated group had only a few seminiferous tubules with eroded germinal epithelium. The germinal epithelia were mostly compact. Pyknotic changes in the germinal epithelium were confined to cell layer closest to the basement membrane of the seminiferous tubules. Lime essential oil-treated groups had less shrunken seminiferous tubules with compact germinal epithelium in a dose-dependent manner. Traces of pyknosis in the germinal epithelium and tubulointerstitial space were present in the medium and low dose groups but were almost absent in the high dose group (Figure 7).

3.7. Effect of Treatments on Liver Histology. The model group showed enlarged hepatocytes with cytoplasmic vacuolations, an enlarged nucleus with the nucleolus and or pyknotic nuclei. Some hepatocytes appeared small and had eosinophilic cytoplasm. Sinusoids separating hepatocytes had bile accumulations and Kupffer cells. Finasteride-treated group had hepatocytes with pale staining cytoplasm, slightly large nuclei with a prominent nucleolus. Low dose LEO-treated group had hepatocytes with cytoplasmic vacuolations and densely-stained nuclei as well as wide sinusoids with moderate bile accumulation. Middle dose LEO-treated group had hepatocytes with a moderate number of pyknotic nuclei and cytoplasmic vacuolations. Sinusoids were relatively narrowed and had moderate bile accumulation. Present also in the blood vessels were karyorrhexis nuclear fragments. High dose LEO-treated group had hepatocytes with cytoplasmic vacuolations, an enlarged nucleus with a prominent nucleolus. Pyknotic nuclei and bile accumulation in the sinusoids were almost absent. Present also in the blood vessels were karyorrhexis nuclear fragments (Figure 8).

3.8. Effect of Treatments on Kidney Histology. Kidney micrographs of the model group showed shrunken tubules and renal corpuscles or diffuse vasodilatation and/or infiltration of inflammatory cells in the glomeruli and tubulointerstitium, tubular necrosis; and dilatation of medullary ray tubules. The finasteride-treated group had mild vasodilation and sparse enlarged renal corpuscles and glomeruli and no dilatation in medullary ray tubules. However, the glomeruli and tubulointerstitium were infiltrated with inflammatory cells, and proximal convoluted tubules had pyknotic nuclei. The lime essential oil-treated group showed a dose-dependent decrease in the severity of these features. High dose LEO-treated group had kidney features comparable to the finasteride-treated group (Figure 9).

4. Discussion

Citrus aurantifolia lime essential oil was evaluated for its ability to ameliorate variables indicative of benign prostatic hyperplasia (BPH) *in vivo*. The effect of lime essential oil on testosterone induced histological changes in selected organs including the testis, the liver, and the kidney was therefore assessed. Thus, benign prostatic hyperplasia was evaluated using serum prostate specific antigen (PSA) levels, weight, and histology of the prostate gland in this study.

Benign prostatic hyperplasia is characterized by prostatic enlargement which culminates into an increase in weight of the prostate gland [20]. In this study, testosterone-induced BPH rat groups showed a significant increase in prostate weight when compared to the sham group. A similar result of prostatic enlargement upon testosterone administration has been reported in a study by Mbaka et al. [21], on the histomorphological changes in induced benign prostatic hyperplasia with exogenous testosterone and estradiol in adult male rats. Testosterone and/or its active form dihydrotestosterone ultimately activate growth factors which regulate cell proliferation and death in cells of the prostate gland including stromal and epithelial cells of the prostate gland [22]. In BPH, TGF-β which promotes cell death in the prostate is downregulated while there is overexpression of KGF, EGF, and IGF which rather promotes epithelial and stromal proliferation [23–28].

When compared to the lime essential oil (LEO) and finasteride-treated groups, the model group showed a significant increase in prostate weight. Among LEO-treated group, the high dose group had significantly lesser mean prostate weight than the model group, indicative of LEO of

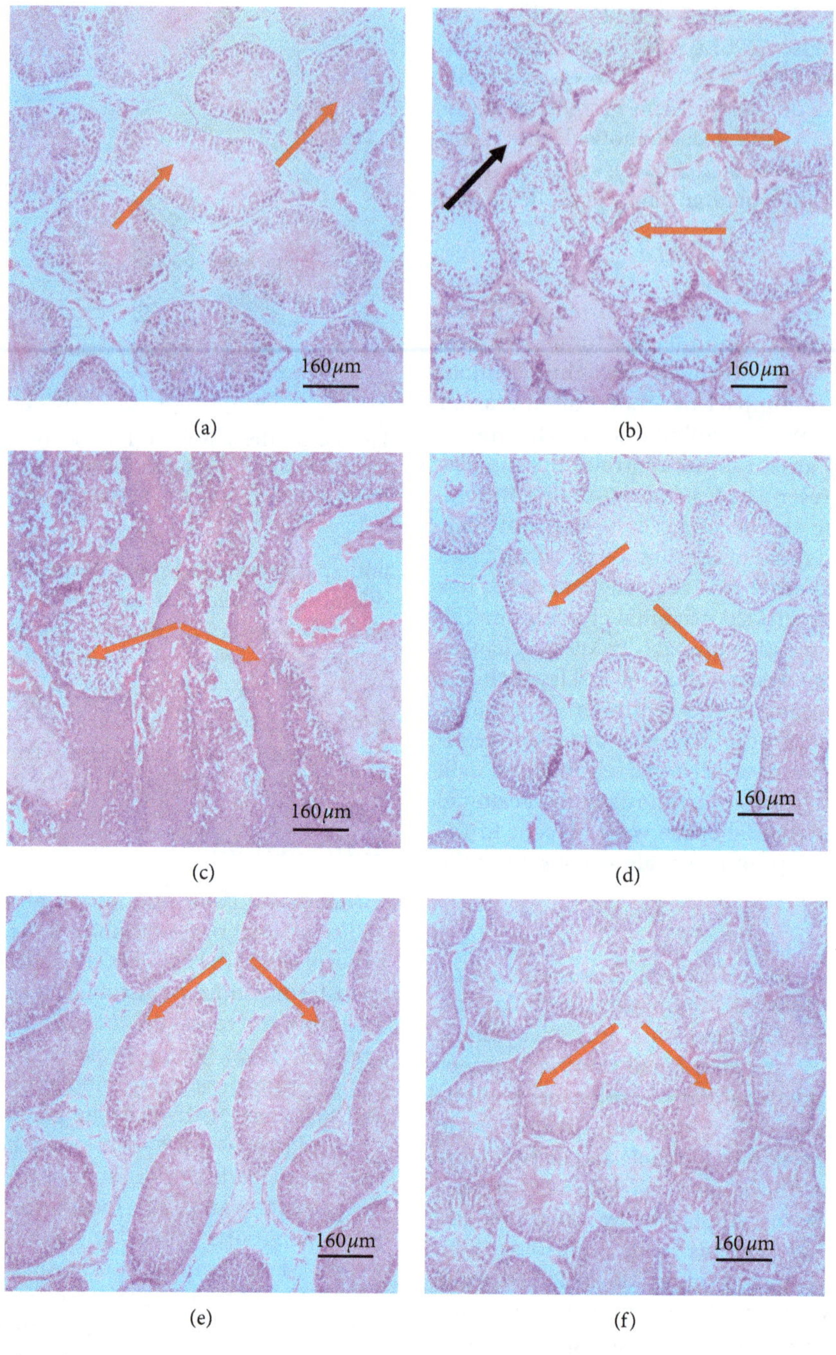

FIGURE 6: Photomicrographs of seminiferous tubules in testis of various experimental groups: (a) sham; (b) model, TE (10 mg/kg)/olive oil injection (i.m.); (c) finasteride, positive control, TE (10 mg/kg)/olive oil injection (i.m. + finasteride administration (15 mg/kg, p.o.); (d) small dose, TE (10 mg/kg) olive oil injection (i.m.) + LEO (30 mg/kg); (e) medium dose, TE (10 mg/kg)/olive oil injection (i.m.) + LEO (100 mg/kg); (f) high dose, TE (10 mg/kg)/olive oil injection (i.m.) + LEO (300 mg/kg). The red arrow represents seminiferous tubules, and blue arrow represents eosinophilic secretion in intertubular space. When compared to the sham group, model group had seminiferous tubules with less compact or eroded germinal epithelium and eosinophilic secretion in the tubulointerstitium. Finasteride-treated group had few seminiferous tubules with vacuolated epithelium. All lime essential oil-treated groups had seminiferous with intact epithelium similar to the sham group.

C. aurantifolia's potential of preventing or delaying prostatic hypertrophy.

Another important biomarker for the diagnosis of BPH is serum prostate specific antigen (PSA) levels. PSA is a serine protease glycoprotein which is naturally produced by epithelial cells of the prostate, and it is produced in minute amounts in the serum, but seen to be greatly elevated in BPH and prostate cancer [29]. Reduction of serum PSA levels is, therefore, indicative of the effectiveness of a trial drug or natural agent in the treatment of BPH. In this study, and

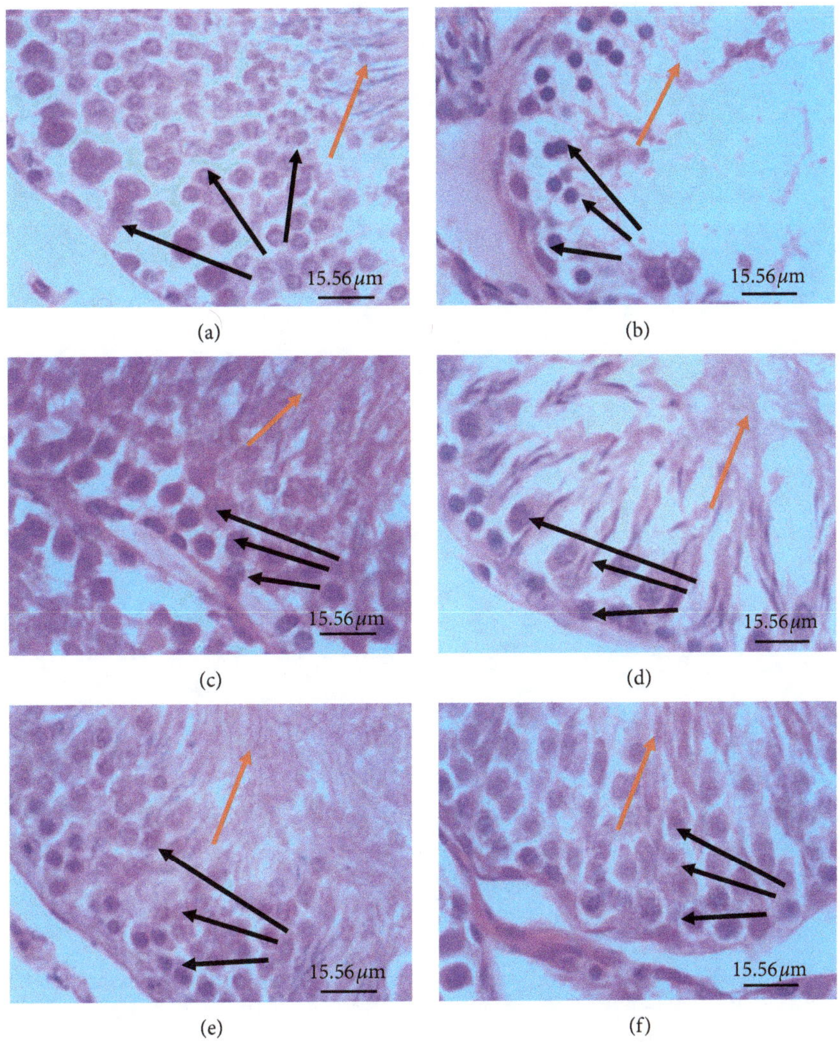

FIGURE 7: Photomicrographs of testis showing spermatogenic series in seminiferous tubules: (a) sham; (b) model, TE (10 mg/kg)/olive oil injection (i.m.); (c) finasteride (positive control), TE (10 mg/kg)/olive oil injection (i.m.) + finasteride administration (15 mg/kg, p.o.); (d) small dose, TE (10 mg/kg)/olive oil injection (i.m.) + LEO (30 mg/kg); (e) medium dose, TE (10 mg/kg)/olive oil injection (i.m.) + LEO (100 mg/kg); (f) high dose, TE (10 mg/kg)/olive oil injection (i.m.) + LEO (300 mg/kg). Red arrow represents spermatozoon in adluminal compartment, black arrows represent germinal epithelium. Model group had less compact germinal epithelium, severe pyknosis in the germinal epithelium (black arrow) and few or no spermatozoa in the adluminal compartment of the seminiferous tubules as well as eosinophilic secretion in the interstitial space. Lime essential oil treatment group had dose dependent decrease in these features.

prior to administration of lime essential oil and or finasteride, serum PSA levels were significantly elevated in rats which received testosterone enanthate injection, unlike the sham group which received no testosterone injection. After treatment, serum PSA levels of the model group were significantly higher than all treatment groups. This result correlates with the findings of a study done on the evaluation of *Cynanchum wilfordii* ability to ameliorate testosterone-induced benign prostatic hyperplasia [30].

The mean serum PSA levels of low and medium dose LEO treatment groups were significantly higher than that of finasteride treatment groups. On the other hand, the mean serum PSA level of the high dose LEO group was not substantially different from the finasteride-treatment group, attesting to its efficacy. One of the effects of testosterone and/or dihydrotestosterone androgen receptor complex's binding to the androgen response element is an expression of the protein PSA [31, 32]. The phytochemicals identified in LEO may actively decrease serum PSA by minimising or preventing the conversion of testosterone to dihydrotestosterone by inhibiting the enzyme 5α-reductase or competitively inhibiting binding of testosterone or dihydrotestosterone to the androgen receptor. Finasteride was more effective than low and medium doses of lime essential oil in terms of its ability to reduce serum PSA levels. Finasteride preferentially inhibits type II 5α-reductase, subsequently blocking peripheral conversion of testosterone to DHT. These resulted in low serum and tissue levels of DHT, minimal to moderate increase in serum testosterone concentrations as well as substantial increases in prostatic testosterone concentrations [33]. Finasteride is a more purified compound, unlike lime essential oil which is a cocktail of variable phytochemicals as

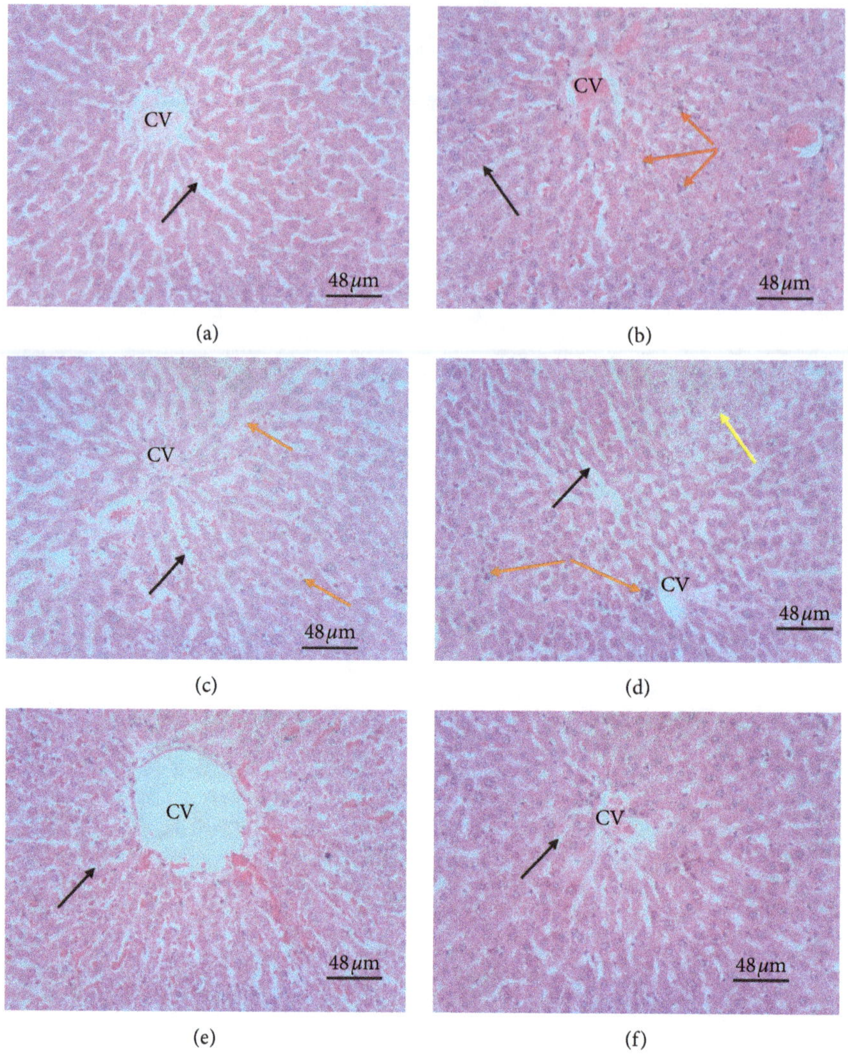

FIGURE 8: Photomicrographs of H&E stained liver sections of experimental groups: (a) sham; (b) model, TE (10 mg/kg)/olive oil injection (i.m.); (c) finasteride, positive control, TE (10 mg/kg)/olive oil injection (i.m.) + finasteride administration (15 mg/kg, p.o.); (d) small dose, TE (10 mg/kg)/olive oil injection (i.m.) + LEO (30 mg/kg); (e) medium dose, TE (10 mg/kg)/olive oil injection (i.m.) + LEO (100 mg/kg); (f) high dose, TE (10 mg/kg)/olive oil injection (i.m.) + LEO (300 mg/kg). Black arrow represents sinusoids separating plates of hepatocytes; red arrow represents Kupffer cells; Yellow arrow represents hepatocytes with fat accumulation, the orange arrow represents inflammatory cells, and CV represents centrilobular vein. The model group showed enlarged hepatocytes with eosinophilic or pale staining cytoplasm or enlarged nucleus and enlarged sinusoids infiltrated with Kupffer cells and inflammatory cells. Finasteride-treated group had dilated sinusoids with few inflammatory cells and normal sized hepatocytes with slightly enlarged nuclei with a prominent nucleolus. Lime essential oil-treated groups showed dose-dependent decrease in sinusoids infiltrated with Kupffer cells or inflammatory cells, dose-dependent increase in hepatocyte fat accumulation. High dose treated group had a presentation close to the sham group.

demonstrated by the GC analyses. Thus, for a particular dose of finasteride, relatively higher doses of lime essential, as observed with the high dose, will be needed to exert a comparable effect. This could account for why low doses of the lime essential oil could not produce results similar to finasteride. This notwithstanding lime essential oil is readily available and relatively cheaper compared finasteride.

Additionally, restoration of prostate histoarchitecture is an important parameter used in various studies to assess the potency of anti-BPH agents. So far, no known study has commented on the association between prostatic secretion and BPH development. In this study, BPH-untreated group produced more prostatic secretions, compared to all BPH-treatment and the sham groups. More so, glandular epithelial thickening of the glands irrespective of the lobes was more pronounced in the model group than lime essential oil- and finasteride-treated groups. Androgens like testosterone and dihydrotestosterone (DHT) are known to be associated with the regulation of cell proliferation, specifically, in androgen-dependent organs like the prostate and seminal vesicles [31]. Exogenous testosterone, administered is often converted to DHT, and after binding to androgen receptors increase transcription of androgen-dependent genes to stimulate protein synthesis. The overall mechanism leads to the proliferation of cells, by stimulating

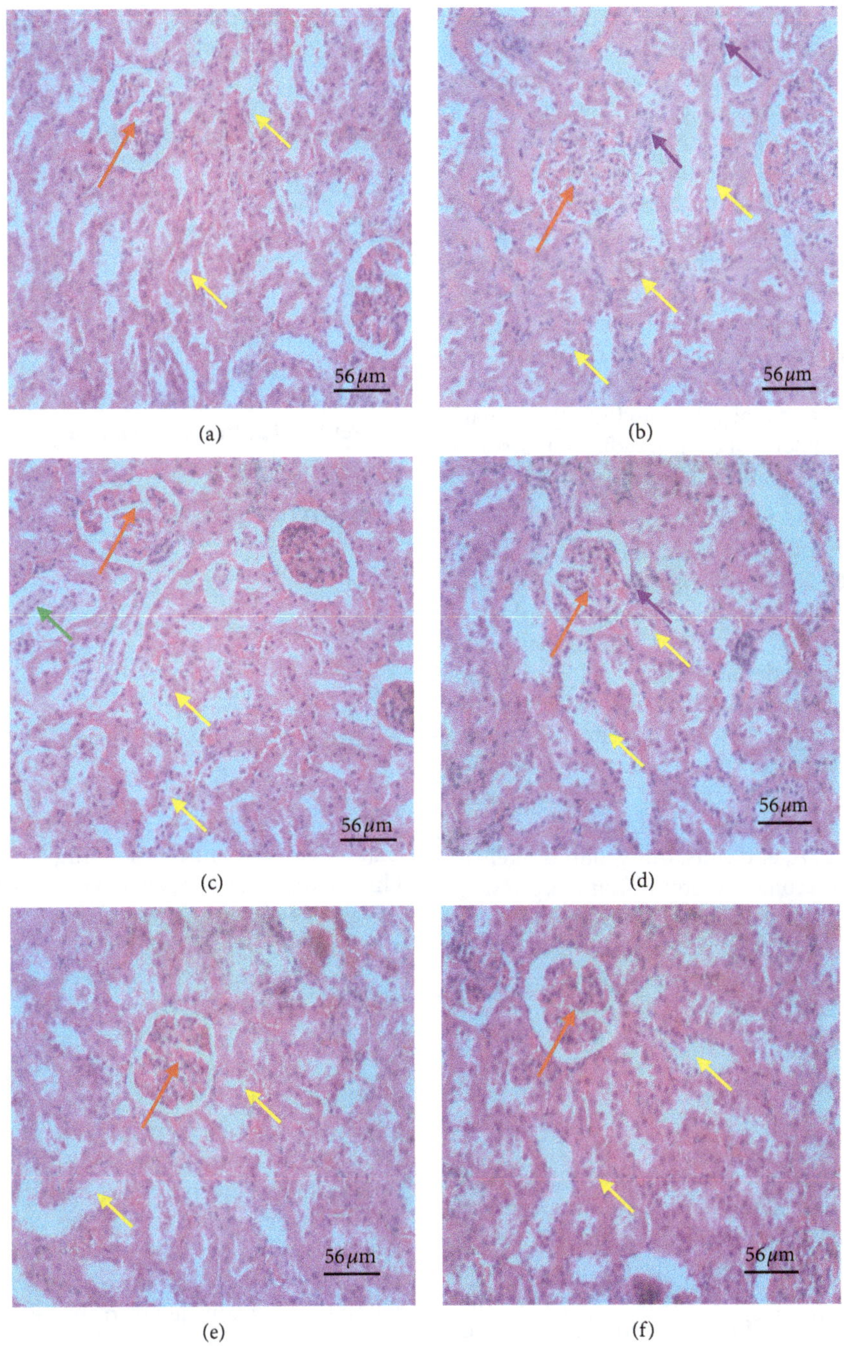

FIGURE 9: Photomicrographs of H&E stained kidney sections of various experimental groups: (a) sham; (b) model, TE (10 mg/kg)/olive oil injection (i.m.); (c) finasteride (positive control), TE (10 mg/kg)/olive oil injection (i.m.) + finasteride administration (15 mg/kg, p.o.); (d) small dose, TE (10 mg/kg)/olive oil injection (i.m.) + LEO (30 mg/kg); (e) medium dose, TE (10 mg/kg)/olive oil injection (i.m.) + LEO (100 mg/kg); (f) high dose, TE (10 mg/kg)/olive oil injection (i.m.) + LEO (300 mg/kg). The red arrow represents glomeruli with surrounding Bowman's space, the yellow arrow represents proximal and distal convoluted tubules, green represents collecting duct, and the purple arrow represents inflammatory cells. Model group showed diffuse vasodilatation and/or infiltration of inflammatory cells in the glomeruli and tubulointerstitium, enlarged glomeruli and reduced Bowman's space, tubular degenerative changes; and dilatation of medullary ray tubules. Finasteride-treated group had mild vasodilation and few enlarged glomeruli, few inflammatory cells, less tubular degenerative changes but enlarged collecting ducts. Lime essential oil-treated group showed a dose-dependent decrease in severity of these features. High dose LEO-treated group had kidney features comparable to the sham group.

transcription of growth factors which are mitogenic for the epithelial and stromal cells of the prostate, hence the thickening of the glandular epithelium [17].

BPH is known to increase the presence of free radicals in serum; therefore, the ability of the investigated plant extract to reduce these free radicals is essential for the treatment of BPH.

Hypotestosteronemia is reported to cause a buildup of oxidative radical species in tissues [32] by impairing the activity of three main antioxidant enzymes, namely, catalase, superoxide dismutase, and glutathione peroxidase in human testes [33], or downregulate the activity of prooxidant enzymes (i.e. NADPH-oxidase) in the prostate [34, 35]. In this study, the total antioxidant capacity (TAC) of serum was used to quantify residual antioxidants in the serum. The model group had the least serum TAC while lime essential oil-treated groups recorded a dose-dependent increase in serum TAC levels. Antioxidant potential of lime essential oil has been confirmed *in vitro* using egg albumin assay and red blood cell model, and thus, ingestion of the oil could add to the plasma antioxidants thereby causing the lime essential oil-treated groups to have higher plasma TAC. The buildup of oxygen radicals in tissue or plasma results in damage to the histology of a tissue [36, 37].

Testosterone has an effect on several body organs including the kidney [16, 38–41], testis, and liver [39, 40]. Therefore the impact of hypotestosteronemia on histology of selected organs of the body was assessed. The model group recorded more histological damages than oil- and finasteride-treated groups. Histological changes observed in the study could be attributable to testosterone engendered oxidative stress-mediated damage. Serum testosterone was not determined, but the serum PSA level has a positive correlation with serum testosterone level. The finasteride-treated group had lesser serum PSA, and thus, this group is likely to record low serum testosterone thereby minimizing testosterone-mediated histological changes. The oil- treated group also recorded a dose dependent decrease in histological changes with the high dose oil-treated group having better histological outcomes than lower and mid-dose groups.

5. Conclusion

Lime essential oil from unripe *Citrus aurantifolia* has demonstrated potent anti-benign prostatic hyperplastic activity by causing significant reduction in serum PSA levels, minimizing prostate gland enlargement and also reverted testosterone-induced histological changes in experimental rats. Lime essential oil from *Citrus aurantifolia* could potentially be used as an alternative drug to manage benign prostatic hyperplasia, and therefore should be investigated further to derive its full potential as a drug. Thus, the individual phytochemicals need to be investigated to establish the particular phytochemical exerting particular bioactivity and the mechanism of action and whether there is a synergy among them.

Ethical Approval

Ethical approval for the study was obtained from the University of Cape Coast Institute Review Board (UCCIRB). ID: UCCIRB/CHAS/2016/13, University of Cape Coast, Cape Coast, Ghana.

Authors' Contributions

This study was carried out with the collaboration of all authors. DOA, EAA, AB, and JFO designed the study. DOA, EAA, JFO, BA, CKA, FAA, and IKB performed the experiment. DOA, EAA, IKB, and AB wrote the first draft of the manuscript. CKA performed the GC-MS analysis and interpreted the data thereof. FAA, AB, RO, IKB, and EAA managed the statistical analysis and the literature searches of the study and edited the final manuscript for intellectual content. All authors read and approved the final manuscript.

Acknowledgments

The authors are grateful to Department of Biomedical Sciences, University of Cape Coast, Ghana, for permitting them to use their laboratory facility during this study. The corresponding author funded the study.

Supplementary Materials

Chemical composition of the unripe lime essential oil GC/MS analysis identified about ten (10) phytochemicals as its major constituents. The single ion monitoring (SIM) chromatograms generated via accurate *m/z* representation of terpenes in literature [1] were employed to identify respective MS spectra of essential oil components and their molecular formulae were also computed on the basis that the isotopic fit ratios (iFit) were assumed to be close to zero as possible (Figures S1–S7). Schemes S1–S7 and Figures S1–S7 depicts fragmentation mechanistic pattern and GC/MS spectra of individual components of the oil detailed explained in the main text. In summary, two isomers of Germacrene isomers were the major components (61.2%) followed by Pineen (14%). The remaining chemical compounds were in trace amounts as listed in Table 1 in the main text. The peaks labeled as **2** and **3** in the GC spectrum with *m/z* 207 are isomers of germacrene with a typical fragmentation pattern depicted in the MS spectrum (Figure S2 and Scheme S2) comparable to literature data [1, 2]. The fragmentation mechanisms of all the compounds were proposed to further confirm their presence (Scheme S2). For germacrene isomers, the first step in fragmentation reactions seems to be breaking a single bond through the loss of an electron from the molecule **2**. Molecule **2** with retention time (Rt) of 6.10 min. (Figure S2) produced a precursor ion at *m/z* 207 [M + H] ($C_{15}H_{26}$) due to completely breakdown of a π-bond by loss of an electron. This led to loss of an isopropyl group. The fragmentation of this molecule (Figure S2, Scheme S2) gave molecular ion at *m/z* 136, derived from the loss of two methyl (−30 Da) groups and isopropyl group (seventy-one mass units (−71 Da) after a possible 1,2 methyl rearrangement of dimethyl derivative of germacrene to a more stable derivative of cyclooctene-dimer (Scheme S2). Products ions at m/z 93 corresponds to the ring opening of the cyclooctene-dimer and the loss of an m/z 44 neutral fragment to form the base peak with 100%. Similarly, fragmentation mechanism of all other components (Pineen, Anisole, Anethole, Safrole and Demitol) were proposed to further confirm their presence (Scheme S1, S4–S7). Table S1: effect of LEO on prostate weight. (*Supplementary Materials*)

References

[1] B. Chughtai, J. C. Forde, D. D. M. Thomas et al., "Benign prostatic hyperplasia," *Nature Reviews Disease Primers*, vol. 2, no. 1, p. 16031, 2016.

[2] M. Kantah, B. Singh, H. Sweed et al., "Beneficial effect of a multifunctional polyphytocompound in experimental prostatic hyperplasia in rats," *Clinical Pharmacology & Biopharmaceutics*, vol. 6, no. 2, pp. 1–7, 2017.

[3] P. Verze, T. Cai, and S. Lorenzetti, "The role of the prostate in male fertility, health and disease," *Nature Reviews Urology*, vol. 13, no. 7, pp. 379–386, 2016.

[4] B. Chughtai, R. Lee, A. Te, and S. Kaplan, "Role of inflammation in benign prostatic hyperplasia," *Reviews in Urology*, vol. 13, no. 3, pp. 147–150, 2011.

[5] P. Vital, P. Castro, and M. Ittmann, "Oxidative stress promotes benign prostatic hyperplasia," *The Prostate*, vol. 76, no. 1, pp. 58–67, 2016.

[6] M. Glover, S. Soni, Q. Ren, G. T. Maclennan, P. Fu, and S. Gupta, "Influence of chronic inflammation on Bcl-2 and PCNA expression in prostate needle biopsy specimens," *Oncology Letters*, vol. 14, no. 4, pp. 3927–3934, 2017.

[7] A. Rahal, A. Kumar, V. Singh et al., "Oxidative stress, prooxidants, and antioxidants: the interplay," *BioMed Research International*, vol. 2014, Article ID 761264, 19 pages, 2014.

[8] W. Jiraungkoorskul and N. Narang, "Anticancer activity of key lime, citrus aurantifolia," *Pharmacognosy Reviews*, vol. 10, no. 20, pp. 118–122, 2016.

[9] E. I. Oikeh, E. S. Omoregie, F. E. Oviasogie, and K. Oriakhi, "Phytochemical, antimicrobial, and antioxidant activities of different citrus juice concentrates," *Food Science & Nutrition*, vol. 4, no. 1, pp. 103–109, 2016.

[10] M. A. Oshaghi, R. Ghalandari, H. Vatandoost et al., "Repellent effect of extracts and essential oils of Citrus limon (Rutaceae) and Melissa officinalis (Labiatae) against main malaria vector, Anopheles stephensi (Diptera: Culicidae)," *Iranian Journal of Public Health*, vol. 32, pp. 47–52, 2003.

[11] M. Nasri, F. Bedjou, D. Porras, and S. Martínez-Flórez, "Antioxidant, anti-inflammatory, and analgesic activities of Citrus reticulata Blanco leaves extracts: an in vivo and in vitro study," *Phytothérapie*, vol. 1–13, 2017.

[12] R. k. Pathan, P. R. Gali, T. Gowtham, and S. Pasupuleti, "In vitro antimicrobial activity of citrus aurantifolia and its phytochemical screening," *Asian Pacific Journal of Tropical Disease*, vol. 2, pp. S328–S331, 2012.

[13] I. U. Nwankwo, R. C. dan Osaro-Matthew, and I. N. Ekpe, "Synergistic antibacterial potentials of citrus aurantifolia (lime) and honey against some bacteria isolated from sputum of patients attending Federal Medical Center Umuahia," *International Journal of Current Microbiology and Applied Sciences*, vol. 4, pp. 534–544, 2015.

[14] J. L. Amorim, D. L. R. Simas, M. M. G. Pinheiro et al., "Anti-inflammatory properties and chemical characterization of the essential oils of four Citrus species," *PLoS One*, vol. 11, pp. 1–18, 2016.

[15] M. R. Loizzo, R. Tundis, M. Bonesi et al., "Evaluation of Citrus aurantifolia peel and leaves extracts for their chemical composition, antioxidant and anti-cholinesterase activities," *Journal of the Science of Food and Agriculture*, vol. 92, no. 15, pp. 2960–2967, 2012.

[16] K. M. Park, J. I. Kim, Y. Ahn, A. J. Bonventre, and J. V. Bonventre, "Testosterone is responsible for enhanced susceptibility of males to ischemic renal injury," *Journal of Biological Chemistry*, vol. 279, no. 50, pp. 52282–52292, 2004.

[17] B. Rostami, M. Nematbakhsh, Z. Pezeshki, and A. Talebi, "Effect of testosterone on cisplatin induced nephrotoxicity in surgically castrated rats," *Nephro-Urology Monthly*, vol. 6, pp. 1–3, 2014.

[18] P. Prieto, M. Pineda, and M. Miguelar, "Spectrophotometric quantitation of antioxidant capacity through the formation of phosphomolybdenum complex: specific application to the determination of Vitamin E," *Analytical Biochemistry*, vol. 269, no. 2, pp. 337–341, 1999.

[19] A. El-Said El-Mehi and N. M. El-Sherif, "Modulating role of Panax ginseng in experimentally induced benign prostatic hyperplasia in adult male albino rats," *Austin Journal of Anatomy*, vol. 2, no. 1, 2015.

[20] National Institute of Standard Technology (NIST), "Material measurement Laboratory NIST chemistry webbook," 2016, http://webbook.nist.gov/cgi/cbook.cgi?ID=C94597&Mask=200.

[21] G. Mbaka, C. Anunobi, S. Ogunsina, and D. Osiagwu, "Histomorphological changes in induced benign prostatic hyperplasia with exogenous testosterone and estradiol in adult male rats treated with aqueous ethanol extract of Secamone afzelii," *Egyptian Journal of Basic and Applied Sciences*, vol. 4, no. 1, pp. 15–21, 2017.

[22] S. K. Bechis, A. G. Otsetov, R. Ge, and A. F. Olumi, "Personalized medicine for management of benign prostatic hyperplasia," *The Journal of Urology*, vol. 192, no. 1, pp. 16–23, 2014.

[23] I. D. McLarena, T. J. Jerdeb, and W. Bushmana, "Role of interleukins, IGF and stem cells in BPH," *Differentiation*, vol. 82, no. 4-5, pp. 237–243, 2011.

[24] W. Li, C.-L. Wu, P. G. Febbo, and A. F. Olumi, "Stromally expressed c-jun regulates proliferation of prostate epithelial cells," *The American Journal of Pathology*, vol. 171, no. 4, pp. 1189–1198, 2007.

[25] C. Carson III and R. Rittmaster, "The role of dihydrotestosterone in benign prostatic hyperplasia," *Urology*, vol. 61, no. 4, pp. 2–7, 2003.

[26] D. O. Acheampong, M. Tang, Y. Wang et al., "A novel fusion antibody exhibits antiangiogenic activity and stimulates NK cell-mediated immune surveillance through fused NKG2D ligand," *Journal of Immunotherapy*, vol. 40, no. 3, pp. 94–103, 2017.

[27] H. Li, W. Cao, Z. Chen et al., "The antiangiogenic activity of a soluble fragment of the VEGFR extracellular domain," *Biomedicine & Pharmacotherapy*, vol. 67, no. 7, pp. 599–606, 2013.

[28] S. D. Mikolajczyk, L. S. Millar, T. J. Wang et al., "A precursor form of prostate-specific antigen is more highly elevated in prostate cancer compared with benign transition zone prostate tissue," *Cancer Research*, vol. 60, no. 3, pp. 756–759, 2000.

[29] G. Lee, J. Shin, H. Choi et al., "Cynanchum wilfordii ameliorates testosterone-induced benign prostatic hyperplasia by

regulating 5α-reductase and androgen receptor activities in a rat model," *Nutrients*, vol. 9, no. 10, p. 1070, 2017.

[30] L. Jia and G. A. Coetzee, "Androgen receptor-dependent PSA expression in androgen-independent prostate cancer cells does not involve androgen receptor occupancy of the PSA-Locus," *Cancer Research*, vol. 65, no. 17, pp. 8003–8008, 2005.

[31] N. C. Bennett, R. A. Gardiner, J. D. Hooper, D. W. Johnson, and G. C. Gobe, "Molecular cell biology of androgen receptor signalling," *The International Journal of Biochemistry & Cell Biology*, vol. 42, no. 6, pp. 813–827, 2010.

[32] E. H. Kim, J. A. Brockman, and G. L. Andriole, "The use of 5-alpha reductase inhibitors in the treatment of benign prostatic hyperplasia," *Asian Journal of Urology*, vol. 5, no. 1, pp. 28–32, 2018.

[33] C. Gonzales, J. Leiva-Revilla, J. Rubio, M. Gasco, and G. F. Gonzales, "Effect of red maca (Lepidium meyenii) on prostate zinc levels in rats with testosterone-induced prostatic hyperplasia," *Andrologia*, vol. 44, pp. 362–369, 2012.

[34] C. Alonso-alvarez, S. Bertrand, B. Faivre, O. Chastel, and G. Sorci, "Testosterone and oxidative stress: the oxidation handicap hypothesis," *Proceedings of the Royal Society B: Biological Sciences*, vol. 274, no. 1611, pp. 819–825, 2007.

[35] G. B. N. Chainy, S. Samantaray, and L. Samanta, "Testosterone-induced changes in testicular antioxidant system," *Andrologia*, vol. 29, no. 6, pp. 343–349, 2009.

[36] N. N. C. Tam, S. Ghatak, and S.-M. Ho, "Sex hormone-induced alterations in the activities of antioxidant enzymes and lipid peroxidation status in the prostate of noble rats," *The Prostate*, vol. 55, no. 1, pp. 1–8, 2003.

[37] N. N. C. Tam, Y. Gao, Y.-K. Leung, and S.-M. Ho, "Androgenic regulation of oxidative stress in the rat prostate: involvement of NAD(P)H oxidases and antioxidant defense machinery during prostatic involution and regrowth," *The American Journal of Pathology*, vol. 163, no. 6, pp. 2513–2522, 2003.

[38] N. Kurita, S. Horie, and S. Yamazaki, "Low testosterone levels and reduced kidney function in Japanese adult men : the locomotive syndrome and health outcome in aizu cohort study," *Journal of the American Medical Directors Association*, vol. 17, no. 4, pp. 371.e1–371.e6, 2016.

[39] G. Filler, A. Ramsaroop, R. Stein et al., "Is testosterone detrimental to renal function?," *Kidney International Reports*, vol. 1, no. 4, pp. 306–310, 2016.

[40] M. T. Bento-silva, M. d. C. d. C. e. Martins, F. L. Torres-Leal et al., "Effects of administering testosterone undecanoate in rats subjected to physical exercise: effects on the estrous cycle, motor behavior and morphology of the liver and kidney," *Brazilian Journal of Pharmaceutical Sciences*, vol. 46, no. 1, pp. 79–89, 2010.

[41] A. A. Samaha, W. Nasser-eddine, E. Shatila, J. J. Haddad, J. Wazne, and A. H. Eid, "Multi-organ damage induced by anabolic steroid supplements : a case report and literature review," *Journal of Medical Case Reports*, vol. 2, no. 1, 2008.

14

Nephrolithiasis and Polycystic Ovary Syndrome: A Case-Control Study Evaluating Testosterone and Urinary Stone Metabolic Panels

Donald Fedrigon III, Kareem Alazem, Sri Sivalingam, Manoj Monga, and Juan Calle

Cleveland Clinic, Glickman Urological & Kidney Institute, 9500 Euclid Avenue, Cleveland, OH 44195, USA

Correspondence should be addressed to Juan Calle; callej@ccf.org

Academic Editor: Kostis Gyftopoulos

Introduction. Both elevated testosterone and polycystic ovary syndrome (PCOS) have been speculated as possible risk factors for kidney stone formation; however, the details of this potential relationship with regards to 24-hour urine metabolic panels and stone composition have not previously been characterized. *Methods*. A total of 74 PCOS patients were retrospectively identified and matched with a cohort of female stone formers at a 3 : 1 ratio (by age and BMI). All patients had 24-hour urinary metabolic panels and stone compositions. These groups were compared using Pearson chi-square and Student t-tests. Additionally, the PCOS group was differentiated based on free testosterone using multivariate analysis. *Results*. The case-control cohort showed that PCOS patients had significantly lower sodium excretion ($p = 0.015$) and hypernatriuria rates (28.9% vs 50.9%, $p = 0.009$). The PCOS-testosterone cohort demonstrated that high testosterone patients had significantly higher citrate values ($p = 0.041$) and significantly lower odds of hypocitraturia (36.7% vs 54.2%, OR = 0.2, $p = 0.042$). The high testosterone group also had higher sodium excretion ($p = 0.058$) with significantly higher odds of having hypernatriuria (40.0% vs 13.6%, OR = 13.3, $p = 0.021$). No significant patterns were revealed based on stone composition analysis. *Conclusions*. Compared to healthy stone formers, PCOS patients did not demonstrate significant differences in 24-hour urine and stone composition values. Elevated free testosterone in PCOS patients has a significant association with higher urinary citrate and sodium values: findings that in and of themselves do not confirm the hypothesized increased risk of stone formation. This patient cohort may provide deeper insight into the interplay between androgens and stone formation; however, further study is needed to fully characterize the possible relationship between PCOS and stone formation.

1. Introduction and Objective

Polycystic ovary syndrome (PCOS) is a common endocrine disorder characterized by oligomenorrhea and androgen excess, which affects 5–10% of women at reproductive-age and has been suggested to be a potential risk factor for stone formation [1, 2]. Elevated testosterone has been implicated as a causal factor in kidney stone formation based on a variety of inferential evidence: the incidence of urolithiasis is 2-3 times higher in men than in women, the risk of stone formation is reduced in castrated rats, as well as male stone formers having higher serum total testosterone levels than stone-free controls [3–8]. Our goal was to evaluate the relationship between PCOS, elevated testosterone, and stone formation from the perspective of stone composition and 24-hour urine metabolic stone panels.

2. Methods

2.1. Study Design. We retrospectively identified 74 patients from the Cleveland Clinic stone registry (ICD-9 592.xx and 594.xx) with diagnosis of PCOS (ICD-9 256.4) who had a recorded free testosterone level and 24-hour urinary collection. A matched cohort of female stone formers, matched by age and BMI on the date of 24-hour urine collection, was generated from our registry at a 3 : 1 ratio, for a total of 222 control patients. Patients were selected from our database in the timeframe from Oct. 2002 to Jul. 2014. If multiple testosterone values were available, the result closest in time to the date of the 24-urine collection was used. The PCOS patients were divided into normal and high (>6.4 pg/mL) testosterone groups based on previously published reference values [9].

2.2. Metabolic and Laboratory Evaluation. Stone composition was analyzed by Fourier transform infrared spectrometry and expressed as the amount of each component in the stone. Studied components were calcium oxalate monohydrate (CaOMH), calcium oxalate dihydrate (CaODH), calcium phosphate (CaPh), calcium hydrogen phosphate (CaHPh), magnesium ammonium phosphate (MAP), and uric acid (UA). A stone was considered pure if 70% or greater of the stone was composed of a single component. Patient urinary risk factors for stone disease were evaluated by 24-hour urine collection with the patient on an unrestricted diet. Urine samples were examined for calcium, sodium, oxalate, citrate, UA, volume, and creatinine. Urinary normal values were set using specific methodologies, including calcium less than 200 mg per day for women by the o-cresolphthalein complexone method, sodium less than 150 mmol per day by ion-selective electrode, oxalate less than 40 mg per day by enzyme immunoassay, citrate greater than 550 mg per day for women by enzyme immunoassay, UA less than 750 mg per day for women by the uricase method, and volume 2,000 ml or greater per day. Urinary creatinine was measured by the enzymatic method. Serum-free testosterone was evaluated by liquid chromatography tandem mass spectrometry (LC/MS/MS).

2.3. Study Endpoints. Primary endpoints for both sets of analysis were 24-hour urinary metabolic panels and stone composition. We compared baseline 24-hour urinary metabolic panels within both the case-control and PCOS-testosterone cohorts by absolute levels of all parameters and the proportion of patients with specific abnormalities. We compared stone composition by the relative amount of each component in the stone, mixed/pure status, and proportion of patients with each pure stone type. When multiple stones or stone fragments were passed or retrieved surgically for a single episode of nephrolithiasis, they were sent for analysis as a single sample.

2.4. Medications and Comorbidities. Registry patients were not included in either the PCOS or control group if their 24-hour urinary metabolic panel overlapped with medications such as thiazides, citrates, or allopurinol that could impact stone formation or urine metabolic panels. Medications commonly used in the treatment of PCOS (i.e., oral contraceptives, spironolactone, and metformin) and common comorbidities (i.e., diabetes mellitus and hypertension) were evaluated for potential confounding effects on free testosterone levels. Only metformin was found to have a potential confounding effect and was therefore included, along with age and BMI, as an adjusted variable in multivariable analysis.

2.5. Statistical Analysis. Statistical analysis was performed using R Statistical Software (R Foundation for Statistical Computing, Vienna, Austria). Case-control and PCOS testosterone group means were compared using Student t-tests and group percentages were compared using Pearson chi-square. Within the PCOS cohort, endpoints were also compared using multivariable linear and logistic regression, adjusted for age, BMI, and metformin status. For all tests, $p < 0.05$ was considered statistically significant.

3. Results

3.1. Urinary Stone Panel: Case-Control Cohort. We identified 88 PCOS patients in our stone registry, of which 14 were excluded based on medications that could impact 24-hour urine results. Demographic characteristics as well as the urinary calcium, citrate, creatinine, oxalate, uric acid, and volume were similar between the PCOS and control groups (Table 1). The 24-hour urine metabolic panels for the case-control cohort revealed that PCOS patients had both significantly lower urinary sodium excretion ($p = 0.015$) and lower frequency of hypernatriuria (28.9% vs 50.9%, $p = 0.009$). Urinary citrate was higher in the PCOS group (624.1 ± 361.9) than that in the control group (527.5 ± 317.8) but this did not reach statistical significance ($p = 0.08$).

3.2. Urinary Stone Panel: PCOS Testosterone Cohort. Within the 74 eligible PCOS patients, 38 (51.3%) were classified as having high free testosterone (>6.4 pg/mL). Diabetes ($n = 11$), hypertension ($n = 25$), spironolactone ($n = 8$), and oral contraceptive ($n = 16$) status were all evaluated as potential confounding variables for both nominal and continuous testosterone values but not found to be statistically significant. High testosterone classification was significantly associated with younger age ($p = 0.008$), higher BMI ($p < 0.001$), and active metformin therapy ($p = 0.05$). PCOS patients on metformin also had significantly higher free testosterone values ($p = 0.026$). Therefore, BMI, age, and metformin status were included as confounding variables in the multivariate analysis. Table 2 shows the original data analysis and significance values for the PCOS testosterone cohort.

Multivariate analysis revealed that high testosterone patients had significantly higher urinary citrate values ($p = 0.041$, Table 3) with significantly lower odds of having hypocitraturia (36.7% vs 54.2%, OR = 0.2, $p = 0.042$). High testosterone PCOS patients also had higher urinary sodium that approached statistical significance ($p = 0.058$) with significantly higher odds of having hypernatriuria (40.0% vs 13.6%, OR = 13.3, $p = 0.021$). Additionally, high testosterone PCOS patients had a higher average urinary volume output ($p = 0.066$) and a decreased frequency of

TABLE 1: Bivariate analysis using PCOS status within case-control cohort.

	PCOS ($n = 74$)		No PCOS ($n = 222$)		p value	N
Mean ± SD age (range)	35.9 ± 11.8	(13–73)	36.0 ± 11.7	(13–73)	0.989	296
Mean ± SD kg/m^2 BMI (range)	31.2 ± 7.4	(17.9–54.5)	31.0 ± 7.3	(18.6–55.0)	0.865	296
Mean ± SD 24 hr urine panel (range):						
Calcium (mg/day)	211.2 ± 128.3	(35.5–913.6)	214.7 ± 119.7	(16.7–817.1)	0.848	251
Citrate (mg/day)	624.1 ± 361.9	(82–1903)	527.5 ± 317.8	(4–1546)	0.083	220
Creatinine (g/day)	1.3 ± 0.4	(0.6–3.2)	1.3 ± 0.41	(0.1–2.9)	0.316	230
Oxalate (mg/day)	38.4 ± 15.2	(17–113)	39.1 ± 20.8	(0–180)	0.777	224
Sodium (mmol/day)	135.7 ± 52.0	(49–283)	158.8 ± 76.3	(28–442)	0.015	211
Uric acid (mg/day)	520.2 ± 194.6	(179–1016)	550.1 ± 210.2	(30.3–1361.3)	0.319	231
Volume (ml/day)	1643 ± 793.6	(581–3440)	1690 ± 789.9	(310–4450)	0.712	188
No. abnormality (%):						
Hypercalciuria (>200 mg/day)	35	(53.9%)	87	(46.8%)	0.402	251
Hypocitraturia (<550 mg/day)	24	(44.4%)	95	(57.2%)	0.139	220
Hyperoxaluria (>40 mg/day)	20	(34.5%)	58	(34.9%)	1.000	224
Hypernatriuria (>150 mmol/day)	15	(28.9%)	81	(50.9%)	0.009	211
Hyperuricosuria (>750 mg/day)	8	(13.3%)	29	(17.0%)	0.650	231
Low volume (<2000 ml/day)	35	(66.0%)	93	(68.9%)	0.839	188
Mean ± SD stone composition % (range):						
CaOMH	45.4 ± 31.2	(0–90)	38.1 ± 31.4	(0–90)	0.286	239
CaODH	16.9 ± 19.0	(0–60)	17.0 ± 20.4	(0–90)	0.985	239
CaPh	25.2 ± 29.0	(0–90)	32.4 ± 34.6	(0–100)	0.270	239
CaHPh	4.6 ± 17.2	(0–80)	2.0 ± 11.7	(0–90)	0.479	239
MAP	2.5 ± 12.3	(0–60)	3.2 ± 12.9	(0–70)	0.791	239
UA	1.7 ± 4.8	(0–20)	3.4 ± 15.9	(0–100)	0.240	239
No. greater than 70% mixed (%)*	11	(45.8%)	94	(43.7%)	1.000	239
No. 70% or greater pure (%)*					0.261	239
CaOMH	9	(69.2%)	48	(39.7%)		
CaODH	0	(0%)	8	(6.6%)		
CaPh	3	(23.1%)	54	(44.6%)		
CaHPh	1	(7.7%)	3	(2.5%)		
MAP	0	(0%)	2	(1.7%)		
UA	0	(0%)	6	(5.0%)		

*Stones qualified as pure if the dominant component made up ≥ 70% of the stone.

low urine volume (63.0% vs 69.2%, $p = 0.079$) but these did not reach statistical significance.

Multivariate analysis of the PCOS patients using continuous free testosterone values did not reveal any statistically significant associations between 24-hour urine and stone composition parameters and free testosterone levels.

3.3. Stone Composition. Stone composition was recorded when present (24/74 PCOS patients, 215/222 controls). Stone composition assessment for the case-control cohort showed calcium oxalate monohydrate as the predominant component in both the PCOS patients and the controls (45.4% and 38.1%, respectively, Table 1). Mixed stone frequency was similar between the groups being present in 45.8% of the PCOS patients and 43.7% of the controls. Calcium oxalate monohydrate was the most frequent pure stone type in the PCOS group, while calcium phosphate was the most frequent amongst controls. Overall, stone composition assessment for both the testosterone and case-control cohorts did not reveal any statistically significant patterns in stone composition for either stone content quantitative or stone type qualitative parameters.

4. Discussion

4.1. PCOS-Nephrolithiasis Relationship. Even though the etiology of PCOS is still unclear, its clinical associations with hypertension, insulin resistance, and abdominal obesity due to androgen excess have been successfully documented [10–13]. However, the potential clinical association with kidney stones is still unexplored. We attempted to characterize the 24-hour urine metabolic and stone composition parameters of PCOS via our case-control cohort. Only sodium showed significant variations between PCOS patients with stones and our control group. Of relevance to this observation, there is evidence that sex differences can impact osmotic regulation of vasopressin and renal sodium handling, most likely due to alterations in testosterone and estrogen levels [14]. While we cannot make any definitive conclusions based on these findings, the broad hormonal changes in PCOS may be driving these differences in sodium excretion; however, menstrual cycle phase can also impact these outcomes that were not able to account for in our sample.

Polycystic ovary syndrome has also been linked to increased rates of the metabolic syndrome with an estimated prevalence of 33–43% in PCOS patients and a statistically

Table 2: Bivariate analysis using categorical testosterone levels within the PCOS cohort.

	High testosterone ($n = 38$)		Normal testosterone ($n = 36$)		p value	N
Mean ± SD age (range)	32.4 ± 8.2	(14.9–57.0)	39.7 ± 13.8	(13.63–73.69)	0.008	74
Mean ± SD kg/m^2 BMI (range)	34.3 ± 7.0	(21.0–54.5)	27.9 ± 6.3	(17.93–48.79)	<0.001	74
Mean ± SD 24 hr urine panel (range)						
Calcium (mg/day)	223.7 ± 158.5	(35.5–913.6)	198.3 ± 87.7	(50.5–366.7)	0.426	65
Citrate (mg/day)	709.6 ± 411.7	(118–1903)	517.1 ± 257.9	(82–956	0.041	54
Creatinine (g/day)	1.3 ± 0.5	(0.6–3.2)	1.2 ± 0.3	(0.6–1.6)	0.224	56
Oxalate (mg/day)	37.6 ± 12.3	(17–66)	39.3 ± 18.3	(19–113)	0.681	58
Sodium (mmol/day)	144.4 ± 54.1	(49–282)	123.8 ± 47.8	(52–283)	0.154	52
Uric acid (mg/day)	565.3 ± 225.2	(179–1016)	461.4 ± 126.9	(208–739)	0.028	60
Volume (ml/day)	1721.8 ± 822.9	(581–3440)	1561.1 ± 769.6	(590–3259)	0.466	53
No. abnormality (%)						
Hypercalciuria (>200 mg/day)	17	(51.5%)	18	(56.3%)	0.893	65
Hypocitraturia (<550 mg/day)	11	(36.7%)	13	(54.2%)	0.312	54
Hyperoxaluria (>40 mg/day)	13	(41.9%)	7	(25.9%)	0.316	58
Hypernatriuria (>150 mmol/day)	12	(40.0%)	3	(13.6%)	0.078	52
Hyperuricosuria (>750 mg/day)	8	(23.5%)	0	(0%)	0.008	60
Low volume (<2000 ml/day)	17	(63.0%)	18	(69.2%)	0.848	53
Mean ± SD stone composition % (range)						
CaOMH	35.7 ± 31.8	(0–80)	59.0 ± 26.0	(0–90)	0.062	24
CaODH	16.4 ± 17.8	(0–60)	17.5 ± 21.5	(0–50)	0.899	24
CaPh	31.4 ± 31.8	(0–90)	16.5 ± 23.3	(0–80)	0.199	24
CaHPh	7.9 ± 22.3	(0–80)	—	—	0.209	24
MAP	4.3 ± 16.0	(0–60)	—	—	0.336	24
UA	0.7 ± 2.7	(0–10)	3.0 ± 6.8	(0–20)	0.332	24
No. greater than 70% mixed (%)*	7	(50%)	4	(40%)	1.000	24

No adjustments made for confounding variables, original analysis only, and therefore, p values not referenced in discussion. *Stones qualified as pure if the dominant component made up ≥70% of the stone.

Table 3: Multivariate analysis using categorical testosterone levels within the PCOS cohort.

Linear regression	β coefficient	Standard error	p value	N
Mean ± SD 24 hr urine panel (range):				
Calcium (mg/day)	−32.4	38.8	0.406	65
Citrate (mg/day)	−246.3	117.4	0.041	54
Creatinine (g/day)	−0.1	0.1	0.691	56
Oxalate (mg/day)	1.8	4.8	0.705	58
Sodium (mmol/day)	−36.7	18.9	0.058	52
Uric acid (mg/day)	−28.4	57.2	0.621	60
Volume (ml/day)	−449.5	238.7	0.066	53
Mean ± SD stone composition % (range):				
CaOMH	11.9	13.6	0.392	24
CaODH	3.6	10.9	0.743	24
CaPh	2.5	12.9	0.851	24
CaHPh	−14.4	9.5	0.144	24
MAP	−9.6	6.3	0.145	24
UA	1.8	2.4	0.481	24
Logistic regression	**Odds ratio**	**95% CI**	**p value**	**N**
No. abnormality (%):				
Hypercalciuria (>200 mg/day)	1.0	0.32–3.33	0.955	65
Hypocitraturia (<550 mg/day)	0.2	0.04–0.94	0.042	54
Hyperoxaluria (>40 mg/day)	1.9	0.50–7.14	0.340	58
Hypernatriuria (>150 mmol/day)	13.3	1.49–100	0.021	52
Hyperuricosuria (>750 mg/day)	6250	4×10^{22}–9×10^{-16}	0.693	60
Low volume (<2000 ml/day)	0.2	0.04–1.19	0.079	53
No. greater than 70% mixed (%)*	1.0	0.11–9.09	0.978	24

Note: confounding variables adjusted for age, BMI, and metformin status with high or normal testosterone classification as an independent variable. Odds ratio is reported as the likelihood of a high testosterone PCOS patient having a given urine or stone analysis finding. Negative β coefficient indicates an elevation of that parameter in the high testosterone cohort. CI = confidence interval.

significantly positive trend with free testosterone levels but only before adjusting for BMI [15, 16]. The metabolic syndrome in turn has been linked to several urological disease processes including nephrolithiasis [17]. Additionally, abdominal adiposity is commonly associated with PCOS and obesity is a well-documented risk factor for kidney stone formation [12, 18, 19].

Both our data and these observations indicate that a potential relationship between PCOS and kidney stones may not be directly related to hyperandrogenism but rather the obesity, metabolic syndrome, and/or insulin resistance that are frequently associated with this syndrome. It seems that urinary metabolic and stone composition data on PCOS patients compared with stone forming controls for age and BMI are not sufficient to determine whether PCOS is an independent risk factor for stone formation. Further prospective data regarding the prevalence of kidney stones in PCOS patients and potential associations within that group for obesity and the metabolic syndrome may shed more light on the issue.

4.2. Testosterone-Nephrolithiasis Relationship. The association between PCOS and hyperandrogenism offers an opportunity to explore the relationship between testosterone and urolithiasis [2]. However, PCOS is also a complex endocrine disorder with a variety of clinical signs, including variations in hyperandrogenism, which makes it heterogenous and difficult to diagnose [10]. Therefore, the lack of significant differences in our case-control cohort may have been due to our sample including a mixture of elevated and normal testosterone PCOS patients. Future studies may choose to look at only a subset of actively hyperandrogenic or newly diagnosed PCOS patients to account for this variation. This clinical variability in androgen levels could be due to both variations in treatment or disease severity. In light of these variations, we also chose to examine the impact of testosterone values within our PCOS group while accounting for antiandrogenic and other medications used in the treatment of PCOS.

Previous studies on the associations between androgens and nephrolithiasis have reached divergent conclusions, possibly due to variations in use of total and/or free testosterone assays. Several investigators have reported that both free and total testosterone are elevated in stone forming patients [4, 7]. However, others reported that only total testosterone is elevated in stone-forming patients [5, 8]. Clouding the discussion further, one study reported an increased risk of stones with lower testosterone levels [20]. A single study found no association with testosterone [21]. Our endocrinologists only evaluate free testosterone due to previous evidence that it is more sensitive than total testosterone for the diagnosis of hyperandrogenic disorders such as PCOS [22]. Our cutoff for high free testosterone classification was set at >6.4 pg/mL due to previously published reference ranges [9].

4.3. Testosterone: Citrate, Natriuria, and Urinary Volume. High free testosterone classification was associated in our multivariable analysis with increased urinary citrate, sodium, and volume (Table 1). Regarding the increase in citrate excretion, previous literature has found that PCOS patients have increased rates of cortisol production as well as insulin-resistance-related increase in serum aldosterone [23, 24]. These two processes may be contributing to a metabolic alkalosis leading in turn to the increased citrate excretion we observed; however, we were not able to obtain a large enough sample of serum bicarbonate values to fully examine this possibility. Higher citrate and urinary volumes have been found to be protective against the formation of kidney stones [25]. This may support a prior study that reported increased urinary stone risk in those with lower testosterone levels [20].

Previous examinations into testosterone's role in hypertension have indicated that testosterone may be driving a rightward shift in the pressure-natriuresis curve as well as contributing to increased interglomerular pressure [26]. Based on these findings, the respective increases in urine volume and sodium excretion among high testosterone PCOS patients could be secondary to this androgen-induced increase in interglomerular pressure and rightward shift in the pressure-natriuresis relationship.

4.4. Testosterone: Oxalate. Population data have shown that men have higher urinary oxalate excretion, an important promoter of lithogenesis [27]. Lee and colleagues noted decreased calcium oxalate stone formation in castrated male rats [3]. More recently, Nath, et al. reported significantly higher 24-hour urinary oxalate excretion in male stone formers and a positive association between free testosterone levels and urinary oxalate [4]. Despite these findings, we did not observe any significant changes in oxalate excretion within 24-hour urine metabolic panels or an increased frequency of calcium oxalate stones based on either PCOS or testosterone status.

4.5. Limitations. One major limitation to our study is its retrospective nature; however, a case-control methodology increases the likelihood that a difference in outcomes would be the result of PCOS. We also were not able to adjust for dietary factors that could impact 24-hour urine results or menstrual cycle timing that could impact free testosterone levels. It is also possible that the impact of androgens on stone risk in women may differ from that in men. Additionally, very few of the PCOS patients selected from the registry had stone composition analysis performed, which limited our analysis. Also, as a registry-based study, there is the possibility of bias regarding the criteria applied by different providers in assigning the diagnosis of polycystic ovarian syndrome.

5. Conclusions

When compared to matched cohort of healthy stone formers, PCOS patients did not demonstrate significant differences in 24-hour urine and stone composition values. It is possible that the potential relationship between PCOS and kidney stones may not be directly related to hyperandrogenism but rather the obesity, metabolic syndrome, and/or insulin resistance that are frequently associated with this syndrome. Elevated free testosterone in PCOS patients demonstrated a significant association with higher sodium and urine volume, possibly secondary to an increased intraglomerular pressure and a rightward shift in the pressure-natriuresis relationship. This patient cohort may provide deeper insight into the interplay between androgens and stone formation; however, further study is needed to fully characterize the possible relationship between PCOS and stone formation.

Abbreviations

CaOMH:	Calcium oxalate monohydrate
CaODH:	Calcium oxalate dihydrate
CaPh:	Calcium phosphate
CaHPh:	Calcium hydrogen phosphate
CI:	Confidence interval
LC/MS/MS:	Liquid chromatography tandem mass spectrometry
MAP:	Magnesium ammonium phosphate
PCOS:	Polycystic ovarian syndrome
UA:	Uric acid.

References

[1] R. S. Legro and J. F. Strauss, "Molecular progress in infertility: polycystic ovary syndrome," *Fertility and Sterility*, vol. 78, no. 3, pp. 569–576, 2002.

[2] I. Kaygusuz, O. F. Karatas, H. Kafali, E. Cimentepe, and D. Unal, "Is polycystic ovarian syndrome a risk factor for urolithiasis?," *Urolithiasis*, vol. 41, no. 4, pp. 361-362, 2013.

[3] Y. H. Lee, W. C. Huang, J. K. Huang, and L. S. Chang, "Testosterone enhances whereas estrogen inhibits calcium oxalate stone formation in ethylene glycol treated rats," *The Journal of Urology*, vol. 156, no. 2, pp. 502–505, 1996.

[4] S. J. Nath, D. Sarma, P. K. Bagchi, S. K. Baruah, R. T. Puthenveetil, and S. J. Baruah, "The role of serum testosterone as a lithogenic factor and its correlation with stone and urine composition amongst male stone formers," *UroToday International Journal*, vol. 6, no. 3, p. 37, 2013.

[5] J. M. Watson, A. B. Shrewsberry, S. Taghechian et al., "Serum testosterone may be associated with calcium oxalate urolithogenesis," *Journal of Endourology*, vol. 24, no. 7, pp. 1183–1187, 2010.

[6] G. C. Curhan, "Epidemiology of stone disease," *Urologic Clinics of North America*, vol. 34, no. 3, pp. 287–293, 2007.

[7] M. R. Naghii, M. Babaei, and M. Hedayati, "Androgens involvement in the pathogenesis of renal stones formation," *PLoS One*, vol. 9, no. 4, pp. 1–4, 2014.

[8] K. Gupta, G. Gill, and R. Mahajan, "Possible role of elevated serum testosterone in pathogenesis of renal stone formation," *International Journal of Applied and Basic Medical Research*, vol. 6, no. 4, pp. 241–244, 2016.

[9] G. D. Braunstein, R. E. Reitz, A. Buch, D. Schnell, and M. P. Caulfield, "Testosterone reference ranges in normally cycling healthy premenopausal women," *The Journal of Sexual Medicine*, vol. 8, no. 10, pp. 2924–2934, 2011.

[10] E. Diamanti-Kandarakis, "Insulin resistance in PCOS," *Endocrine*, vol. 30, no. 1, pp. 13–18, 2006.

[11] M.-J. Chen, W.-S. Yang, J.-H. Yang, C.-L. Chen, H.-N. Ho, and Y.-S. Yang, "Relationship between androgen levels and blood pressure in young women with polycystic ovary syndrome," *Hypertension*, vol. 49, no. 6, pp. 1442–1447, 2007.

[12] H. F. Escobar-Morreale and J. L. S. Millán, "Abdominal adiposity and the polycystic ovary syndrome," *Trends in Endocrinology & Metabolism*, vol. 18, no. 7, pp. 266–272, 2007.

[13] M. Luque-Ramírez, D. Martí, E. Fernández-Durán, M. Alpañés, F. Álvarez-Blasco, and H. F. Escobar-Morreale, "Office blood pressure, ambulatory blood pressure monitoring, and echocardiographic abnormalities in women with polycystic ovary syndrome," *Hypertension*, vol. 63, no. 3, pp. 624–629, 2014.

[14] N. S. Stachenfeld, A. E. Splenser, W. L. Calzone, M. P. Taylor, and D. L. Keefe, "Selected contribution: sex differences in osmotic regulation of AVP and renal sodium handling," *Journal of Applied Physiology*, vol. 91, no. 4, pp. 1893–1901, 2001.

[15] P. Essah and J. Nestler, "Metabolic syndrome in women with polycystic ovary syndrome," *Fertility and Sterility*, vol. 86, pp. S18–S19, 2006.

[16] D. A. Ehrmann, D. R. Liljenquist, K. Kasza, R. Azziz, R. S. Legro, and M. N. Ghazzi, "Prevalence and predictors of the metabolic syndrome in women with polycystic ovary syndrome," *The Journal of Clinical Endocrinology & Metabolism*, vol. 91, no. 1, pp. 48–53, 2006.

[17] I. Gorbachinsky, H. Akpinar, and D. G. Assimos, "Metabolic syndrome and urologic diseases," *Reviews in Urology*, vol. 12, no. 4, pp. e157–e180, 2010.

[18] E. N. Taylor, M. J. Stampfer, and G. C. Curhan, "Obesity, weight gain, and the risk of kidney stones," *JAMA*, vol. 293, no. 4, pp. 455–462, 2005.

[19] M. J. Semins, A. D. Shore, M. A. Makary, T. Magnuson, R. Johns, and B. R. Matlaga, "The association of increasing body mass index and kidney stone disease," *Journal of Urology*, vol. 183, no. 2, pp. 571–575, 2010.

[20] A. Otunctemur, E. Ozbek, S. S. Cakir et al., "Urolithiasis is associated with low serum testosterone levels in men," *Archivio Italiano di Urologia e Andrologia*, vol. 87, no. 1, pp. 83–86, 2015.

[21] J. J. Knoedler, A. E. Krambeck, W. Astorne, E. Bergstralh, and J. Lieske, "Sex steroid hormone levels may not explain gender differences in development of nephrolithiasis," *Journal of Endourology*, vol. 29, no. 12, pp. 1341–1345, 2015.

[22] R. Azziz, E. Carmina, D. Dewailly et al., "The androgen excess and PCOS society criteria for the polycystic ovary syndrome: the complete task force report," *Fertility and Sterility*, vol. 91, no. 2, pp. 456–488, 2009.

[23] T. Cascella, S. Palomba, L. Tauchmanovà et al., "Serum aldosterone concentration and cardiovascular risk in women with polycystic ovarian syndrome," *The Journal of Clinical Endocrinology & Metabolism*, vol. 91, no. 11, pp. 4395–4400, 2006.

[24] T. Tsilchorozidou, J. W. Honour, and G. S. Conway, "Altered cortisol metabolism in polycystic ovary syndrome: insulin enhances 5α-reduction but not the elevated adrenal steroid production rates," *The Journal of Clinical Endocrinology & Metabolism*, vol. 88, no. 12, pp. 5907–5913, 2003.

[25] O. W. Moe, "Kidney stones: pathophysiology and medical management," *The Lancet*, vol. 367, no. 9507, pp. 333–344, 2006.
[26] J. F. Reckelhoff and J. P. Granger, "Role of androgens in mediating hypertension and renal injury," *Clinical and Experimental Pharmacology and Physiology*, vol. 26, no. 2, pp. 127–131, 1999.
[27] K. K. Stamatelou, M. E. Francis, C. A. Jones, L. M. Nyberg, and G. C. Curhan, "Time trends in reported prevalence of kidney stones in the United States: 1976–1994," *Kidney International*, vol. 63, no. 5, pp. 1817–1823, 2003.

15

Recent Pathophysiological Aspects of Peyronie's Disease: Role of Free Radicals, Rationale and Therapeutic Implications for Antioxidant Treatment

Gianni Paulis,[1,2] Gennaro Romano,[3] Luca Paulis,[4] and Davide Barletta[5]

[1]*Regina Apostolorum Hospital, Andrology Center, Albano Laziale, Rome, Italy*
[2]*Castelfidardo Medical Team, Peyronie's Disease Care Center, Rome, Italy*
[3]*Italian League against Cancer, Department of Urologic Oncology, Section of Avellino, Avellino, Italy*
[4]*Faculty of Pharmacy, University of Rome "La Sapienza", Rome, Italy*
[5]*Department of Urology, Andrology Center, San Matteo Hospital, Pavia, Italy*

Correspondence should be addressed to Gianni Paulis; paulisg@libero.it

Academic Editor: Matthew Rutman

Peyronie's disease (PD) is a chronic inflammation of tunica albuginea of the corpora cavernosa that causes an inelastic plaque resulting in penis deformation. Although its etiology is not completely known, there is general consensus that PD is genetically transmitted and secondary to penile trauma. In recent years, numerous studies demonstrated the role played by oxidative stress in PD pathogenesis, and other studies have described successful use of antioxidants in PD treatment. Oxidative stress is an integral part of this disease, influencing its progression. In the early stages of PD, the inflammatory infiltrate cells produce high quantities of free radicals and proinflammatory and profibrotic cytokines, with consequent activation of transcription factor NF-κB. While conservative therapies commonly used in the early stages of PD include oral substances (Potaba, tamoxifen, colchicine, and vitamin E), intralesional treatment (verapamil, interferon, steroids, and more recently collagenase clostridium histolyticum-Xiaflex), and local physical treatment (iontophoresis, extracorporeal shock wave therapy, and penile extender), the significant results obtained by emerging treatments with the antioxidants cited in this article suggest these therapeutic agents interfere at several levels with the disease's pathogenetic mechanisms. Antioxidants therapy outcomes are interesting for good clinical practice and also confirm the fundamental role played by oxidative stress in PD.

1. Introduction

Peyronie's disease (PD), a chronic inflammation of the tunica albuginea of the corpora cavernosa, causes formation of a hard, inelastic plaque, often resulting in penis deformation. Prevalence varies between 3.2% and 13%; it generally affects males around 50 years of age, but recently a rise in frequency has been recorded in younger patients [1, 2]. Like Dupuytren's contracture, PD more frequently affects white men, more rarely black, and Asian men [3]. Although its etiology is not completely known, there is general consensus that PD is genetically transmitted and secondary to penile trauma [4, 5]. Familiar aggregation and genetic transmission through HLA-B7 antigens had been amply described and understood [6–8]. Recently, a genetic locus that PD shares with Dupuytren's contracture was identified; WNT2 is the locus involved in genetic predisposition for both Dupuytren's disease and PD [9]. Previously, some studies had already observed the analogy and strong affinity between the two diseases: Dupuytren's contracture's typical cells with "cross-banded" nuclei had been observed in PD plaques in 1976; in 1989, Somers et al., after histological examination of PD plaques, proved an increase in type III collagen content, similarly to what occurs in Dupuytren's contracture [10, 11].

PD symptoms include penile pain (20%–70% of cases), penile curvature or deformation (94% of cases), erectile dysfunction (31.5% of cases), depressive state (48% of cases), and presence of a more or less palpable penile nodule [12–14]. Penile distortion occurs because the area of disease (plaque) has a tendency to gradually become less elastic; histological analysis of penile plaques unfailingly detects an alteration and disorganization of collagen associated with a reduction in elastin density [15].

The disease has three stages: acute posttraumatic period > inflammatory remodeling phase > stabilization phase.

The first stage of the disease is characterized by a brief acute posttraumatic period, lasting about 2 weeks, during which, after blood extravasation and fibrin and platelet accumulation, powerful recruitment of inflammatory cells, macrophages, and lymphocytes occurs [16]. During this brief period, no penile nodule is palpable and no plaque is visible on ultrasound. The next stage which lasts about 12–18 months is the inflammatory remodeling phase [16, 17]. In this stage various growth factors start to be produced, initially causing tissue degradation, production of a new extracellular matrix (ECM), and tissue remodeling; in this stage, rapid growth of plaque occurs, often associated with pain and penile curvature; the plaque then tends to gradually consolidate and become increasingly more fibrous, until one or more areas of calcification, which tend to grow larger, make their appearance. Pain (when present) then usually disappears, but an increase in curvature angle is almost always observed. At the end of this inflammatory phase, the disease stabilizes. In this third phase (stabilization), pain is typically absent, penis deformation is stable, and fibrocalcification of the plaque is practically complete; consequently, nodules are always clearly palpable in this phase.

1.1. Premises of Microscopic and Functional Anatomy. The tunica albuginea of the corpora cavernosa is made up of both collagen fibers (the majority) and elastic fibers. Whereas collagen fibers have greater resistance to traction and are inelastic, elastic fibers can be extended up to 150% of their normal length [18]. With no elastic fibers in the tunica albuginea, the penis would not be able to grow in length and size during erection. In normal conditions and in the absence of disease, the elastic fibers along the penile shaft, within the tunica albuginea, appear as a net interwoven with collagen fibers. However, in the penile crura and distal part of the corpora cavernosa (apex), the tunica albuginea is only or almost exclusively made up of collagen fibers [18, 19]. Thus, any local change in elastic fiber content can cause penile deformation.

The purpose of this article is to clarify and explain the significant role of the oxidative stress in PD pathogenesis; the other important objective of the article is to explain the resulting role of antioxidants in PD treatment.

2. Pathophysiology of Peyronie's' Disease (Figure 1)

2.1. Mechanism of Plaque Formation. Following trauma, delamination of the tunica albuginea occurs, with extravasation and accumulation of fibrin between the layers, due to insufficient activation of fibrinolysis [6]. Presence of the platelet thrombus and fibrin is responsible for the subsequent cascade of events. Fibrin acts as a strong chemotactic factor, recruiting inflammatory cells like neutrophil granulocytes, macrophages, mast cells, and so forth [20]. These cells immediately begin to produce proinflammatory cytokines, particularly transforming-growth-factor-beta-1 (TGF-ß1); platelets, too, along with the macrophages already present in the area after the posttraumatic extravasation, release TGF-ß1 cytokines and platelet-derived-growth-factor (PDGF) [17, 21]. Fibrin accumulation also promotes the influx of fibroblasts, already attracted by TGF-ß1 and PDGF [20, 21]. Macrophages and inflammatory cells are also responsible for the production of elastase, an enzyme that can cause degradation of the tunica albuginea's elastic fibers [20, 22]. Enhanced elastase activity and elastin-derived peptides act chemotactically, contributing to both the increase in the inflammatory cellular infiltrate and the influx of fibroblasts [20].

2.2. Role of the Disease's Most Important Biological Mediators

2.2.1. Transforming-Growth-Factor-Beta-1 (TGF-ß1). TGF-ß1, produced by platelets, macrophages, neutrophils, and T-lymphocytes, is considered the most important profibrotic factor associated with PD.

TGF-ß1 possesses chemotactic activity on blood neutrophils, monocytes, lymphocytes, and fibroblasts [6, 17, 22–24]. TGF-ß1 activity includes the following: inducing fibroblasts to produce collagen; influencing ECM deposition, stimulating synthesis of individual components of the matrix, such as proteoglycans and fibronectin; promoting fibroblast proliferation and differentiation into myofibroblasts, that is, mesenchymal cells that share the same phenotype as smooth muscle cells and fibroblasts and therefore have the capacity both to contract and to synthesize collagen [6, 22, 23, 25]. In addition, TGF-ß1 has the following actions: induces *reactive oxygen species* (ROS) production; inhibits production of certain *matrix metalloproteinases* (MMPs), particularly MMP-1, MMP-8, and MMP-13, which have collagenolytic activity, increasing synthesis of *tissue inhibitors of matrix metalloproteinase* (TIMPs, specifically TIMP-1); increases synthesis of MMP-10, which can degrade elastin; activates the *nuclear factor kappa-light-chain-enhancer of activated B cells* (NF-κB); inhibits fibrinolysis by inducing synthesis of *plasminogen activator inhibitor-1* (PAI-1); induces osteogenesis [17, 22, 26–32]. However, it has been shown that during the progression of disease the plaque undergoes calcification or ossification in 15%–25% of PD cases [32].

2.2.2. Platelet-Derived Growth Factor (PDGF). Produced mainly by platelets, but even by macrophages, PDGF, too, is profibrotic. Like TGF-ß1, PDGF has chemotactic activity on fibroblasts [6]. Furthermore, PDGF induces TIMP-1 synthesis, collagen biosynthesis, fibroblast proliferation, and differentiation into myofibroblasts, and it contributes to plaque calcification and ossification, also recruiting osteoblasts [6, 21, 22, 26, 33, 34].

2.2.3. Interleukin (IL-1). Proinflammatory cytokine IL-1 is produced by macrophages and fibroblasts [35, 36]. One of PD's numerous profibrotic factors is that it is strongly chemotactic for fibroblasts; it stimulates collagen synthesis;

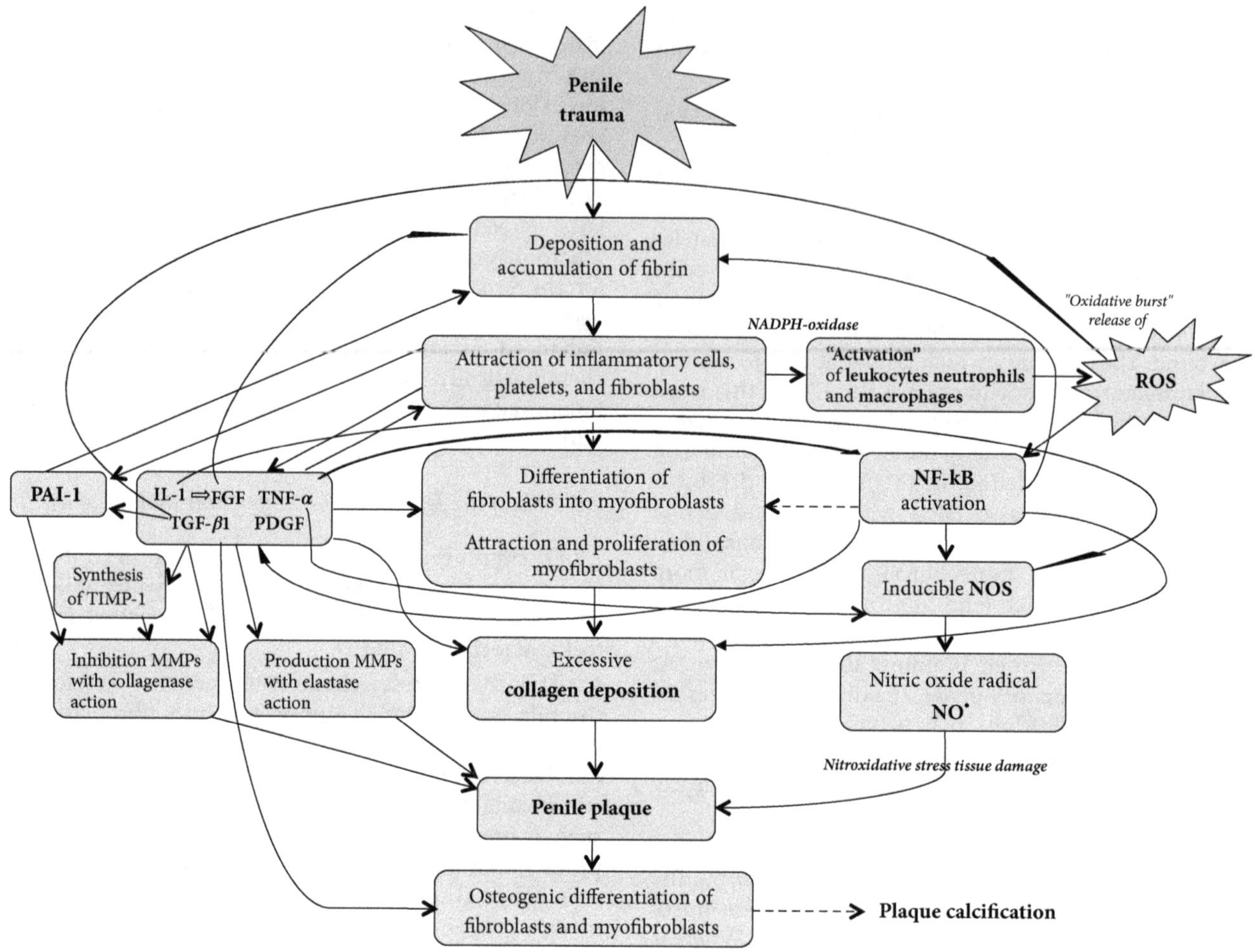

FIGURE 1: Pathogenetic mechanisms of Peyronie's disease.

it increases fibroblast production of MMP-1, MMP-2, MMP-8, MMP-9, MMP-10, and MMP-13; it promotes synthesis of MMP-9 and MMP-3 and basic fibroblast growth factor; it stimulates production of *inducible nitric oxide synthase* (iNOS), an enzyme that plays a fundamental role in oxidative stress; it activates NF-κB [6, 12, 17, 34, 35, 37, 38].

2.2.4. Basic Fibroblast Growth Factor (bFGF). This typically profibrotic growth factor is mainly produced by fibroblasts and myofibroblasts; it attracts fibroblasts in the area and induces their proliferation, stimulates collagen synthesis, increases synthesis of MMP-1 and MMP-9 (with elastic activity) and TIMP-1, and causes further local fibrin deposit [6, 33, 34, 37].

2.2.5. Plasminogen Activator Inhibitor-1 (PAI-1). Another important profibrotic factor produced mainly by platelets is that PAI-1 inhibits fibrinolysis, causing fibrin to remain at the site, triggering recruitment of inflammatory cells and subsequent release of profibrotic factors (cytokines, etc.); it also hinders collagenolysis and inhibits MMPs [39, 40].

2.2.6. Tumor Necrosis Factor (TNF-α). Produced by monocytes and macrophages, in the course of the disease its activity involves the following: recruiting fibroblasts and stimulating their proliferation; stimulating iNOS production; inducing cellular apoptosis; stimulating production of MMP-9 (elastase); activating nuclear factor NF-κB; inducing PAI-1 synthesis [6, 34, 37, 41–43].

In PD, therefore, we have a preponderance of profibrotic factors causing excessive deposition of collagen and ECM; this leads to extreme disorganization of the collagen fibers, loss of elastic fibers, and consequent elasticity loss in the tissues involved. Although both type I collagen and type III collagen have been shown to be present in PD, the latter is much more plentiful in PD plaque [11, 30]. Microscopic studies have shown that besides an increased number of fibroblasts, a haphazard arrangement is present, with random orientation of collagen bands and a marked reduction in elastic fibers, which appear disrupted, with excessive accumulation of elastin [20]. Consequently, a thickening of the tissue (plaque) forms, resulting in elasticity loss and inevitable onset of penile deformation.

2.3. Free Radicals and Oxidative and Nitrosative Stress as Fundamental Component of Peyronie's Disease. In the last fifteen years, oxidative stress has been shown to play a decisive

TABLE 1: Chemical reactions during oxidative stress and direct reactions of vitamin E and coenzyme Q10 with reactive species.

Superoxide anion ($O_2^{\bullet-}$)	$NADPH + O_2 \rightarrow NADP^+ + H^+ + O_2^{\bullet-}$
Hydrogen peroxide (H_2O_2)	SOD $2H^+ + 2O_2^{\bullet-} \rightarrow O_2 + H_2O_2$
Hydroxyl radical ($HO^\bullet$)	$Fe^{2+} + H_2O_2 \rightarrow Fe^{3+} + HO^- + HO^\bullet$ (Fenton's reaction)
Hydroxyl radical ($HO^\bullet$)	$O_2^{\bullet-} + H_2O_2 \rightarrow O_2 + HO^- + HO^\bullet$ (Haber-Weiss reaction)
Hypochlorous acid (HOCl)	MPO $Cl^- + H_2O_2 \rightarrow HO^- + HOCl$
Singlet oxygen ($^1O_2^\bullet$)	$H_2O_2 + HOCl \rightarrow H_2O + Cl^- + {}^1O_2^\bullet$
Nitric oxide ($NO^\bullet$)	NOS L-Arginine + NADPH + O_2 → L-Citrulline + $NO^\bullet$
Peroxynitrite ($ONOO^-$)	$O_2^{\bullet-} + NO^\bullet \rightarrow ONOO^-$
Peroxynitrous acid (HOONO)	$ONOO^- + H^+ \rightarrow HOONO$
Hydroxyl radical ($HO^\bullet$) and nitrogen dioxide radical ($NO_2^\bullet$)	$HOONO \rightarrow HO^\bullet + NO_2^\bullet$
Antioxidant activity of *vitamin E*(α-tocopherol-OH)	$R^\bullet$ (reactive species) + α-tocopherol-OH → RH + α-tocopherol-$O^\bullet$ $HO^\bullet$ (hydroxyl radical) + α-tocopherol-OH → H_2O + α-tocopherol-$O^\bullet$ $LOO^\bullet$ + α-tocopherol-OH → LOOH + α-tocopherol-$O^\bullet$
Antioxidant activity of *coenzyme Q10*	Q10H2 + $LOO^\bullet$ → $Q10^{\bullet-}$ + H^+ + LOOH

role in the physiopathological mechanisms of PD [6, 22, 26, 30, 32, 34, 35, 39].

At the disease site, ROS hyperproduction occurs in addition to cytokine production. The oxidative stress process begins very early, in the first 24–48 hours: through fibrin's chemotactic activity, an inflammatory cellular infiltrate is produced. Oxidation is truly triggered at this stage of the disease [30]. After leukocyte activation, neutrophil granulocytes and macrophages at the inflammatory site undergo degranulation and release lysosomal enzymes (collagenase, elastase, etc.); at the same time, a "respiratory burst" (or oxidative burst) occurs, which consists in rapid release of ROS (specifically, superoxide radicals and hydrogen peroxide) by neutrophils and macrophages [22]. The activation mechanism is supported by intracellular enzyme *nicotinamide adenine dinucleotide phosphate* (NADPH) oxidase, present in neutrophils, eosinophils, and macrophages. NADPH-oxidase catalyzes electron transfer from the cytoplasmic NADPH donor to molecular oxygen (acceptor), forming *superoxide anion* ($O_2^{\bullet-}$) (Table 1). The inflammatory cells then produce high quantities of $O_2^{\bullet-}$ that is dismutated to *hydrogen peroxide* (H_2O_2) thanks to the presence of the *superoxide dismutase* (SOD) enzyme (Table 1). SOD, a part of the endogenous antioxidant defense system, then intervenes as primary cellular defense against $O_2^{\bullet-}$, causing catalytic removal of the superoxide radical. Extracellular SOD plays an essential role in maintaining the redox state, blocking negative local effects of $O_2^{\bullet-}$. The superoxide anion also has a direct vasoconstrictive effect through mobilization of calcium ions and can therefore cause erectile dysfunction [44]. The existence of H_2O_2 produced via SOD, and simultaneous presence of metal cations such as iron (Fe^{2+}), causes Fenton's reaction, which produces another highly toxic reactive species, the *hydroxyl radical* ($HO^\bullet$) (Table 1). However, H_2O_2 can also react with $O_2^{\bullet-}$ through *the Haber-Weiss reaction* to produce $HO^\bullet$ (Table 1). H_2O_2 may also be transformed into *hypochlorous acid* (HOCl), given the presence of *myeloperoxidase* (MPO) in neutrophils and macrophages (Table 1). Subsequently, HOCl and H_2O_2 react to form *singlet oxygen* ($^1O_2^\bullet$), another highly toxic reactive species (Table 1). Production of large amounts of proinflammatory cytokines and ROS hyperproduction cause NF-κB activation, a central event in the inflammatory response and further production of inflammatory cytokines [34, 35, 38]. NF-κB, present in almost all cell types is a protein complex controlling DNA transcription; in PD, it regulates the expression of genes encoding for FGF, TGF-ß1, iNOS, fibrin, collagen, and so forth [30]. In the course of PD, the iNOS enzyme is mainly produced by macrophages, smooth muscle cells, and myofibroblasts [22]. Induction of an upregulation of iNOS therefore produces high local levels of *nitric oxide* and a series of its metabolites called *reactive nitrogen species* (RNS), which are free radicals like ROS but can cause greater cell and tissue damage [34]. In normal conditions, *nitric oxide* (NO) is the main mediator of penile erection and acts as a nonadrenergic and noncholinergic neurotransmitter, causing release of the smooth muscles of the corpora cavernosa. NO was also known as *endothelium-derived relaxing factor* (EDRF), and long-standing widespread prejudice held that EDRF could not be identified with unconventional gaseous molecule NO [45]. The chemical reaction producing NO occurs thanks to the presence of amino acid L-arginine via *nitric oxide synthase (NOS)* activity and leads to final synthesis of *L-citrulline* and NO (Table 1). The chemical process requires molecular oxygen and proceeds via synthesis of an intermediate, Nω-hydroxyarginine [46]. Furthermore, the presence of certain cofactors is necessary: *NADPH, flavin adenine dinucleotide* (FAD), *flavin mononucleotide* (FMN), *tetrahydrobiopterin (BH_4),* and *calmodulin (CaM)* [34]. Whereas in normal conditions penile erection is mediated by the action of the two "constitutive" enzyme forms, *neuronal* (nNOS) and *endothelial NOS* (eNOS), which cause normal NO amounts to be produced, in pathological conditions and in PD high local *nitric oxide radical* ($NO^{\bullet -}$) concentrations occur, due to mediation of the inducible enzyme form (iNOS) [34]. While isoforms eNOS and nNOS are Ca^{2+}- and calmodulin-dependent, iNOS is Ca^{2+}- and calmodulin-independent and can be induced by inflammatory cytokines. $NO^{\bullet -}$ is synthesized by monocytes, macrophages, and fibroblasts. $NO^{\bullet -}$ production from iNOS activity is 100 to 1,000 times greater and has longer duration than $NO^{\bullet -}$ production from nNOS or eNOS [34]. It must be stressed that the effects of *nitric oxide radical* ($NO^{\bullet -}$) depend on its concentration, so when local $NO^{\bullet -}$ levels increase significantly (as in PD) a high oxidation state is produced. In these conditions, $NO^{\bullet -}$ starts to compete with SOD, removing *superoxide anion* ($O_2^{\bullet -}$) and causing the formation of peroxynitrite (Table 1) [37]. Therefore, synthesis of peroxynitrite depends on the balance between $O_2^{\bullet -}$ and SOD production and NO synthesis/consumption [34]. Peroxynitrite is a highly toxic, reactive molecule, which can cause cell damage (by lipid peroxidation and DNA fragmentation), tissue damage depletion of plasmatic antioxidants, endothelial smooth muscle relaxation impairment, vascular tone change, and organ dysfunction [34]. When peroxynitrite is protonated, peroxynitrous acid (HOONO) forms, another highly toxic reactive molecule which rapidly breaks down into *hydroxyl radical* ($HO^{\bullet}$) and *nitrogen dioxide radical* ($NO_2^{\bullet}$), two other highly reactive cytotoxic molecules (Table 1). During the inflammatory process, some of these reactive species, such as $HO^{\bullet}$, can chemically react with lipids (lipid peroxidation) generating radicals, for example, *lipid alkyl radical* ($L^{\bullet}$), *lipid alkoxyl radical* ($LO^{\bullet}$), and *lipid peroxyl radical* ($LOO^{\bullet}$); these toxic substances can also react with $NO^{\bullet -}$ producing less reactive substances *(lipid nitrite/LONO, lipid peroxynitrite/LOONO)* which can play a role as diagnostic indicators of lipid peroxidation [30].

2.4. Mechanisms of Action of Antioxidants Used in the Treatment of Peyronie's Disease (Table 2)

2.4.1. Vitamin E. This liposoluble substance was first suggested for PD treatment in 1948 by Scott and Scardino [47]. It has many properties. Antioxidant properties: vitamin E generally reacts with reactive species ($R^{\bullet}$), but its best-known reaction is with *hydroxyl radical* ($HO^{\bullet}$), with donation of a hydrogen ion (H^+) and formation of a stable, no longer reactive molecule *(hydrogen peroxide)* [30]. Furthermore, when vitamin E reacts with *lipid peroxyl radical*, it leads to formation of a tocopheroxyl radical, a relatively stable, poorly reactive molecule that does not cause a new lipid peroxidation process (Table 1); the tocopheroxyl radical soon reacts with any available H^+ molecule, going back to the stable form of vitamin E (α-tocopherol-OH). Vitamin E inhibits inflammatory cell ROS release (respiratory burst) [48].

Antifibrotic Properties. Vitamin E inhibits TGF-ß1 production; D-alpha-tocopherol and α-tocopherol succinate have been shown to inhibit cellular proliferation of fibroblasts in human pathological fibrosis [49, 50].

Anti-Inflammatory Properties. Vitamin E interferes with factor NF-κB, also hindering proinflammatory cytokine transcription; vitamin E has an anti-COX-2 mechanism; it inhibits cell proliferation through a protein kinase C (PKC) inhibition mechanism [51–53].

Furthermore, vitamin E inhibits platelet adhesion and aggregation, improves endothelial function, and can repair DNA [54, 55].

Literature Review. Vitamin E is the oldest substance still currently in use in PD treatment. Scardino and Scott (1948-49) and Steinberg (1951) pioneered the use of vitamin E in medical treatment of PD [56, 57]. In their 1948 study, after treating 23 patients with tocopherol, Scardino and Scott obtained a plaque size reduction in 91% of cases, curvature improvement in 78% of cases, and resolution of pain in all cases. Pryor and Farell (1983) and Safarinejad et al. (2007) observed no significant improvement after treating PD patients with tocopherol compared to placebo treatment [58, 59]. However, several studies have shown that vitamin E is effective only when combined with other treatments (combination or multimodal therapy) [60–62]. In particular, our 2012 controlled study demonstrated the superiority of treatment results when adding vitamin E (600 mg/daily = group A) to a combination therapy (verapamil injection and iontophoresis + blueberries oral + propolis oral + topical Diclofenac/for 6 months = group B): (group A versus group B) success in reducing plaque size 97.14% versus 68.57% ($p = 0.004$); actual plaque size reduction 50.2% versus 35.8% ($p = 0.027$); penile curvature improvement 96.6% versus 48.4% ($p = 0.0001$); mean penile curvature decrease of 12.25° versus 6.73° ($p = 0.01$) [62].

2.4.2. Carnitine. This molecule is very similar to an amino acid; in humans, it is synthesized in the liver, brain, and kidneys from essential amino acids lysine and methionine by ALC transferase. The carnitine system is comprised of L-carnitine, its esters (acetyl L-carnitine, propionyl-L-carnitine), and a complex enzymatic system located in the mitochondrial membrane. It has been estimated that carnitine produced endogenously is 1.2 μmol per day per kg of body weight, but in omnivorous human beings about 75% of carnitine in the body comes from diet, while 25% comes from de novo biosynthesis [63].

Meat is the main external source of carnitine, but it is present in lower concentrations in cod and dairy and in even lower concentrations in plant-based products. Its main role is that of mitochondrial long-chain fatty acid transport; therefore it works to convert fat to energy.

Antioxidant Properties. It is scavenger and neutralizer of *superoxide anion, hydrogen peroxide,* and *peroxynitrite* [64].

L-Carnitine inhibits proliferation and osteoblastic differentiation of fibroblasts [65].

Anti-Inflammatory Properties. L-Carnitine is able to reduce blood levels of C-reactive protein (CRP), interleukin-6 (IL-6),

TABLE 2: Biological properties and mechanisms of action of antioxidants used in the treatment of Peyronie's disease.

Active substance	Biological properties	Mechanisms of action
Vitamin E	Antioxidant	(i) Scavenger activity against hydroxyl radical and lipid peroxyl radical
		(ii) Inhibition of respiratory/oxidative burst and relative release of ROS
	Anti-inflammatory	(i) Inhibition of NF-kappa-B activation and proinflammatory cytokine expression
		(ii) Inhibition of COX-2 activity
	Antifibrotic	(i) Inhibition of TGF-beta-1
		(ii) Inhibition of fibroblast proliferation
		(iii) Inhibition of PDGF activity
	Antiproliferative	(i) Inhibition of protein kinase C activity
		(ii) DNA repair activity
	Antiplatelet	(i) Antiadhesive and antiaggregating activity
Carnitine	Antioxidant	(i) Scavenger activity against super oxide, hydrogen peroxide, and peroxynitrite
		(ii) Suppresses iNOS protein expression and nitric oxide radical production
		(iii) Increase in eNOS expression (counteracting the negative effects of the nitric oxide radical)
	Anti-inflammatory	(i) Downregulation of C-reactive protein, IL-6, and TNF-α expression
		(ii) Inhibition of NF-kappa-B activation and proinflammatory cytokine expression
		(iii) Upregulation of PPARγ
	Antifibrotic	(i) Inhibition of fibroblast proliferation
	Anticalcific	(i) Inhibition of osteogenic differentiation of fibroblasts
Pentoxifylline	Antioxidant	(i) Inhibition of respiratory/oxidative burst and relative release of ROS
		(ii) Hydroxyl radical scavenger
		(iii) Inhibition of lipid oxidation
		(iv) Downregulation of iNOS protein expression
	Anti-inflammatory	(i) Inhibition of NF-kappa-B activation and proinflammatory cytokine expression
		(ii) Inhibition of COX-2 expression
		(iii) Inhibition of TNF-α expression
	Antifibrotic	(i) Reduction of collagen deposition
		(ii) Inhibition of fibroblast proliferation
		(iii) Inhibition of myofibroblastic differentiation of fibroblasts
		(iv) Inhibition of TGF-beta-1 and PAI-1 expression
		(v) Stimulation of fibroblast apoptosis
		(vi) Nonspecific PDE inhibitory activity
	Antiplatelet	(i) Antiaggregating activity
Coenzyme Q10	Antioxidant	(i) Inhibition of increased production of ROS by blocking mitochondrial membrane depolarization
		(ii) Scavenger activity against hydrogen peroxide and singlet oxygen
		(iii) Downregulation of iNOS protein expression
		(iv) Inhibition of excess of nitric oxide production
		(v) Inhibition of lipid peroxidation
		(vi) Regeneration activity of antioxidants vitamin E and vitamin C
	Anti-inflammatory	(i) Inhibition of NF-kappa-B expression
		(ii) Downregulation of IL-6, TNF-α, MCP-1 protein, and IL-1-beta expression
	Antifibrotic	(i) Inhibition of TGF-beta-1

TABLE 2: Continued.

Active substance	Biological properties	Mechanisms of action
Propolis	Antioxidant	(i) Inhibition of release of NADPH-oxidase and myeloperoxidase (quercetin) (ii) Inhibition of xanthine oxidase activity responsible for superoxide anion production (chrysin, pinocembrin, pinobanksin, and apigenin) (iii) Inhibition of respiratory/oxidative burst and relative release of ROS (quercetin, CAPE, and chrysin) (iv) Scavenger activity against superoxide anion, hydroxyl radical, singlet oxygen, peroxynitrite, and lipid peroxyl radicals (quercetin) (v) Scavenger activity against superoxide anion, hydrogen peroxide, and hypochlorous acid (CAPE) (vi) Inhibition of lipid peroxidation (galangin, CAPE, pinocembrin, and pinobanksin) (vii) Regeneration activity of antioxidants vitamin E and vitamin C (galangin) (viii) Downregulation of iNOS protein expression (galangin, quercetin, CAPE, chrysin, and pinocembrin)
	Anti-inflammatory	(i) Inhibition of NF-kappa-B activation (galangin, quercetin, CAPE, chrysin, and apigenin) (ii) Inhibition of IL-1-beta and TNF-α expression (galangin, quercetin, CAPE, chrysin, pinocembrin, and apigenin) (iii) Inhibition of IL-6 expression (galangin, quercetin, CAPE, pinocembrin, and apigenin) (iv) Inhibition of IL-8 expression (quercetin, apigenin) (v) Inhibition of COX-2 (quercetin, CAPE, chrysin, pinocembrin, and apigenin) (vi) Inhibition of lipoxygenase (quercetin) (vii) Inhibition of neutrophil migration to the inflammatory site (apigenin)
	Antifibrotic	(i) Downregulation of TGF-beta-1 expression (galangin, quercetin, CAPE, chrysin, pinocembrin, and apigenin) (ii) Inhibition of MMP-2 and MMP-9 (both with elastase activity) expression (quercetin, galangin, and pinocembrin) (iii) Inhibition of myofibroblastic differentiation of fibroblasts (CAPE, apigenin) (iv) Capacity to reverse myofibroblasts into fibroblasts and reverse collagen formation (CAPE) (v) Inhibition of PDGF activity (chrysin, apigenin) (vi) Inhibition of PAI-1 and fibronectin expression (chrysin)
	Antiplatelet	(i) Antiaggregating activity (apigenin)
Bilberry (*Vaccinium myrtillus* L.)	Antioxidant	(i) Inhibition of release of NADPH-oxidase and myeloperoxidase (quercetin) (ii) Inhibition of respiratory/oxidative burst and relative release of ROS (quercetin) (iii) Scavenger activity against superoxide anion, hydroxyl radical, singlet oxygen, peroxynitrite, and lipid peroxyl radicals (quercetin) (iv) Scavenger activity against superoxide anion, hydroxyl radical, and peroxynitrite (anthocyanins) (v) Scavenger activity against nitrogen species/RNS (delphinidin) (vi) Downregulation of iNOS protein expression (quercetin, cyanidin) (vii) Increase in eNOS expression (delphinidin, cyanidin)
	Anti-inflammatory	(i) Inhibition of NF-kappa-B activation (quercetin, anthocyanins) (ii) Inhibition of IL-1-beta and TNF-α expression (quercetin, anthocyanins) (iii) Inhibition of IL-6 expression (quercetin) (iv) Inhibition of IL-8 expression (quercetin) (v) Inhibition of COX-2 (quercetin, delphinidin, and cyanidin) (vi) Inhibition of lipoxygenase (quercetin) (vii) Downregulation of MCP-1 expression (anthocyanins)
	Antifibrotic	(i) Downregulation of TGF-beta-1 expression (quercetin, anthocyanins) (ii) Inhibition of MMP-2 and MMP-9 (both with elastase activity) expression (quercetin) (iii) Inhibition of PDGF and FGB activity (catechins)
	Antiproliferative	(i) Antiproliferative and proapoptotic activity (catechins)

and TNF-α [66]. It can inhibit factor NF-κB, also suppressing *nitric oxide radical* production and iNOS protein expression [67]. The anti-inflammatory and antifibrotic properties of L-carnitine derive from its ability to cause upregulation of *peroxisome proliferator-activated receptor-γ* (PPARγ) which can inhibit expression of proinflammatory cytokines (TGF-ß1, TNF-α, and IL-1) [68]. L-Carnitine also increases eNOS expression, contrasting the negative effects of *nitric oxide radical* and related *reactive nitrogen species* production (peroxynitrite, etc.) [69]. It is important to mention that L-carnitine is a peripheral antagonist of thyroid hormone action: L-carnitine inhibits triiodothyronine (T3) and thyroxine (T4) entry into the cell nuclei. A randomized study proved that 2 and 4 grams/oral/daily of L-carnitine are capable of reversing hyperthyroidism symptoms [70]. Therefore, if at therapeutic doses (<2 grams) there is no problem for euthyroid patients, hyperthyroid patients, or hypothyroid patients treated with thyroid hormones, caution should be exercised if patients to be treated with carnitine are hypothyroid. In case of long-term therapy with carnitine (at high doses) mild euphoria is possible as a side effect, as it negatively interferes with γ-aminobutyric acid (GABA), causing an antidepressant-excitatory effect.

Literature Review. Carnitine has been successfully used to treat PD. In their 2001 randomized controlled study, Biagiotti and Cavallini, after administering acetyl-L-carnitine (ALC) (1 g twice daily for 3 months) to patients with active-phase PD, compared results with a control group (tamoxifen 20 mg twice daily for 3 months): (ALC group versus tamoxifen controlled-group) erectile pain improvement 92% versus 50% of cases ($p < 0.01$); mean penile curvature decrease, 7.5° versus 0.5° ($p < 0.01$); plaque size reduction (mm2), 48.8 versus 26.9 mm^2 ($p < 0.01$); inhibiting disease progression, 92% versus 46% [71].

In a subsequent controlled randomized study on patients with advanced resistant PD, Cavallini and Biagiotti (2002) administered propionyl-L-carnitine (PLC) (1 g twice daily) + 10 intraplaque infiltrations (one/week) with verapamil 10 mg for 3 months and compared results with those of the control group (tamoxifen 20 mg twice/day + 10 intraplaque infiltrations once weekly with verapamil 10 mg for 3 months); they demonstrated that the PLC + verapamil association (versus tamoxifen + verapamil control group) was able to significantly reduce both plaque volume ($p < 0.01$) and penile curvature ($p < 0.01$) [72].

2.4.3. Pentoxifylline. PTX is a synthetic xanthine derivative structurally related to theophylline and caffeine. As hemorheologic agent, it was initially used to treat peripheral vascular diseases, cerebrovascular insufficiency, sickle cell disease, and diabetic neuropathy. PTX inhibits platelet aggregation and improves blood flow by increasing erythrocyte and leukocyte deformability [73].

Antioxidant Properties. They include inhibiting ROS release (respiratory burst) by neutrophils, inhibiting lipid oxidation, and interfering with oxygen-radical-mediated activation of proinflammatory transcription factor NF-κB [74, 75]. Furthermore, PTX has been shown to have *hydroxyl radical* scavenging activity [76].

Anti-Inflammatory Properties. PTX reduces proinflammatory cytokines (TNF-α, TGF-ß1, and IL-1), NF-κB, and COX-2 expression [77–79].

Antifibrotic Properties. Due mainly to its capacity to inhibit production of TGF-ß1, FGF, and PDGF [77–80], PTX can reduce collagen deposition, as well as having strong inhibitory effects on fibroblast proliferation, ECM synthesis, and myofibroblastic differentiation. Thanks to its capacity to inhibit TGF-ß1 and TNF-α production, PTX can also hinder production of PAI-1. PTX is also a nonspecific phosphodiesterase (PDE) inhibitor and therefore has further antifibrotic activity by reducing iNOS and collagen expression and stimulating fibroblast apoptosis within the tunica albuginea [81, 82].

Literature Review. Besides treatment of peripheral artery disease, PTX has been used multiple times in man to treat various inflammatory conditions associated with fibrosis (radiation-induced and pulmonary fibrosis, scleroderma, etc.). A 2003 article by Valente et al. described an experimental study which included PTX administration (10 mg/kg/day/oral in drinking water for 45 days) in rats with PD-like plaque elicited by injection of TGF-β1 into the penile tunica albuginea [82]. PTX monotherapy resulted in an 80%–95% reduction in both plaque size and collagen/fibroblast ratio. The authors concluded that PTX was effective in stimulating fibroblast apoptosis in the tunica albuginea and therefore suggested PTX may be effective in reversing PD fibrosis [82]. The first article in which PTX was proposed as treatment for PD was published in 2006 [83]. It was a report about a 51-year-old Caucasian patient suffering from PD, treated with PTX, who suffered from moderate erectile dysfunction associated with two calcifications of the corpora cavernosa and 30-degree penile curvature; after treatment with PTX 400 mg/three times daily for 6 months, curvature had decreased to about 10 degrees. The patient continued the same therapy for 2 more years; at follow-up the dorsal plaque had decreased in volume and consistency, erectile function had significantly improved, and ultrasound confirmed disappearance of dorsal calcification with persistence of ventral calcific plaque. In 2010, Lin et al. published in two articles appearing in the same journal, one shortly after the other, a study divided into two parts, concerning the effects of TGF-ß1 and PTX on cultures of samples of *tunica albuginea-derived fibroblasts* (TADFs) from men with and without PD; in particular, it focused on the effects on collagen metabolism, elastin expression, and elastogenesis [77, 78]. The specimens of plaque containing tunica albuginea were harvested from 12 patients with chronic PD, during surgery for curvature correction. Biopsy samples of healthy tunica albuginea were taken from 6 patients during surgery for penile prosthesis positioning. The study yielded the following results: TGF-β1 stimulates collagen and elastin production; treatment of

TADF with PTX reduces the TGF-β1-mediated increase in elastogenesis and collagen deposition. In 2011, the first cohort study was published in which PTX was used to treat a group of 62 patients with PD and sonographic evidence of penile calcification [84]. The study's control group did not receive PTX. Treatment consisted in PTX 400 mg/three times daily (mean duration of treatment = 1.2 years). After treatment, patients were reassessed with a clinical exam and gray-scale or duplex ultrasound. Compared to the no-treatment group, patients who took PTX had a reduction in calcification volume (69.4% versus 33.3%, $p = 0.03$). Moreover, PTX-treated patients were much more likely to have stabilization (no change) or improvement in their calcium burden compared to patients of the control group (91.9% versus 44.4%, $p < 0.001$).

In 2012, a study assessed PTX efficacy in 74 PD patients using a combined therapy which included oral PTX (400 mg/three times daily) associated with oral L-arginine (1 g/twice daily) and verapamil injections (12 in total, every 2 weeks). Seventy-four PD patients were divided into two treatment groups: group I (39 patients), verapamil injections + oral therapy (L-arginine + PTX) + daily penile traction therapy (PTT) for 6 months; group II (35 patients), like group I but without PTT. Mean penile curvature improvement was 26.9° in group I versus 20.9° in group II. Although PTX was not used exclusively, the study demonstrated that combined treatment without PTT still led to significant penile curvature improvement [85]. In 2013, another report was published about a young PD patient who was treated successfully (significant plaque volume reduction) with a 2-year combined therapy (oral PTX/400 mg/3 times daily + oral tadalafil/5 mg/3 times a week + oral L-arginine/2500 mg/daily + oral PLC/250 mg/daily + oral vitamin B3/20 mg/daily + penile extender) [86]. Another report about exclusive use of PTX was published in 2014, describing PTX treatment in a 35-year-old PD patient with a large plaque in the distal third of the penis. Even though he had no bending, the patient complained of difficulty in coital penetration due to a lack of rigidity and tumescence in the terminal part of the penis. After oral PTX therapy (400 mg/oral/3 times daily) for 6 months, the patient had significant improvement of erectile function and glans tumescence, which made penetration possible [87]. In 2014, Alizadeh et al. published a study using PTX for treatment of PD. Ninety PD patients were randomized and divided into three treatment groups: group 1, oral PTX/1200 mg/day; group 2, verapamil injection/10 mg for up to 12 injections; group 3, oral PTX/1200 mg/day + intralesional verapamil injection. The outcomes were the following: (oral PTX versus intralesional verapamil versus oral PTX + intralesional verapamil) % of patients with plaque size reduction = 30 versus 33 versus 33; % of patients with improvement in penile curvature = 26.7 versus 36.7 versus 36.7; % of patients with improvement in erectile dysfunction = 46.7 versus 66.7 versus 86.7; % of patients with pain reduction = 73.3 versus 76.7 versus 80.0. Even in this study, PTX appeared effective in treating PD [88].

We published a controlled study last year in which PTX was used for 6 months in association with other antioxidant and anti-inflammatory substances for PD treatment [89]. All 307 patients of the study had PD in its evolutionary phase; the control group (group C, no treatment) included 101 patients.

The 206 treated patients were divided into two groups and differed only in whether they received penile PTX injections. Group A received PTX 100 mg 12 perilesional injections (twice a month for 6 months) + oral PTX 400 mg/twice a day + oral propolis 600 mg/daily + oral blueberry (*Vaccinium myrtillus* L., see below for a detailed description) 160 mg/daily + oral vitamin E 600 mg/daily + Diclofenac sodium 4% gel twice daily, as topical treatment for 6 months; group B received the same therapy as group A, but without PTX injections. The most significant results were as follows: (group A versus group B) % of patients with plaque size reduction = 100 versus 79.7 ($p < 0.001$); actual mean plaque size reduction = −46.9% versus −24.8% ($p < 0.001$); % of patients with improvement in penile curvature = 96.8 versus 56.4 ($p < 0.001$); actual mean penile curvature reduction = −10.1° versus −4.8° ($p < 0.001$); mean variation in % of penile curve angle = −40.7 versus −21.7 ($p < 0.001$); % of patients with complete disappearance of penile curvature = 6.3 versus 1.2 ($p = 0.128$); % of recovery of penile rigidity in patients with erectile dysfunction = 56.0 versus 23.5 ($p = 0.005$); % of patients with reduction in calcification size = 96.7 versus 70.8 ($p = 0.01$); actual mean reduction in calcification size = −54.0% versus −40.2% ($p < 0.131$); % of patients with complete disappearance of penile calcification = 9.6 versus 8.33 ($p = 0.863$). Incidence of side-effects after oral administration of PTX: blood pressure drop 0.46%, tachycardia 1.38%, dizziness 0.92%, skin rash 1.85%, headache 0.97%, hot flashes 0.97%, vomiting 0.48%, dyspepsia 2.42%, nausea 2.91%, meteorism 3.88%, and cumulative gastrointestinal adverse effects 9.69%. The only adverse effect of the penile PTX injection was local bruising at the infiltration site (3.57% incidence) [89]. The most important outcome was that PTX via perilesional penile injection was shown to be effective in treating PD and greatly statistically significantly improved the (already positive) results obtained with combined oral therapy alone. This study confirmed a peculiarity of PTX already mentioned in previous studies: a capacity to cause almost complete clearance of penile calcifications [83, 84].

2.4.4. Coenzyme Q10 (CoQ10). CoQ10, also known as ubiquinone, ubidecarenone, coenzyme Q, CoQ, or Q10, is a fat-soluble molecule involved in mitochondrial electron transport and oxidative phosphorylation and necessary for cellular respiration and *adenosine triphosphate* (ATP) production. The molecule exists in both reduced (ubiquinol, CoQ10H2) and oxidized (ubiquinone, CoQ10) form. CoQ10 inhibits increased ROS production, by blocking mitochondrial membrane depolarization. In its reduced form, CoQ10 acts as a potent endogenous antioxidant, interacting with oxygen-related radicals, hydrogen peroxide, and singlet oxygen and inhibiting lipid peroxidation (Table 1) [90]. CoQ10 prevents nitrosative stress by inhibition of excess nitric oxide radical production, and it participates in vitamin E and C regeneration [91, 92]. CoQ10 has a strong anti-inflammatory and antifibrotic activity, producing a decrease of proinflammatory cytokines TNF-α, IL-6, TGF-ß1, and *monocyte chemoattractant protein-1* (MCP-1), one of the cytokines that regulate migration and infiltration of monocytes-macrophages; furthermore, higher MCP-1 expression was found in PD-fibroblasts [93]. In addition, CoQ10 decreases gene expression of IL-1β, NF-κB, and iNOS [94].

Literature Review. A single study exists where CoQ10 was used to treat PD; this prospective, double-blind placebo-controlled randomized clinical trial demonstrated significant positive results: 186 patients affected by early chronic PD were divided into two groups of 93 patients each (treatment group and no-medication control group) [95]. Patients in the treatment group were treated with CoQ10, 300 mg/daily for 24 weeks. At the end of treatment, results were the following: (CoQ10 group versus placebo group) change in plaque size = −40.0% versus +35.7%; % of patients with objective curvature improvement = 54.3 versus 12.2; % of patients with increased curvature = 14.8 versus 69.5; % of patients with improvement of sexual function = 51.9 versus 8.6 [95].

2.4.5. Propolis. Propolis has been used by mankind since ancient times for its curative properties. It is plant-based and consists in a mixture of compounds which bees *(Apis mellifera L.)* extract from tree bark and buds. The resinous substances extracted by the bees are then processed with the addition of wax, pollen, and saliva enzymes. The final product is a resinous mixture with a color varying in shade from yellow to black. Bees produce propolis to seal any small opening in their beehives, protecting themselves from the cold, rain, wind, and possible attacks by other insects. The most interesting property of propolis is that of preventing disease, protecting the bees in the beehive from parasites, bacteria, viruses, and microbes in general. Many polyphenolic compounds, flavonoids, phenolic acids (caffeic acid and cinnamic acid), and esters and fatty acids have been found in propolis. Flavonoids commonly contained in propolis are acacetin, apigenin, catechin, chrysin, galangin, kaempferol, luteolin, myricetin, naringenin, pinocembrin, quercetin, and rutin. Propolis also contains resveratrol (a natural stilbene derivative) and several minerals (Mg, Ca, I, K, Na, Cu, Zn, Mn, and F), as well as vitamins (B1, B2, B6, C, and E) [96]. Since propolis indirectly derives from plants, its composite content varies depending on the geographical position and climate of the area of production. For instance, the characteristic compounds of Chinese propolis are caffeic acid, caffeic acid phenethyl ester (CAPE), caffeic acid benzyl ester, 5-methoxy pinobanksin, pinobanksin, pinobanksin-3-O-acetate, pinocembrin, chrysin, and galangin [97]. Brazilian propolis contains the following: liquiritigenin, daidzein, dalbergin, isoliquiritigenin, formononetin, biochanin A, galangin, kaempferol, pinostrobin, and pinocembrin [98]. Geographical differences of propolis are significant. CAPE is present in amounts greater than 10 mg/g in propolis extracts from Australia, China (up to 29 mg/g), Hungary, New Zealand, Uruguay, and Uzbekistan. Less than 10 mg/g of CAPE is found instead in propolis extracts from Argentina, Bulgaria, Chile, Ukraine, and USA [99]. CAPE is scarcely present or even absent in propolis extracts from Brazil, South Africa, and Thailand. Poplars, and their buds in particular, are considered the main indirect source of propolis in Europe and North America, nontropical Asia, New Zealand, and North Africa (especially the Nile delta) [100]. Considering the heterogeneous nature of the composition of propolis, pharmaceutical industries use standard quantities of the individual compounds by chemical extraction, choosing the substances based on their particular properties.

(i) Properties of the Most Common Substances Contained in Propolis

Galangin

Antioxidative Properties. It affects lipid peroxidation and helps preserve other antioxidants such as vitamin E and vitamin C [101, 102].

Antifibrotic Properties. It diminishes gene expression of TGF-ß1, MMP-2, and MMP-9 [103].

Anti-Inflammatory Properties. It inhibits factor NF-κB and reduces production of IL-1β, TNF-α, IL-6, and iNOS [104].

Quercetin

Antioxidant Properties. Quercetin decreases neutrophil activity (respiratory burst and degranulation) and inhibits release of NADPH-oxidase and MPO by decreasing generation of superoxide and derived ROS [105]. It is able to scavenge highly reactive species such as peroxynitrite, hydroxyl radical, superoxide anion, singlet oxygen, and lipid peroxyl radicals [106].

Anti-Inflammatory Properties. It inhibits production of TNF-α, IL-8, IL-1α, IL-1β, and IL-6 through inhibition of NF-κB activation [107]. Moreover quercetin inhibits inflammatory enzymes cyclooxygenase (COX), lipoxygenase (LOX), and iNOS [108].

Antifibrotic Properties. It suppresses TGF-β-induced collagen production and inhibits matrix metalloproteinases (MMP-2 and MMP-9), which are normally inhibited by PAI-1 [109].

Caffeic Acid Phenethyl Ester (CAPE). CAPE exhibits a stronger antioxidant activity than galangin [102]. It hinders oxidative burst and related polymorphonuclear neutrophil production of superoxide anion, hydrogen peroxide, and hypochlorous acid (HOCl) by activated leukocytes; moreover, it suppresses lipid peroxidation activity [110].

Anti-Inflammatory Properties. CAPE is a potent, specific inhibitor of NF-κB-dependent transcriptional activity, as well as cyclooxygenase (COX-1 and COX-2) and lipoxygenase activity [110–112]. Moreover, CAPE inhibits iNOS, TNF-α, IL-1β, and IL-6 production [110, 111].

Antifibrotic Properties. CAPE attenuates TGF-β-mediated collagen synthesis, inhibits peroxynitrite-augmented TGF-β1 release, counteracts TGF-β-induced differentiation of fibroblasts into myofibroblasts, and the concurrent formation of collagen; it is capable of partially reversing myofibroblasts into fibroblasts and reversing collagen formation [112, 113].

Chrysin

Antioxidant Properties. It inhibits xanthine oxidase activity, which is responsible for superoxide anion production; it also inhibits the release of NADPH-oxidase and the oxidative burst of neutrophils [105].

Anti-Inflammatory Properties. It inhibits NF-κB and iNOS enzyme activity and cyclooxygenase- (COX-) 2 and IL-1β gene expression, significantly inhibiting the release of NO, TNF-α, and related increase in PAI-1 [114, 115].

Antifibrotic Properties. It suppresses TGF-β and fibronectin expression; it also inhibits the profibrotic activity of PDGF [116, 117].

Pinocembrin. Pinocembrin possesses a high oxygen radical antioxidant capacity and nitrite scavenging capacity, inhibiting xanthine oxidase activity, which usually induces the generation of superoxide radicals; it also inhibits lipid peroxidation [118, 119].

Anti-Inflammatory Properties. It inhibits production of TNF-α, IL-1β, and IL-6, as well as iNOS and COX-2 expression [120].

Antifibrotic Properties. It inhibits TGF-β and MMP-2 and MMP-9 expression [121].

Pinobanksin

Antioxidant Capacity. It inhibits xanthine oxidase activity, which is responsible for superoxide radical production; it can also inhibit lipid peroxidation [118, 119]. Pinobanksin also has antiproliferative and proapoptotic activity [122].

Apigenin. Apigenin is an antioxidant; it inhibits xanthine oxidase activity responsible for ROS and hydrogen peroxide production.

Anti-Inflammatory Activity. It prevents migration of neutrophils toward the inflammatory site; it inhibits platelet aggregation, hindering the cyclooxygenase (COX) pathway; it also inhibits production of proinflammatory cytokines (IL-1β, TNF-α, IL-6, and IL-8) through inhibition of the activation of factor NF-κB [123–125].

Antifibrotic Properties. It inhibits the expression of TGF-β1 and PDGF, therefore blocking collagen production; apigenin also inhibits differentiation of fibroblasts into myofibroblasts [125].

Literature Review. Cuban urologists (Lemourt et al., 1998) were the first authors to publish a study on the use of propolis in the treatment of PD, as they discovered by serendipity that propolis could cure the disease: they had noticed that a patient suffering from PD who had been treated with propoleum (oil of propolis) due to giardiasis had reported a “spontaneous” improvement in his penile curvature; they therefore began to administer propolis to several PD patients, subsequently publishing various studies reporting excellent clinical results [126–129]. In one of their studies, they analyzed the effects of propolis on 34 PD patients, assessing after 6 months two different daily doses of propolis (300 and 900 mg) in two respective groups (each made up of 17 patients) and concluded that patients treated with 900 mg/daily had superior clinical results; furthermore, clinical improvement and plaque volume reduction occurred earlier in this group [128]. In another study, the same authors studied the effects of propolis on PD in three treatment groups: (group 1) propoleum 900 mg/daily for over six months (10 patients); (group 2) 10 laser sessions every 2 months for over six months (8 patients); (group 3) propoleum 900 mg/daily + 10 laser sessions every 2 months (10 patients). The best outcomes in terms of curvature reduction were obtained in the group of patients treated only with propolis (mean penile curvature improvement: −10.8°); in the patients of the propolis + laser group, the curvature improvement was slightly inferior (−10.3°); only a few patients in the laser group referred to improvement (−8.0°) while a progression in curvature was observed in the remaining patients in this group, with a mean increase of 12.6°; as to plaque volume, mean US-measured reduction was 2.3 mm (only propolis group) and 12.16 mm (propolis + laser group); the laser group ultrasound results were not comparable due to the low number of patients compared to the other groups [129]. Another study where propolis was used to treat PD was published by Favilla et al. (2014); the authors used propolis in combination with other antioxidants and verapamil in patients with initial-phase PD, assessing in particular the efficacy of associating intralesional verapamil injection (10 mg weekly for 12 weeks) and oral antioxidants (group B) compared with verapamil injection monotherapy (group A). The oral antioxidant therapy consisted in a tablet/daily (for 3 months) with the following composition formula: propolis 100 mg, blueberry anthocyanins 80 mg, para-aminobenzoic acid 100 mg, Muira Puama 25 mg, soya isoflavones 50 mg, *Persea americana* 50 mg, vitamin E 36 mg, and Damiana 25 mg [61]. Although no significant differences were observed between the two groups in mean plaque size change (group A versus group B = −0.38 cm3 versus −0.29 cm3) and mean penile curvature improvement (−10.86° versus −11.97°), statistically significant results were obtained in group B in regard to orgasmic function (subdomain of 15-question International Index of Erectile Function, IIEF), intercourse satisfaction (subdomain of IIEF), overall satisfaction (subdomain of IIEF), and pain/visual analogue score (VAS) [61]. We ourselves have published five controlled studies in which we used propolis associated with other substances, always with excellent, statistically significant results; the most recent one of these studies is discussed in detail above in the section on pentoxifylline, and the others are in the following paragraph on bilberry [62, 89, 130–132].

2.4.6. Bilberry (Vaccinium myrtillus L.). Bilberry is also known as “European wild blueberry” and “Whortleberry.” Bilberry grows in forest undergrowth, generally in mountainous areas in North America and Northern and Central Europe. It contains numerous flavonoids, including anthocyanins, pigments that give fruit its color. Anthocyanins contained in bilberry are cyanidin, delphinidin, petunidin, malvidin, and peonidin; cyanidin is present in higher concentrations compared to the other anthocyanins (mean amount 0.053 μg/mL); delphinidin and petunidin are present 2.5 times less, while malvidin and peonidin are present in very low concentrations (mean amount 0.011–0.012 μg/mL) [133]. Although anthocyanins are the most preponderant substances in bilberry, it contains a variety of phenolic compounds, including quercetin, tannins, ellagitannins, and flavonols such as catechin, epicatechin, gallocatechin, and epigallocatechin (the latter two only in unripe fruit), and small quantities of vitamin C [134, 135]. Since it contains quercetin (already mentioned above when discussing propolis) bilberry has antioxidant, anti-inflammatory, and antifibrotic properties [105–109]. Due to its high anthocyanin content, bilberry has powerful antioxidant effects against superoxide anion, hydroxyl radical, and peroxynitrite [136]. Anthocyanins, especially delphinidin, quickly reacts with extended oxidation products of nitric oxide radical (RNS) [137]. Anthocyanins also reduce the levels of NF-κB, TNF-α, and MCP-1, which regulates migration and infiltration of monocytes-macrophages [138]. Furthermore, delphinidin and cyanidin inhibit COX-2 and increase the protein level of eNOS; cyanidin is also able to cause downregulation of iNOS [139–141]. Anthocyanins can also inhibit phosphodiesterase (PDE) [142]. Bilberries (thanks to their high content of anthocyanins) also have antifibrotic action, suppressing TGF-β-induced collagen production [109]. Catechins contained in bilberries inhibit PDGF and FGF; moreover catechins show antiproliferative and proapoptotic activity [143].

Literature Review. In six controlled studies bilberry was used in combined PD therapy (see PTX and propolis sections above). Statistically significant results after treatment were found in all these studies [61, 62, 89, 130–132]. In particular, in our 2013 study, European blueberry was administered to 41 patients (group A) for 18 months, 160 mg/daily + verapamil 10 mg penile perilesional injections (twice monthly for 6 months and then once monthly for 12 months, for a total of 24 injections) + iontophoresis with verapamil 5 mg daily + propolis 600 mg/daily + vitamin E 600 mg/daily + topical Diclofenac 4%/daily. The control group (group B) was made up of 41 patients who received no treatment [132]. After 18 months of treatment, plaque size reduction occurred in 100.0% of patients in group A and none in group B ($p < 0.0001$); on the contrary, in group B plaque size always increased; in group A, mean plaque size reduction was −73.6%, while in group B, there was a mean increase in plaque size = +118.7% ($p = 0.000$); in group A, penile curvature improvement occurred in 81.5% of cases versus only 8.1% in group B; in group A, mean decrease of penile curvature angle was −16.74° while in group B it was −4.0° ($p = 0.019$) [132]. In the no-treatment group, penile curvature improved in only a few cases (8.1% = 3/41 cases); actually, in these cases the disease had progressed with an increase in plaque size which resulted in changes of the architectural structure of the penis that led to a paradoxical improvement in curvature.

3. Discussion and Conclusions

As can be gathered from the number of references in our article, numerous studies have demonstrated the fundamental role played by oxidative stress in PD pathogenesis, and several studies have described successful use of various antioxidants in PD treatment. Oxidative stress is an integral part of the disease, influencing its progression; in the very early stages of PD, the inflammatory infiltrate cells begin to produce high quantities of ROS and proinflammatory and profibrotic cytokines, with consequent activation of transcription factor NF-κB which induces iNOS production and subsequent release of high nitric oxide radical concentrations. The next chemical reaction cascade leads to production of high amounts of reactive nitrogen species, particularly peroxynitrite, which can damage cells and tissue by lipid peroxidation and DNA fragmentation. As described above, inflammatory cytokine- and NF-κB-induced expression of iNOS leads to overproduction of nitric oxide radical, which reacting with superoxide anion causes peroxynitrite production [34]. Oxidative stress, furthermore, is an important factor in the possible onset of erectile dysfunction in PD, as hyperproduction of superoxide anion and peroxynitrite reduces nitric oxide concentration available for cavernosal muscle relaxation, resulting in long-term endothelial damage; superoxide anion is also reported to have a direct vasoconstriction effect [44, 144]. The presence of high iNOS concentrations has been proven in the cavernous tissue of men with PD [34]. The exact role of iNOS was long unclear, and a number of authors attributed a protective, antifibrotic role to it [39, 145]. Other authors, instead, proved that iNOS inhibition and peroxynitrite scavenging suppressed evolution of the inflammatory response and the normal course of collagen-induced diseases [146, 147]. Moreover, numerous studies listed in our literature review proved that iNOS inhibition after treatment with antioxidants (in PD patients) can have antifibrotic effects, resulting in significant clinical improvement [60–62, 71, 72, 82–89, 95, 128–132].

Since ROS damage occurs during the early stages of the disease, the treatment with antioxidants is only indicated in the initial stages of PD and not in the stabilization phase. For the same reason, the antioxidant therapy should be started immediately at the earliest diagnosis of the disease. Therefore, a "watchful waiting behavior" is not justified at the first time of PD diagnosis.

While conservative therapies commonly used in the early stages of PD include oral substances (Potaba, tamoxifen, colchicine, and vitamin E), intralesional treatment (verapamil, interferon, steroids, and more recently collagenase clostridium histolyticum-Xiaflex), and local physical treatment (iontophoresis, extracorporeal shock wave therapy-ESWT, and penile extender), the significant results obtained by emerging treatments with the antioxidants cited in this article suggest these therapeutic agents (which are also antifibrotic and anti-inflammatory) interfere at several levels with the disease's pathogenetic mechanisms (Table 2); combination therapy is therefore an effective treatment strategy today, capable of curing early-stage PD, yielding better results than those traditionally obtained with a single substance.

Combination therapy outcomes are interesting for good clinical practice and also confirm the fundamental role played by oxidative stress in PD. However, further prospective randomized placebo-controlled studies are needed to evaluate the efficacy of emerging antioxidant therapies.

References

[1] U. Schwarzer, F. Sommer, T. Klotz, M. Braun, B. Reifenrath, and U. Engelmann, "The prevalence of Peyronie's disease: results of a large survey," *BJU International*, vol. 88, no. 7, pp. 727–730, 2001.

[2] D. B. DiBenedetti, D. Nguyen, L. Zografos, R. Ziemiecki, and X. Zhou, "A Population-based study of peyronie's disease: prevalence and treatment patterns in the United States," *Advances in Urology*, vol. 2011, Article ID 282503, 9 pages, 2011.

[3] A. P. Saboeiro, J. J. Pokorny, S. I. Shehadi, K. S. Virgo, and F. E. Johnson, "Racial distribution of dupuytren's disease in department of veterans affairs patients," *Plastic & Reconstructive Surgery*, vol. 106, no. 1, pp. 71–75, 2000.

[4] J. P. Jarow and F. C. Lowe, "Penile trauma: an etiologic factor in Peyronie's disease and erectile dysfunction," *The Journal of Urology*, vol. 158, no. 4, pp. 1388–1390, 1997.

[5] C. J. Devine Jr., K. D. Somers, G. H. Jordan, and S. M. Schlossberg, "Proposal: trauma as the cause of the Peyronie's lesion," *Journal of Urology*, vol. 157, no. 1, pp. 285–290, 1997.

[6] A. I. El-Sakka, E. Salabas, M. Dinçer, and A. Kadioglu, "The pathophysiology of Peyronie's disease," *Arab Journal of Urology*, vol. 11, no. 3, pp. 272–277, 2013.

[7] R. Rompel, G. Mueller-Eckhardt, I. Schroeder-Printzen, and W. Weidner, "HLA antigens in Peyronie's disease," *Urologia Internationalis*, vol. 52, no. 1, pp. 34–37, 1994.

[8] A. S. Herati and A. W. Pastuszak, "The Genetic Basis of Peyronie Disease: A Review," *Sexual Medicine Reviews*, vol. 4, no. 1, pp. 85–94, 2016.

[9] G. H. Dolmans, P. M. Werker, I. J. de Jong, R. J. Nijman, C. Wijmenga, and R. A. Ophoff, "WNT2 Locus Is Involved in Genetic Susceptibility of Peyronie's Disease," *Journal of Sexual Medicine*, vol. 9, no. 5, pp. 1430–1434, 2012.

[10] J. Byström and C. Rubio, "Induratio penis plastica (peyronie's disease): Clinical features and etiology," *Scandinavian Journal of Urology and Nephrology*, vol. 10, no. 1, pp. 12–20, 1976.

[11] K. D. Somers, E. N. Sismour, G. L. Wright Jr., C. J. Devine Jr., D. A. Gilbert, and C. E. Horton, "Isolation and characterization of collagen in Peyronie's disease," *Journal of Urology*, vol. 141, no. 3 I, pp. 629–631, 1989.

[12] J. P. Pryor and D. J. Ralph, "Clinical presentations of Peyronie's disease," *International Journal of Impotence Research*, vol. 14, no. 5, pp. 414–417, 2002.

[13] C. J. Nelson, C. Diblasio, M. Kendirci, W. Hellstrom, P. Guhring, and J. P. Mulhall, "The chronology of depression and distress in men with peyronie's disease," *Journal of Sexual Medicine*, vol. 5, no. 8, pp. 1985–1990, 2008.

[14] W. Weidner, I. Schroeder-Printzen, W.-H. Weiske, and R. Vosshenrich, "Sexual dysfunction in Peyronie's disease: An analysis of 222 patients without previous local plaque therapy," *Journal of Urology*, vol. 157, no. 1, pp. 325–328, 1997.

[15] E. Akkus, S. Carrier, K. Baba et al., "Structural alterations in the tunica albuginea of the penis: Impact of Peyronie's disease, ageing and impotence," *British Journal of Urology*, vol. 79, no. 1, pp. 47–53, 1997.

[16] LA. Levine and S. Larsen, "Diagnosis and management of peyronie disease," in *Campbell-Walsh Urology*, A. J. Wein, L. R. Kavoussi, A. W. Partin, and C. A. Peters, Eds., vol. 1, Chap 31, pp. 722–748, Elsevier Saunders, Philadelphia, Pa, USA, 11th edition, 2015.

[17] G. Garaffa, L. W. Trost, E. C. Serefoglu, D. Ralph, and W. J. G. Hellstrom, "Understanding the course of Peyronie's disease," *International Journal of Clinical Practice*, vol. 67, no. 8, pp. 781–788, 2013.

[18] G. Brock, G.-L. Hsu, L. Nunes, B. von Heyden, and T. F. Lue, "The anatomy of the tunica albuginea in the normal penis and Peyronie's disease," *Journal of Urology*, vol. 157, no. 1, pp. 276–281, 1997.

[19] G.-. Hsu, G. Brock, B. Von Heyden, L. Nunes, T. F. Lue, and E. A. Tanagho, "The distribution of elastic fibrous elements within the human penis," *British Journal of Urology*, vol. 73, no. 5, pp. 566–571, 1994.

[20] K. D. Somers and D. M. Dawson, "Fibrin deposition in Peyronie's disease plaque," *Journal of Urology*, vol. 157, no. 1, pp. 311–315, 1997.

[21] V. Gentile, A. Modesti, G. La Pera et al., "Ultrastructural and immunohistochemical characterization of the tunica albuginea in Peyronie's disease and veno-occlusive dysfunction," *Journal of Andrology*, vol. 17, no. 2, pp. 96–103, 1996.

[22] N. F. Gonzalez-Cadavid, T. R. Magee, M. Ferrini, A. Qian, D. Vernet, and J. Rajfer, "Gene expression in Peyronie's disease," *International Journal of Impotence Research*, vol. 14, no. 5, pp. 361–374, 2002.

[23] S. K. Agarwal, "Integrins and cadherins as therapeutic targets in fibrosis," *Frontiers in Pharmacology*, vol. 5, article 131, 2014.

[24] S. M. Wahl, G. L. Costa, D. E. Mizel, J. B. Allen, U. Skaleric, and D. F. Mangan, "Role of transforming growth factor beta in the pathophysiology of chronic inflammation.," *Journal of Periodontology*, vol. 64, no. 5, pp. 450–455, 1993.

[25] J.-K. Ryu, W.-J. Kim, M.-J. Choi et al., "Inhibition of histone deacetylase 2 mitigates profibrotic TGF-$\beta 1$ responses in fibroblasts derived from Peyronie's plaque," *Asian Journal of Andrology*, vol. 15, no. 5, pp. 640–645, 2013.

[26] R. B. Moreland and A. Nehra, "Pathophysiology of Peyronie's disease," *International Journal of Impotence Research*, vol. 14, no. 5, pp. 406–410, 2002.

[27] M. Del Carlo, A. A. Cole, and L. A. Levine, "Differential Calcium Independent Regulation of Matrix Metalloproteinases and Tissue Inhibitors of Matrix Metalloproteinases by Interleukin-1β and Transforming Growth Factor-β in Peyronie's Plaque Fibroblasts," *Journal of Urology*, vol. 179, no. 6, pp. 2447–2455, 2008.

[28] D. R. Edwards, K. J. Leco, P. P. Beaudry, P. W. Atadja, C. Veillette, and K. T. Riabowol, "Differential effects of transforming growth factor-$\beta 1$ on the expression of matrix metalloproteinases and tissue inhibitors of metalloproteinases in young and old human fibroblasts," *Experimental Gerontology*, vol. 31, no. 1-2, pp. 207–223, 1996.

[29] JP. Mulhall, "The clinical implications of basic science research in Peyronies disease, a guide to clinical management," in *Current clinical urology: Peyronie's disease*, LA. Levine, Ed., pp. 39–58, Humana Press, Totowa, NJ, USA, 2007.

[30] S. C. Sikka and W. J. G. Hellstrom, "Role of oxidative stress and antioxidants in Peyronie's disease," *International Journal of Impotence Research*, vol. 14, no. 5, pp. 353–360, 2002.

[31] H. Sakurai, N. Shigemori, K. Hasegawa, and T. Sugita, "TGF-β-activated kinase 1 stimulates NF-κB activation by an NF-κB-inducing kinase-independent mechanism," *Biochemical and Biophysical Research Communications*, vol. 243, no. 2, pp. 545–549, 1998.

[32] D. Vernet, G. Nolazco, L. Cantini et al., "Evidence that osteogenic progenitor cells in the human tunica albuginea may originate from stem cells: implications for peyronie disease," *Biology of Reproduction*, vol. 73, no. 6, pp. 1199–1210, 2005.

[33] E. Lambert, E. Dassé, B. Haye, and E. Petitfrère, "TIMPs as multifacial proteins," *Critical Reviews in Oncology/Hematology*, vol. 49, no. 3, pp. 187–198, 2004.

[34] T. J. Bivalacqual, H. C. Champion, and W. J. G. Hellstrom, "Implications of nitric oxide synthase isoforms in the pathophysiology of Peyronie's disease," *International Journal of Impotence Research*, vol. 14, no. 5, pp. 345–352, 2002.

[35] G. Paulis and T. Brancato, "Inflammatory mechanisms and oxidative stress in Peyronie's disease: Therapeutic "rationale" and related emerging treatment strategies," *Inflammation and Allergy - Drug Targets*, vol. 11, no. 1, pp. 48–57, 2012.

[36] M. Huleihel, A. Douvdevani, S. Segal, and R. N. Apte, "Regulation of interleukin 1 generation in immune-activated fibroblasts," *European Journal of Immunology*, vol. 20, no. 4, pp. 731–738, 1990.

[37] K. Sasaki, T. Hattori, T. Fujisawa, K. Takahashi, H. Inoue, and M. Takigawa, "Nitric oxide mediates interleukin-1-induced gene expression of matrix metalloproteinases and basic fibroblast growth factor in cultured rabbit articular chondrocytes," *Journal of Biochemistry*, vol. 123, no. 3, pp. 431–439, 1998.

[38] R. J. Van't Hof, K. J. Armour, L. M. Smith et al., "Requirement of the inducible nitric oxide synthase pathway for IL-1- induced osteoclastic bone resorption," *Proceedings of the National Academy of Sciences of the United States of America*, vol. 97, no. 14, pp. 7993–7998, 2000.

[39] H. H. Davila, T. R. Magee, D. Vernet, J. Rajfer, and N. F. Gonzalez-Cadavid, "Gene transfer of inducible nitric oxide synthase complementary DNA regresses the fibrotic plaque in an animal model of Peyronie's disease," *Biology of Reproduction*, vol. 71, no. 5, pp. 1568–1577, 2004.

[40] H. H. Davila, T. R. Magee, F. I. Zuniga, J. Rajfer, and N. F. Gonzalez-Cadavid, "Peyronie's disease associated with increase in plasminogen activator inhibitor in fibrotic plaque," *Urology*, vol. 65, no. 4, pp. 645–648, 2005.

[41] M. Sasaki, M. Kashima, T. Ito et al., "Differential regulation of metalloproteinase production, proliferation and chemotaxis of human lung fibroblasts by PDGF, interleukin-1β and TNF-α," *Mediators of Inflammation*, vol. 9, no. 3-4, pp. 155–160, 2000.

[42] M. M. Chaturvedi, M. Higuchi, and B. B. Aggarwal, "Effect of tumor necrosis factors, interferons, interleukins, and growth factors on the activation of NF-κB: Evidence for lack of correlation with cell proliferation," *Lymphokine and Cytokine Research*, vol. 13, no. 5, pp. 309–313, 1994.

[43] R.-M. Liu, "Oxidative stress, plasminogen activator inhibitor 1, and lung fibrosis," *Antioxidants and Redox Signaling*, vol. 10, no. 2, pp. 303–319, 2008.

[44] A. Agarwal, K. C. Nandipati, R. K. Sharma, C. D. Zippe, and R. Raina, "Role of oxidative stress in the pathophysiological mechanism of erectile dysfunction," *Journal of Andrology*, vol. 27, no. 3, pp. 335–347, 2006.

[45] E. Nava and S. Llorens, "The paracrine control of vascular motion. A historical perspective," *Pharmacological Research*, vol. 113, pp. 125–145, 2016.

[46] R. M. J. Palmer, D. S. Ashton, and S. Moncada, "Vascular endothelial cells synthesize nitric oxide from L-arginine," *Nature*, vol. 333, no. 6174, pp. 664–666, 1988.

[47] W. W. Scott and P. L. Scardino, "A new concept in the treatment of peyronie's disease," *Southern Medical Journal*, vol. 41, no. 2, pp. 173–177, 1948.

[48] O. Cachia, J. El Benna, E. Pedruzzi, B. Descomps, M.-A. Gougerot-Pocidalo, and C.-L. Leger, "α-Tocopherol inhibits the respiratory burst in human monocytes: Attenuation of p47(phox) membrane translocation and phosphorylation," *Journal of Biological Chemistry*, vol. 273, no. 49, pp. 32801–32805, 1998.

[49] A. Tasanarong, S. Kongkham, S. Duangchana, S. Thitiarchakul, and S. Eiam-Ong, "Vitamin E ameliorates renal fibrosis by inhibition of TGF-beta/Smad2/3 signaling pathway in UUO mice," *Journal of the Medical Association of Thailand*, vol. 94, Supplement 7:S1-9, 2011.

[50] A. L. Haas, D. Boscoboinik, D. S. Mojon, M. Böhnke, and A. Azzi, "Vitamin E inhibits proliferation of human Tenon's capsule fibroblasts in vitro," *Ophthalmic Research*, vol. 28, no. 3, pp. 171–175, 1996.

[51] J. P. Godbout, B. M. Berg, C. Krzyszton, and R. W. Johnson, "α-Tocopherol attenuates NFκB activation and pro-inflammatory cytokine production in brain and improves recovery from lipopolysaccharide- induced sickness behavior," *Journal of Neuroimmunology*, vol. 169, no. 1-2, pp. 97–105, 2005.

[52] Q. Jiang, X. Yin, M. A. Lil, M. L. Danielson, H. Freiser, and J. Huang, "Long-chain carboxychromanols, metabolites of vitamin E, are potent inhibitors of cyclooxygenases," *Proceedings of the National Academy of Sciences of the United States of America*, vol. 105, no. 51, pp. 20464–20469, 2008.

[53] A. Fazzio, D. Marilley, and A. Azzi, "The effect of α-Tocopherol and β-tocopherol on proliferation, protein kinase C activity and gene expression in different cell lines.," *IUBMB Life*, vol. 41, no. 1, pp. 93–101, 1997.

[54] E. Kakishita, A. Suehiro, Y. Oura, and K. Nagai, "Inhibitory effect of vitamin E (α -tocopherol) on spontaneous platelet aggregation in whole blood," *Thrombosis Research*, vol. 60, no. 6, pp. 489–499, 1990.

[55] J. J. Hu, G. C. Roush, M. Berwick et al., "Effects of dietary supplementation of alpha-tocopherol on plasma glutathione and DNA repair activities," *Cancer Epidemiol Biomarkers Prev*, vol. 5, no. 4, pp. 263–270, 1996.

[56] P. L. Scardino and W. W. Scott, "THE use of tocopherols in the treatment of peyronie's disease," *Annals of the New York Academy of Sciences*, vol. 52, no. 3, pp. 390–396, 1949.

[57] C. L. Steinberg, "Tocopherols in treatment of primary fibrositis; including Dupuytren's contracture, periarthritis of the shoulders, and Peyronie's disease," *A.M.A. Archives of Surgery*, vol. 63, no. 6, p. 824, 1951.

[58] J. P. Pryor and C. R. Farell, "Controlled clinical trial of vitamin E in Peyronies disease," *Prog Reprod Biol Med*, vol. 9, pp. 41–45, 1983.

[59] M. R. Safarinejad, S. Y. Hosseini, and A. A. Kolahi, "Comparison of Vitamin E and Propionyl-L-Carnitine, Separately or in Combination, in Patients With Early Chronic Peyronie's Disease: A Double-Blind, Placebo Controlled, Randomized Study," *Journal of Urology*, vol. 178, no. 4, pp. 1398–1403, 2007.

[60] A. A. Halal, P. Geavlete, and E. Ceban, "Pharmacological therapy in patients diagnosed with Peyronie's disease.," *Journal of medicine and life*, vol. 5, no. 2, pp. 192–195, 2012.

[61] V. Favilla, G. I. Russo, and S. Privitera, "Combination of intralesional verapamil and oral antioxidants for Peyronie's disease: a prospective, randomised controlled study," *Andrologia*, vol. 46, no. 8, pp. 936–942, 2014.

[62] G. Paulis, T. Brancato, R. D'Ascenzo et al., "Efficacy of vitamin E in the conservative treatment of Peyronie's disease: legend or reality? A controlled study of 70 cases.," *Andrology*, vol. 1, no. 1, pp. 120–128, 2013.

[63] F. M. Vaz and R. J. A. Wanders, "Carnitine biosynthesis in mammals," *Biochemical Journal*, vol. 361, no. 3, pp. 417–429, 2002.

[64] I. Gülçin, "Antioxidant and antiradical activities of L-carnitine," *Life Sciences*, vol. 78, no. 8, pp. 803–811, 2006.

[65] P. Ge, Y. Cui, F. Liu, J. Luan, X. Zhou, and J. Han, "L-carnitine affects osteoblast differentiation in NIH3T3 fibroblasts by the IGF-1/PI3K/Akt signalling pathway," *BioScience Trends*, vol. 9, no. 1, pp. 42–48, 2015.

[66] B.-J. Lee, J.-S. Lin, Y.-C. Lin, and P.-T. Lin, "Antiinflammatory effects of l-carnitine supplementation (1000 mg/d) in coronary artery disease patients," *Nutrition*, vol. 31, no. 3, pp. 475–479, 2015.

[67] A. Koc, T. Ozkan, A. Z. Karabay, A. Sunguroglu, and F. Aktan, "Effect of L-carnitine on the synthesis of nitric oxide in RAW 264·7 murine macrophage cell line," *Cell Biochemistry and Function*, vol. 29, no. 8, pp. 679–685, 2011.

[68] F. Jiang, Z. Zhang, Y. Zhang, J. Wu, L. Yu, and S. Liu, "L-carnitine ameliorates the liver inflammatory response by regulating carnitine palmitoyltransferase I-dependent PPARγ signaling," *Molecular Medicine Reports*, vol. 13, no. 2, pp. 1320–1328, 2016.

[69] M. Alvarez De Sotomayor, R. Bueno, C. Pérez-Guerrero, and M. D. Herrera, "Effect of L-carnitine and propionyl-L-carnitine on endothelial function of small mesenteric arteries from SHR," *Journal of Vascular Research*, vol. 44, no. 5, pp. 354–364, 2007.

[70] S. Benvenga, A. Amato, M. Calvani, and F. Trimarchi, "Effects of carnitine on thyroid hormone action," *Annals of the New York Academy of Sciences*, vol. 1033, pp. 158–167, 2004.

[71] G. Biagiotti and G. Cavallini, "Acetyl-L-carnitine vs tamoxifen in the oral therapy of Peyronie's disease: A preliminary report," *BJU International*, vol. 88, no. 1, pp. 63–67, 2001.

[72] G. Cavallini, G. Biagiotti, A. Koverech, and G. Vitali, "Oral propionyl-L-carnitine and intraplaque verapamil in the therapy of advanced and resistant Peyronie's disease," *BJU International*, vol. 89, no. 9, pp. 895–900, 2002.

[73] J. P. De La Cruz, M. M. Romero, P. Sanchez, and F. Sanchez de la Cuesta, "Antiplatelet effect of pentoxifylline in human whole blood," *General Pharmacology*, vol. 24, no. 3, pp. 605–609, 1993.

[74] T. W. Costantini, J. Deree, C. Y. Peterson et al., "Pentoxifylline modulates p47phox activation and downregulates neutrophil oxidative burst through PKA-dependent and -independent mechanisms," *Immunopharmacology and Immunotoxicology*, vol. 32, no. 1, pp. 82–91, 2010.

[75] V. R. Sunil, K. N. Vayas, J. A. Cervelli et al., "Pentoxifylline attenuates nitrogen mustard-induced acute lung injury, oxidative stress and inflammation," *Experimental and Molecular Pathology*, vol. 97, no. 1, pp. 89–98, 2014.

[76] J. P. Freitas and P. M. Filipe, "Pentoxifylline - A hydroxyl radical scavenger," *Biological Trace Element Research*, vol. 47, no. 1-3, pp. 307–311, 1995.

[77] G. Lin, A. W. Shindel, L. Banie et al., "Pentoxifylline attenuates transforming growth factor-β1-stimulated elastogenesis in human Tunica albuginea-derived fibroblasts part 2: Interference in a TGF-β1/smad-dependent mechanism and downregulation of AAT1," *Journal of Sexual Medicine*, vol. 7, no. 5, pp. 1787–1797, 2010.

[78] A. W. Shindel, G. Lin, H. Ning et al., "Pentoxifylline attenuates transforming growth factor-β1-stimulated collagen deposition and elastogenesis in human tunica albuginea-derived fibroblasts part 1: impact on extracellular matrix," *The Journal of Sexual Medicine*, vol. 7, no. 6, pp. 2077–2085, 2010.

[79] Q. Ji, L. Zhang, H. Jia, and J. Xu, "Pentoxifylline inhibits endotoxin-induced NF-kappa B activation and associated production of proinflammatory cytokines," *Annals of Clinical & Laboratory Science*, vol. 4, pp. 427–436, 2004.

[80] R. A. Isbrucker and T. C. Peterson, "Platelet-derived growth factor and pentoxifylline modulation of collagen synthesis in myofibroblasts," *Toxicology and Applied Pharmacology*, vol. 149, no. 1, pp. 120–126, 1998.

[81] J.-M. Anaya and L. R. Espinoza, "Phosphodiesterase inhibitor pentoxifylline: an antiinflammatory/immunomodulatory drug potentially useful in some rheumatic diseases," *Journal of Rheumatology*, vol. 22, no. 4, pp. 595–599, 1995.

[82] E. G. A. Valente, D. Vernet, M. G. Ferrini, A. Qian, J. Rajfer, and N. F. Gonzalez-Cadavid, "L-Arginine and phosphodiesterase (PDE) inhibitors counteract fibrosis in the Peyronie's fibrotic plaque and related fibroblast cultures," *Nitric Oxide - Biology and Chemistry*, vol. 9, no. 4, pp. 229–244, 2003.

[83] W. O. Brant, R. C. Dean, and T. F. Lue, "Treatment of Peyronie's disease with oral pentoxifylline," *Nature Clinical Practice Urology*, vol. 3, no. 2, pp. 111–115, 2006.

[84] J. F. Smith, A. W. Shindel, Y.-C. Huang et al., "Pentoxifylline treatment and penile calcifications in men with Peyronie's disease," *Asian Journal of Andrology*, vol. 13, no. 2, pp. 322–325, 2011.

[85] M. R. Abern, S. Larsen, and L. A. Levine, "Combination of penile traction, intralesional verapamil, and oral therapies for peyronie's disease," *Journal of Sexual Medicine*, vol. 9, no. 1, pp. 288–295, 2012.

[86] F. Ciociola and G. M. Colpi, "Peyronie's disease: A triple oxygenant therapy," *Archivio Italiano di Urologia e Andrologia*, vol. 85, no. 1, pp. 36–40, 2013.

[87] L. Dell'Atti and G. Ughi, "Efficacy of pentoxifylline in Peyronie's disease: clinical case of a young man," *Archivio Italiano di Urologia e Andrologia*, vol. 86, no. 3, pp. 237-237, 2014.

[88] M. Alizadeh, F. Karimi, and M. R. Fallah, "Evaluation of verapamil efficacy in Peyronie's disease comparing with pentoxifylline," *Global journal of health science*, vol. 6, no. 7, pp. 23–30, 2014.

[89] G. Paulis, D. Barletta, P. Turchi et al., "Efficacy and safety evaluation of pentoxifylline associated with other antioxidants in medical treatment of Peyronie's disease: a case-control study," *Research and Reports in Urology*, vol. 8, pp. 1–10, 2015.

[90] B. Frei, M. C. Kim, and B. N. Ames, "Ubiquinol-10 is an effective lipid-soluble antioxidant at physiological concentrations," *Proceedings of the National Academy of Sciences of the United States of America*, vol. 87, no. 12, pp. 4879–4883, 1990.

[91] H.-J. Jung, E.-H. Park, and C.-J. Lim, "Evaluation of anti-angiogenic, anti-inflammatory and antinociceptive activity of coenzyme Q10 in experimental animals," *Journal of Pharmacy and Pharmacology*, vol. 61, no. 10, pp. 1391–1395, 2009.

[92] G. López-Lluch, M. P. Barroso, S. F. Martín et al., "Role of plasma membrane coenzyme Q on the regulation of apoptosis," *BioFactors*, vol. 9, no. 2-4, pp. 171–177, 1999.

[93] C. Szardening-Kirchner, L. Konrad, E. W. Hauck, S. M. Haag, O. Eickelberg, and W. Weidner, "Upregulation of mRNA expression of MCP-1 by TGF-β1 in fibroblast cells from Peyronie's disease," *World Journal of Urology*, vol. 27, no. 1, pp. 123–130, 2009.

[94] M. Ebadi, S. K. Sharma, S. Wanpen, and A. Amornpan, "Coenzyme Q10 inhibits mitochondrial complex-1 down-regulation and nuclear factor-kappa B activation," *Journal of Cellular and Molecular Medicine*, vol. 8, no. 2, pp. 213–222, 2004.

[95] M. R. Safarinejad, "Safety and efficacy of coenzyme Q 10 supplementation in early chronic Peyronie's disease: A double-blind, placebo-controlled randomized study," *International Journal of Impotence Research*, vol. 22, no. 5, pp. 298–309, 2010.

[96] M. L. Khalil, "Biological activity of bee propolis in health and disease," *Asian Pacific Journal of Cancer Prevention*, vol. 7, no. 1, pp. 22–31, 2006.

[97] C. Sun, Z. Wu, Z. Wang, and H. Zhang, "Effect of ethanol/water solvents on phenolic profiles and antioxidant properties of Beijing propolis extracts," *Evidence-Based Complementary and Alternative Medicine*, vol. 2015, Article ID 595393, 9 pages, 2015.

[98] C. S. Machado, J. B. Mokochinski, T. O. de Lira et al., "Comparative study of chemical composition and biological activity of yellow, green, brown, and red Brazilian propolis," *Evidence-Based Complementary and Alternative Medicine*, vol. 2016, Article ID 6057650, 11 pages, 2016.

[99] S. Kumazawa, T. Hamasaka, and T. Nakayama, "Antioxidant activity of propolis of various geographic origins," *Food Chemistry*, vol. 84, no. 3, pp. 329–339, 2004.

[100] S. Huang, C.-P. Zhang, K. Wang, G. Li, and F.-L. Hu, "Recent advances in the chemical composition of propolis," *Molecules*, vol. 19, no. 12, pp. 19610–19632, 2014.

[101] M. Khalil and S. Sulaiman, "The potential role of honey and its polyphenols in preventing heart disease: a review," *African Journal of Traditional, Complementary and Alternative Medicines*, vol. 7, no. 4, pp. 315–321, 2010.

[102] A. Russo, R. Longo, and A. Vanella, "Antioxidant activity of propolis: role of caffeic acid phenethyl ester and galangin," *Fitoterapia*, vol. 73, supplement 1, pp. S21–S29, 2002.

[103] X. Wang, G. Gong, W. Yang, Y. Li, M. Jiang, and L. Li, "Antifibrotic activity of galangin, a novel function evaluated in animal liver fibrosis model," *Environmental Toxicology and Pharmacology*, vol. 36, no. 2, pp. 288–295, 2013.

[104] Y. C. Jung, M. E. Kim, J. H. Yoon et al., "Anti-inflammatory effects of galangin on lipopolysaccharide-activated macrophages via ERK and NF-κB pathway regulation," *Immunopharmacology and Immunotoxicology*, vol. 36, no. 6, pp. 426–432, 2014.

[105] D. Ribeiro, M. Freitas, S. M. Tomé, A. M. S. Silva, G. Porto, and E. Fernandes, "Modulation of human neutrophils' oxidative burst by flavonoids," *European Journal of Medicinal Chemistry*, vol. 67, pp. 280–292, 2013.

[106] A. W. Boots, G. R. M. M. Haenen, and A. Bast, "Health effects of quercetin: from antioxidant to nutraceutical," *European Journal of Pharmacology*, vol. 585, no. 2-3, pp. 325–337, 2008.

[107] Y.-D. Min, C.-H. Choi, H. Bark et al., "Quercetin inhibits expression of inflammatory cytokines through attenuation of NF-κB and p38 MAPK in HMC-1 human mast cell line," *Inflammation Research*, vol. 56, no. 5, pp. 210–215, 2007.

[108] G. M. Raso, R. Meli, G. di Carlo, M. Pacilio, and R. di Carlo, "Inhibition of inducible nitric oxide synthase and cyclooxygenase-2 expression by flavonoids in macrophage J774A.1," *Life Sciences*, vol. 68, no. 8, pp. 921–931, 2001.

[109] T. Nakamura, M. Matsushima, Y. Hayashi et al., "Attenuation of transforming growth factor-β-stimulated collagen production in fibroblasts by quercetin-induced heme oxygenase-1," *American Journal of Respiratory Cell and Molecular Biology*, vol. 44, no. 5, pp. 614–620, 2011.

[110] L. C. Paracatu, C. M. Faria, C. Quinello et al., "Caffeic acid phenethyl ester: consequences of its hydrophobicity in the oxidative functions and cytokine release by leukocytes," *Evidence-Based Complementary and Alternative Medicine*, vol. 2014, Article ID 793629, 13 pages, 2014.

[111] F. Armutcu, S. Akyol, S. Ustunsoy, and F. F. Turan, "Therapeutic potential of caffeic acid phenethyl ester and its anti-inflammatory and immunomodulatory effects (Review)," *Experimental and Therapeutic Medicine*, vol. 9, no. 5, pp. 1582–1588, 2015.

[112] W.-X. Zhao, L. Wang, J.-L. Yang, L.-Z. Li, W.-M. Xu, and T. Li, "Caffeic acid phenethyl ester attenuates pro-inflammatory and fibrogenic phenotypes of LPS-stimulated hepatic stellate cells through the inhibition of NF-kB signaling," *International Journal of Molecular Medicine*, vol. 33, no. 3, pp. 687–694, 2014.

[113] M. M. Mia and R. A. Bank, "The pro-fibrotic properties of transforming growth factor on human fibroblasts are counteracted by caffeic acid by inhibiting myofibroblast formation and collagen synthesis," *Cell and Tissue Research*, vol. 363, no. 3, pp. 775–789, 2016.

[114] K. J. Woo, Y.-J. Jeong, H. Inoue, J.-W. Park, and T. K. Kwon, "Chrysin suppresses lipopolysaccharide-induced cyclooxygenase-2 expression through the inhibition of nuclear factor for IL-6 (NF-IL6) DNA-binding activity," *FEBS Letters*, vol. 579, no. 3, pp. 705–711, 2005.

[115] H. Cho, C.-W. Yun, W.-K. Park et al., "Modulation of the activity of pro-inflammatory enzymes, COX-2 and iNOS, by chrysin derivatives," *Pharmacological Research*, vol. 49, no. 1, pp. 37–43, 2004.

[116] A. Ahad, A. A. Ganai, M. Mujeeb, and W. A. Siddiqui, "Chrysin, an anti-inflammatory molecule, abrogates renal dysfunction in type 2 diabetic rats," *Toxicology and Applied Pharmacology*, vol. 279, no. 1, pp. 1–7, 2014.

[117] H.-M. Lo, M.-W. Wu, S.-L. Pan, C.-Y. Peng, P.-H. Wu, and W.-B. Wu, "Chrysin restores PDGF-induced inhibition on protein tyrosine phosphatase and reduces PDGF signaling in cultured VSMCs," *Journal of Nutritional Biochemistry*, vol. 23, no. 6, pp. 667–678, 2012.

[118] Y. Dong, H. Huang, M. Zhao, D. Sun-Waterhouse, L. Lin, and C. Xiao, "Mechanisms underlying the xanthine oxidase inhibitory effects of dietary flavonoids galangin and pinobanksin," *Journal of Functional Foods*, vol. 24, pp. 26–36, 2016.

[119] A. C. Santos, S. A. Uyemura, J. L. C. Lopes, J. N. Bazon, F. E. Mingatto, and C. Curti, "Effect of naturally occurring flavonoids on lipid peroxidation and membrane permeability transition in mitochondria," *Free Radical Biology and Medicine*, vol. 24, no. 9, pp. 1455–1461, 1998.

[120] L.-T. Zhou, K.-J. Wang, L. Li, H. Li, and M. Geng, "Pinocembrin inhibits lipopolysaccharide-induced inflammatory mediators production in BV2 microglial cells through suppression of PI3K/Akt/NF-κB pathway," *European Journal of Pharmacology*, vol. 761, pp. 211–216, 2015.

[121] K.-S. Chen, M.-D. Shi, C.-S. Chien, and Y.-W. Shih, "Pinocembrin suppresses TGF-β1-induced epithelial-mesenchymal transition and metastasis of human Y-79 retinoblastoma cells through inactivating $\alpha v\beta 3$ integrin/FAK/p38α signaling pathway," *Cell and Bioscience*, vol. 4, no. 1, article 41, 2014.

[122] E. Alday, D. Valencia, A. L. Carreño et al., "Apoptotic induction by pinobanksin and some of its ester derivatives from Sonoran propolis in a B-cell lymphoma cell line," *Chemico-Biological Interactions*, vol. 242, pp. 35–44, 2015.

[123] W.-W. Jung, "Protective effect of apigenin against oxidative stress-induced damage in osteoblastic cells," *International Journal of Molecular Medicine*, vol. 33, no. 5, pp. 1327–1334, 2014.

[124] R. Landolfi, R. L. Mower, and M. Steiner, "Modification of platelet function and arachidonic acid metabolism by bioflavonoids. Structure-activity relations," *Biochemical Pharmacology*, vol. 33, no. 9, pp. 1525–1530, 1984.

[125] L. Chen and W. Zhao, "Apigenin protects against bleomycin-induced lung fibrosis in rats," *Experimental and Therapeutic Medicine*, vol. 11, no. 1, pp. 230–234, 2016.

[126] Lemourt O. M., Filgueiras L. E., Rodríguez B. A., González O. E., and Bordonado R., "Clinical evaluation of the use of propoleum in Peyronie's disease," *Archivos Españoles de Urología*, vol. 51, no. 2, pp. 171–176, 1998.

[127] Lemourt O. M., Rodríguez B. A., Puente G. M., Vega G. C., Navarro C. M., and Pérez M. A., "Peyronie's disease and propoleum," *Archivos Espanoles de Urologia*, vol. 56, no. 7, pp. 805–813, 2003.

[128] Lemourt O. M., Rodríguez B. A., Bordonado R. R., González O. E., and Molina C. F., "Dose study with propoleum in Peyronie's disease," *Archivos Espanoles de Urologia*, vol. 56, no. 7, pp. 814–819, 2003.

[129] Lemourt O. M., Fragas V. R., Bordonado R. R., J. L. Santana, González O. E., and A. Merino, "Peyronie's disease. Evaluation of three therapeutic methodologies: Propoleum, laser and propoleum-laser," *Archivos Espanoles de Urologia*, vol. 58, no. 9, pp. 931–935, 2005.

[130] G. Paulis, R. D'Ascenzo, P. Nupieri et al., "Effectiveness of antioxidants (propolis, blueberry, vitamin E) associated with verapamil in the medical management of Peyronie's disease: A study of 151 cases," *International Journal of Andrology*, vol. 35, no. 4, pp. 521–527, 2012.

[131] G. Paulis, G. Cavallini, T. Brancato, and R. Alvaro, "Peironimev-plus® in the treatment of chronic inflammation of tunica albuginea (peyronie's disease). Results of a controlled study," *Inflammation and Allergy - Drug Targets*, vol. 12, no. 1, pp. 61–67, 2013.

[132] G. Paulis, G. Cavallini, G. De Giorgio, S. Quattrocchi, T. Brancato, and R. Alvaro, "Long-term multimodal therapy (Verapamil associated with propolis, blueberry, vitamin E and local Diclofenac) on patients with peyronie's disease (chronic inflammation of the tunica albuginea). results of a controlled study," *Inflammation and Allergy - Drug Targets*, vol. 12, no. 6, pp. 403–409, 2013.

[133] D. Burdulis, L. Ivanauskas, V. Dirse, S. Kazlauskas, and A. Razukas, "Study of diversity of anthocyanin composition in bilberry (Vaccinium myrtillus L.) fruits.," *Medicina (Kaunas, Lithuania)*, vol. 43, no. 12, pp. 971–977, 2007.

[134] N. P. Seeram, "Berry fruits for cancer prevention: current status and future prospects," *Journal of Agricultural and Food Chemistry*, vol. 56, no. 3, pp. 630–635, 2008.

[135] A. Fleuriet, "The Main Phenolics of Fruit," in *Fruit Phenolics*, J. J. Macheix, A. Fleuriet, and J. Billot, Eds., pp. 1–99, CRC Press, Inc, Boca Raton, Fla, USA, 1990.

[136] M. M. Rahman, T. Ichiyanagi, T. Komiyama, Y. Hatano, and T. Konishi, "Superoxide radical- and peroxynitrite-scavenging activity of anthocyanins; structure-activity relationship and their synergism," *Free Radical Research*, vol. 40, no. 9, pp. 993–1002, 2006.

[137] T. Ichiyanagi, Y. Hatano, S. Matsuo, and T. Konishi, "Simultaneous comparison of relative reactivities of twelve major anthocyanins in bilberry towards reactive nitrogen species," *Chemical and Pharmaceutical Bulletin*, vol. 52, no. 11, pp. 1312–1315, 2004.

[138] S. Roth, M. R. Spalinger, C. Gottier et al., "Bilberry-derived anthocyanins modulate cytokine expression in the intestine of patients with ulcerative colitis," *PLoS ONE*, vol. 11, no. 5, Article ID e0154817, 2016.

[139] D.-X. Hou, T. Yanagita, T. Uto, S. Masuzaki, and M. Fujii, "Anthocyanidins inhibit cyclooxygenase-2 expression in LPS-evoked macrophages: Structure-activity relationship and molecular mechanisms involved," *Biochemical Pharmacology*, vol. 70, no. 3, pp. 417–425, 2005.

[140] M. C. Lazzè, R. Pizzala, P. Perucca et al., "Anthocyanidins decrease endothelin-1 production and increase endothelial nitric oxide synthase in human endothelial cells," *Molecular Nutrition and Food Research*, vol. 50, no. 1, pp. 44–51, 2006.

[141] N. Xia, A. Pautz, U. Wollscheid, G. Reifenberg, U. Förstermann, and H. Li, "Artichoke, cynarin and cyanidin downregulate the expression of inducible nitric oxide synthase in human coronary smooth muscle cells," *Molecules*, vol. 19, no. 3, pp. 3654–3668, 2014.

[142] C. Artaria, R. Pace, G. Maramaldi, and G. Appendino, "Different brands of bilberry extract: a comparison of selected components," *NUTRAfoods*, vol. 6, no. 4, pp. 13–18, 2007.

[143] I. Gouni-Berthold and A. Sachinidis, "Molecular mechanisms explaining the preventive effects of catechins on the development of proliferative diseases," *Current Pharmaceutical Design*, vol. 10, no. 11, pp. 1261–1271, 2004.

[144] T. J. Bivalacqua, H. C. Champion, S. Leungwattanakij et al., "Evaluation of nitric oxide synthase and arginase in the induction of a Peyronie's-like condition in the rat," *Journal of Andrology*, vol. 22, no. 3, pp. 497–506, 2001.

[145] M. G. Ferrini, D. Vernet, T. R. Magee et al., "Antifibrotic role of inducible nitric oxide synthase," *Nitric Oxide*, vol. 6, no. 3, pp. 283–294, 2002.

[146] M. Bentz, C. Zaouter, Q. Shi et al., "Inhibition of inducible nitric oxide synthase prevents lipid peroxidation in osteoarthritic chondrocytes," *Journal of Cellular Biochemistry*, vol. 113, no. 7, pp. 2256–2267, 2012.

[147] J.-P. Pelletier, D. Jovanovic, J. C. Fernandes et al., "Reduced progression of experimental osteoarthritis in vivo by selective inhibition of inducible nitric oxide synthase," *Arthritis and Rheumatism*, vol. 41, no. 7, pp. 1275–1286, 1998.

16

The Modified Gil-Vernet Antireflux Surgery: A Successful Technique for High-Grade Vesicoureteral Reflux Correction in Children —Long-Term Follow-Up

Mahmoudreza Moradi,[1] Abolhassan Seyedzadeh,[2] Saeed Gharakhloo,[3] Aref Teymourinezhad,[3] Kaveh Kaseb,[3] and Haress Rezaee[3]

[1]*Professor in Pediatric Urology, Chairman of Urology Department in Imam Reza Hospital, Chairman of Regenerative Medicine Research Center (RMRC), Kermanshah University of Medical Sciences, Kermanshah, Iran*
[2]*Professor in Pediatric Nephrology, Kermanshah University of Medical Sciences, Kermanshah, Iran*
[3]*Urology Resident in Kermanshah University of Medical Sciences, Kermanshah, Iran*

Correspondence should be addressed to Mahmoudreza Moradi; drmrmoradi@gmail.com

Academic Editor: Darius J. Bagli

Introduction. Vesicoureteral reflux (VUR) is a common urologic anomaly in children. Many techniques have been offered to manage this condition, in which one of them is modified Gil-Vernet antireflux surgery. The study fullfiled to evaluate the efficacy and safety of modified Gil-Vernet antireflux surgery in correction of high-grade VUR. *Materials and Methods.* A retrospective study in which we evaluated efficacy, safety, and complications of modified Gil-Vernet antireflux surgery as a choice procedure for high-grade reflux in all patients who underwent it since 2000 to 2016 at 2 hospitals of Kermanshah University of medical sciences that all of them were done by one surgeon. *Results.* 183 patients with 290 high-grade refluxing units (grade IV or V) were reviewed. 182 refluxing units were grade IV, and 108 units were grade V. There were 76 (41.54%) patients with unilateral and 107 (58.46%) patients with bilateral VUR. Reflux in high-grade group corrected completely in 278 (95.86%) refluxing units and 175 patients (95.62%). *Conclusions.* Our results are remarkable and compatible with other techniques' results. This simple and safe technique can correct bilateral VURs simultaneously; thus, it is rational to be considered for high-grade VUR correction. According to our results, we suggest the modified Gil-Vernet antireflux procedure for high-grade VUR correction as a simple, safe, and successful technique. This trial is registered with 67145/86/1233.

1. Introduction

Vesicoureteral reflux (VUR) has been defined as non-physiologic retrograde flow of urine from the bladder up the ureter into the kidney as the result of an insufficient vesicoureteral junction [1]. It is a common urologic anomaly in children. The prevalence of VUR is 0.4–1.8% of normal children and 30–50% among children with urinary tract infection [2, 3]. Untreated VUR can be associated with pyelonephritic scaring [4, 5]. The aims of management of a child with VUR are prevention of renal injury, recurrent febrile UTI, minimization of treatment morbidities, and follow-up duration [6]. Preferred therapy for a selected patient with VUR depends on different parameters as age, gender, VUR grade, symptoms, renal damage and function, laterality, bladder and bowel problems, compliance, and parents' choice [7]. Despite all of advancements, voiding cystourethrography (VCUG) is the gold standard of VUR which can demonstrate timing and laterality of the reflux, reflux grade, exact anatomy of the upper and lower urinary tracts, voiding phase, and anatomy of the bladder outlet and urethra [8]. High-grade VUR by IRS is defined as grade IV or V [1].

Treatment modalities include conservative (medical management and waiting for spontaneous resolution or downgrading) and interventional (open surgical, laparoscopic, or endoscopic approaches) [9]. Selecting surgical or medical management is of high controversy. Low-dose prophylactic antibiotic is the first line of treatment, and the cases of VUR should be permitted to resolve spontaneously [9]. However, in some conditions, surgical approach is inevitable. Multiple surgical procedures have been described to correct VUR. The surgeon can select the appropriate technique. The selective procedure is individualized according to the surgeon and patient condition [9]. The open surgical approaches can be classified as extravesical or intravesical based on the approach to the ureter. Gil-Vernet antireflux surgery is one of the intravesical approaches. Other conventional techniques such as Cohen and Leadbetter have high success rate, but stenosis of ureteral orifices, long time operation, long days of hospitalization, difficulty in catheterization, and malpositioning of ureteral orifices are their disadvantages. Gil-Vernet antireflux surgery is a useful and less invasive method that was introduced in 1983 and with fewer complications, bilaterally correction of VUR by one operation and prevention of reflux relapse in contralateral side which can occur in 10% of cases [10, 11].

It has many advantages such as shorter operating time and high success with lower complication rate; but in some literatures, this method has been accused of inefficacy in high-grade reflux [4]. In this study, the efficacy of Gil-Vernet antireflux technique in primary high-grade vesicoureteral reflux is assessed.

2. Methods

This study was a retrospective one in which we evaluated all the patients who underwent modified Gil-Vernet antireflux surgery as for their high-grade reflux from 2000 to 2016 in 2 hospitals of the Kermanshah University of Medical Sciences, and all of them were done by one surgeon. The study group was selected from patients with primary high-grade vesicoureteral reflux (grade IV or V) diagnosed by VCUG (X-ray contrast) with various complaints. The grading of vesicoureteral reflux was based on IRS radiologic classification of VCUG which was evaluated by a radiologist. *Indications for surgery were the failure of medical management, breakthrough UTI despite antibiotic prophylaxis, and the occurrence of new scars or worsening of renal function.* The exclusion criteria were relapsing reflux after other procedures or secondary reflux and patients with neurogenic bladder. The modified Gil-Vernet antireflux procedure was performed for all patients.

2.1. Surgical Technique. A pfannenstiel skin incision was made. After splitting muscles and vertically opening the anterior bladder wall, two ureteral orifices were catheterized. A transverse incision is made through mucosa across superior aspect of trigone between ureteral orifices. The mucosa is then elevated off the bladder wall muscle carefully. Medial aspects of ureters gently dissected from surrounding tissues till hiatus and trigonal muscles up to advantis layer without damage to ureters in order to make the orifices free; in other words, waldeyer's sheath of bladder dissected completely from medial aspect of intramural ureter carefully so that by this action, approximation of ureter to midline would be tension free. It is an essential step to prevent lateral displacement of ureter orifice in future. One 5-0 vicryl suture was placed in a mattress fashion exactly near the orifice at the medial wall of each ureter to fix ureteral orifices in the midline, encompassing the periureteral sheath and muscle. This suture advances the ureters toward the midline tension freely, increasing their intramural length. The place of this suture is very important and must be on the edge of ureter's orifice, to prevent angulation of distal ureter near to the orifice. In addition to this, to prevent lateralization of ureters in future, 2 anchoring sutures were placed above and below the first suture. Mucosa repaired vertically with the 5-0 vicryl suture (Figure 1). Then, ureteral catheters were removed, and by intravenous injection of furosemide and observing the jet of urine from the ureteral orifices, their patency was confirmed. Surgery was ended by insertion and fixation of urethral catheter and repair of bladder water tight in two layers. No kind of drains was applied.

On the second postoperation day, if urine was clear, urethral catheter was removed and patient was discharged from the hospital. All patients visited one week after surgery and were followed by ultrasonography one month and radionuclide cystography (RNC) 3 months after surgery; if RNC was normal, follow-up imaging was done by using ultrasonography at 6 and 12 months after operation and then annually. If VUR was not resolved after 1 year, the patient was undergone reoperation by injection or different technique according to age, reflux grade, and the time passed from primary surgery. Also during annual follow-up sonography, if hydronephrosis or UTI was detected, the patient was evaluated by VCUG or RNC once again. Data of postoperative outcomes including days of hospitalization, reflux downgrading, complications, and the need of reoperation were collected and analyzed by SPSS-23.

3. Results

183 patients with 290 high-grade refluxing units were studied: 114 (68.3%) female and 69 (31.7%) male patients with mean age of 4.8 years (range 1–13 years). There were 76 (41.54%) patients with unilateral and 107 (58.46%) ones with bilateral VUR. 182 refluxing units were grade IV, and 108 were grade V. Mean operation time was 50 ± 10 minutes and mean hospitalization was 2.56 days (range 2–9 days). Mean follow-up time was 65 months (range 1–15 years). Reflux in the high-grade group had been corrected completely in 278 (95.86%) refluxing units and 175 patients (95.62%) (Table 1). The failure rate with persistent reflux was 8 patients (5 unilateral with grade IV VUR and 2 bilateral VUR with 1 side grade IV and other side grade V and 3 patients with unilateral grade V) with 12 refluxing units (4.1%). Six patients were retreated by ureteral submucosal injection of vantris which resolved finally. Two patients were managed by prophylactic antibiotic prescription. One postoperative complication occurred, and it was bladder dehiscence which at end repaired successfully. We had no complication, such

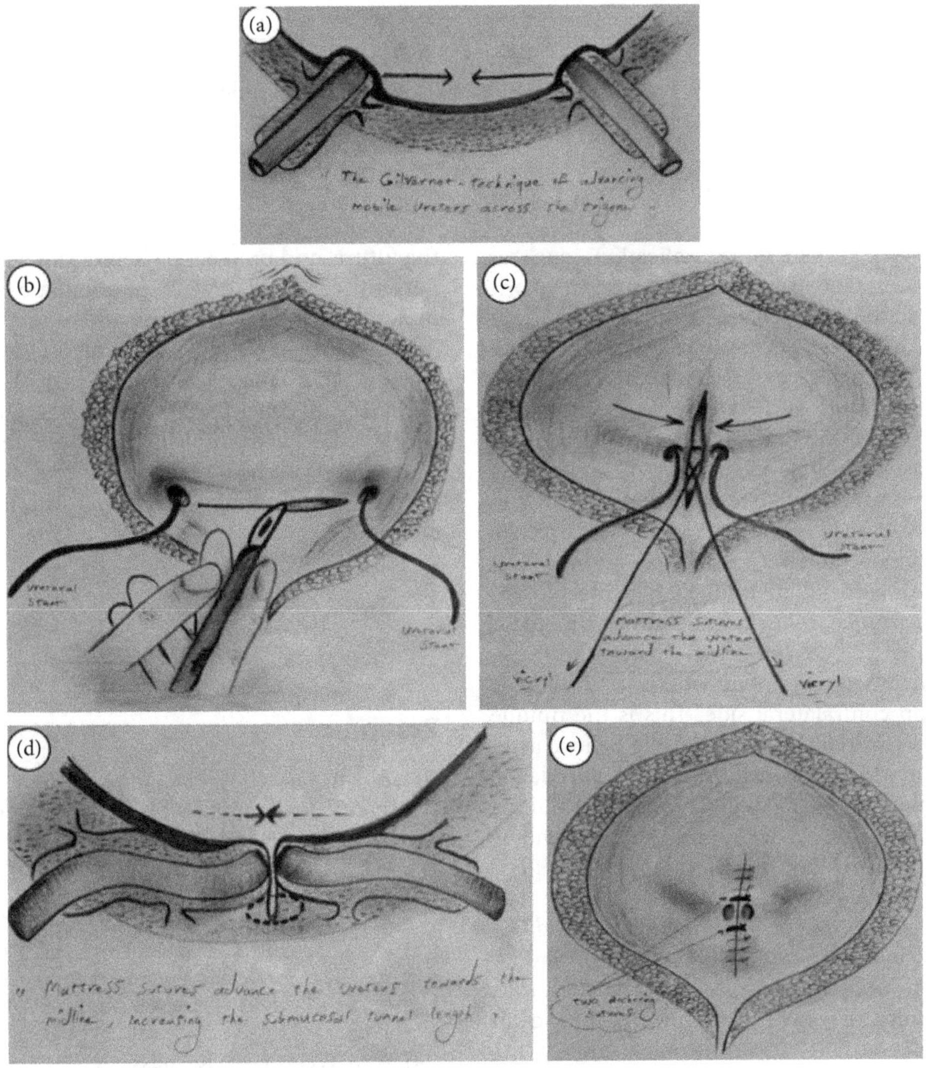

FIGURE 1: Schematic representation of the modified Gil-Vernet antireflux technique (drawn by Kaveh Kaseb).

as stenosis of ureteral orifices or ureteral obstruction, voiding dysfunction, contralateral VUR, urinary retention, and laboratory abnormalities.

4. Discussion

Vesicoureteral reflux is a common urologic anomaly in children. Untreated VUR can be associated with pyelonephritic scaring. Multiple surgical and medical procedures have been described to correct VUR. The basic steps of reimplantation are ureterolysis, creation of a new ureteral tunnel, the ureteral advancement, and anastomosis of the ureter with the bladder. In conventional open surgical techniques, despite high success rate, some complications are common and these procedures are invasive. The Gil-Vernet antireflux surgery has been accused of low efficacy in elimination reflux due to following reasons which are not effective especially in high-grade VUR [12]. And, in the latest edition of *Campbell-Walsh Textbook of Urology*, it has been cited "this procedure has been accomplished laparoscopically with limited success. Okamura and colleagues (1999) and Cartwright and colleagues (1996) reported success rates of 59% and 62.5%, respectively" [4]. Because of the relation between submucosal length and ureteral diameter in high-grade reflux, it is logical that the efficacy of Gil-Vernet operation may decrease [13]. The high success rate of other intravesical procedures has been cited in comparison to Gil-Vernet technique.

In Mirshemirani et al.'s study, 72 patients with VUR underwent Gil-Vernet antireflux surgery; success rate was 96.15%, and there was no postoperative complication [14]. Sharifi and Akhavizadegan reported that 39 women (18–65 years) underwent Gil-Vernet antireflux surgery with 97.95% success rate [15].

We believe modified Gil-Vernet antireflux surgery is simple with high success rate that has not gained attention and is a neglected operation in urology. Most conventional methods are more invasive, and many complications can occur. Contralateral VUR, urinary retention, voiding dysfunction, long operation time, long day's hospitalization, and obstruction are anticipated complications of different techniques of VUR repairment [4, 10, 15], that rarely occur

Table 1: The basic statistics of the present study.

Gender	Side and grade				
	Left side and grade IV	Left side and grade V	Right side and grade IV	Right side and grade V	Bilateral high-grade
Female	18	10	16	7	63
Male	9	2	7	7	44

in Gil-Vernet surgery. We had no complications such as mentioned one or ureteral obstruction; however, just in one case, we observed bladder dehiscence. Applying this modified technique resulted in high success rate, compatible with Gil-Vernet report [16]; however, Sharifiaghdas et al. have recently reported the lower success rate with long-term follow-up by trigonoplasty [17]. This technique is simple, safe, and least invasive. We had failure in 6 high grade refluxing units only. The relapse after operation occurred in patients with grade 4 VUR that managed with ureteral submucosal injection of vantris (promedon) and/or conservatively. In addition to all mentioned benefits of Gil-Vernet antireflux technique, other advantages of this technique are management of contralateral VUR without excessive intervention, and in cases of unilateral VUR, there is no need to follow-up contralateral side. This is the unique feature of Gil-Vernet antireflux technique. We believe as in high-grade VURs in which the orifices are lateralized, the maximum approximation of orifices is achieved by modified Gil-Vernet, and subsequently, more favorable results will be obtained. *Actually, it seems that more lateral ureter orifices more effective results for modified Gil-Vernet technique; thus as in high-grade VURs, lateral ectopia is more, and modified Gil-Vernet is more effective* . Our high success rate of modified Gil-Vernet antireflux surgery in contrast with previous studies results, may be, is due to the difference in our technique with classic Gil-Vernet antireflux surgery (the classic description by Gil-Vernet uses a single 3–0 nylon or prolene suture while we use 5-0 vicryl suture with 2 anchoring sutures higher and lower the cornerstone suture) and with more dissection of ureters till hiatus more submucosal ureteral length with approximation sheath technique of lateralized ureteral orifice is achieved.

In our personal experience, as we do and have done other antireflux techniques, it is obvious that "Gil-Vernet antireflux technique" has shorter operation time; however, though we emphasize the various advantages of the Gil-Vernet technique, as we did not compare different techniques related to their exact operation time, we cannot prove it statistically. In a recent study, Sarhan et al. have reported the necessity of surgical intervention in 89% of patient with primary high-grade VURs with success rate of 60% and 100% following endoscopic and surgical reimplantation, respectively [18].

Summarily, Gil-Vernet antireflux technique in contrast with Politano-Leadbetter technique is less invasive, with lower possibility of damage to adjacent organs and bilaterally operable simultaneously. Also in contrary to Cohen technique, there is no likelihood of ureteral angulation, and ureteral orifices are closer to their natural site which results in the easier retrograde catheterization and ureteroscopy in the future, and unlike the Glenn-Anderson technique, in the present technique, by less manipulation of trigone and less ureteral mobilization, the limitations of favorable submucosal ureter length creation are not present. Overall present technique is much easier than other one. Our experience indicates that the modified Gil-Vernet antireflux surgery is a very simple, safe, rapid, and highly successful procedure. We believe in its efficacy for high-grade VUR correction and thus suggest its application by other surgeon colleagues.

References

[1] R. L. Lebowitz, H. Olbing, K. V. Parkkulainen, J. M. Smellie, and T. E. Tamminen-MÖbius, "International system of radiographic grading of vesicoureteric reflux," *Pediatric Radiology*, vol. 15, no. 2, pp. 105–109, 1985.

[2] D. G. Bundy and J. R. Serwint, "Vesicoureteral reflux," *Pediatrics in Review*, vol. 28, no. 2, pp. e6–e8, 2007.

[3] J. M. Smellie and I. C. Normand, "Clinical features and significance of urinary tract infection in children," *Proceedings of the Royal Society of Medicine*, vol. 59, no. 5, pp. 415-416, 1966.

[4] J. A. Wein, L. R. Kavoussi, A. W. Patrin, and C. A. Peters, *Campbell-Walsh Urology*, Chapter 137, 11th edition, 2016.

[5] M. Moradi and D. A. Diamond, "Summary of recent AUA guidelines for the management of vesicoureteral reflux in children," *African Journal of Urology*, vol. 19, no. 4, pp. 155–159, 2013.

[6] C. A. Peters, S. J. Skoog, B. S. Arant et al., "Summary of the AUA guideline on management of primary vesicoureteral reflux in children," *Journal of Urology*, vol. 184, no. 3, pp. 1134–1144, 2010.

[7] W. H. Rosch and V. Geyer, "Vesikoureterale refluxerkrankung," *Der Urologe*, vol. 50, no. 6, pp. 725–734, 2011.

[8] G. A. Bogaert and K. Slabbaert, "Vesicoureteral reflux," *European Urology Supplements*, vol. 11, no. 2, pp. 16–24, 2012.

[9] N. Simfroosh, "A new approach to vesicoureteral reflux persisting after posterior urethral valve ablation using Gil-Vernet anti reflux technique," *MJRI*, vol. 2, pp. 249–254, 1988.

[10] J. Maria and G. Vernet, "A new technique for surgical correction of vesicoureteral reflux," *Journal of Urology*, vol. 131, no. 3, pp. 456–458, 1984.

[11] K. E. Sparr, A. H. Balcom, and H. G. Mesrobian, "Incidence and natural history of contralateral vesicoureteral reflux in patients presenting with unilateral disease," *Journal of Urology*, vol. 160, no. 3, pp. 1023–1025, 1998.

[12] A. Atala and M. A. Keating, "Vesicoureteral reflux and megaureter," in *Campbell's Urology*, P. C. Walsh, A. B. Retik, E. D. Vaugen Jr., and A. J. Wein, Eds., pp. 1859–1916, W.B

Saunders Co., Philadelphia, PA, USA, Chapter 61, 7th edition, 1997.

[13] R. Minervini, G. Morelli, L. Vigano, and P. Gadducci, "Trigonoplasty by Gil Vernet in the treatment of vesicoureteral reflux in adult patients," *European Urology*, vol. 24, no. 2, pp. 201-202, 1993.

[14] A. Mirshemirani, A. Khaleghnejad Tabari, F. Roshanzamir, and S. Shayeghi, "Gil-Vernet antireflux surgery in children's primary vesicoureteral reflux," *Pediatric Surgery International*, vol. 26, no. 10, pp. 981–984, 2010.

[15] F. S. Aghdas and H. Akhavizadegan, "Gil-Vernet anti-reflux surgery and primary vesicoureteral reflux in women," *Scandinavian Journal of Urology and Nephrology*, vol. 41, no. 1, pp. 72–74, 2007.

[16] A. C. McCool, L. M. Perez, and D. B. Joseph, "Contralateral vesicoureteral reflux after simple and tapered unilateral ureteroneocystostomy revisited," *Journal of Urology*, vol. 158, no. 3, pp. 1219-1220, 1997.

[17] F. Sharifiaghdas, N. Mahmoudnejad, A. H. Kashi, M. H. Ramezani, and B. Narouie, "Long-term follow-up of trigonoplasty antireflux operation," *Urologia Journal*, vol. 84, no. 1, pp. 48–50, 2016.

[18] O. Sarhan, M. Al Ghanbar, A. El Helaly, A. Al Otay, and Z. Nakshabandi, "Primary bilateral high grade vesicoureteral reflux: management perspective," *European Urology Supplements*, vol. 17, no. 2, p. e1192, 2018.

17

Treatment of Priapism Secondary to Drugs for Erectile Dysfunction

José Pablo Saffon Cuartas, Carolina Sandoval-Salinas, Juan M. Martínez, and Héctor A. Corredor

Clinical Research Group, Boston Medical Group, Bogotá 110111, Colombia

Correspondence should be addressed to Carolina Sandoval-Salinas; carolina_ss81@yahoo.es

Academic Editor: Kostis Gyftopoulos

Priapism may present as a side effect in patients treated with medications for erectile dysfunction, in which it should be controlled in a timely manner to avoid complications. There is little information regarding the use of local measures for the treatment of this condition. This study was done with the objective to describe the management of priapism secondary to erectile dysfunction drugs in a cohort of men. Records of emergencies and adverse events were reviewed by two researchers to identify patients diagnosed with erectile dysfunction who received oral or intracavernosal drugs for their illness and presented priapism. Sociodemographic data, clinical background, and information on the duration, management, and evolution of the priapism were extracted. Priapism incidence, percentage of improvement by type of treatment subgroups, and frequency of complications were estimated. 698 patients were treated with PDE-5 inhibitors and 2,135 with intracavernosal drugs. Thirty-one patients (1.4%) reported at least one priapism event during treatment, all with intracavernosal drugs. Treatment with local measures was effective for 10 (32.2%) patients, 1 (3.2%) required terbutaline, 19 (61.2%) used intracavernosal etilefrine, and 1 (3.2%) required drainage and flushing of cavernous bodies. After the priapism episode, 3 (9.6%) patients required an increased dose of the drug in order to achieve satisfactory erection. The results suggest that in men treated for priapism secondary to the use of sexual impotence drugs, initial treatment with local measures and etilefrine can achieve detumescence, decreasing the need for invasive procedures or surgery as a first-line therapy alternative. It is necessary to carry out research studies to confirm this hypothesis.

1. Introduction

Priapism is defined as an erection for more than four hours after the erotic stimulation ends or in the absence of stimulation. It is classified as ischemic and nonischemic, the former being more frequent [1, 2]. Its etiology varies and can include blood dyscrasia, metabolic or neurological disorders, infections, toxins, and some drugs including those used to treat erectile dysfunction (ED) [1–4]. Priapism is a very rare event for patients who use phosphodiesterase-5 inhibitors (iPDE-5). An incidence of 0 to 35% has been reported for patients receiving intracavernosal drugs, depending on the drug used and how the studies define priapism [5–10].

It is widely known that inadequate and late treatment of priapism has irreversible consequences for the patient, secondary to anatomical and functional changes in the cavernous bodies of the penis, which can range from erectile dysfunction to penile fibrosis [1, 2, 4, 11–14]. Lesions are due to the absence of arterial blood flow, which produces an ischemic process that improves only by reducing the erection. Hypoxic and inflammatory changes are evident 12 hours after onset of erection, observing destruction of the sinusoidal endothelium. The exact point at which irreversible damage occurs is difficult to determine [15]. Zacharakis et al. have reported extensive necrosis of cavernous smooth muscle in patients with over 48 hours of priapism [16]. Therefore, timely treatment of this urological emergency is highly important.

There is very little scientific evidence for the use of local measures to treat priapism [10, 17]. The last European guidelines for male sexual dysfunction recommended intracavernosal sympathomimetic drugs as a first line of treatment for priapism secondary to intracavernosal injections of vasoactive drugs, while local measures such as ice and exercise, although named, are not recommended because of a lack of scientific support [2].

The aim of this study was to describe the experience in the treatment of priapism secondary to pharmacological treatment of erectile dysfunction in a men cohort attended in a specialized health centre in different cities of Colombia.

2. Materials and Methods

This was an observational retrospective study. Institutional records were reviewed to identify patients diagnosed with erectile dysfunction who received oral or intracavernosal treatment, between January 1 and December 31, 2017. In order to determine the priapism cases related with the use of medication, two researchers reviewed: (1) records from call centre emergency services, which describe cases of priapism when patients call to request medical care for this event, and (2) records of adverse events reported by physicians, which describe cases treated at the centers or at other institutions and identified at a follow-up visit.

A priapism case related with the use of medication was defined as an erection for more than 4 hours after sexual stimulation ended after taking a phosphodiesterase-5 inhibitor or intracavernosal injection composed of alprostadil, papaverine, atropine, and phentolamine (QuadMix) or alprostadil, papaverine, and phentolamine (Trimix); with or without pain, without a history of sickle cell anemia.

After identifying the cases, the researchers reviewed the clinical register of the patients and, entered information regarding duration, treatment, and evolution of priapism in an Excel® database. They also reviewed the records posterior to the presentation of the priapism episode and until the present, as the follow-up period for verifying sequels.

The data was validated before the analysis by a third investigator. When extreme or incoherent data were found, the clinical history was reviewed to confirm the information. Absolute and relative frequency measurements were calculated for categorical variables, and measures of central tendency and dispersion were estimated for numerical variables, globally and by subgroups of interest according to the duration of priapism. Only the information of the first episode of priapism was included. The incidence of priapism was estimated considering the population at risk as all patients with dysfunction who were treated from January 1 to December 31, 2017, who received pharmacological treatment. Stata 15.1® software was used for statistical analysis.

The study was approved by the institution's research committee and was conducted in accordance with ethical considerations for human research described by the Declaration of Helsinki and by national norms, respecting the rights and confidentiality of the research subjects.

3. Results

During the period of interest, 2,833 patients with erectile dysfunction were treated with medication, of which 698 (24.7%) received PDE-5 inhibitors as a first line of treatment. Another 2,135 (75.3%) received intracavernosal drugs as a second-line therapy option. Thirty-one (1.4%) patients with intracavernosal treatment reported at least one priapism event; thirty with QuadMix and one with Trimix. Four patients presented two episodes of priapism and one man presented 3 incidents. None of the patients receiving oral drugs reported an erection for more than 4 hours after sexual stimulus. One patient presented priapism with the first application of the drug on the erection test; in the other cases, patients presented this condition during the treatment.

For the group of men who presented priapism, the average age was 48.6 years (SD 11.7 years). The most frequent comorbidity was high blood pressure (eight patients), nineteen patients consumed alcohol occasionally, and seven were smokers. The median duration of the ED was 4.4 years, and the median IIEF-5 score at the time of diagnosis was 14 points. The dose of the medication varied between 6 and 54 units (Table 1).

Regarding to the first priapism event related with the use of medications, the median erection time was 4.5 hours (range 4 to 14.5 hours), 4 patients (12.9%) had priapism for more than 12 hours. The application of local measures (cold water or ice on the penis, and perianal area) or exercising, resulted in detumescence in 10 patients (32.3%), all of whom had an erection lasting less than 5 hours. One patient (3.2%) required additional terbutaline after 6 hours of priapism, which resulted in detumescence 4 hours after taking the drug (this was used due to a lack of access to etilefrine). Nineteen subjects (61.3%) required intracavernosal administration of etilefrine, 68.4% of this took a dose of 10 mg or less to reverse priapism. One patient (3.2%) required drainage and flushing of cavernous bodies after 11 hours of erection, since etilefrine and terbutaline were not available given the remote region where he was located and it is not possible to know if it would have responded to less invasive measures ass etilefrine. No patients underwent surgical intervention (Figure 1).

In the follow-up, the medication dose was increased or the treatment formula was changed in 3 patients (9.7%), which may suggest deterioration in erectile function. Twenty-seven patients (87.1%) did not report any event and continued their treatment with a dose equal to or less than before the event (Figure 2). Follow-up information was not obtained from 1 patient.

4. Discussion

Priapism secondary to erectile dysfunction medications is an event of great interest to patients and physicians, especially because of the consequences when not treated early or adequately, such as fibrosis of cavernous bodies and permanent erectile dysfunction [14].

Table 1: Clinical characteristics of patients with priapism secondary to erectile dysfunction drugs.

	N	%
Comorbidities		
Arterial hypertension	8	25.8
Diabetes	5	16.1
Hyperlipidemia	6	19.4
Peyronie's disease	1	3.2
Consumption history		
Alcohol	19	61.3
Tobacco	7	22.6
Recreational drugs	1	3.2
Characterization of erectile dysfunction	Median	Range
Duration of dysfunction (years)	4.4	4–14
IIEF-5 score	14	2–21

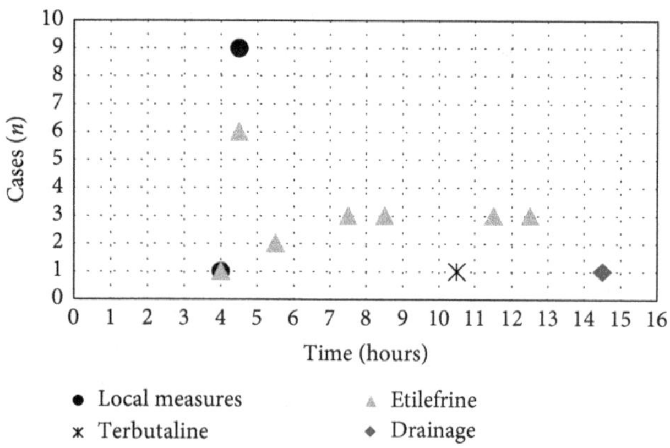

Figure 1: Number of patients by measures applied and duration of priapism.

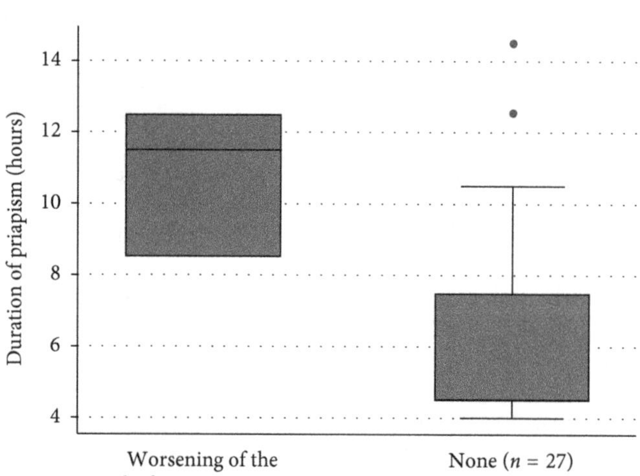

Figure 2: Sequels and duration of priapism.

In the present study, 1.4% incidence of priapism posterior to the use of intracavernous medication was found and 0% after the daily use of phosphodiesterase-5 inhibitors, similar to reports by other studies [6–9, 13].

Current clinical guidelines recommend the use of etilefrine as a first line of treatment for patients with iatrogenic priapism [12]. There is very little evidence to support the use of local measures or exercise to treat this type of priapism, and it is limited to case reports and case series [5, 10, 17]; the majority of the studies focus on pharmacological and surgical treatment [18–21]. We began treatment with local measures, which included exposure to cold water or ice and vigorous physical activity. This was effective in 32.3% of the individuals in the study, a finding that is similar to a report by Habous et al., who indicated decreased erection after climbing up and down stairs for 30 minutes in 39.6% of patients who had prolonged erections (3 hours) after intracavernosal administration of QuadMix for a Doppler [10]. It is important to evaluate whether this option to treat priapism during the first few hours of presentation is being undervalued, given that it can benefit some patients, especially those living in rural areas that are far from a health centre, thereby avoiding the risk of invasive interventions and decreasing medical costs. Regarding intracavernosal etilefrine, this was effective in 61.3% of the cases in our study, including patients with priapism lasting 11.5 to 12. 5 hours.

With regard to sequels, 3 patients experienced increased dysfunction. Nevertheless, given the data recorded, it is not possible to infer as to whether those cases were a consequence of the priapism event or the evolution of the illness itself resulting from a lack of check-ups or other factors, such as diabetes or hypertension, which were presented by 2/3 patients. A limitation of this study was that diagnostic images were not taken to confirm vascular integrity, given that no change was detected by the physical exam and the patients did not report curvatures or masses.

The main limitation of this study was the retrospective collection of data, which can possibly generate information bias [22]. Besides events that are not recorded, this affects the analysis of other variables not found in the historical records and that could be related with priapism or its resolution. In addition, although clinical evaluation did not find fibrous plaque or penile deviations after priapism in any of the patients, Doppler ultrasound was not performed to confirm that there were no sequels of this type.

The results presented herein are limited to the description of our experience, and given the design of the study, causal effects of these interventions cannot be confirmed.

5. Conclusions

In patients with priapism secondary to the use of sexual impotence drugs, initial treatment in the first hours with local measures or etilefrine can achieve detumescence, decreasing the need for invasive procedures or surgery as a first-line therapy. It is necessary to carry out studies with more patients and appropriate designs to confirm this hypothesis.

Acknowledgments

This research was funded with resources from the Boston Medical Group Research Center.

References

[1] J. Ridgley, N. Raison, M. I. Sheikh, P. Dasgupta, M. S. Khan, and K. Ahmed, "Ischaemic priapism: a clinical review," *Türk Üroloji Dergisi/Turkish Journal of Urology*, vol. 43, no. 1, pp. 1–8, 2017.

[2] K. Hatzimouratidis, F. Giuliano, I. Moncada et al., "EAU-ESTRO-SIOG guidelines on male sexual dysfunction," April 2018, https://uroweb.org/guideline/male-sexual-dysfunction.

[3] R. Berger, K. Billups, G. Brock et al., "Report of the American Foundation for Urologic Disease (AFUD) Thought Leader Panel for evaluation and treatment of priapism," *International Journal of Impotence Research*, vol. 13, no. 5, pp. S39–S43, 2001.

[4] F. O. Ugwumba, H. C. Ekwedigwe, K. N. Echetabu, A. D. Okoh, I. Nnabugwu, and E. S. Ugwuidu, "Ischemic priapism in South-East Nigeria: presentation, management challenges, and aftermath issues," *Nigerian Journal of Clinical Practice*, vol. 19, no. 2, pp. 207–211, 2016.

[5] G. A. Broderick, A. Kadioglu, T. J. Bivalacqua, H. Ghanem, A. Nehra, and R. Shamloul, "Priapism: pathogenesis, epidemiology, and management," *The Journal of Sexual Medicine*, vol. 7, no. 1, pp. 476–500, 2010.

[6] P. Perimenis, A. Athanasopoulos, I. Geramoutsos, and G. Barbalias, "The incidence of pharmacologically induced priapism in the diagnostic and Therapeutic management of 685 men with erectile dysfunction," *Urologia Internationalis*, vol. 66, no. 1, pp. 27–29, 2001.

[7] O. I. Linet and F. G. Ogrinc, "Efficacy and safety of intracavernosal alprostadil in men with erectile dysfunction," *New England Journal of Medicine*, vol. 334, no. 14, pp. 873–877, 1996.

[8] P. G. Coombs, M. Heck, P. Guhring, J. Narus, and J. P. Mulhall, "A review of outcomes of an intracavernosal injection therapy programme," *BJU International*, vol. 110, no. 11, pp. 1787–1791, 2012.

[9] The European Alprostadil Study Group, "The long-term safety of alprostadil (prostaglandin-E1) in patients with erectile dysfunction. The European Alprostadil Study Group," *British Journal of Urology*, vol. 82, no. 4, pp. 538–543, 1998.

[10] M. Habous, M. Elkhouly, O. Abdelwahab et al., "Noninvasive treatments for iatrogenic priapism: do they really work? A prospective multicenter study," *Urology Annals*, vol. 8, no. 2, pp. 193–196, 2016.

[11] D. Pal, D. Biswal, and B. Ghosh, "Outcome and erectile function following treatment of priapism: an institutional experience," *Urology Annals*, vol. 8, no. 1, pp. 46–50, 2016.

[12] M. Ahmed, B. Augustine, M. Matthew et al., "Prognostic factors and outcome of management of ischemic priapism in Zaria, Nigeria," *Nigerian Journal of Surgery*, vol. 23, no. 1, pp. 15–19, 2017.

[13] H. Porst, "The rationale for prostaglandin E1 in erectile Failure: a survey of worldwide experience," *The Journal of Urology*, vol. 155, no. 3, pp. 802–815, 1996.

[14] M. A. Spycher and D. Hauri, "The ultrastructure of the erectile tissue in priapism," *Journal of Urology*, vol. 135, no. 1, pp. 142–147, 1986.

[15] M. Falcone, A. Gillo, M. Capece, A. Raheem, D. Ralph, and G. Garaffa, "El manejo del priapismo isquémico agudo: una revisión actualizada," *Actas Urológicas Españolas*, vol. 41, no. 10, pp. 607–613, 2017.

[16] E. Zacharakis, A. A. Raheem, A. Freeman et al., "The efficacy of the T-shunt procedure and intracavernous tunneling (snake maneuver) for refractory ischemic priapism," *Journal of Urology*, vol. 191, no. 1, pp. 164–168, 2014.

[17] J. Gravel, C. Leblanc, C. Varner et al., "Management of priapism with a trial of exercise in the emergency department," *Canadian Journal of Emergency Medicine*, vol. 21, no. 1, pp. 150–153, 2019.

[18] F. C. Lowe and J. P. Jarow, "Placebo-controlled study of oral terbutaline and pseudoephedrine in management of prostaglandin E1-induced prolonged erections," *Urology*, vol. 42, no. 1, pp. 51–53, 1993.

[19] F. J. Martinez, J. Hoang-Boehm, J. Weiss et al., "Methylene blue as a successful treatment alternative for pharmacologically induced priapism," *European Urology*, vol. 39, no. 1, pp. 20–23, 2001.

[20] C. Martin and C. Cocchio, "Effect of phenylephrine and terbutaline on ischemic priapism: a retrospective review," *The American Journal of Emergency Medicine*, vol. 34, no. 2, pp. 222–224, 2016.

[21] D. G. Ridyard, E. A. Phillips, W. Vincent, and R. Munarriz, "Use of high-dose phenylephrine in the treatment of ischemic priapism: five-year experience at a single institution," *The Journal of Sexual Medicine*, vol. 13, no. 11, pp. 1704–1707, 2016.

[22] M. Hernández-Avila, F. Garrido, and E. Salazar-Martínez, "Bias in epidemiological studies," *Salud Pública de México*, vol. 42, no. 5, pp. 438–446, 2000.

18

Management of the Uncommon Bladder Cancers: A Single-Center Experience over 10 Years

Youssef Kadouri, Salim Lachkar, Hamza Dergamoun, Hachem El Sayegh, Lounis Benslimane, and Yassine Nouini

[1]*Mohammed V University, Faculty of Medicine and Pharmacy of Rabat, Ibn Sina Hospital, Department of Urology A, Rabat, Morocco*

Correspondence should be addressed to Youssef Kadouri; youcef.kadouri@gmail.com

Academic Editor: Jason M. Hafron

Background. Under the name of uncommon bladder cancers are gathered rare histological entities which represent less than 5% of bladder tumors. There is not a clear and consensual therapeutic management for these entities. *Purpose.* To review a single-institution 10-year experience with rare form of bladder cancers detailing the diagnosis, treatment, and patient outcome. *Materials and Methods.* We performed a retrospective review of 27 medical records of rare bladder cancer form treated at our center between February 2006 and February 2015. The clinicopathologic features are reported with emphasis on treatment and survival. *Results.* Mean patient age was 65.5 ± 20 yr and 70% of patients were males. Smoking background was found in 16 cases, chronic bladder irritation factors were found in 12 cases, and past urinary tract infection was found in 11 cases. The main symptom was total hematuria (93%) causing an anemia in 16 cases. The two mean histological forms were epidermoid carcinoma (37%) and adenocarcinoma (22%). 26% of patients were found to have extended invasive tumors (T4) at diagnosis. Metastatic disease was confirmed in 8 cases. Our patients were managed by a wide range of therapeutic modalities as total cystectomy with bilateral lymph node dissection (63%), palliative chemotherapy (30%), or concomitant radiochemotherapy (7%). 55.6% of patients were alive one year after diagnosis. Epidermoid carcinoma has the best prognosis followed by leiomyosarcoma and sarcomatoid carcinoma. Neuroendocrine carcinoma has the worst outcome. The overall 5-year survival rate is 33.3%. *Conclusion.* The rarity and small size of these tumors justify the absence of clear and consensual therapeutic management. No role of total cystectomy concerning the conclusions could be drawn but elements suggest this may be the treatment of choice. The highly aggressive nature of those lesions justifies an aggressive and fast therapy when feasible which gives the best outcomes.

1. Introduction

Bladder cancer is the 2nd urological cancer by frequency with 2.7 million people diagnosed worldwide each year and an incidence constantly increasing by about 1% per year [1, 2]. 95% of histological types are urothelial carcinoma. Rare form of bladder tumor does exist, including heterogeneous histological groups. They can constitute the main part of the tumor process or coexist with other more frequent components. There is not a specific genetic predisposition. Rare bladder tumors have some main risk factors: tobacco, exposition to aniline or alkylating agent (as cyclophosphamide), and pelvic irradiation. Their relative rarity provides difficulty to gain experience in the management of these tumors and could justify the lack of a clear and consensual therapeutic management. A review of our center experience over a 10-year period was undertaken to try to define more clearly their clinical features and response to treatment.

2. Materials and Methods

We performed a retrospective review of 27 medical records of rare bladder cancer form treated at our center, Urology « A » department of Ibn Sina Hospital in Rabat, between February 2006 and February 2015. The clinicopathologic features are reported with emphasis on treatment and survival.

The data collected for carrying out this work comes from patient files in the department's archives and operating reports.

After histological confirmation, 27 out of a total of 574 patients with bladder tumors were seen to have rare bladder carcinoma, an incidence of 4.1%. Under the "rare bladder carcinoma" term, all histological forms that are not urothelial carcinoma were included.

Patient age, sex, medical background, clinical history, physical examination data, histology, radiology and biology, treatment technique, and outcomes data were collected and summarized here.

The discussion is about a review of the literature, using the PubMed database and guidelines from urological and oncological learned societies. We detail many aspects of the diagnosis and treatment of bladder's rare tumors and we emphasize their prognostic factors and evolution.

3. Results

Over the data collecting period, there were 574 cases of bladder cancer. 27 were not urothelial carcinoma, with an incidence of 4.1%.

3.1. Epidemiology. There were 19 men (70%) and 8 women for an average age of 65.5 ± 20 years. Men were diagnosed earlier than women, respectively, at 60 and 71 years of age.

Regarding the medical background, 16 cases (59.3%) of smoking habits were found, whether active (14 cases) or passive (2 cases). The average consumption was 27 pack-year and 7 patients were not weaned at the diagnosis.

3.2. Medical Background. Chronic irritation factors were found in 12 cases (44%), as urolithiasis (6 cases), perineostomy due to a urethra trauma (2 cases), a four-time endoscopic urethrotomy due to a postinfectious urethra stenosis (1 case), urinary incontinence (2 cases), and a treated bilharzia infection (1 case). Bacteria's urinary tract infections were found in 11 cases (40.7%).

3.3. Presenting Symptoms. The presenting symptoms in the group are summarized in Table 1. Total hematuria was the main symptom, found in 25 cases (93%). Hematuria was painless in 14 patients (51.9%), with the remaining 11 (40.7%) having associated symptoms of bladder irritation (frequency, urgency, nocturia, or dysuria). The pathology was also revealed by an acute urinary retention (1 case) or a hypogastric budding lesions (1 case).

3.4. Physical Examination. The results of physical examination are grouped in Tables 1 and 2. On general physical examination, vitals were stable in all cases. 21 patients (77%) had abnormality as a hypogastric mass (4 cases), a mattery hypogastric fistula (2 cases), a bladder globe (4 cases), a hypogastric sensitivity (3 cases), a previous laparotomy scar (1 case), and groans on auscultation (3 cases).

TABLE 1: Presenting symptoms and physicals examinations' results.

	Number of patients	%
Total hematuria	25	93
(i) Painless hematuria	14	51.9
(ii) Hematuria and frequency/ dysuria	11	40.7
Acute urinary retention	1	3.7
Hypogastric budding lesions	1	3.7
Normal physical examination	6	37
Abnormal physical examination	21	77

TABLE 2: Physical examination abnormal sign.

Abnormal physical examination sign	29	—
(i) Hypogastric mass	4	13.8
(ii) Mattery hypogastric fistula	2	6.9
(iii) Bladder globe	4	13.8
(iv) Hypogastric sensitivity	3	10.3
(v) Previous laparotomy scar	1	3.4
(vi) Groans on auscultation	3	10.3
(vii) Enlarged prostate	7	24.1
(viii) Pelvic shield	1	3.4
(ix) Anterior vaginal wall's infiltration	4	13.8

More specifically, the urogenital and pelvic examination showed an enlarged prostate (7 cases), a pelvic shield (1 case), and an anterior vaginal wall's infiltration (4 cases), that is to say, 50% of the female patients.

3.5. Biological and Bacteriological Findings. The complete blood counts were often abnormal mainly due to anemia (16 cases, 60%), with a hemoglobin level ranging from 6.7 g/dl to 11.2 g/dl., caused either by the neoplastic disease or hematuria spoliation. Blood transfusion was required in 11 cases, therefore 62% of anemic patients. There were 6 cases of renal acute failure, twice treated by percutaneous nephrostomy. Significant bacteriuria (greater than 10^5 organisms per ml) was identified at presentation in 18 (66.7%) of 27 patients where the midstream specimen of urine MSU results was available.

3.6. Radiology and Endoscopic Findings. 24 patients had an abdominal ultrasonography examination (Figure 1). Ultrasonography of abdomen revealed a parietal tissue mass in 23 cases (85.2%) and a pyelocaliceal cavities dilation (10 cases), completed 1 time by an intravenous urography showing a lacunar image amputating right bladder horn and vesical dome with left ureterohydronephrosis.

A unique transurethral resection of the bladder (TURB) was performed for all patients. TURB was incomplete in 18 cases (66.7%) due to an endoscopically uncontrollable tumor. The diagnosis was made at endoscopy in all cases. Tumors were recorded as solitary in 21 patients and multiple in 6. The sites occupied by tumor were very variable (Table 3)

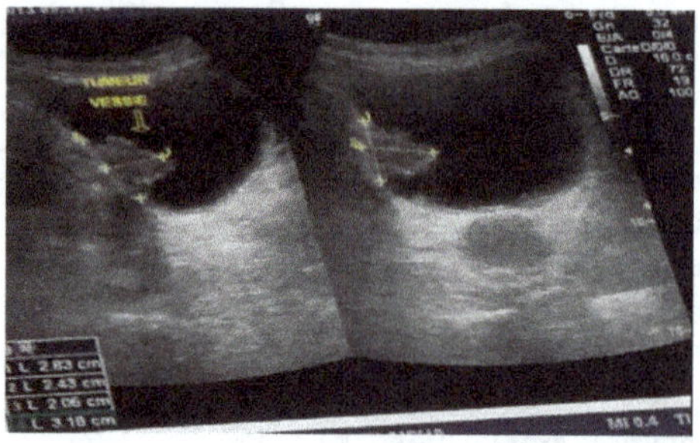

Figure 1: Bladder ultrasound showing a hyperechoic image of the right lateral wall.

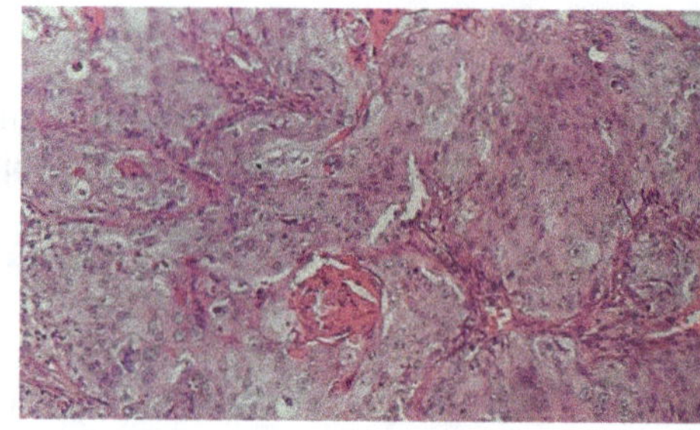

Figure 2: Moderately differentiated and keratinizing squamous cell carcinoma of the bladder mucosa (HEx100).

Table 3: Cumulative distribution of tumors at endoscopy.

Localization	Number	%
Anterior wall	4	7.8
Vault	6	11.8
Right wall	9	17.6
Left wall	12	23.5
Trigonal	14	27.5
Posterior wall	5	9.8
Bladder neck	1	2.0

but there appeared to be a slight predilection for the trigonal area and lateral walls. Tumors were usually described as solid, necrotic, or sessile and were frequently extensive, in 20 patients occupying 2 or more of the bladder areas listed in Table 3.

3.7. Anatomopathology. The anatomopathological examination of resection shavings is the key for the diagnosis (Figures 2 and 3). Figure 4 shows the histological results. The two mean histological forms were the epidermoid carcinoma (37%) and the adenocarcinoma (22%), followed by neuroendocrine carcinoma (19%), sarcomatoid carcinoma (11%), and leiomyosarcoma (11%).

3.8. Tumor Grading. The tumor extension staging is based on thoracoabdominopelvic scanner. The CT scan was performed for all patients and revealed a perivesical fat tumor extension in 21 cases (78%). 78% of patients were found to have extended invasive tumors (T4) at diagnosis. The others found were an iliac lymphadenopathy (10 cases, 37%), intraparenchymal pulmonary nodules considered as pulmonary metastasis (6 cases), a case of rectosigmoid junction tumoral invasion, and a case of hepatic and retroperitoneal nodules (Figure 5). Bones scintigraphy was performed 3 times without revealed abnormality. Metastatic disease was confirmed in 8 cases. Table 4 summarizes the tumor's grading.

3.9. Treatment and Survival. Our patients were managed by a wide range of therapeutic modalities. Total cystectomy associated with a bilateral ilioobturator lymph node dissection was performed for 17 patients (63%) whether male treated by total cystoprostatectomy (11 cases) or female by anterior pelvectomy (6 cases). Urinary diversion consisted in a wide range of techniques: enterocystoplasty (1 case) for a T2N0M0 young male, Bricker construction (9 cases), and cutaneous ureterostomy (7 cases) for altered general condition or patients appearing severely malnourished. Sometimes radical surgery was completed by adjuvant chemotherapy (5 cases). Two patients (7%) were treated with concomitant radiochemotherapy after refusing surgery.

As indicated 8 times (30%), palliative chemotherapy was not performed twice either for patient's refusal or for altered general condition.

Immediate postoperative complications were a day 6 abdominal collection, a hemorrhagic shock requiring intensive care (2 cases), and a case of day 7 death following respiratory distress and ischemic stroke.

The average long-term follow-up was 5 years. Favorable evolution occurred in 16 cases (60%). 55.55% of patients were alive one year after diagnosis. There were 4 patients with an unfavorable becoming: metastatic relapse at 5 months with hepatic, right adrenal and retroperitoneal metastases (1 case), and death at month 5 due to palliative treatment refusal (1 case) and death after the start of the chemotherapy (2 cases) at day 14 and month 4.

Survival at 1 and 5 years was heterogeneous depending on the tumor histological type. The epidermoid carcinoma has the best prognosis with a 70% 1-year survival and a 50% at 5-year survival. Leiomyosarcoma and sarcomatoid carcinoma has the second best outcomes with same results: 66.6% at 1 year and 33.3% at 5 years. Neuroendocrine carcinoma has the worst outcome with a 0% of 5-year survival. The overall survival rate of our series is 55.6% at 1 year and 33.3% at 5 years. Six patients were lost to follow-up.

Table 5 summarizes the survival depending on tumor histological type.

4. Discussion

Uncommon bladder tumors are very heterogeneous histological entities. Their aggressive nature and poor prognosis are a challenge for the medical team. However, because of their low incidence, there is not a clear consensual therapeutic management.

4.1. Vesical Epidermoid Carcinoma. It is the second more frequent type after urothelial carcinoma, with an overall average frequency of 2 to 5%. Epidermoid carcinomas are

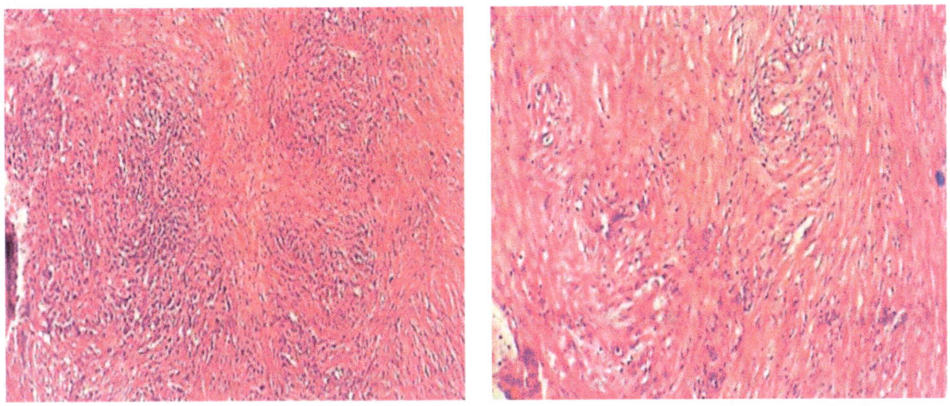

(a) (b)

FIGURE 3: Sarcomatoid carcinoma presenting round cells, giant pleomorphic cells, and spindle-shaped anisokaryocytic cells. (A) HE original magnification ×100. (B) HE original magnification ×200.

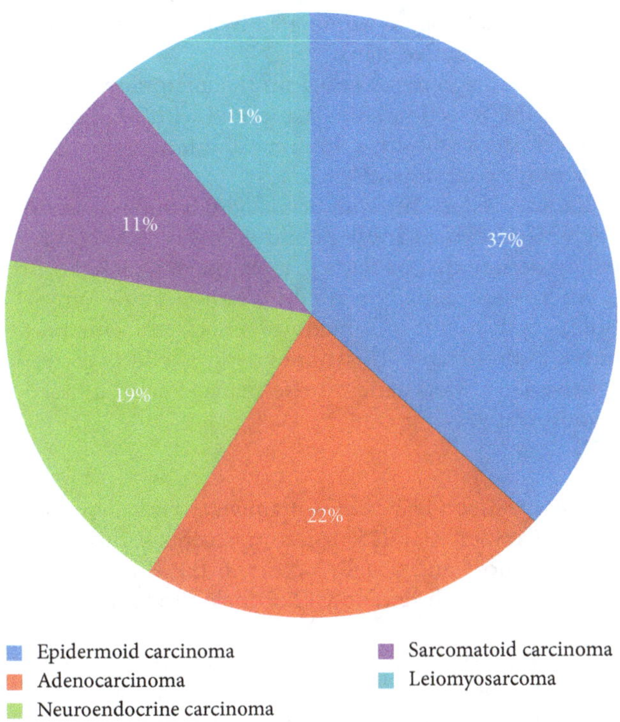

FIGURE 4: Distribution of cases collected in the department according to the histological type.

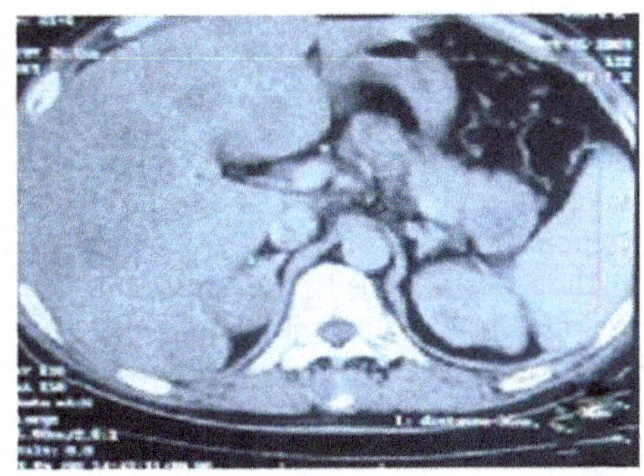

FIGURE 5: Abdominal CT showing diffuse secondary hepatic locations.

TABLE 4: Tumor's grading at the diagnosis.

	Number	%
T1	3	11
T2	10	37
T3	7	26
T4	7	26
Tx	0	0

more common in the Middle East countries, Southeast Asia, and South America where its frequency can reach 20 to 30% of all bladder tumors. Its event is the first histological subtype in Egypt, before urothelial carcinoma. A possible explanation is the endemic bilharzia state in those countries. Links between bilharzia and epidermoid carcinoma have been widely proved, especially by Mostofi et al. with the chronic bladder epithelium irritation theory [3]. Other risk factors are smoking, neurological bladders, radiotherapy, chronic urinary tract infections, and intravesical foreign bodies. In our studies, 70% of patients had a chronic bladder irritation.

Hematuria is the main clinical sign. Other possible symptoms are voiding disorders as pollakiuria, voiding burns, pelvic pain, and low back pain related to tumor extension. Bladder irritants leading to tumor carcinogenesis are themselves sources of previous clinical sign. A physician has to avoid being falsely reassured by a too obvious clinical sign explanation that could hide a beginning tumor process.

Cystoscopy generally finds a compact nodule or plaque tumor. Bilharzia origin has a pearly coating and non-bilharzia forms an ulcerating appearance. Lesion is most often unique. Some diffuse cases have been reported.

Diagnosis is based on anatomopathological bladder tissue examination obtained by TURB. Epidermoid nature is confirmed by finding keratinizing differentiation and/or intercellular bridges. A transitional cell contingent can

Table 5: Survival depending on tumor histological type at 1 and 5 years.

Histological type	Number of cases	%	1-year survival %	5-year survival %	Patient lost to follow-up
Adenocarcinoma	6	22	50.0	33.3	2
Leiomyosarcoma	3	11	66.6	33.3	0
Neuroendocrine carcinoma	5	19	20	0	1
Sarcomatoid carcinoma	3	11	66.6	33.3	1
Epidermoid carcinoma	10	37	70.0	50.0	2
Overall	27	100	55.6	33.3	6

coexist, leading to the urothelial carcinoma with epidermoid inflection diagnosis.

Radical cystectomy with pelvic lymph node dissection and urinary diversion is the main treatment for such tumor type. Béjany and al. observed 40% urethral recurrences after cystectomy. Their team recommends a systematic urethrectomy [4]. Concomitant radiochemotherapy is an alternative for no-resectable tumor or surgery refusal. Immunotherapy appears to be a future possible promising approach as complement to surgery.

4.2. Primary Vesical Adenocarcinoma (PVA). This is the third histological type with a 2% average frequency.

PVA generally appears between 60 and 70 years [5, 6]. The etiopathogenesis remains hypothetical. Adenocarcinoma development on an epithelium without glandular structure has led to many theories. The metaplastic theory seems to unite many authors.

Mechanical or chemical irritant factors lead to a metaplastic transformation of urothelial lining [5, 6].

Histologically tumor lesions form a glandular structure similar to colonic adenocarcinoma. Grignon proposed a classification into 6 histological types [6]: enteric ADK, mucinous ADK, kitten ring cell ADK, clear-cell ADK, mixed ADK, and undifferentiated ADK.

In our study we found a cell-ring kitten variant (1 case), mucinous adenocarcinoma (4 cases), and clear-cell ADK (1 case).

Macroscopic hematuria remains the main sign found in 90% of cases. Irritation bladder sign as pollakiuria or urinary burns can be found. Mucosuria is a very suggestive sign reported in 25% of the cases [7].

Cystoscopy shows often a trigonal or posterior wall single solid or ulcerative lesion.

TURB followed up by histological study confirms the diagnosis. An immunhistochemical analysis by markers is important to differentiate a primary bladder adenocarcinoma from a secondary adenocarcinoma. Such markers are cytokeratin CK7- CK 20- CDX2 and especially β-catenin.

Total cystectomy with extensive lymph node dissection remains the gold standard. Partial cystectomy is an option for mobile bladder part tumor, with often disappointing results [8, 9]. Based on results obtained with colonic adenocarcinomas, some authors propose 5-fluorouracil (5-FU) chemotherapy, with fickle results [10–12]. Neoadjuvant chemotherapy based on platinum salts can be used for locally advanced tumors.

4.3. Sarcomatoid Bladder Carcinoma. Rare type represents less than 0.5% of bladder tumors.

Histologically we found the coexistence of an epithelial urothelial contingent and spindle cells with sarcomatous connective appearance predominant contingent.

It is a very aggressive type, often diagnosed at an advanced stage. It mainly affects men with an average age of 66.4 years [13, 14]. Three etiological factors have been suggested: radiation, smoking, and cyclophosphamide.

Symptomatology is dominated by hematuria associated or not with irritative signs.

Positive diagnosis is based on the anatomopathological study of the resection chips associated with immunohistochemical study: positive immunostaining with epithelial markers (cytokeratins, EMA).

Radical cystectomy with pelvic lymph node dissection is widely described in most published cases [13, 14]. Perret et al. underline that patients that survived the longer (up to 12 years) were initially treated by radical cystectomy [14]. Radical cystectomy is sometimes associated with postoperative radiotherapy. This tumor type is effectively radiosensitive [13]. Metastatic disease management is based on chemotherapy.

4.4. Neuroendocrine Vesical Carcinoma. First described in 1981 by Cramer et al. [15, 16], it represents 0.5 to 1% of all bladder tumors and usually occurs in the elderly, between the fifth and ninth decade with a male predominance (sex ratio of 3.6) [15].

Pathogenesis hypothesis is as follows: a malignant transformation of neuroendocrine cells normally presents urothelium, a totipotent stem cell, and a urothelial metaplasia.

Tumors with a neuroendocrine contingent are classified into two groups:

(i) Pure NET: more than 90% of tumor cells express neuroendocrine differentiation.

(ii) Mixed NET: the neuroendocrine contingent represents between 10 and 90% of the tumor. The presence of neuroendocrine cells dispersed within a tumor (neuroendocrine contingent <10%) has no particular prognostic value.

Smoking was reported in 67% of the cases. However, correlation between tobacco and bladder small cell carcinoma is not as important as for small cell lung carcinoma.

Macroscopic hematuria is the main sign, associated with irritative urinary signs. Some cases report paraneoplastic syndrome as Lambert Eaton syndrome, Cushing's syndrome, etc.

Anatomopathological examination shows small cells with an irregular hyperchromatic nucleus, often in mitosis, arranged in elongated spans with necrosis.

Immunohistochemistry confirms the diagnosis and reveals the expression of at least one neuroendocrine marker: NSE (+), chromogranin (+), and synaptophysin (+).

In our series, synaptophysin immunostaining was positive in all cases, associated with positive labeling with chromogranin (3 cases) or cytokeratin in the urothelial component (1 case) or CD56 (1 case).

4.5. The Bladder Sarcomas. Rare entities represent less than 1% of bladder cancers [17, 18]. Those are very aggressive tumors with grim prognosis. The most common types are leiomyosarcoma and rhabdomyosarcoma. There were 3 cases of leiomyosarcoma in our series.

4.5.1. Leiomyosarcoma. It is a malignant mesenchymal tumor with smooth muscle differentiation. Bladder location is extremely rare and occurs in both children and adults with a maximum incidence beyond 60 years and a male preference with a sex ratio 3/1.

Etiopathogenesis remains unknown. Several factors have been described as malignant transformation of a leiomyoma into leiomyosarcoma [19], chronic bladder irritation, some chemical carcinogens, the mutation of the retinoblastoma gene, radiation [20], and hereditary factors in 1% of cases, as well as long-term chemotherapy with cyclophosphamide [21].

Leiomyosarcoma has a significant local extension potential, before metastasis.

Positive diagnosis based on anatomopathological study reveals tangled bundles of spindle cells with more or less marked nuclear atypia. Immunohistochemistry usually shows strong expression of muscle markers as smooth muscle α-actin and HHF35. Surprisingly the desmin is less frequently positive.

Total cystectomy preceded by neoadjuvant chemotherapy seems to be the best option. Radiotherapy can be used as adjuvant to surgery for high grade tumor (2-3), size >5 cm, or R1-R2 marging with no possibility of recovery [22].

4.5.2. Rhabdomyosarcoma. Exceptional tumor with no sex ratio or age predilection: there are many reports on rhabdomyosarcomas radiation induced case especially after other cancer treatments.

Hematuria is the main symptom. Abdominal mass or dysuria can lead to the diagnosis.

The embryonic histological type is most frequent. The botryoid forms with intraluminal polypoid growth have better prognosis than invasive growth form.

Treatment is based on surgery and irradiation. Chemotherapy is here used to facilitate local treatment rather than to prevent metastases [23].

4.5.3. Angiosarcomas. Bladder localization of angiosarcomas is exceptional. It occur at endothelial vessels cells expense. Those are very aggressive tumors often diagnosed at locally advanced or metastatic stage, with a male predilection. Some risk factors have been described like pelvic irradiation, exposition to vinyl chloride, and arsenic.

Anatomopathological study shows structures resembling anastomosed vessels, filled with blood and bordered by atypical endothelial cells [24].

4.5.4. Other Sarcomas. Cases of osteosarcomas, malignant fibrous histiocytomas, liposarcomas, and primary neuroectodermal tumors have been described [25].

5. Conclusion

Bladder tumors arouse particular interest in urological carcinology because they represent a diagnosis challenge due to their frequency, pathological polymorphism, precise staging difficulty, and grim prognosis.

Rare bladder tumors include histological entities which represent for each of them less than 5% of bladder tumors. The rarity and small size of these tumors justify the absence of clear and consensual therapeutic management.

Hematuria is the main common clinical sign. Diagnosis should be done as soon as possible due to the poor prognosis, with a 5-year overall survival rate of 33.3% in our study.

Diagnosis is based on an anatomopathological bladder tissue examination obtained by TURB.

No role of total cystectomy concerning the conclusions could be drawn from this series because of the small number of patients undergoing the operation, but a review of the literature suggests this may be the treatment of choice. Our data reaffirm the highly aggressive nature of those lesions. Therefore, aggressive and fast therapy is justified when feasible and gives the best outcomes.

Abbreviations

MRI: Magnetic resonance imaging
IVU: Intravenous urography
TURB: Transurethral resection of the bladder
ADK: Adenocarcinoma
CK: Cytokeratin
CDX2: Caudal-type homeobox 2
5-FU: 5-Fluorouracil
EMA: Epithelial Membrane Antigen
NET: Neuroendocrine tumor
NSE: Neuron-specific enolase
CD 56: Cluster of differentiation 56.

Consent

The patients included in this study gave verbal consent to participate in this research and to publish the data contained within this study.

Authors' Contributions

All authors have contributed to this work and have read and approved the final version of the manuscript.

References

[1] R. L. Siegel, K. D. Miller, and A. Jemal, "Cancer statistics," *Cancer Journal for Clinicians*, vol. 68, pp. 7–30, 2018.

[2] Z. Uhry, L. Remontet, M. Colonna et al., "Cancer incidence estimation at a district level without a national registry: a validation study for 24 cancer sites using French health insurance and registry data," *Cancer Epidemiology*, vol. 37, no. 2, p. 99, 2013.

[3] J. S. H. Rundle, A. J. L. Hart, A. McGeorge, J. S. Smith, A. J. Malcolm, and P. M. Smith, "Squamous cell carcinoma of bladder. A review of 114 patients," *British Journal of Urology*, vol. 54, no. 5, pp. 522–526, 1982.

[4] D. E. Bejany, J. L. Lockhart, and R. K. Rhamy, "Malignant vesical tumors following spinal cord injury," *Journal of Urology*, vol. 138, no. 6, pp. 1390–1392, 1987.

[5] A. Debbagh, S. Bennani, M. Hafiani, M. el Mrini, and S. Benjelloun, "Primary adenocarcinoma of the bladder: report of a case," *Annales d'Urologie*, vol. 34, no. 1, pp. 20–27, 2000.

[6] D. J. Grignon, J. Y. Ro, A. G. Ayala, D. E. Johnson et al., "« Primary adenocarcinoma of the urinary bladder: a clinicopathologic analysis of 72 cases," *Cancer*, vol. 67, no. 8, pp. 2165–2172, 1991.

[7] M. Zerbib and O. Bouchot, "Adenocarcinoma of the bladder," *Progrès en Urologie*, vol. 12, no. 5, pp. 1121–1127, 2002.

[8] D. G. ThomasA. M. Ward et al., "A study of 52 cases of adenocarcinoma of the bladder," *BJU International*, vol. 43, no. 1, pp. 4–15, 1971.

[9] J. K. Bennett, J. K. Wheatley, and K. N. Walton, "10-year experience with adenocarcinoma of the bladder," *The Journal of Urology*, vol. 131, no. 2, pp. 262-263, 1984.

[10] J. E. Nevin, I. Melnick, J. T. Baggerly, C. A. Easley, and R. Landes, "Advanced carcinoma of bladder: treatment using hypogastric artery infusion with 5-fluorouracil, either as a single agent or in combination with bleomycin or adriamycin and supervoltage radiation," *The Journal of Urology*, vol. 112, no. 6, pp. 752–758, 1974.

[11] C. J. Logothetis, M. L. Samuels, and S. Ogden, "Chemotherapy for adenocarcinomas of bladder and urachal origin: 5-Fluorouracil, doxorubicin, and mitomycin-C," *Urology*, vol. 26, no. 3, pp. 252–255, 1985.

[12] T. R. Hatch and E. F. Fuchs, "Intra-arterial infusion of 5-fluorouracil for recurrent adenocarcinoma of bladder," *Urology*, vol. 33, no. 4, pp. 311-312, 1989.

[13] A. Lopez-Beltran, A. Pacelli, H. J. Rothenberg et al., "Carcinosarcoma and sarcomatoid carcinoma of the bladder: clinicopathological study of 41 cases," *Journal of Urology*, vol. 159, no. 5, pp. 1497–1503, 1998.

[14] L. Perret, P. Chaubert, D. Hessler, and L. Guillou, "Primary heterologous carcinosarcoma (Metaplastic carcinoma) of the urinary bladder," *Cancer*, vol. 82, no. 8, pp. 1535–1549, 1998.

[15] M. Ghadouane, M. Zannoud, M. Alami et al., "Tumeur neuroendocrine à petites cellules de la vessie. Une nouvelle observation," *Annales d'Urologie*, vol. 37, no. 2, pp. 75–78, 2003.

[16] S. Navarra, C. Pfister, F. Gobet, O. Cappele, M. Planet, and P. Grise, "Tumeur neuroendocrine maligne de vessie: une entité à ne pas méconnaître," *Progrès en Urologie*, vol. 9, no. 1, pp. 129–132, 1999.

[17] P. Dahm and J. E. Gschwend, "Malignant non-urothelial neoplasms of the urinary bladder: a review," *European Urology*, vol. 44, no. 6, pp. 672–681, 2003.

[18] A. Manunta, S. Vincendeau, G. Kiriakou, B. Lobel, and F. Guillé, "Non-transitional cell bladder carcinomas," *BJU International*, vol. 95, no. 4, pp. 497–502, 2005.

[19] B. M. Stigssen, "Leiomyosarcoma of the bladder in a patient with von Recklinghausen disease," *Ugeskr Laeger*, vol. 161, no. 45, pp. 6203-6204, 1999.

[20] C. C. Berdjis, *Pathology of Irradiation*, The williamso et Wilkins CO, Baltimore, MD, USA, 1971.

[21] J. B. Trasher, "Bladder leiomyosarcoma following cyclophosphamide therapy for lupus nephritis," *Journal of Urology*, vol. 143, no. 1, pp. 119–121, 1990.

[22] Group EESNW, "Soft tissue and visceral sarcomas: ESMO Clinical Practice Guidelines for diagnosis, treatment and follow-up," *Annals of Oncology*, vol. 25, 2014.

[23] Y. Atmani, "les tumeurs de vessie chez l'enfant à propos de 05 cas," 2017.

[24] H. Boyle, A. Fléchon, and J.-P. Droz, "Tumeurs rares de la vessie," *Bulletin du Cancer*, vol. 97, no. 3, pp. S51–S7, 2010.

[25] S. Lott, A. Lopez-Beltran, R. Montironi, G. T. MacLennan, and L. Cheng, "Soft tissue tumors of the urinary bladder," *Human Pathology*, vol. 38, no. 7, pp. 963–977, 2007.

19

Adjuvant Therapy for Stage IB Germ Cell Tumors: One versus Two Cycles of BEP

Robert A. Huddart and Alison M. Reid

Institute of Cancer Research and Royal Marsden Hospital FT, Sutton, Surrey, UK

Correspondence should be addressed to Robert A. Huddart; robert.huddart@icr.ac.uk

Academic Editor: Timothy A. Masterson

Testicular germ cell tumours are the commonest tumours of young men and are broadly managed either as pure seminomas or as 'nonseminomas'. The management of Stage 1 nonseminomatous germ cell tumours (NSGCTs), beyond surgical removal of the primary tumour at orchidectomy, is somewhat controversial. Cancer-specific survival rates in these patients are in the order of 99% regardless of whether surveillance, retroperitoneal lymph node dissection, or adjuvant chemotherapy is employed. However, the toxicities of these treatment modalities differ. Undertreating those destined to relapse exposes them to the potentially significant toxicities of 3-4 cycles of bleomycin, etoposide, and cisplatin (BEP) chemotherapy. Conversely, giving adjuvant chemotherapy to all patients following orchidectomy results in overtreatment of a significant proportion. Therefore, the challenge lies in delineating the patient population who require adjuvant chemotherapy and in determining how much chemotherapy to give to adequately reduce relapse risk. This chapter reviews the factors to be considered when adopting a risk-adapted strategy for giving adjuvant chemotherapy in Stage 1B NSGCT sand discusses the data regarding the number of BEP cycles to administer.

1. Background

Testicular germ cell tumours (TGCTs) are the commonest tumours of young men aged between 20 and 35 years. They are divided into those of pure seminoma subtype (that histologically resemble primordial germ cells) and those with elements that resemble extra embryonic tissue (with or without seminoma components), generally termed "nonseminomas." Nonseminomatous germ cell tumours (NSGCT) make up roughly 50% of cases and are common in a younger age group than seminomas (median age around 25 years). A characteristic of TGCT is their sensitivity to cisplatin-based chemotherapy which means that, in contrast to most solid tumours, patients with metastasis are usually cured. The most commonly used schedule is "BEP," consisting of bleomycin, etoposide, and cisplatin. This is highly successful chemotherapy and will cure around 85–90% of patients with metastatic disease and over 95% of those with good prognostic features (i.e., absence of visceral metastasis and low tumour markers) [1]. The cost of this is the risk of significant toxicity, both acute and late (e.g., renal damage, peripheral neuropathy, hearing damage, increased risk of cardiovascular disease, and second cancer; summarised in Table 1). Management of these patients is supported by monitoring tumour markers such as alpha fetoprotein (AFP) and human chorionic gonadotrophin (HCG), which are elevated in patients with metastatic NSGCT in around two-thirds of cases [2].

Around 75–80% of patients diagnosed with NSGCT present with no other clinical evidence of disease outside the testis on examination, imaging, or on tumour markers. These patients are termed Stage I and have excellent outcomes, with 5-year disease-specific survival over 98% [3]. Without additional treatment though, relapse occurs in around 30%.

Histopathological markers have been used to help predict the risk of recurrence. The best validated of these prognostic markers has been the presence or absence of lymphovascular invasion (LVI). Patients without LVI have around 15–20% risk of relapse, and if LVI is present, there is a 40–50% risk of recurrence [4]. This finding has been consistent across

Table 1: Toxicities of BEP chemotherapy.

Dose-related toxicities of BEP	Non dose related	Unknown relationship to dose
Infertility	Febrile neutropenia	Second malignancy
Peripheral neuropathy	Alopecia	Cardiovascular disease
Ototoxicity	Nausea/vomiting	
Raynaud's phenomena		
Fatigue		
Skin toxicity		
Avascular necrosis hip		
Pneumonitis/lung fibrosis		
Renal damage		
Anaemia		
Metabolic syndrome		

a number of large studies and is current standard of care in dividing patients into higher risk groups despite the modest predictive power; that is, even in low-risk group, 15–20% of patients will relapse and 50% of high-risk patients will remain in remission [1].

Other markers such as proportion of embryonal carcinoma (EC), rete testis invasion, and MIB-1 staining have been proposed, but results have not been fully validated. Tumours with no embryonal components generally have a low rate of recurrence [5–7]. Absence of undifferentiated embryonal carcinoma was one of the original MRC risk factors identified in the first MRC surveillance studies [6]. Some studies have suggested that the proportion of embryonal carcinoma may increase relapse risk [4, 8] though this does correlate with LVI and so has not been fully validated. MIB-1 has also been suggested to be associated with increased relapse risk, but in a recent study [8], an association could not be validated. Recently, CXCL12 expression has been proposed as a prognostic marker and validated in two data sets. On the basis of this marker and vascular invasion, three risk groups have been proposed including low (10% risk), intermediate (30–40% risk), and high (70%) risk groups though this remains to be validated.

A number of different approaches have been utilised in this patient group. In the past, removing the retroperitoneal lymph nodes has been practiced particularly in the United States and parts of Europe. Patients who are node negative (pN0) have a lower rate of subsequent recurrence (~10–15%). Node-positive patients (pN1) may be cured by this approach but continue to have a significant rate of recurrence (~30%). These patients have often been offered subsequent adjuvant chemotherapy (see below). Though undoubtedly some patients may avoid chemotherapy, this is at the cost of a major surgical procedure with the risk of attendant morbidity both immediate and long term. Patients still require follow-up as there remains a significant risk of relapse even in the pN0 group, and even without the use of adjuvant chemotherapy, a substantial number of patients will still be exposed to chemotherapy.

An alternative approach, based on pioneering work of Peckham and colleagues and subsequent MRC trials is to watch patients closely a policy termed active surveillance. This approach watches carefully with the aim of early relapse detection and treatment of recurrence by BEP chemotherapy. This approach has the virtue of avoiding treatment (and its attendant toxicities) except when necessary. The use of surveillance has grown over the years but is not necessarily trouble free. Patients who relapse require the use of full-dose chemotherapy [3]. The surveillance phase can cause psychological stress and can make it difficult for some patients to return to a normal lifestyle for fear of recurrence. Finally, there remains a concern regarding compliance. Several studies have shown a degree of noncompliance with follow-up in GCT patients. The fear is that noncompliers can relapse with more advanced disease with a poorer prognosis. This is a concern as a priori identification of noncompliance is difficult. For these reasons, the role of adjuvant chemotherapy has been explored especially in those at high risk of recurrence.

2. Adjuvant BEP Chemotherapy

An alternative approach to surveillance is to use adjuvant chemotherapy following treatment. This was first explored in the early 1990s after the success of using BEP chemotherapy in metastatic disease. It was argued that using more limited chemotherapy in those at high risk would restrict exposure to chemotherapy and prevent relapse. The key study of this approach was the MRC TE05 study. 114 patients were recruited with a predicted recurrence risk based on MRC risk factors of >50% [9]. Two patients recurred but one patient on histology review was proven to have a non-germ cell cancer, so in the 108 patients with centrally reviewed NSGCT, 1 relapsed and the 95% CI excluded a risk of relapse of 5%. This study was supported by similar smaller studies from Bern and Vienna [10, 11]. These data have been replicated in a number of reported studies totalling almost 1000 patients and a combined risk of relapse of <2% (summarised in Table 2). Most of the studies have used BEP for adjuvant treatment though a few studies have used variants of BEP. MD Anderson reported on substituting carboplatin for cisplatin [12], and the MRC replaced etoposide with vincristine [13], both achieving results similar to that achieved by BEP. The lower efficacy of carboplatin in metastatic disease and concerns regarding neurotoxicity, respectively, has meant that these approaches have not been adopted.

Following this work, adjuvant BEP has become an option for high-risk stage 1 NSGCT. Its use has been the subject of

Table 2: Studies of 2 cycles of adjuvant chemotherapy in testicular nonseminomatous germ cell tumours.

Study	Institution	Chemotherapy	Eligibility	Median follow-up (months)	N	Number of malignant relapses (all relapses)
Cullen et al. [9]	MRC, UK	BEP	MRC >50% risk	NS	104	1 (1)
Pont et al. [11]	Vienna	BEP	VI	79 (range, 27 to 119)	40	1 (2)
Bohlen et al. [10]	Berne	BEP/PVB	≥pT2/EC	93 (range 32 to 146).	58	0 (1)
Germa-Lluch et al. [14]	Spanish germ cell group	BEP (90%)	≥pT2	NS	168	1
Chevreau et al. [15]	Toulouse	BEP	VI or EC	113.2 (range 63–189)	40	0
Oliver et al. [16]	Anglia, UK	BEP BOP	MRC >30% risk	NS	28 74	1 (1) 2 (2)
Amato et al. [12]	MD Anderson	CEB	*MDA high risk	38	68	0 (1)
Guney et al. [17]	Istanbul	BEP	*MDA high risk	26 (range 10–60)	71	3 (4)
Dearnaley et al. [13]	MRC, UK	BOP	VI	70	115	2 (2)
Bamias et al. [18]	Hellenic germ cell group	BEP	≥pT2/EC	79	142	1 (1)
Mezvrishvili and Managadze [19]	Tbilisi	BEP/EP	VI	NS	41	0 (1)
Total					949	12 (17) 1.3% (1.8%)

*MDA high risk: pre-op AFP > 80 ng/ml, VI or >pT2. Chemotherapy drugs: B, bleomycin; C, carboplatin; E, etoposide; O, vincristine; P, cisplatin; V, vinblastine. MRC, Medical Research Council; VI, lymphovascular invasion present; EC, embryonal carcinoma.

much debate. This is centered on the issue of late toxicity from BEP. The acute toxicities of BEP (Table 1) have been recognised for many years. Over the last decade, the risk of long-term effects have been better appreciated especially neuropathy, cardiovascular disease, and second malignancy. This has meant that opponents of adjuvant chemotherapy have advocated avoiding exposure of patients to the hazards of chemotherapy unless there is evidence of defined disease. On the other hand, proponents of adjuvant chemotherapy point to the lower doses used, and assuming this means less risk of toxicity. They also note the benefit of lower use of retroperitoneal lymph node surgery. Originally, the 2 cycles of BEP used adjuvantly was half of the dose of that used for metastatic disease. So, with a ~50% relapse risk, the total number of cycles of chemotherapy needed to be delivered ("burden" of chemotherapy) was similar with either approach, though distributed differently in the population. However, with a MRC/EORTC randomised trial [12] showing that 3 cycles of BEP was sufficient for most patients, the balance in terms of burden of chemotherapy was in favour of a surveillance approach (i.e., assuming a 50% relapse risk); for every 100 adjuvant patients, 200 cycles of BEP would be delivered compared to 150 cycles for 100 surveillance patients undergoing 50 relapses. This has led to the exploration as to whether less adjuvant chemotherapy may be sufficient.

3. Single-Cycle Adjuvant BEP

At the Royal Marsden, we initially investigated a single cycle of BEP in patients with intermediate risk of recurrence. In 22 patients with approximately 20% risk of recurrence (i.e., 4-5 patients expected to recur), no active recurrences were noted though 1 patient required resection for teratoma differentiated [20]. In a similar higher risk group (defined as presence of vascular invasion or predominant embryonal carcinoma) in 42 patients, Westermann and colleagues reported a single active relapse compared to an expected rate of around 15 patients [21] (updated in [22]).

This approach has now been tested in 3 larger studies (Table 3). In the first of these, Albers and colleagues in the German germ cell cancer study group conducted a randomised trial comparing a single cycle of BEP versus RPLND [23]. In 191 patients randomised to BEP, 2 relapses were seen (1 of which was mature teratoma). In the RPLND arm, 32/173 patients were node positive and received adjuvant chemotherapy, and 15 node-negative patients relapsed (equating to 47 patients with active disease, 27%). The Scandinavian Swenoteca [24] group adopted a single cycle of BEP for intermediate- and high-risk patients as a population-based treatment protocol. In their latest report on 571 patients and a median follow-up of 7.9 years, 3.2% of patients with lymphovascular invasion ($n = 258$) and 1.6% patients with no lymphovascular invasion ($n = 255$) have relapsed with only one patient dying of multiply relapsed TGCT.

The latest study to report is the UK 111 study [25]. This large prospective nonrandomised study was designed to specifically exclude a relapse risk of over 5% after a single cycle of BEP. This study recruited 246 patients and reported after a median follow-up of 39.9 months and with a minimum follow-up of 2 years in 91% of patients. Four patients have had a malignant recurrence and 3 a TD recurrence. The primary end point was 2-year malignant recurrence rate which was 1.3% (95% CI 0.4–4.0%) and thus met its aim to exclude a 2-year recurrence rate of 5%. A full publication is awaited.

Table 3: Summary of studies of single-cycle adjuvant BEP chemotherapy.

Study	Eligibility	Median follow-up (months)	N	Number of malignant relapses (all relapses)	Predicted relapse risk	Predicted number of relapses
Gilbert (RMH) [20]	1 or 2 MRC RF	120	22	0 (1)	20%	4
Westermann (Switzerland) [21]	VI+ >50% EC	99	13 29	1	30%	13
Albers (GCSCG) [23]	Any	56	191	1 (2)	26%	50
Tandstad [24] (SWENOTECA)	VI+	95	258	7 (8)	42%	108
	VI−		255	3 (4)	12%	31
111 study [25]	VI+	40	236	4 (7)	42%	99
Total			**1004**	**16 (23)** **1.6% (2.3%)**		**305***

*23/305 equals 7.5% of predicted relapses.

4. Current Perspectives

It is our opinion that the data discussed are now robust enough to conclude that 1 cycle of BEP can successfully reduce the risk of recurrence to less than 5%. The additional benefit of adding a second cycle in terms of risk reduction of relapse is small and, in our judgement, is not sufficient to justify the additional toxicity. Using a single cycle of BEP would reduce the overall use of chemotherapy in the "high-risk" vascular invasion population. Using the model described above, treating 100 patients with single-cycle adjuvant BEP would give 100 cycles to this population compared to 150 cycles if it is assumed that 50% relapse on surveillance. In addition to amount of chemotherapy, the balance of who receives is very different either spread across the whole population or concentrating, with greater exposure, in those with proven disease. There is no evidence in any of the studies of adjuvant chemotherapy or surveillance that use of either approach affects overall survival. This has prompted a vigorous debate between supporters [26–28] of adjuvant chemotherapy and surveillance as to the optimal approach, both in seminoma and nonseminoma. To our mind, to exclusively offer either approach, given lack of survival difference, is inappropriate. We attempt to present a balanced argument of the pros and cons of the two approaches stressing the impact on relapse and discussing what is known regarding immediate- and long-term toxicity (including risk of cardiovascular disease and second malignancy). The idea of adjuvant toxicity seems intrinsically attractive to many, with the wish to get treatment over with and avoid future uncertainty of relapse as common levers for deciding on adjuvant chemotherapy.

4.1. Future Approaches. Adjuvant chemotherapy has usually been used for patients found to be at higher risk of recurrence. The adoption of single-cycle adjuvant chemotherapy raises the question of whether patients with lower risk should be offered this treatment. The Swenoteca group allowed patients with lower risk of recurrence to receive adjuvant BEP in their protocols and reported a less than 2% relapse risk [24]. We do not offer this approach routinely as this would expose 80% or more of patients to BEP who would not have relapsed and increases the overall burden of chemotherapy. There may be exceptional instances such as when surveillance or full course of BEP would be difficult when it might be considered.

The landscape of adjuvant therapy could be changed if there was better prognostication. We recently reported a new prognostic index that could split stage 1 NSGCT patients into 3 broad groups based on vascular invasion and whether they had expression of CXCL12 or had near 100% embryonal content [8]. Using these criteria, we identified a small group (10–15%) with a very high recurrence risk (>70%) and a significant group (~40–50%) with a low risk of recurrence (~10%) with the remainder having a 30–40% recurrence risk. This index needs further validation but may have implications for decision making regarding adjuvant therapy. We believe most clinicians would agree the low-risk group should be surveyed and the high-risk group would benefit from adjuvant therapy. The intermediate group may be more controversial. The total burden of chemotherapy for surveillance and adjuvant chemotherapy would be roughly similar. These patients might reasonably be surveyed but many may consider the risk high enough to justify adjuvant chemotherapy if a single cycle of BEP is used.

This landscape is not static. More sophisticated genetic profiling may be on the horizon [29], and whilst data are emerging, that microRNA analysis may be a sensitive indicator of subclinical disease [2, 30]. Any impact on prognostication may affect the balance between surveillance and adjuvant therapy.

It is possible that the increasing confidence in the use of adjuvant BEP could change the treatment algorithm in other areas. For instance, could single-cycle BEP with less-invasive surgical techniques lead to a resurgence of surgical management of low-volume (stage 2) NSGCT [31]?

5. Conclusion

Single-cycle BEP is effective at reducing the risk of recurrence of stage 1 NSGCT to less than 5% and should be the preferred over two cycles of BEP if adjuvant therapy is chosen rather than surveillance. However, surveillance approaches can legitimately still be offered to all patients.

Acknowledgments

The authors acknowledge support of The Royal Marsden/Institute of Cancer Research NIHR Biomedical Research Centre and the Josh Carrick Foundation.

References

[1] A. Horwich, D. Nicol, and R. Huddart, "Testicular germ cell tumours," *BMJ*, vol. 347, p. f5526, 2013.
[2] M. J. Murray, R. A. Huddart, and N. Coleman, "The present and future of serum diagnostic tests for testicular germ cell tumours," *Nature Reviews Urology*, vol. 13, no. 12, pp. 715–725, 2016.
[3] M. Chovanec, N. Hanna, K. C. Cary, L. Einhorn, and C. Albany, "Management of stage I testicular germ cell tumours," *Nature Reviews Urology*, vol. 13, no. 11, pp. 663–673, 2016.
[4] Y. Vergouwe, E. W. Steyerberg, M. J. Eijkemans, P. Albers, and J. D. Habbema, "Predictors of occult metastasis in clinical stage I nonseminoma: a systematic review," *Journal of Clinical Oncology*, vol. 21, no. 22, pp. 4092–4099, 2003.
[5] G. Daugaard, M. G. Gundgaard, M. S. Mortensen et al., "Surveillance for stage I nonseminoma testicular cancer: outcomes and long-term follow-up in a population-based cohort," *Journal of Clinical Oncology*, vol. 32, no. 34, pp. 3817–3823, 2014.
[6] L. S. Freedman, M. C. Parkinson, W. G. Jones et al., "Histopathology in the prediction of relapse of patients with stage I testicular teratoma treated by orchidectomy alone," *The Lancet*, vol. 2, no. 8554, pp. 294–298, 1987.
[7] C. A. Lago-Hernandez, H. Feldman, E. O'Donnell et al., "A refined risk stratification scheme for clinical stage 1 NSGCT based on evaluation of both embryonal predominance and lymphovascular invasion," *Annals of Oncology*, vol. 26, no. 7, pp. 1396–1401, 2015.
[8] D. C. Gilbert, R. Al-Saadi, K. Thway et al., "Defining a new prognostic index for stage I nonseminomatous germ cell tumors using CXCL12 expression and proportion of embryonal carcinoma," *Clinical Cancer Research*, vol. 22, no. 5, pp. 1265–1273, 2016.
[9] M. H. Cullen, S. P. Stenning, M. C. Parkinson et al., "Short-course adjuvant chemotherapy in high-risk stage I nonseminomatous germ cell tumors of the testis: a Medical Research Council report," *Journal of Clinical Oncology*, vol. 14, no. 4, pp. 1106–1113, 1996.
[10] D. Bohlen, M. Borner, R. W. Sonntag, M. F. Fey, and U. E. Studer, "Long-term results following adjuvant chemotherapy in patients with clinical stage I testicular nonseminomatous malignant germ cell tumors with high risk factors," *Journal of Urology*, vol. 161, no. 4, pp. 1148–1152, 1999.
[11] J. Pont, W. Albrecht, G. Postner, F. Sellner, K. Angel, and W. Holtl, "Adjuvant chemotherapy for high-risk clinical stage I nonseminomatous testicular germ cell cancer: long-term results of a prospective trial," *Journal of Clinical Oncology*, vol. 14, no. 2, pp. 441–448, 1996.
[12] R. de Wit, J. T. Roberts, P. M. Wilkinson et al., "Equivalence of three or four cycles of bleomycin, etoposide, and cisplatin chemotherapy and of a 3- or 5-day schedule in good-prognosis germ cell cancer: a randomized study of the European Organization for Research and Treatment of Cancer Genitourinary Tract Cancer Cooperative Group and the Medical Research Council," *Journal of Clinical Oncology*, vol. 19, no. 6, pp. 1629–1640, 2001.
[13] D. P. Dearnaley, S. D. Fossa, S. B. Kaye et al., "Adjuvant bleomycin, vincristine and cisplatin (BOP) for high-risk stage I non-seminomatous germ cell tumours: a prospective trial (MRC TE17)," *British Journal of Cancer*, vol. 92, no. 12, pp. 2107–2113, 2005.
[14] J. R. Germa-Lluch, X. Garcia del Muro, P. Maroto et al., "Clinical pattern and therapeutic results achieved in 1490 patients with germ-cell tumours of the testis: the experience of the Spanish Germ-Cell Cancer Group (GG)," *European Urology*, vol. 42, no. 6, pp. 553–562, 2002.
[15] C. Chevreau, C. Mazerolles, M. Soulie et al., "Long-term efficacy of two cycles of BEP regimen in high-risk stage I nonseminomatous testicular germ cell tumors with embryonal carcinoma and/or vascular invasion," *European Urology*, vol. 46, no. 2, pp. 209–214, 2004.
[16] R. T. Oliver, J. Ong, J. Shamash et al., "Long-term follow-up of Anglian Germ Cell Cancer Group surveillance versus patients with stage 1 nonseminoma treated with adjuvant chemotherapy," *Urology*, vol. 63, no. 3, pp. 556–561, 2004.
[17] S. Guney, N. Guney, N. C. Sonmez, and E. Ergenekon, "Risk-adapted management for patients with clinical stage I non-seminomatous germ cell tumour of the testis," *Medical Oncology*, vol. 26, no. 2, pp. 136–142, 2009.
[18] A. Bamias, G. Aravantinos, I. Kastriotis et al., "Report of the long-term efficacy of two cycles of adjuvant bleomycin/etoposide/cisplatin in patients with stage I testicular nonseminomatous germ-cell tumors (NSGCT): a risk adapted protocol of the Hellenic Cooperative Oncology Group," *Urologic Oncology*, vol. 29, no. 2, pp. 189–193, 2011.
[19] Z. Mezvrishvili and L. Managadze, "Is bleomycin necessary in adjuvant chemotherapy of clinical stage I non-seminomatous testicular cancer?," *Georgian Medical News*, vol. 134, pp. 25–28, 2006.
[20] D. C. Gilbert, A. R. Norman, J. Nicholl, D. P. Dearnaley, A. Horwich, and R. A. Huddart, "Treating stage I nonseminomatous germ cell tumours with a single cycle of chemotherapy," *BJU International*, vol. 98, no. 1, pp. 67–69, 2006.
[21] D. H. Westermann, H. Schefer, G. N. Thalmann, E. Karamitopoulou-Diamantis, M. F. Fey, and U. E. Studer, "Long-term followup results of 1 cycle of adjuvant bleomycin, etoposide and cisplatin chemotherapy for high risk clinical stage I nonseminomatous germ cell tumors of the testis," *Journal of Urology*, vol. 179, no. 1, pp. 163–166, 2008.
[22] A. D. Vidal, G. N. Thalmann, E. Karamitopoulou-Diamantis, M. F. Fey, and U. E. Studer, "Long-term outcome of patients with clinical stage I high-risk nonseminomatous germ-cell tumors 15 years after one adjuvant cycle of bleomycin, etoposide, and cisplatin chemotherapy," *Annals of Oncology*, vol. 26, no. 2, pp. 374–377, 2015.
[23] P. Albers, R. Siener, S. Krege et al., "Randomized phase III trial comparing retroperitoneal lymph node dissection with one course of bleomycin and etoposide plus cisplatin chemotherapy in the adjuvant treatment of clinical stage I nonseminomatous testicular germ cell tumors: AUO trial AH 01/94 by the German Testicular Cancer Study Group," *Journal of Clinical Oncology*, vol. 26, no. 18, pp. 2966–2972, 2008.
[24] T. Tandstad, O. Dahl, G. Cohn-Cedermark et al., "Risk-adapted treatment in clinical stage I nonseminomatous germ cell testicular cancer: the SWENOTECA management program," *Journal of Clinical Oncology*, vol. 27, no. 13, pp. 2122–2128, 2009.

[25] R. A. Huddart, J. D. White, P. Hutton et al., "111: a single-arm trial evaluating one cycle of BEP as adjuvant chemotherapy in high-risk, stage 1 non-seminomatous or combined germ cell tumors of the testis (NSGCTT)," *Journal of Clinical Oncology*, vol. 35, no. 6, p. 400, 2017.

[26] J. Oldenburg, J. Aparicio, J. Beyer et al., "Personalizing, not patronizing: the case for patient autonomy by unbiased presentation of management options in stage I testicular cancer," *Annals of Oncology*, vol. 26, no. 5, pp. 833–838, 2015.

[27] C. R. Nichols, B. Roth, P. Albers et al., "Active surveillance is the preferred approach to clinical stage I testicular cancer," *Journal of Clinical Oncology*, vol. 31, no. 28, pp. 3490–3493, 2013.

[28] R. de Wit and G. J. Bosl, "Optimal management of clinical stage I testis cancer: one size does not fit all," *Journal of Clinical Oncology*, vol. 31, no. 28, pp. 3477–3479, 2013.

[29] J. E. Korkola, S. Heck, A. B. Olshen et al., "Development and validation of a gene-based model for outcome prediction in germ cell tumors using a combined genomic and expression profiling approach," *PLoS One*, vol. 10, no. 12, article e0142846, 2015.

[30] K. P. Dieckmann, A. Radtke, M. Spiekermann et al., "Serum levels of microRNA miR-371a-3p: a sensitive and specific new biomarker for germ cell tumours," *European Urology*, vol. 71, no. 2, pp. 213–220, 2017.

[31] M. Behnia, R. Foster, L. H. Einhorn, J. Donohue, and C. R. Nichols, "Adjuvant bleomycin, etoposide and cisplatin in pathological stage II non-seminomatous testicular cancer. The Indiana University experience," *European Journal of Cancer*, vol. 36, no. 4, pp. 472–475, 2000.

20

Traumatic Bladder Ruptures: A Ten-Year Review at a Level 1 Trauma Center

John Barnard,[1] **Tyler Overholt**,[2] **Ali Hajiran**,[1] **Chad Crigger**,[1] **Morris Jessop**,[1] **Jennifer Knight**,[3] **and Chad Morley**[1]

[1]*West Virginia University Hospitals, Department of Urology, Morgantown, USA*
[2]*West Virginia University, School of Medicine, Morgantown, USA*
[3]*West Virginia University Hospitals, Department of Surgery, Morgantown, USA*

Correspondence should be addressed to John Barnard; jbarnar4@hsc.wvu.edu

Academic Editor: Darius J. Bagli

Bladder rupture occurs in only 1.6% of blunt abdominopelvic trauma cases. Although rare, bladder rupture can result in significant morbidity if undiagnosed or inappropriately managed. AUA Urotrauma Guidelines suggest that urethral catheter drainage is a standard of care for both extraperitoneal and intraperitoneal bladder rupture regardless of the need for surgical repair. However, no specific guidance is given regarding the length of catheterization. The present study seeks to summarize contemporary management of bladder trauma at our tertiary care center, assess the impact of length of catheterization on bladder injuries and complications, and develop a protocol for management of bladder injuries from time of injury to catheter removal. A retrospective review was performed on 34,413 blunt trauma cases to identify traumatic bladder ruptures over the past 10 years (January 2008–January 2018) at our tertiary care facility. Patient data were collected including age, gender, BMI, mechanism of injury, and type of injury. The primary treatment modality (surgical repair vs. catheter drainage only), length of catheterization, and post-injury complications were also assessed. Review of our institutional trauma database identified 44 patients with bladder trauma. Mean age was 41 years, mean BMI was 24.8 kg/m^2, 95% were Caucasian, and 55% were female. Motor vehicle collision (MVC) was the most common mechanism, representing 45% of total injuries. Other mechanisms included falls (20%) and all-terrain vehicle (ATV) accidents (13.6%). 31 patients had extraperitoneal injury, and 13 were intraperitoneal. Pelvic fractures were present in 93%, and 39% had additional solid organ injuries. Formal cystogram was performed in 59% on presentation, and mean time to cystogram was 4 hours. Gross hematuria was noted in 95% of cases. Operative management was performed for all intraperitoneal injuries and 35.5% of extraperitoneal cases. Bladder closure in operative cases was typically performed in 2 layers with absorbable suture in a running fashion. The intraperitoneal and extraperitoneal injuries managed operatively were compared, and length of catheterization (28 d vs. 22 d, $p = 0.46$), time from injury to normal fluorocystogram (19.8 d vs. 20.7 d, $p = 0.80$), and time from injury to repair (4.3 vs. 60.5 h, $p = 0.23$) were not statistically different between cohorts. Patients whose catheter remained in place for greater than 14 days had prolonged time to initial cystogram (26.6 d vs. 11.5 d) compared with those whose foley catheter was removed within 14 days. The complication rate was 21% for catheters left more than 14 days while patients whose catheter remained less than 14 days experienced no complications. The present study provides a 10-year retrospective review characterizing the presentation, management, and follow-up of bladder trauma patients at our level 1 trauma center. Based on our findings, we have developed an institutional protocol which now includes recommendations regarding length of catheterization after traumatic bladder rupture. By providing specific guidelines for initial follow-up cystogram and foley removal, we hope to decrease patient morbidity from prolonged catheterization. Further study will seek to allow multidisciplinary trauma teams to standardize management, streamline care, and minimize complications for patients presenting with traumatic bladder injuries.

1. Introduction

Urogenital tract injury occurs in approximately 10% of all abdominopelvic traumatic injuries with bladder rupture representing just 1.6% of these cases [1, 2]. Due to the structural protection from the bony pelvis, injury to the bladder is rare and usually associated with a high-impact injury [2, 3]. Bladder rupture can be classified as either extraperitoneal (EP) or intraperitoneal (IP). EP ruptures are more common and usually result from forceful impact to the anterior bladder [2, 3]. IP ruptures usually result from a rise in intravesicular pressure following an abdomino pelvic impact that causes rupture of one of the weaker points of the bladder such as the dome [2, 3].

The clinical presentation of bladder trauma patients may vary based on injury severity, but most patients have gross hematuria, difficulty with or painful voiding, and suprapubic pain [3]. Pelvic fractures are very common in patients with bladder injury. Pelvic fractures have been found to be associated with increased morbidity and mortality in bladder trauma patients, and identification of a pelvic fracture should raise clinical suspicion to assess for urogenital injury [4]. Although bladder rupture is rare, it is associated with significant patient morbidity and a mortality rate of approximately 22% [5]. In studies assessing mortality trends in patients with bladder rupture, it has been shown that there has been no improvement in the mortality rate in these patients over the last two decades [4].

The American Urological Association (AUA) has guidelines in place regarding the management of urogenital trauma [6]. The guidelines recommend formal retrograde cystography in stable patients with gross hematuria and/or a pelvic fracture or any other patient with signs and symptoms suspicious of bladder injury [6]. The guidelines state that urethral catheter drainage is the standard of care for both EP and IP bladder ruptures [6]. The AUA guidelines also recommend surgical repair for all IP bladder ruptures for prevention of peritonitis following intraperitoneal exposure to bladder contents [6].

Although guidelines recommend catheterization for all patients with bladder rupture, no specific recommendations regarding length of catheterization are in place. Additionally, there are no recommendations on ideal operative technique for management of intraperitoneal and/or complicated extraperitoneal bladder ruptures. The present study seeks to summarize the patients with bladder trauma at our center using 10 years of data. Herein, we assess the management of these patients including the impact of length of catheterization on bladder injuries and associated complications.

2. Methods

Following IRB approval, we performed a retrospective review of 34,413 blunt trauma cases using a database provided by the trauma registry at our institution during the last ten years (January 2008–January 2018). Patients included in the study all had an ICD-9 diagnosis of bladder injury. Patients were excluded if they were less than 18 years old.

Table 1: 10-year summary of contemporary bladder trauma.

Demographics	
Age	41.8 years (8–87)
Gender	55% female
Ethnicity	95% Caucasian/Nonhispanic
BMI	24.8 kg/m^2 (16.6–35.3)
Mechanism	$N = 44$
MVC	45.5% (20)
Fall	20.5% (9)
ATV	13.6% (6)
Pedestrian vs automobile	9.1% (4)
Crush	6.8% (3)
GSW	2.3% (1)
Others	2.3% (1)
Injury type	
Intraperitoneal	29.5% (13)
Extraperitoneal	70.5% (31)
Pelvic fracture	93.1% (41)
Gross hematuria	95.5% (42)

Patient data collected included age, ethnicity, gender, BMI, mechanism of injury, type of injury, any associated additional injuries, and complications. We additionally assessed management of patients including imaging studies performed, catheterization length, and surgical modalities used. Two-tailed T-test was utilized via Microsoft Excel for comparison of means with $p < 0.05$ being considered significant.

3. Results

3.1. Demographic Data. Chart review identified 44 total patients with a bladder injury in the last ten years. Of these patients, the mean age was 41.8 years old, and the mean body mass index (BMI) was 24.8 kg/m^2. Demographic data also showed that 55% identified as female, 45% identified as male, and 95% were of Caucasian ethnicity. Motor vehicle collisions (MVC) were the most common mechanism of injury representing 45% of total cases. Other common mechanisms of injury were falls (20%) and ATV accidents (14%) (Table 1).

3.2. Characterization of Injuries. Of the 44 identified injuries, 31 cases were classified as EP injuries (70.1%), and 13 were classified as IP injuries (29.5%). Pelvic fractures were present in 93% of cases, and gross hematuria was present in 95%. Additional solid organ injuries were present in 39% of cases. The most common additional solid organ injured was the lung, followed by the spleen and the brain. Interestingly, 18% of all bladder trauma cases had a concomitant second genitourinary organ injury with kidney being most commonly followed by the urethra.

3.3. Management. Formal retrograde cystography was performed in 59% of bladder trauma cases during the initial hospitalization. Of these patients, mean time from presentation at our facility to cystogram was 4 hours. All patients were catheterized following initial presentation and/or

Table 2: Summary of complications in patients with catheter dwell time >14 days.

Patient	Catheter dwell time (d)	Complication(s)	Treatment/outcome
1	38	Continuous urinary extravasation	Bilateral percutaneous nephrostomy placement Resolved after 11 weeks of maximal urinary diversion
2	43	Multiple UTIs/pyelonephritis	Neurogenic bladder requiring chronic intermittent catheterization
3	96	Urinary retention/UTIs	Neurogenic bladder requiring chronic intermittent catheterization
4	30	Lower extremity DVT	Resolved with anticoagulation therapy
5	34	Hematuria, calcification of catheter	Resolved with foley removal
6	27	Hematuria with clot retention	Resolved with bedside irrigation and foley removal
7	33	*E fecalis* UTI	Resolved with PO antibiotics

diagnosis of bladder injury. Operative management was performed for all intraperitoneal injuries as well as 35.5% of extraperitoneal injuries. Bladder closure in operative cases was typically performed in 2 layers with absorbable suture in a running fashion.

3.4. Outcomes. The intraperitoneal and extraperitoneal injuries managed operatively were compared, and length of catheterization (28 d vs. 22 d, $p = 0.46$), time from injury to normal fluorocystogram (19.8 d vs. 20.7 d, $p = 0.80$), and time from injury to repair (4.3 h vs. 60.5 h, $p = 0.23$) were not statistically different between cohorts. Of the extraperitoneal injury patients who were managed operatively, the indications included planned orthopedic open fixation with permanent hardware to be exposed to the area of injury ($n = 8$), presence of a bony spicule within the bladder ($n = 3$), concomitant bladder neck or rectal injury ($n = 1$), and initial concern for intraperitoneal injury ($n = 1$).

In patients with catheter dwell time less than or equal to 14 days, the average time to fluorocystogram was 11.5 days. There were no complications in this cohort. In patients with catheter dwell time greater than 14 days, the average time to fluorocystogram was 26.6 days. Complications were present in 21% of these cases including urinary tract infection, DVT, and gross hematuria with clot retention (Table 2). Mortality during initial hospitalization was noted in 3 patients (6.8%).

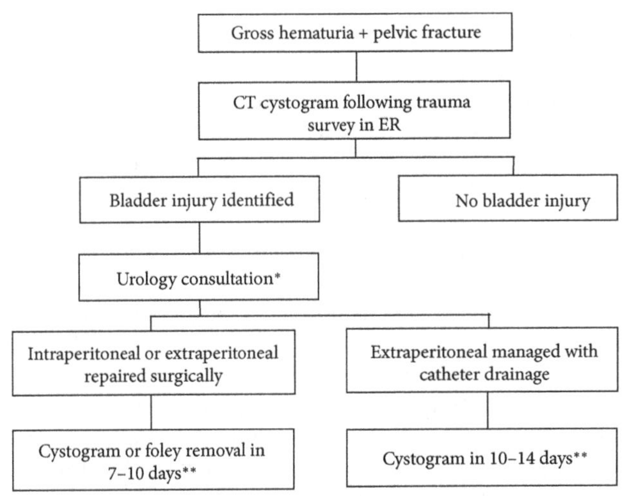

Figure 1: Revised institutional bladder trauma protocol. *Surgical repair is performed in all intraperitoneal injuries and extraperitoneal injuries involving the bladder neck, concomitant rectal or vaginal injury, exposure to orthopedic hardware (i.e., pelvic fixation), or nonhealing state after management with catheter drainage. **Revisions to our institutional protocol reflect standardization of length of catheterization based on the finding that catheterization less than 14 days resulted in decreased morbidity. Previously, there was no institutional consensus or protocol on length of catheterization, and it was highly variable.

4. Discussion

Over the past ten years, nearly all bladder injuries identified were associated with both gross hematuria and pelvic fractures. This finding falls in agreement with the AUA Urotrauma Guidelines that recommend formal bladder imaging for all patients with both findings [4]. However, only 59% of these patients received appropriate bladder imaging on initial presentation in the Emergency Department (ED) indicating an opportunity for improvement. Prior studies have also demonstrated weaker compliance with imaging recommendations of a CT cystogram or plain cystogram in patients with suspected bladder trauma. At a level 1 trauma center in Utah, only 24% of bladder injuries in a 15-year time span were diagnosed with cystogram or CT cystogram [7]. Additionally, they found that in bladder injury patients who only received standard CT imaging on presentation, 13% were missed or incorrectly diagnosed on initial presentation. and some cases were inappropriately operatively explored as a result [7]. Another study assessed patients with traumatic pelvic and acetabular fractures and found that only 47% of patients with pelvic or acetabular fractures that also had hematuria had a formal urologic evaluation on initial presentation [8]. These findings emphasize that although guidelines are in place for appropriate bladder imaging, they are not always being followed.

We additionally found that 39% of patients with bladder injuries had an additional solid organ injury. In another study of outcomes following genitourinary injury in United States (US) military members, it was found that genitourinary injury patients had a high incidence of concurrent traumatic brain injury as well as trends between

GU injury and PTSD [9]. This emphasizes the significant morbidity of bladder trauma and the need for thorough evaluation for any additional injuries in all bladder injury patients.

Patients with catheterization longer than 14 days had a longer time to follow-up imaging as well as an increased complication rate. When assessing reasons for delayed catheter removal, it was often found that the delay was due to coordination of follow-up appointments rather than any medical indication for longer catheterization. The increased catheter dwell time and associated complications emphasize the need for sooner follow-up and imaging to allow catheter removal as soon as clinically indicated to minimize the risk of complications in these patients.

Based on the findings of this study, our institution generated a standardized treatment algorithm which we plan to integrate into our institutional trauma protocols (Figure 1). House staff members covering the trauma service are provided with a written handbook containing all pertinent solid organ protocols to promote adherence to established protocols and homogeneity in treatment for all trauma patients in our high volume, level 1 trauma center. To date, length of catheterization after bladder injury was a metric that was not included or addressed at an institutional level or a national level as evidenced by no specific AUA Urotrauma recommendations. Given the results of our study, we aim to limit catheterization to less than 14 days for all bladder injuries given the higher complication rate observed for patients with catheter dwell times exceeding this metric.

5. Implications

The present study provides a 10-year retrospective review characterizing the presentation, management, and follow-up of bladder trauma patients at a tertiary care facility. Following this investigation, we introduced an institutional protocol for the management of bladder trauma patients hoping to increase adherence to Urotrauma Guidelines and to strictly define length of catheterization prior to initial follow-up cystogram. In patients with both gross hematuria and pelvic fracture, formal retrograde cystography should be performed in the emergency department following the primary trauma survey. If bladder injury is identified, urology consultation should be obtained promptly to guide management. Bladder catheterization should be performed, and if the injury is IP, operative management will follow. When possible, follow-up cystogram and urinary catheter removal should be performed within 10–14 days to limit the risk of complications in those patients who have a normal initial follow-up cystogram. Further study will seek to allow multidisciplinary trauma teams to standardize management, streamline care, and minimize complications for patients presenting with traumatic bladder injuries.

Supplementary Materials

The supplementary data file is a table which has all of the demographic and clinical data for bladder trauma patients listed in a deidentified manner. Demographic data include age, gender, ethnicity, and BMI. The clinical variables include date and time of initial injury, mechanism of injury, concomitant injuries, and imaging studies. Additional data regarding length of catheterization, complications, and follow-up studies are also included. (*Supplementary Materials*)

References

[1] D. J. Bryk and L. C. Zhao, "Guideline of guidelines: a review of urological trauma guidelines," *BJU International*, vol. 117, no. 2, 2015.

[2] R. G. Gomez, L. Ceballos, M. Coburn et al., "Consensus statement on bladder injuries," *BJU International*, vol. 94, no. 1, pp. 27–32, 2004.

[3] I. Guttmann and H. A. Kerr, "Blunt bladder injury," *Clinics in Sports Medicine*, vol. 32, no. 2, pp. 239–246, 2013.

[4] B. M. T. Pereira, C. C. C. de Campos, T. R. A. Calderan, L. O. Reis, and G. P. Fraga, "Bladder injuries after external trauma: 20 years experience report in a population-based cross-sectional view," *World Journal of Urology*, vol. 31, no. 4, pp. 913–917, 2013.

[5] A. S. Cass and M. Luxenberg, "Features of 164 bladder ruptures," *Journal of Urology*, vol. 138, no. 4 Part 1, pp. 743–745, 1987.

[6] A. F. Morey, S. Brandes, D. D. Dugi et al., "Urotrauma: AUA guideline. American Urologic Association," 2014, https://www.auanet.org/guidelines/urotrauma-(2014-amended-2017)#x3277.

[7] J. B. Myers, M. B. Taylor, W. O. Brant et al., "Process improvement in trauma," *Journal of Trauma and Acute Care Surgery*, vol. 74, no. 1, pp. 264–269, 2013.

[8] N. R. Bhatt, R. Merchant, N. F. Davis et al., "Incidence and immediate management of genitourinary injuries in pelvic and acetabular trauma: a 10-year retrospective study," *BJU International*, vol. 122, no. 1, pp. 126–132, 2018.

[9] N. S. Nnamani, M. J. Pugh, M. E. Amuan et al., "Outcomes of genitourinary injury in U.S. Iraq and Afghanistan war veterans receiving care from the veterans health administration," *Military Medicine*, vol. 184, no. 3-4, pp. e297–e301, 2018.

21

Ultrasound Guided Percutaneous Nephrolithotomy in Mesh-Repaired Incisional Hernia

Seyed Hassan Inanloo ,[1] Mohammad Reza Nikoobakht ,[1] Hamed Akhavizadegan ,[1] and Mojgan Karbakhsh [2]

[1]*Department of Urology, Sina Hospital, Tehran University of Medical Sciences, Tehran, Iran*
[2]*Department of Community Medicine, Tehran University of Medical Sciences, Tehran, Iran*

Correspondence should be addressed to Hamed Akhavizadegan; h-akhavizadegan@tums.ac.ir

Academic Editor: Paddy Dewan

Objectives. To describe our technique of percutaneous nephrolithotomy (PNL) in patients with mesh-repaired flank incisional hernia. Polypropylene mesh which is used for fascia strengthening in hernia repair elicits intense inflammatory reaction and the consequent fibrosis alters the characteristics of abdominal wall. Thus, prior history of flank hernia repair with mesh may result in percutaneous nephrolithotomy failure. *Materials and Methods.* Demographic data, renal stones characteristics, and any complication during surgery and follow-up of patients who were treated by PNL during 2011 to 2020 and had mesh in their flank region were collected. *Results.* Percutaneous nephrolithotomy was performed without any problem in 8 patients with guide of ultrasonography. *Conclusion.* Based on our experience, ultrasound-guided PNL is feasible and hypothetically superior to fluoroscopy in such circumstances.

1. Introduction

Introduction of polypropylene mesh was a great step in successful management of hernia and significantly decreased the likelihood of recurrence [1]. However, reoperation may be challenging in the mesh-covered regions due to intense inflammatory reaction and the consequent fibrosis alters the characteristics of abdominal wall [2]. Presence of scar tissue interferes with appropriate surgical access and the required tract dilatation during percutaneous nephrolithotomy (PNL) [3]. In these occasions, ultrasound can serve as a guide, visualizing the region, including the scar and fibrotic tissues. In this article, we report application of ultrasound for facilitating surgical access during PNL in a patient with history of mesh-based flank hernia repair.

2. Materials and Methods

During years 2011 to 2020, a total of 8 patients with history of flank incisional hernia which had been repaired by propylene mesh have been managed with ultrasound-guided percutaneous nephrolithotomy in our center. Age, gender, stones size and place, surgery adverse happenings, length of hospital stay, imaging after surgery, and follow-up visit 2 weeks and 2 months after surgery were recorded from their files anonymously.

All of them had history of mesh-repaired flank incisional hernia due to previous nephrolithotomy. The main diagnostic modality before surgery was spiral CT scanning without contrast [4] (Figure 1(a)). Ultrasound was used to avoid puncture through the mesh in percutaneous

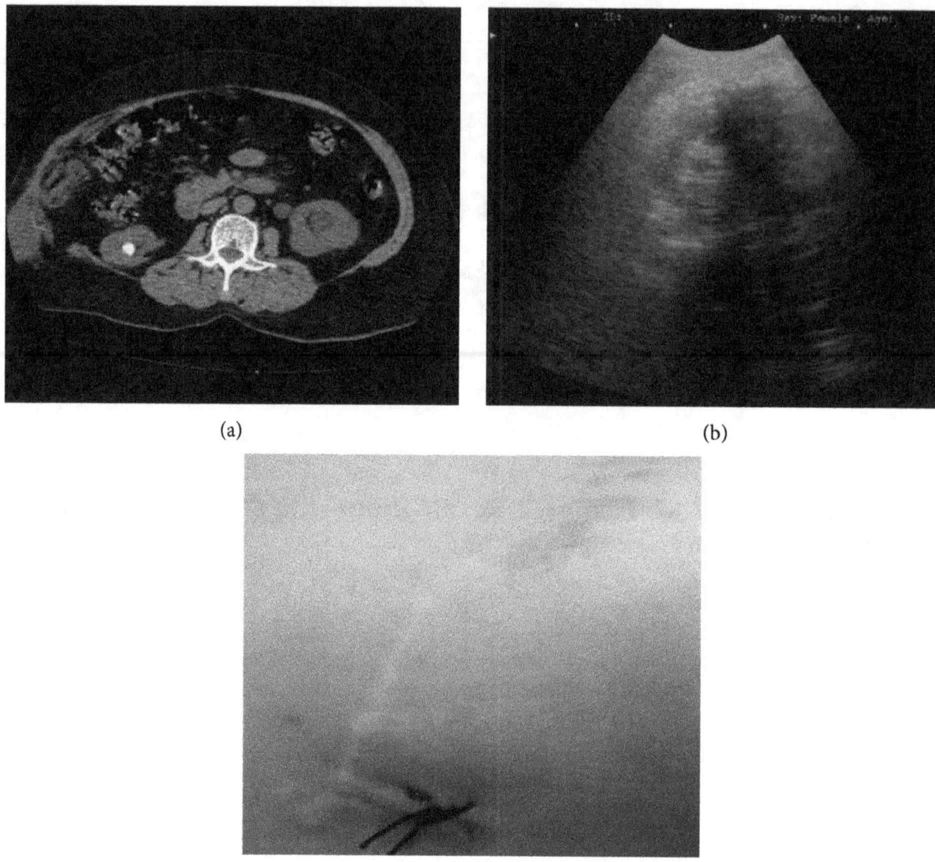

(a) (b) (c)

Figure 1: A 54-year-old woman with history of mesh-repaired right incisional flank hernia with right inferior calyx stone and left hydronephrosis; (a) CT scanning view, (b) ultrasound view of hypoechoic shadow of mesh, and (c) surgical hole of PNL and 2 incision lines in flank position for nephrolithotomy and hernia repair.

nephrolithotomy in flank position [5, 6]. The mesh shadow on the right side of Figure 1(b) is seen as the hypoechoic area, while the kidney is clearly visible on the mesh-free side (i.e., the left side of the photo). Then, the mesh area was marked and the kidney was accessed successfully from lateral using the ultrasound guide. The puncture site in relation to the other two previous incisions (the old one in anterior and the recent one in posterior) is shown in Figure 1(c).

3. Results

3 males and 5 females, 48 to 65 year old were found. Three patients with a stone in the pelvis, 3 with inferior calyx stone, and the last 2 with stones in the inferior and middle calyx.

There was no complication during operation and 6 were stone free on follow-up imaging and 2 had residue smaller than 1 cm which were managed by extracorporeal shock wave lithotripsy. The patients were discharged as usual (2 and 3 days). There was no sign of infection of the mesh at early postoperative visit (2 weeks) and no sign of hernia recurrence at late postoperative visit (2 months).

4. Discussion

Percutaneous nephrolithotomy is a minimally invasive procedure which can be life-threatening in case of complications. Therefore, in order for the patient to enjoy the benefits of this minimally invasive method, it must be done with maximum observance of safety principles [7].

Following the use of mesh in incisional hernia repair, the abdominal wall becomes very stiff and fibrous and the intestines can be pulled to the location of the mesh in case of contact with the peritoneum [8]. Dilatation through the fibrotic area requires increased pressure on the dilators and Amplatz Sheath, which can damage the equipment or lead to loss of access and sudden/uncontrolled advancement of equipment into the kidney region through perforation [3].

For these reasons, approaching the area through access from the mesh-free zones is preferable. The areas affected by mesh fibrosis might not be easily discernible based on the external location of recent surgical scar, as the mesh sometimes extends to wider areas than the incision itself. As in our case, the mesh was radiolucent, using the C-arm, which was not useful either. Therefore, we decided to use ultrasound, which is an acceptable method of access in percutaneous nephrolithotomy [3].

Ultrasound not only has the ability to show if the bowels are pulled under the mesh but also provides a good view of the area covered by the mesh [9]. After finding a suitable, mesh-free site for the puncture, both C-arm and ultrasound can be used for the rest of the procedure. Due to the appropriate experience, we continued to work under the ultrasound guide [3].

Our study has its limitations. Inclusion criteria including history of open nephrolithotomy, herniation of the incision site, and the need for reoperation of the stone are the factors that reduce the number of patients. Another limitation of our study was the type of mesh used [10]. Because the patients had been operated on long ago in other centers, we did not know the exact type of mesh used except that the available mesh for incisional hernia repair at that time in our country was only nonabsorbable propylene mesh. However, due to the fibrosis and scar of the mesh site, which causes the strength of the surgical site and is visible in all types of meshes, the effect of the mesh type on the surgery will not be great and tract dilatation will be difficult in all types of meshes.

5. Conclusion

Based on our experience, ultrasound-guided PNL is feasible and hypothetically superior to fluoroscopy in case of percutaneous interventions with earlier mesh placement/involvement.

References

[1] K. Najjari, H. Zabihi Mahmoudabadi, S. Z. Seyedjavadeyn, and R. Hajebi, "Reduction en masse of inguinal hernia after self-reduction: a case report," *Journal of Medical Case Reports*, vol. 15, no. 1, p. 251, 2021.

[2] S. Mehrabi, M. J. Yavari Barhaghtalab, and M. Babapour, "Renal pelvis and ureteropelvic junction incarceration in a grynfeltt-lesshaft hernia: a case report and review of the literature," *BMC Urology*, vol. 20, no. 1, p. 74, 2020.

[3] S. H. Inanloo, S. R. Yahyazadeh, S. Rashidi et al., "Feasibility and safety of ultrasonography guidance and flank position during percutaneous nephrolithotomy," *The Journal of Urology*, vol. 200, no. 1, pp. 195–201, 2018.

[4] A. Mohammadi, M. R. Nikoobakht, H. Akhavizadegan, S. M. Kazem Aghamir, S. H. Inanloo, and F. Nosrati, "How a renal artery aneurysm may mimic renal stone?" *Urology Case Reports*, vol. 37, Article ID 101621, 2021.

[5] A. Tabibi, H. Akhavizadegan, K. Nouri-Mahdavi, M. Najafi-Semnani, M. Karbakhsh, and A. R. Niroomand, "Percutaneous nephrolithotomy with and without retrograde pyelography: a randomized clinical trial," *International Brazilian Journal of Urology*, vol. 33, no. 1, pp. 19–24, 2007.

[6] S. R. Hosseini, B. Fatahi, and A. M. Fakhr Yasseri, "Comparison outcomes of percutaneous nephrolithotomy in prone and flank position in obese patients: a randomized clinical trial," *Urologia Journal*, 2021.

[7] S. M. K. Aghamir, A. Salavati, M. Hamidi, M. Hamidi, and A. FallahNejad, "A primary report of totally tubeless percutaneous nephrolithotomy despite pelvi-calyceal perforations," *Urology Journal*, vol. 14, no. 4, pp. 4020–4023, 2017.

[8] A. Yazdankhah Kenary, S. N. Afshin, H. Ahmadi Amoli et al., "Randomized clinical trial comparing lightweight mesh with heavyweight mesh for primary inguinal hernia repair," *Hernia*, vol. 17, no. 4, pp. 471–477, 2013.

[9] S. G. Gavrilov, D. A. Son, D. A. Churikov, and G. D. Shuliak, "Ultrasound appearance of mesh after transabdominal preperitoneal inguinal hernia repair," *Journal of Laparoendoscopic & Advanced Surgical Techniques*, vol. 30, no. 4, pp. 395–401, 2020.

[10] H. Mahmoudvand, S. Forutani, and S. Nadri, "Comparison of treatment outcomes of surgical repair in inguinal hernia with classic versus preperitoneal methods on reduction of postoperative complications," *BioMed Research International*, vol. 2017, Article ID 3785302, 4 pages, 2017.

Open Partial Nephrectomy with Zero Ischaemia Using a Supra 12th Rib Miniflank Incision: A Minimally Invasive Open Approach for Small Renal Masses

Syed Ali Ehsanullah,[1] Abida Sultana,[2] Brian Kelly,[1] Charlotte Dunford,[1] and Zaheer Shah[1]

[1]*Worcestershire Acute Hospitals NHS Trust, Redditch, UK*
[2]*University Hospitals Birmingham NHS Foundation Trust, Birmingham, UK*

Correspondence should be addressed to Syed Ali Ehsanullah; sehsanullah@nhs.net

Academic Editor: Kostis Gyftopoulos

Introduction. To assess a minimally invasive open technique for partial nephrectomy with zero ischaemia time. *Methods.* A review was performed in a prospectively maintained database of a single surgeon series of all patients undergoing partial nephrectomy using a supra 12th rib miniflank incision with zero ischaemia. Data of seventy one patients who underwent a partial nephrectomy over an 82-month period were analyzed. Data analyzed included operative time, estimated blood loss, pre and postoperative renal function, complications, final pathological characteristics, and tumour size. *Results.* Seventy one partial nephrectomies were performed from February 2009 to October 2015. None were converted to radical nephrectomy. Mean operative time was 72 minutes (range 30–250), and mean estimated blood loss was 608 mls (range 100–2500) with one patient receiving blood transfusion. The mean pre and postoperative haemoglobin levels were 144 and 112 g/l. The mean pre and postoperative creatinine levels were 82 and 103 Umol/L. There were 8 Clavian-Dindo Grade 2 complications and 1 major complication (Clavian IIIa). Histology confirmed 24 benign lesions and 47 malignant lesions, 46 cT1a lesions, 24 cT1b lesions, and 1 cT2 lesion. Median follow-up was 38 months with no local recurrence or progression of disease with 5 patients having a positive margin (7%). *Conclusion.* Our results demonstrate that a supra 12th miniflank incision open partial nephrectomy with zero ischaemic time for SRMs has satisfactory outcomes with preservation of renal function. A minimally invasive open partial nephrectomy remains an important option for units that cannot offer patients a laparoscopic or a robotic procedure.

1. Introduction

There has been an increase over the past few decades of the incidental diagnosis of small renal masses (SRM) coinciding with the increasing use of computed tomography (CT) and magnetic resonance imaging (MRI). The diagnosis and treatment of small renal masses continues to evolve with advancements in imaging techniques and surgical approaches [1]. Nephron sparing surgery (NSS) or partial nephrectomy (PN) is now recommended by many international guidelines when patients elect to undergo surgical management of a small renal mass (SRM) [2, 3]. The management of SRMs has evolved over time from an open technique to minimal access approaches including laparoscopic and robotic-assisted techniques. Open nephrectomy (ON) was initially considered the "gold standard," but laparoscopic and robotic approaches now have comparable oncological outcomes [2]. However, open PN still remains an important surgical option for high risk tumours.

The TRIFECTA criteria states that regardless of the technique employed, there should be a safe excision of the lesion, with minimal warm ischaemia time (<25 minutes) and no perioperative complications [4–6]. As such, clinical T1a lesions are best managed by PN, yet debate remains how best to manage larger renal masses. The European Association of Urology recommends PN for T1b lesions, while the

American Association of Urology recommends a radical nephrectomy [2, 3]. The TRIFECTA criteria advocated a warm ischaemia time of less than 25 minutes. However, many would argue that "time is tissue" and that "every minute counts" to reduce the risk of long-term renal impairment [7, 8].

Our minimal access open technique includes insertion of a ureteric stent in all patients and a supra 12th rib flank incision of 6–8 cm without renal artery ischaemia for high-risk renal masses (e.g., with a high RENAL nephrometery scores). We present a series of 71 open partial nephrectomies.

2. Methods

Data were prospectively collected and maintained in our departmental database for a single surgeon series of partial nephrectomies. Data of 71 patients who underwent a partial nephrectomy over an 81/82 month period were analyzed (Feb 2009–Nov 2015). Data analyzed included operative time, estimated blood loss, pre- and postoperative renal function, complications as per Clavien–Dindo classification, final histopathological characteristics, and tumour size. Inclusion criteria were all cT1 and cT2 lesions which were amenable to PN. TNM was assigned according to the 2009 UICC Classification of Malignant Tumours 7th Edition version. Three histological subtypes were classed according to the World Health Organization (WHO) classification [9]. The nuclear grade was classified according to the Fuhrman grading system [10]. A positive surgical margin was defined as the presence of cancer cells at the level of the inked parenchymal excision surface.

All patients underwent a triphasic CT to assess both the renal and tumour anatomy. All patients were subjected to a preoperative assessment by an anaesthetist to assess suitability for surgery. Medical charts were reviewed for patient demographics, tumour characteristics, and intraoperative data. Patient demographic data included age, sex, BMI, ASA status, and comorbidities. Tumour characteristics included tumour size, tumour site, number of tumours, solitary kidney, and histological subtype. Intraoperative data included operative time, estimated blood loss, pelvicalyceal system repair, pre- and postoperative haemoglobin, and renal function. Postoperative complications were assessed and classified according to Clavien–Dindo's classification [11]. Statistical analysis was performed using SPSS. The student's T-test was employed to assess the differences in pre- and postoperative creatinine and haemoglobin levels. ANOVA and Pearson's correlation were performed to assess postoperative findings and tumour characteristics. All tests were two-sided with a statistical significance set at $p < 0.05$.

2.1. Surgical Technique. Under general anesthetic, all patients have a ureteric stent inserted prior to undergoing a partial nephrectomy. Patients are placed in a lateral decubitus position, and a supra 12th rib flank incision of 6–8 cm is made (Figure 1) and used to access the retroperitoneum (Figure 2). The kidney is exposed, and a number of small swabs are placed underneath the kidney to deliver the tumour as high as possible in the wound (Figure 3). This is a zero ischaemic technique with no clamping of the renal vessels. The tumour and a suitable margin of paratumour tissue (5–10 mm) is demarcated with the use of diathermy and the lesion resected from the kidney. Any bleeding vessels are tied with polyfilament sutures (Figure 4) and any opening made in the collecting system is closed with monofilament suture material. No bolster or haemostatic patch is applied, and an argon laser is used to aid in coagulation of the tumour bed. The perirenal fat is suitably replaced around the kidney and closed in layers, and no drain is placed as part of the enhanced recovery protocol. Apart from a ureteric stent, a ropivacaine local anaesthetic pump is placed underneath the external intercostal muscle and removed at 48 hours. The patients also follow our departmental enhanced recovery protocol.

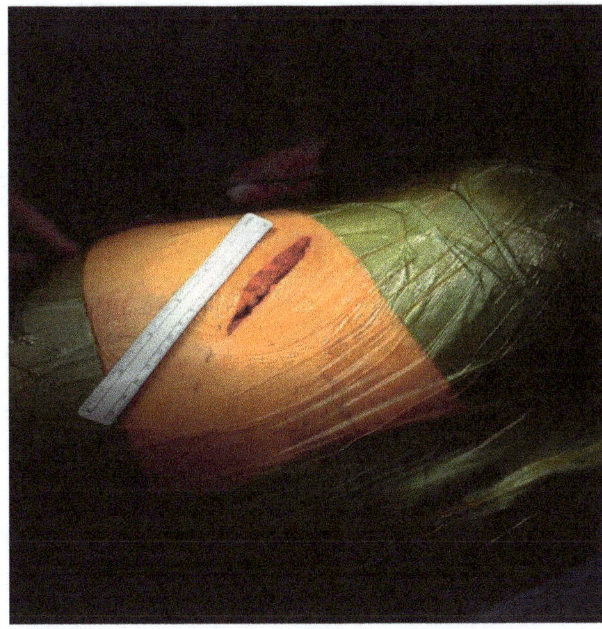

Figure 1: 8 cm supra 12th rib miniflank incision.

3. Resultsx

Seventy-one partial nephrectomies were performed by a single surgeon from February 2009 to October 2015. None were converted to a radical nephrectomy (see Table 1). Mean operative time was 72 minutes (range 30–250 minutes), and mean estimated blood loss was 608 ml (range 100–2500 ml) with one patient (1.4%) receiving a blood transfusion intraoperatively. Mean tumour size was 3.69 cm (range 1.8–7.1 cm). The mean pre- and postoperative haemoglobin levels were 144 and 112 g/l (p = 0.19) with a mean drop in haemoglobin levels of 31 g/l. The mean pre- and postoperative creatinine levels were 82 and 103 Umol/L (p = 0.07) with a mean increase of 20 Umol/L.

There were 8 (11.3%) Grade 2 (Clavien-Dindo) complications and 1 (1.4%) major complication (Clavien IIIa). Histology confirmed 24 benign lesions and 47 malignant lesions, 46 cT1a lesions, 24 cT1b lesions, and 1 cT2 lesion. Median follow-up was 38 months with no local recurrence or progression of disease with 5 patients (7.0%) having a positive margin. 15 patients (21.1%) had a low renal

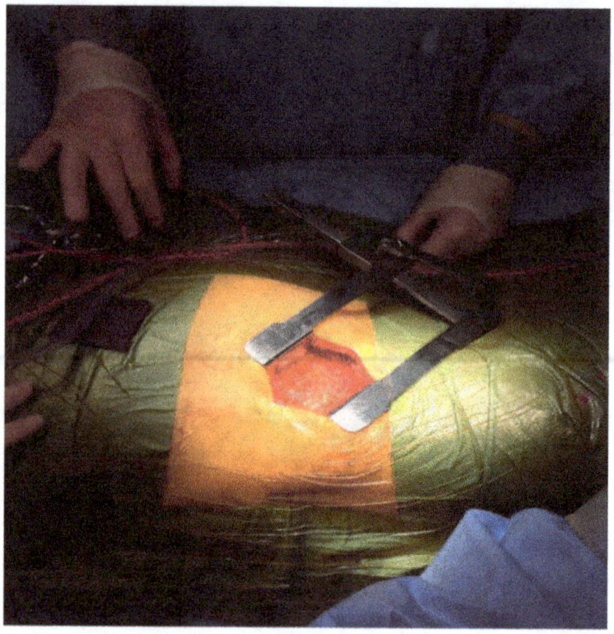

FIGURE 2: Gerota fascia exposed.

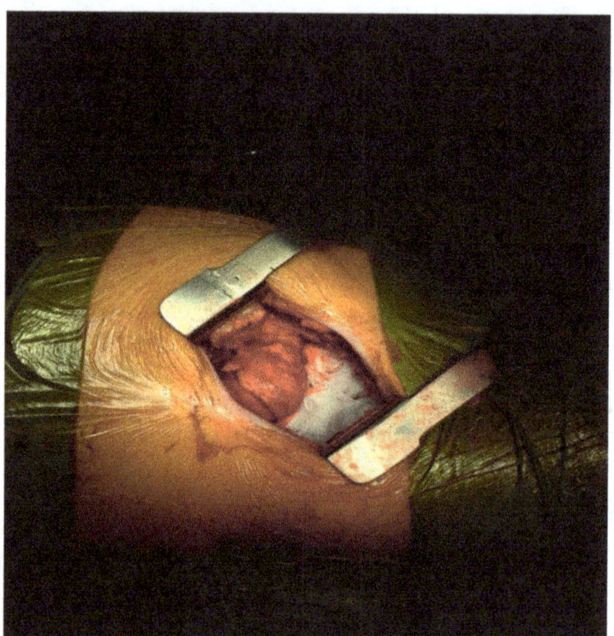

FIGURE 3: Kidney exposed: tumor delivered high in the wound.

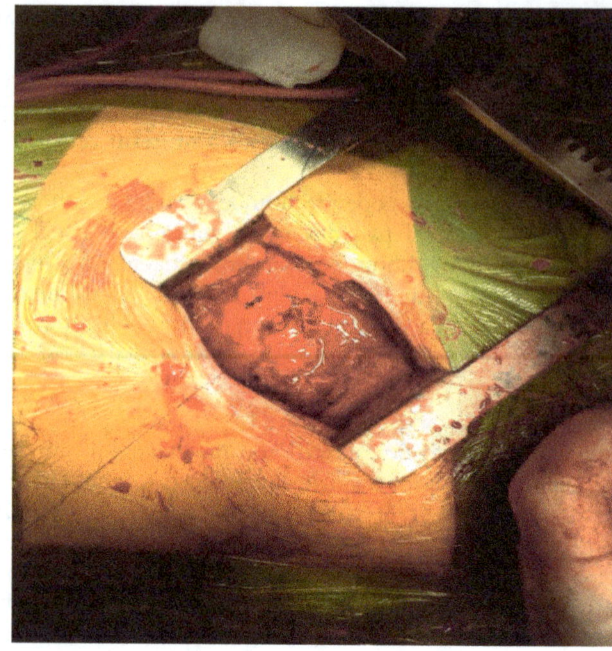

FIGURE 4: Bleeding vessels tied with polyfilament.

TABLE 1: Demographics, tumour characteristics, renal nephrometry score, estimated blood loss, and complications.

Benign		Duration	
Oncocytoma	8	<1 hr	4
Cystic nephroma	5	1-2 hrs	51
Renal cyst	9	2-3 hrs	14
Angiomyolipoma	2	3-4 hrs	1
	24	<4 hrs	1
Malignant		Mean	72 minutes
Clear cell	39	Estimated blood loss	
Chromophobe	6	<500 ml	42
Papillary type 1	2	5–1000	23
	47	1000–2500	6
Fuhrman/nuclear grade		Mean	608 ml
Grade 1	10	Clavien–Dindo complications	
Grade 2	24	Grade 2	8
Grade 3	13	Grade 3a	1
Grade 4	0	Total	**9**
	47	Size	
RENAL nephrometry score		<4 cm	46
4–6	15	4–7 cm	24
7–9	26	>7 cm	1
10–12	30	Mean	3.69 cm

nephrometry score, 26 patients (36.6%) had an intermediate score, and 30 patients (42.3%) had a high score. There was no significant correlation between renal score and haemoglobin change, estimated blood loss, tumour size, operative time, or creatinine increase postoperatively.

4. Discussion

Open PN has become the standard surgical approach for SRMs and cT1b renal lesions. Due to the increase in diagnosis of SRMs in clinical practice, the open PN technique remains an important technique for surgical oncologists [2].

All patients having open partial nephrectomy had a ureteric stent inserted to facilitate urinary drainage which is of particular importance in cases where the collecting system was opened during excision of tumour. Placement of a ureteric stent also makes the insertion of an abdominal drain unnecessary and prevents associated complication, e.g., pain, dislodgement, and or premature removal of drain. The main risk of a zero ischaemic PN is haemorrhage [12]. In our series, the EBL was 608 mls with no cases of urinomas. Clamping the renal vessels could have dramatically reduced the bleeding; however, this may increase the risk of long-term renal impairment. One of our patients required a transfusion (1.4%). The literature suggests that the rate of transfusion for PN varies between 4 and 20% [13]. A recent publication of a series of 40 open zero ischaemia PN had a comparable estimated blood loss of 521 ml [13]. There are laparoscopic and robotic series that employed a zero ischaemic technique with a lower EBL (206 ml); however, they had quite a high transfusion rate of 21% and longer mean operating time of 4.4 hours and a range of up to 8 hours [14].

Similarly, one study in 2018 of 308 patients in a single-centre undergoing robotic off-clamp partial nephrectomies had an overall transfusion rate of 6.2% ($n = 19$). Clavien–Dindo ≥3 grade complications occurred in 4 (1.3%) of patients. Mean EBL was 280 mls (range 50–800) which is less compared to our cohort, and mean creatinine increase was 13% at discharge [15]. Another study looking at laparoscopic and robot-assisted partial nephrectomy with off-clamp technique and controlled hypotension followed 60 patients with a median tumour size of 3.6 cm. Median EBL was 200 ml (range 30–700 ml) with 4 patients (6.6%) requiring postoperative blood transfusions. Due to controlled hypotension, only ASA grade 1-2 patients were selected in this cohort [16].

We always attempted to remove the lesion with a 5–10 mm paratumour safety margin. Given limited anatomical landmarks, this provides a challenge for complex lesions whilst striving to preserve as much benign renal parenchyma as possible. Median follow-up was 38 months with no local recurrence or progression of disease with 5 patients having a positive margin (7%) which is a similar rate to a UK national partial nephrectomy audit of 7% [17]. Other international publications have positive surgical margin rates of 0–31% [18, 19].

Another study from the UK employed an open partial nephrectomy technique. Although they used soft bowel clamps to the kidney to reduce bleeding, with an estimated blood loss of 400 ml, but a statistically significant deterioration in postoperative renal function. In this series of 100 patients, there was 1 case with a positive surgical margin, and there were 2 cases of tumour recurrence [20]. In our series, there is neither a clinically nor a statistically significant change in postoperative renal function or haemoglobin levels.

From a medico-economical perspective, an open PN would have significant cost savings relative to a robotic approach due to the financial outlay necessary to purchase the technology, which may only be cost-effective in large, high volume centres. Our enhanced recovery pathway also aids in our ability to efficiently and safely discharge patients and keep length of stay to a minimum. Patient education is crucial for an efficient discharge and requires regular communication with the patient and family pre-, peri-, and postoperatively to maintain compliance with the enhanced recovery pathway.

The debate will continue as to whether the optimum option for patients requiring a PN is a robotic, laparoscopic, or an open approach. Conventional wisdom has taught us that there are many complex tumours that are technically easier and safer to perform with an open approach. However, surgeon skill and experience as well as an efficient theatre team are paramount for a safe, efficient, open PN regardless of the technique employed.

In the era of robotic and laparoscopic techniques for PN, our supra 12th rib miniflank incision is a suitable alternative for high risk tumours. The 6–8 cm incision leaves the patients with a small, cosmetically acceptable scar. This remains a suitable option for patients who are managed in centres which are not in a position to offer patients a laparoscopic or robotic approach.

5. Conclusion

Our results demonstrate that a supra 12th rib miniflank incision open partial nephrectomy with zero ischaemia time for small renal masses have satisfactory outcomes with preservation of renal function and a small satisfactory cosmetic scar. A minimal access open partial nephrectomy is a fast, safe, and technically easy approach for small renal masses and remains an important and viable treatment option.

References

[1] J.-J. Patard, A. Rodriguez, N. Rioux-Leclercq, F. Guillé, and B. Lobel, "Prognostic significance of the mode of detection in renal tumours," *BJU International*, vol. 90, no. 4, pp. 358–363, 2002.

[2] B. Ljungberg, K. Bensalah, S. Canfield et al., "EAU guidelines on renal cell carcinoma: 2014 update," *European Urology*, vol. 67, no. 5, pp. 913–924, 2015.

[3] S. C. Campbell, A. C. Novick, A. Belldegrun et al., "Guideline for management of the clinical T1 renal mass," *The Journal of Urology*, vol. 182, no. 4, pp. 1271–1279, 2009.

[4] A. J. Hung, J. Cai, M. N. Simmons, and I. S. Gill, ""Trifecta" in partial nephrectomy," *The Journal of Urology*, vol. 189, no. 1, pp. 36–42, 2013.

[5] F. Porpiglia, R. Bertolo, D. Amparore, and C. Fiori, "Margins, ischaemia and complications rate after laparoscopic partial nephrectomy: impact of learning curve and tumour anatomical characteristics," *BJU International*, vol. 112, no. 8, pp. 1125–1132, 2013.

[6] A. Khalifeh, R. Autorino, S. P. Hillyer et al., "Comparative outcomes and assessment of trifecta in 500 robotic and laparoscopic partial nephrectomy cases: a single surgeon experience," *The Journal of Urology*, vol. 189, no. 4, pp. 1236–1242, 2013.

[7] W. C. Huang, A. S. Levey, A. M. Serio et al., "Chronic kidney disease after nephrectomy in patients with renal cortical tumours: a retrospective cohort study," *The Lancet Oncology*, vol. 7, no. 9, pp. 735–740, 2006.

[8] R. H. Thompson, B. R. Lane, C. M. Lohse et al., "Every minute counts when the renal hilum is clamped during partial nephrectomy," *European Urology*, vol. 58, no. 3, pp. 340–345, 2010.

[9] J. N. Eble, G. Sauter, J. Epstein, and I. Sesterhenn, "Pathology and genetics of tumors of the urinary system and male genital organs," *World Health Organization Classification of Tumors*, IARC Press, Lyon, France, 2004.

[10] S. A. Fuhrman, L. C. Lasky, and C. Limas, "Prognostic significance of morphologic parameters in renal cell carcinoma," *The American Journal of Surgical Pathology*, vol. 6, no. 7, pp. 655–664, 1982.
[11] P. A. Clavien, J. Barkun, M. L. de Oliveira et al., "The clavien-dindo classification of surgical complications," *Annals of Surgery*, vol. 250, no. 2, pp. 187–196, 2009.
[12] T. Klatte, V. Ficarra, C. Gratzke et al., "A literature review of renal surgical anatomy and surgical strategies for partial nephrectomy," *European Urology*, vol. 68, no. 6, pp. 980–992, 2015.
[13] M. C. Kriegmair, D. Pfalzgraf, A. Häcker, and M. S. Michel, "ZIRK-technique: zero ischemia resection in the kidney for high-risk renal masses: perioperative outcome," *Urologia Internationalis*, vol. 95, no. 2, pp. 216–222, 2015.
[14] I. S. Gill, M. B. Patil, A. L. de Castro Abreu et al., "Zero ischemia anatomical partial nephrectomy: a novel approach," *The Journal of Urology*, vol. 187, no. 3, pp. 807–815, 2012.
[15] G. Simone, L. Misuraca, G. Tuderti et al., "Purely off-clamp robotic partial nephrectomy: preliminary 3-year oncological and functional outcomes," *International Journal of Urology*, vol. 25, no. 6, pp. 606–614, 2018.
[16] R. Papalia, R. Papalia, G. Simone et al., "Laparoscopic and robotic partial nephrectomy with controlled hypotensive anesthesia to avoid hilar clamping: feasibility, safety and perioperative functional outcomes," *Journal of Urology*, vol. 187, no. 4, pp. 1190–1194, 2012.
[17] A. Fernando, S. Fowler, and T. O'Brien, "Nephron-sparing surgery across a nation—outcomes from the British association of urological surgeons 2012 national partial nephrectomy audit," *BJU International*, vol. 117, no. 6, pp. 874–882, 2015.
[18] M. Peycelon, C. Vaessen, V. Misraï et al., "Résultats de la néphrectomie partielle pour les carcinomes à cellules rénales de plus de 4 cm," *Progrès en Urologie*, vol. 19, no. 2, pp. 69–74, 2009.
[19] R. Schiavina, S. Serni, A. Mari et al., "A prospective, multicenter evaluation of predictive factors for positive surgical margins after nephron-sparing surgery for renal cell carcinoma: the RECORd1 Italian project," *Clinical Genitourinary Cancer*, vol. 13, no. 2, pp. 165–170, 2015.
[20] Z. Cheema, M. Alsinnawi, R. G. Casey, and J. Corr, "A single United Kingdom center experience of open partial nephrectomy using regional ischemia," *The Canadian Journal of Urology*, vol. 21, no. 3, pp. 7277–7282, 2014.

23

Analysis of the Learning Curve of Surgeons without Previous Experience in Laparoscopy to Perform Robot-Assisted Radical Prostatectomy

Felipe Monnerat Lott,[1] Deborah Siqueira,[1] Hermano Argolo,[1] Bernardo Lindberg Nóbrega,[1] Franz Santos Campos,[1] and Luciano Alves Favorito[2]

[1]Brazilian National Cancer Institute, Rio de Janeiro, Brazil
[2]Urogenital Research Unit, State University of Rio de Janeiro (UERJ), Rio de Janeiro-RJ, Brazil

Correspondence should be addressed to Luciano Alves Favorito; lufavorito@yahoo.com.br

Guest Editor: Rajesh Nair

Objective. To assess the learning curve in robot-assisted radical prostatectomy (RARP) performed by surgeons without previous experience in laparoscopic prostatectomy. *Materials and Methods.* We analyzed 119 patients submitted to RARP performed by two surgeons without previous experience in laparoscopic prostatectomy, with emphasis on the relevant outcomes such as continence, erectile function, and oncologic control with a minimum follow-up of 24 months. We used Fisher's exact test and the chi-square test to investigate the existence of a relationship between the variables and analysis of variance (ANOVA) to verify possible statistically significant differences between groups, at the 5% level. *Results.* The patients' age varied from 41 to 72 years (mean = 61.09), with 68 (57.14%) cases having intermediate or high risk. There was a consistent decline in operative time. Of the 119 patients, 80.67% were continent 6 months after surgery and 89.07% 12 months afterward, while 35.29% were potent 6 months after surgery and 60.50% 12 months following surgery. Twelve months after surgery, the trifecta outcome rate was 51.26% and the pentafecta rate was 31.09%. There was progressive postoperative improvement and maintenance of continence and sexual potency until the last patient was operated in our sample. *Conclusions.* Robot-assisted radical prostatectomy does not require previous experience in laparoscopic radical prostatectomy, but the learning curve is not short to achieve the plateau.

1. Introduction

Prostate cancer is the most common tumor other than nonmelanoma skin tumors and the second-leading cause of death due to cancer among men [1]. Robot-assisted radical prostatectomy (RARP) is well established around the world but is still in the implementation phase in various treatment centers in Brazil. Globally, the number of robotic procedures to treat prostate cancer has been growing since its introduction. In 2004, 8% of radical prostatectomies in the United States involved robot assistance [2]. This rate climbed to 53% in 2008 [2] and to 67% in 2010 [3]. Nevertheless, the learning curve of surgeons is highly variable.

To calculate the learning curve, it is necessary to have a complete or nearly complete record of the operations performed by each surgeon in his initial cases. For this reason, we collected data on 40 demographic parameters and the outcomes in our sample.

There is growing evidence that the results of various types of surgery are associated with the characteristics of the surgeon. The discussion of the surgical learning curve is extensive and controversial, with conflicting findings. The articles in general are retrospective, involving analysis only of groups of patients, with evaluation of customary postoperative data: time of hospitalization, bleeding, and time of surgery. A multicentric and prospective study compared 30 initial cases of RARP performed by surgeons with prior fellowship in robotics and by surgeons only with experience in conventional open surgery. There was a statistically significant difference in the compromised surgical margins in favor of surgeons with prior training in robot-assisted surgery (15% versus 34%, $p = 0.008$), but this did not occur after the first 30 cases [4]. Another article, published in 2010, reported that the patients of inexperienced surgeons presented higher recurrence rates [5].

According to Evans et al., recurrence varies among surgeons even when they have performed a similar number of procedures [6]. The biochemical recurrence after surgical treatment of prostate cancer is a good model to analyze the association between characteristics of the surgeon and the outcomes, since adjuvant therapy is not commonly offered and recurrence is not strongly affected by other post-operative aspects.

Our hypothesis was that lack of previous experience in laparoscopic prostatectomy surgery does not interfere in the learning of RARP. To test this hypothesis, the objective of this study was to examine postoperative data to obtain the most relevant functional and oncological outcomes to construct an initial RARP learning curve, with two surgeons without prior experience in LRP, evaluating the rates of postoperative continence, erection, compromised surgical margin, and oncological control of the disease.

2. Patients and Methods

The experimental protocol described here was approved by our university's committee for ethical human experimentation and the ethical standards of the hospital's institutional committee on human experimentation (IRB-65099217.1.0000.5274).

We studied 133 patients who had prospectively undergone radical robotic prostatectomy to treat prostate adenocarcinoma, from June 12, 2012, to July 7, 2015, at the same institution. The patients had been submitted to RARP using the da Vinci Si system (Intuitive Surgical Inc., Sunnyvale, CA) with an average follow-up time of 45 months (varying from 27 to 64 months). It was not possible to obtain all the necessary data on 14 of those patients due to their failure to appear regularly for follow-up consultations, so they were excluded from the study. The diagnosis of cancer was done by transrectal ultrasound-guided biopsy by entities associated with the Brazilian National Health System (SUS).

All the RARP procedures were performed by two surgeons without previous LRP experience, but with more than 10 years of practice in open radical prostatectomy. The technique used was transperitoneal with bilateral opening of the endopelvic fascia.

There were no changes in the surgical technique during the study period. All the patients were first examined by fellows of our institution. The operation time was recorded by the head nurse of robotic surgery, and the data were extracted from the hospital's intranet database. The blood loss was measured at the end of each procedure, deducting the volume of physiological serum possibly administered for washing the surgical field (a bottle of physiological serum with volume markings) and also subtracting the estimated volume of urine after opening the bladder neck (estimated at 5 ml/h—by the hypotensive technique routinely used by the anesthesiology service).

The pathology analyses were performed by pathologists with extensive experience in urooncology and were in all cases reviewed by an experienced uropathologist, although according to the literature, the variation between observers regarding the surgical margin and extraprostatic extension tends to be small. [6] After this review, the extension and location of the compromised surgical margins were recorded, according to the Working Group 5 Consensus of the International Society of Urology Pathology (ISUP) [7].

To assess continence, each patient was questioned whether he used some type of the absorbent, with an additional follow-up of the pelvic physiotherapy service. If the patient had stated no use of absorbent and no contrary report was found in the physiotherapeutic records, the patient was considered continent (totally or socially continent).

The patients were considered potent if they reported successful sexual intercourse (erection degrees 3 or 4) even with the use of oral medication (phosphodiesterase type 5 inhibitor) but without intracavernous drug injection.

For statistical analysis of the learning curve, the patients were divided into four groups (according to the year of surgery), where group 1 contained patients operated in 2012, group 2 in 2013, group 3 in 2014, and group 4 in 2015.

3. Statistical Analysis

We used Fisher's exact text and the chi-square test to investigate the existence of a relation between the variables and analysis of variance (ANOVA) to verify a statistically significant difference between the groups, at the 5% level. For further analysis, the variables that were significant in the ANOVA were investigated by the Tukey test.

4. Results

The age of our patients varied from 41 to 72 years (mean= 61.09), with 68 (57.14%) being cases of intermediate or high risk. The surgery lasted for an average of 238.49 minutes (average console time of 189.28 minutes), and the average hospital stay was 2.43 days. The mean PSA level was 8.23 ng/ml (ranging from 1 to 23 ng/ml). The means and medians of the prostate weight, BMI, and postoperative bleeding and the comparisons of the means can be seen in Table 1.

In 25.21% of the cases, we observed extraprostatic extension, and in 38.65%, we noted compromised surgical margin. Of these compromised margins, 42.55% were unique, and of these, 75% were focal (<3 mm), and 69.38% were radially located. In the anatomopathological review, one case was downgraded and one was upgraded regarding the pathological staging, and there were four alterations in the report from compromised surgical margin (SM+) to free surgical margin (SM−), and vice versa. We observed 4.54% pT3 rate in group 1, 23.07% in group 2, 20% in group 3, and 39.13% in group 4.

Of the 119 patients, 80.67% were continent 6 months after surgery and 89.07% after 12 months. With respect to sexual potency, 15% of the patients had no interest in engaging in sex before the surgery. We observed that 35.29%

TABLE 1: The table shows the descriptive analysis and comparison of the means of the 4 groups of patients submitted to robotic radical prostatectomy. Group 1 contained patients operated in 2012, group 2 in 2013, group 3 in 2014, and group 4 in 2015.

Variable	X	Median	SD	CV	Minimum	Maximum	X of group 1	X of group 2	X of group 3	X of group 4	*p* value
Age (years)	61.09	62.00	5.71	9.34	41.00	72.00	61.28	59.62	61.89	62.30	0.2290
Body mass index	24.8	25	2.68	10.8	18.09	33.00	21.23	24.11	25.75	19.30	0.6570
Prostate weight (g)	29.71	31.00	11.70	39.40	7.00	52.00	27.41	29.31	31.03	30.57	0.6960
PSA density (%)	24.80	25.00	2.69	10.84	18.00	33.00	23.55	24.11	25.75	25.71	0.0017
Probability of extraprostatic extension (PARTIN) (%)	20.29	22.00	4.39	21.63	9.00	25.00	21.23	20.31	20.34	19.30	0.5440
Follow-up (months)	45.30	46.00	10.92	24.10	27.00	64.00	60.68	51.15	39.06	30.17	0.0001
Hospitalization time (days)	2.44	2.00	2.25	92.32	1.00	21.00	3.09	2.23	2.09	2.70	0.3450
Bleeding (milliliters)	207.48	150.00	174.34	84.03	10.00	1200.00	245.00	153.33	277.71	156.52	0.0049
Console time (minutes)	189.29	180.00	63.14	33.36	100.00	470.00	265.23	177.56	178.86	152.39	0.0001
Surgery time (minutes)	238.50	220.00	71.59	30.02	140.00	570.00	324.59	218.08	234.29	197.17	0.0001

X = mean; CV = coefficient of variation; SD = standard deviation.

were potent 6 months after surgery and 60.50% after 12 months. Twelve months after surgery, 51.26% of the outcomes were trifecta and 31.09% were pentafecta.

Regarding complications, 7.56% of the patients presented mild complications (Clavien I-II) and 4.20% suffered more severe ones (Clavien III-IV). In 29.41% of the cases, there was persistence of the disease, high or increasing PSA associated with compromised surgical margin, or biochemical recurrence 24 months after surgery.

Of the 119 patients, 52 were operated by surgeon A and 67 by surgeon B. There was no significant difference between the variables studied when comparing the two surgeons, confirming that their patients had the same profile regarding quantitative variables.

We observed that HAS had a statistically significant relation with erectile function two years after surgery. The majority of the patients did not have HAS and mainly had erection degree of 3. For the other variables, "seeking sexual relations?" and "trifecta 12 m," the p values were lower than 0.05, indicating the existence of a relation between the variables.

The ANOVA presented a p value lower than 0.05 for the variables PSAD, follow-up time, bleeding, console time, and surgery time. Of particular note was the reduction of surgery time between the years: it was 64% shorter in group 4 (most recent) than in group 1.

The number of minutes at the console also declined markedly with the passage of years. The lowest was in group 4, operated in 2015, with $p < 0.0001$, compared with the surgeries performed in 2012, 2013, and 2014, even with worse PSA density in the cases of surgery in 2014 compared to the cases operated in 2012 and 2013 ($p = 0.01$ and 0.03, respectively). Average bleeding was lowest in group 2, and the reductions between groups 3 and 2 ($p = 0.009$) and between groups 4 and 3 ($p = 0.03$) were most notable. In our sample, the patients were operated when presenting higher PSA levels in relation to prostate volume, and even with this adverse prognostic factor, the operative factors progressively improved. Figure 1 shows the learning curve along the series regarding the outcomes surgery time, urinary continence, and sexual potency 12 months after surgery, along with the multiple surgical margin rates in pT2 and pT3 cases along with the multiple surgical margin rates.

The R^2 values of the learning curve were 0.33 for surgical time, 0.02 for continence 12 months after surgery, 0.06 for erection, 0.01 for compromised surgical margin in pT2 and 0.02 for compromised surgical margin in pT3 after that time lapse, and 0.07 for compromised surgical margins. The best value was quantified as 1. In other words, continent = 1, level 4 erection = 1, and so on for all the variables. Therefore, the nearer the lines are to 1, the better the performance was for that variable. The graphs show a progressive improvement and maintenance of postoperative continence and sexual potency until the last patient was operated in our sample. This indicates that the plateau to be reached, after which there is no further significant improvement in the postoperative outcomes, was not attained. The same happened about the surgical margins. The results were better in pt3 than in pT2 cases along the cases done. This was expected due to the low number of cases operated by each surgeon.

For the surgical margin, we attributed a score of "0" to no compromise, so the trend line is inclined and near 0, indicating the margin tended not to be compromised as the surgeon gained experience.

5. Discussion

Postoperative morbidly and mortality are not good parameters to analyze the learning curve because they can be influenced not only by the surgeon's experience but also by the skill of the anesthesiologist and the training and experience of the postoperative intensive care team. A previous study found that the learning curve for LRP to reach a plateau was about 250 cases, with little improvement regarding recurrence after the surgeon had reached 250 procedures [8]. The biochemical recurrence rate after five years was 17.9% (surgeons with 10 cases) versus 10.7% (surgeons with more than 250 cases). When comparing surgeons with fewer than 10 cases against those with more than 250 cases, there was a reduction in the relative risk of 7.2%, meaning that for each 14 patients operated by the surgeon with less experience in comparison with the same

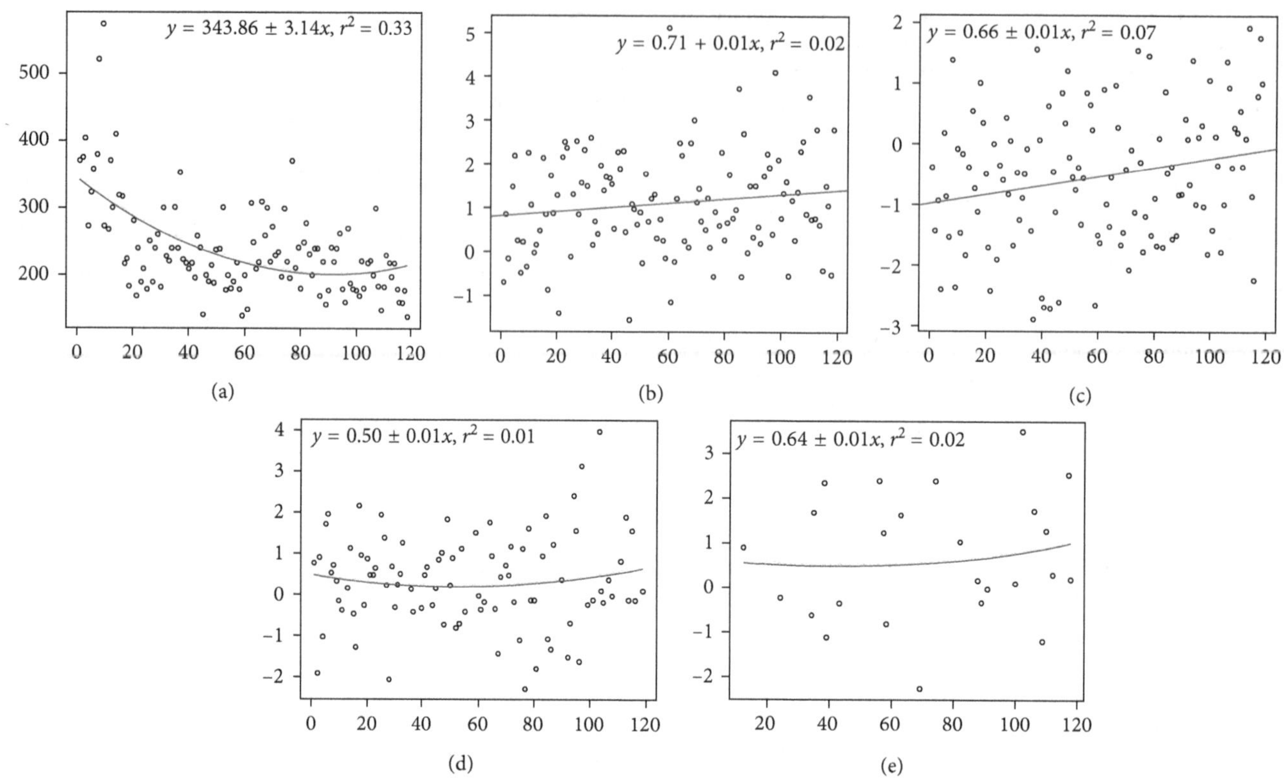

FIGURE 1: The figure shows the linear regressions of the learning curve along the series regarding the outcomes surgery time, urinary continence, and sexual potency 12 months after surgery, along with the multiple surgical margin rates. (a) Surgery time (in minutes–y axis) with progression of cases (number–x axis). The arrow marks the start of the performance of obturator lymphadenectomy, followed later by extended lymphadenectomy; $R^2 = 0.33$; (b) continence 12 months after surgery; the best results approach line 1, $R^2 = 0.06$; (c) erection 12 months after surgery; the best results approach line 1; $R^2 = 0.02$; (d) compromised surgical margins in pT2 cases; the best results approach line 1; $R^2 = 0.01$; (e) compromised surgical margins in pT3 cases; the best results approach line 1; $R^2 = 0.02$.

measure for the more experienced surgeon, one patient will present recurrence.

In another study working with the same database as the one described above, but instead of correlating SM with BCR, the authors found a SM+ rate of 36% for surgeons with fewer than 50 cases versus 11% for surgeons with more than 1,000 cases ($p = 0.017$) [9]. Despite the natural assumption that the surgeon with fewer compromised SM outcomes would have lower BCR, the data from that study indicated independence of these variables. There was a correlation between SM+ and BCR HR of 2.1 ($p < 0.0005$) [10], but this association is weak. A SM+ has 1/4 of the effect of a primary Gleason grade, 1/3 of the effect of a seminal vesicle invasion, and 50% of the effect of an extraprostatic extension to BCR. Obviously, SM is important, but it is questionable to employ it to assess the change in the surgical technique or as feedback to surgeons.

Vickers and colleagues, in a multicentric and retrospective cohort study of 4,702 patients, adopting recurrence criteria of PSA > 0.2 ng/ml (4 institutions) and PSA > 0.1 ng/ml (3 institutions), found that these recurrence criteria did not affect the probability of the same outcome for a surgeon individually. They also found the learning curve to be longer for pure laparoscopic surgery was compared to the open technique, and the results improved up to 750 procedures, when they reached a plateau. When the surgeon already had experience in open surgery, the results were better [11].

Another important point to consider is the fact that few surgeons manage to perform a large enough number of operations to reach a proficiency plateau. More than 80% of American surgeons performed fewer than 10 radical prostatectomies in 2005. Considering that the working life of a surgeon is around 25–30 years, it is estimated that the large majority do not reach this minimum of 250 operations. This means that the majority of patients receive treatment from surgeons that are not experienced enough to have fully hone their skills. Only around 4% of surgeons would reach the plateau in 10 years. In New York City, a metropolis with several quaternary hospitals, 84% of the surgeons in 2005 performed fewer than 10 radical prostatectomies, with only 3.4% performing 50 or more [12].

Another study, with 400 patients submitted to RARP between 2012 and 2015 by a single surgeon with experience of 600 cases of LRP, found an average surgery time of 187.2 minutes, with an estimated blood loss of 240.9 ml. The SM+ rate was 20% (64.6% at pT3 and 35.4% at pT2). With respect to location, 52.4% of the SM+ cases were apical, while we found that the majority of the compromised surgical margins were radial, perhaps due to an exaggerated attempt to achieve good neural preservation. In that other study, there was no significant difference in the SM+ rate as the number of cases progressed, possibly because the surgeon already had good experience in LRP [13].

Machado and colleagues [14] reported that surgeons with more than 200 LRP cases obtained similar oncological results in the first 60 cases using RARP. They found mean operating time of 236 minutes and blood loss of 245.6 ml. They also observed a complication rate of 6.6%, pT2 of 81.6%, pT3 of 18.4%, continence after 6 months of 93.3%, potency after 6 months of 70%, and SM+ rate of 21.6%, with the complications of RARP varying from 1.5% to 17.8%. We observed similar values for surgery time, blood loss, and complications, even though the surgeons had no previous experience in laparoscopic radical prostatectomy.

A recent study compared the results of a surgeon experienced in the use of robot assistance (with analysis after 70 procedures) against those of a surgeon only with experience in open radical prostatectomy [15]. The result reported for operation time was similar to that found in our sample (238 min), and the SM+ rate was 24% in the patients operated with the da Vinci platform.

A cohort study with prospective data collection on 500 patients operated between 2005 and 2012 (RARP) revealed a significant decline in operation time and bleeding rates between group I (1–250 cases) and group II (251–500 cases), even though group II had more advanced cases. There was no significant difference regarding SM+ rates, even though there was a decrease from 38.4% to 30.0% between the two groups ($p = 0.059$). There was a reduction from 49% (group I) to 32.6% (group II) in the SM+ rate at pT3 ($p = 0.007$) [16]. We did not obtain similar reduction in the rates of compromised surgical margin, probably because of the smaller sample.

A meta-analysis comparing RARP with LRP [17] found the following outcome values for the latter procedure: continence at 12 months of 91.5%, potency at 12 months of 81% (results similar to ours), SM+ of 14.4% in a sample with 44% rate of extraprostatic disease, and a biochemical recurrence rate of 9.8%. The authors stated that various factors might have influenced the postoperative continence (patient's age, prostate weight, BMI, nerve sparing, preservation of the bladder neck, sparing of the pubovesical complex, reconstruction/preservation of the anatomical structures, urethral length, and comorbidities) [18].

An analysis of cases initially operated by four surgeons showed that the learning curve to obtain postoperative continence did not reach a plateau even after 200 cases [19], which would also explain what happened in our cases.

Another retrospective study analyzed the learning curve with a total sample of 500 patients operated by two surgeons, where the patients were divided into sequential groups of 25 patients. The authors found a statistically significant reduction in operation time, blood loss, and hospital stay at each 25 procedures. There was a significant decrease for one surgeon and a declining trend for the second one regarding postoperative complications. There was no difference regarding the rates of compromised surgical margins between the groups of patients [20].

The rates of SM+ in robot-assisted radical prostatectomy are variable in the literature, from 6.5 to 32% in general, as described by Yossepowitch [21] and Novarra and colleagues [22], with an average rate of 15% or up to 36% for surgeons with an experience of fewer than 50 cases and 16.7% for surgeons with a background of 51 to 140 cases. In turn, Atug et al. [23] reported that a surgeon's skill increases after the first 30 cases, with rates of compromised surgical margin falling from 45.4% to between 21.2 and 11.7%. Our findings for compromised SM rates are therefore within the parameters found previously in the literature. The total positive surgical margin rate in our sample was 38,65% (34,8% of the PSM occurred in pT3 and 65,2% in pT2). In contrast, Patel and colleagues [24] reported lower SM+ rates: 12.2% for from 1 to 300 cases operated, 6.6% for 301–600 cases, 13.6% for 601–900 cases, 11% for 901–1,200 cases, and 1.8% with an experience of 1201–1500 procedures.

Another retrospective study (2002–2012) in a hospital in the United Kingdom analyzed 592 minimally invasive radical prostatectomies. The SM+ rate was 30.6%, with demographic data and follow-up times similar to those of our sample. The authors found BCR in 10.7% of the cases with SM+ and in 5.1% of the cases with SM−, with an average follow-up time of 30.3 months [25]. An analysis of the initial series of the first 100 cases of three surgeons over a period of nine years [26] observed an increase in the number of pT3 cases in the second group of 50 cases operated, with only a small increase in the occurrence of SM+, similar to our findings.

Finally, Thompson and colleagues [27] conducted a comparative analysis of the initial cases of robot-assisted radical prostatectomy with the cases of open radical prostatectomy of the same surgeon, who had performed more than 3,000 open surgeries and more than 2,000 robot-assisted operations. The results of sexual potency, continence, and compromised surgical margin were significantly better in the cases of open surgery compared to the initial robotic ones, which was reverted soon thereafter. The plateau of the RARP learning curve was 330 cases for sexual potency, 365 for early return of continence, 659 for complete resolution of incontinence, 484 for reduction of the compromised surgical margin rate, and 226 cases for biochemical recurrence.

We should mention the most important weak points of this study: the very small sample, the short follow-up interval for a secure analysis of biochemical recurrence and compromised surgical margin, the lack of analysis based on quality of life questionnaires, and the fact that some patients were submitted to complementary radiotherapy before the PSA exceeded the barrier of 0.2 ng/ml (a traditional threshold considered for biochemical recurrence).

6. Conclusion

Our results and their comparison with other reports in the literature demonstrate that the learning curve for robot-assisted radical prostatectomy is extended, not reaching a plateau with fewer than 100 surgery cases, despite the progressive improvement during the course of the series and the good general results.

In light of the very long learning curve, we recommend regionalization of prostate cancer treatment because surgeons with a larger number of cases under their belts reduce the hospital expenses by lowering the rates of complications and costs for adjuvant treatments.

Abbreviations

ASA:	American Association and Anesthesiology (classification of the physical state)
BCR:	Biochemical recurrence
BMI:	Body mass index
CLAVIEN:	Clavien–Dindo classification of surgical complications
cT:	Clinical staging
HAS:	Systemic arterial hypertension
INCA:	National Cancer Institute
LRP:	Laparoscopic radical prostatectomy
ORP:	Open radical prostatectomy
Pentafecta:	Oncological control of the disease + urinary continence + sexual potency + negative surgical margin + absence of postoperative complications
PSAD:	PSA density
pT:	Pathological staging
RARP:	Robot-assisted radical prostatectomy
SHIM:	Sexual Health Inventory for Men
SM+:	Compromised surgical margin
Trifecta:	Oncological control of the disease + urinary continence + sexual potency
USA:	United States of America
XRT:	X-ray therapy.

References

[1] W. J. Catalona, "Prostate cancer screening," *Medical Clinics of North America*, vol. 102, no. 2, pp. 199–214, 2018.

[2] H.-Y. Yu, N. D. Hevelone, S. R. Lipsitz, K. J. Kowalczyk, and K. C. Hu, "Use, costs and comparative effectiveness of robotic assisted, laparoscopic and open urological surgery," *Journal of Urology*, vol. 187, no. 4, pp. 1392–1398, 2012.

[3] T. J. Leroy, D. D. Thiel, D. A. Duchene et al., "Safety and peri-operative outcomes during learning curve of robot-assisted laparoscopic prostatectomy: a multi- institutional study of fellowship-trained robotic surgeons versus experienced open radical prostatectomy surgeons incorporating robot-assisted laparoscopic prostatectomy," *Journal of Endourology*, vol. 24, no. 10, pp. 1665–1669, 2010.

[4] A. J. Vickers and A. M. Cronin, "Data and programming code from the studies on the learning curve for radical prostatectomy," *BMC Research Notes*, vol. 3, no. 1, p. 234, 2010.

[5] F. J. Bianco, A. J. Vickers, A. M. Cronin et al., "Variations among experienced surgeons in cancer control after open radical prostatectomy," *Journal of Urology*, vol. 183, no. 3, pp. 977–982, 2010.

[6] A. J. Evans, P. C. Henry, T. H. Van der Kwast et al., "Interobserver variability between expert urologic pathologists for extraprostatic extension and surgical margins status in radical prostatectomy specimens," *American Journal of Surgical Pathology*, vol. 32, no. 10, pp. 1503–1512, 2008.

[7] Edge SB, American Joint Committee on Cancer, and American Cancer Society, *AJCC Cancer Staging Handbook: From the AJCC Cancer Staging Manual*, Springer, New York, NY, USA, 7th edition, 2010.

[8] F. P. Secin, C. Savage, C. Abbou et al., "The learning curve for laparoscopic radical prostatectomy: an International Multicenter Study," *Journal of Urology*, vol. 184, no. 6, pp. 2291–2296, 2010.

[9] A. J. Vickers, F. J. Bianco, A. M. Cronim et al., "The learning curve for surgical margins after open radical prostatectomy: implications for the use of margin status as an oncologic endpoint," *Journal of Urology*, vol. 183, no. 4, pp. 1360–1365, 2010.

[10] A. J. Stephenson, P. T. Scardino, J. A. Eastham et al., "Postoperative nomogram predicting the 10-year probability of prostate cancer recurrence after radical prostatectomy," *Journal of Clinical Oncology*, vol. 23, no. 28, pp. 7005–7012, 2005.

[11] A. J. Vickers, C. J. Savage, M. Hruza et al., "The surgical learning curve for laparoscopic compared to open radical prostatectomy: a retrospective cohort study," *The Lancet Oncology*, vol. 10, no. 5, pp. 475–480, 2009.

[12] C. J. Savage and A. J. Vickers, "Low annual caseloads in US surgeons conducting radical prostatectomy," *Jorunal of Urology*, vol. 182, no. 6, pp. 2677–2679, 2009.

[13] A. F. Adili, J. Di Giovanni, E. Kolesar et al., "Positive surgical margin rates during the robot-assisted laparoscopic radical prostatectomy learning curve of an experienced laparoscopic surgeon," *Canadian Urological Association Journal*, vol. 11, no. 11, pp. E409–E413, 2017.

[14] M. Tobias-Machado, A. I. Mitre, M. Rubinstein, E. F. Costa, and A. K. Hidaka, "Robotic-assisted radical prostatectomy learning curve for experienced laparoscopic surgeons: does it really exist?," *International Brazilian Journal of Urology*, vol. 42, no. 1, pp. 83–89, 2016.

[15] L. O. Gagnon, S. L. Goldenberg, K. Lynch, A. Hurtado, and M. E. Gleave, "Comparison of open and robotic-assisted prostatectomy: the University of British Columbia experience," *Canadian Urological Association*, vol. 8, no. 3-4, pp. 92–97, 2014.

[16] Y. C. Ou, C. K. Yang, K. S. Chang et al., "The surgical learning curve for robotic-assisted laparoscopic radical prostatectomy: experience of a single surgeon with 500 cases in Taiwan, China," *Asian Journal of Andrology*, vol. 16, no. 5, pp. 728–734, 2014.

[17] S. H. Lee, H. J. Sei, N. R. Lee, S. K. Son, D. K. Kim, and K. H. Rha, "Robot-assisted radical prostatectomy has lower biochemical recurrence than laparoscopic radical prostatectomy: systematic review and meta-analysis," *Investigative and Clinical Urology*, vol. 58, no. 3, pp. 152–163, 2017.

[18] F. Lott and L. Favorito, "Urinary continence after robot-assisted radical prostatectomy: a systematic review," *International Journal of New Technology and Research*, vol. 2, no. 3, pp. 20–25, 2016.

[19] N. Fossati, E. D. Trapani, G. Gandaglia et al., "Assessing the impact of surgeon experience on urinary continence recovery after robot-assisted radical prostatectomy: results of four high-volume surgeons," *Journal of Endourology*, vol. 31, no. 9, pp. 872–877, 2017.

[20] S. Mason, M. V. Hemeirijck, A. Chandra, C. Brown, and D. Cahil, "Laparoscopic radical prostatectomy outcome data: how should surgeons' performance be reported? A retrospective learning curve analysis of two surgeons," *Ecancermedicalscience*, vol. 10, p. 651, 2016.

[21] O. Yossepowitch, A. Briganti, J. A. Eastham et al., "Positive surgical margins after radical prostatectomy: a systematic review and contemporary update," *European Urology*, vol. 65, no. 2, pp. 303–313, 2014.

[22] G. Novara, V. Ficarra, S. Mocellin et al., "Systematic review and meta-analysis of studies reporting oncologic outcome after robot-assisted radical prostatectomy," *European Urology*, vol. 62, no. 3, pp. 382–404, 2012.

[23] F. Atug, E. P. Castle, S. K. Srivastav, S. V. Burgess, R. Thomas, and R. Davis, "Positive surgical margins in robotic-assisted radical prostatectomy: impact of learning curve on oncologic outcomes," *European Urologyc*, vol. 49, no. 5, pp. 866–871, 2006.

[24] V. R. Patel, K. J. Palmer, G. Coughlin, and S. Samavedi, "Robot-assisted laparoscopic radical prostatectomy: perioperative outcomes of 1500 cases," *Journal of Endourology*, vol. 22, no. 10, pp. 2299–2305, 2008.

[25] A. Sachdeva, R. Veeratterapillay, A. Voysey et al., "Positive surgical margins and biochemical recurrent following minimally-invasive radical prostatectomy—an analysis of outcomes from a UK tertiary referral center," *BMC Urology*, vol. 17, no. 1, p. 91, 2017.

[26] A. Jaulim, A. Srinivasan, S. Hori et al., "A comparison of operative and margin outcomes from surgeon learning curves in robot assisted radical prostatectomy in a changing referral practice," *Annals of The Royal College of Surgeons of England*, vol. 100, no. 3, pp. 226–229, 2018.

[27] J. E. Thompson, S. Egger, M. Bohm et al., "After a long learning curve-updated analysis of a prospective single-surgeon cohort of 2206 consecutive cases," *European Urology*, vol. 73, no. 5, pp. 664–671, 2018.

Randomized Controlled Trial of Laparoscopic versus Open Radical Cystectomy in a Laparoscopic Naïve Center

Waleed Mohamed Fadlalla,[1] **Ayman Hanafy**,[1] **Mahmoud Abdelhakim**,[2] **Hatem Aboulkassem**,[1] **El Sayed Ashraf**,[1] **and Ahmed Abdelbary**[1]

[1]*National Cancer Institute, Cairo University, Department of Surgical Oncology, Cairo, Egypt*
[2]*Department of Urology, Faculty of Medicine, Cairo University, Cairo, Egypt*

Correspondence should be addressed to Ahmed Abdelbary; ahmed.abdelbary@nci.cu.edu.eg

Academic Editor: Fabio Campodonico

Background. Laparoscopic radical cystectomy is a challenging surgical procedure; however, it has been largely abandoned in favor of the more intuitive robotic-assisted cystectomy. Due to the prohibitive cost of robotic surgery, the adoption of laparoscopic cystectomy is of relevance in low-resource institutes. *Methodology.* This is a randomized controlled trial comparing laparoscopic radical cystectomy (LRC) to open radical cystectomy (ORC) at a single institute. Each group included thirty patients. The trial was designed to compare both approaches regarding operative time, blood loss, transfusion requirements, length of hospital stay, time to oral intake, requirement of opioid analgesia, and complications. *Results.* LRC was associated with less hospital stay (9.8 vs. 13.8 days, $P = 0.001$), less time to oral solid intake (6 vs. 8.6 days, $P = 0.031$), and lower opioid requirements (23.3% vs. 53.3%, $P = 0.033$). There was a trend towards lower blood loss and transfusion requirements, but this did not reach statistical significance. Overall complication rates were comparable. *Conclusion.* Laparoscopic radical cystectomy was associated with comparable postoperative outcomes when compared to ORC in the first laparoscopic cystectomy experience in our center. Benefitting from the assistance of an experienced laparoscopic surgeon is recommended to shorten the learning curve.

1. Introduction

In Egypt, bladder cancer is the third most common solid malignancy and the second most common cancer in males after liver cancer [1], representing a major health problem. The standard for the surgical management of muscle invasive bladder cancer (MIBC) and selected cases of non-muscle invasive bladder cancer (NMIBC) is open radical cystectomy. Radical cystectomy is associated with 30–68% complication rates in contemporary series [2, 3]. Few procedures in urology (if any) are associated with the morbidity of radical cystectomy; improvement of results in that domain represents a priority in urologic literature.

The first laparoscopic radical cystectomy was performed in 1992 [4]. The adoption of laparoscopic radical cystectomy was slow due to the challenging nature of the procedure. In addition, the introduction of robotic surgery as a minimally invasive interface for radical cystectomy was a more appealing option, as the robot was designed to remedy the difficulties of conventional laparoscopy and shorten the learning curve required to master the procedure [5]. Laparoscopic cystectomy is performed within a confined space with little room for surgical manipulation; this adds to the difficulty when attempting bladder surgery which is surrounded by a rich vascular network, as well as dissection around great vessels during lymphadenectomy, with the potential for life-threatening injury.

While the robot is an extremely valuable tool, alternatives should be sought after, especially in a low-resource setting. Ideally, these alternatives should not compromise the quality of care provided to the patients. In this study, we explore the feasibility, safety, and postoperative outcome of laparoscopic radical cystectomy in a laparoscopic-naïve center.

2. Methodology

2.1. Study Design. This is a randomized, controlled, unblinded interventional clinical trial comparing open radical cystectomy to laparoscopic radical cystectomy. Operations in the intervention arm were performed by the same surgical team with one of three experienced open surgeons as the operator and the others assisting. One of two expert oncosurgeons performed all the procedures in the control arm (open radical cystectomy). A parallel assignment intervention model with 1 : 1 allocation was used in this study. The trial was registered with ClinicalTrials.gov (NCT04838873).

2.2. Pilot Study. A pilot of 10 patients was performed utilizing the presence of a urologist having an immense experience with laparoscopic radical cystectomy. This helped organize the team, adjust the setup, troubleshoot early problems, and build up confidence.

2.3. Participants. Patients scheduled for radical cystectomy at the National Cancer Institute, Cairo University, between January 25th, 2019, and July 30th, 2019, were recruited and randomized to one of two study groups (a control group and an intervention group) (Figure 1). Both groups were matched in terms of preoperative parameters, including preoperative serum creatinine levels, hemoglobin values, and clinical T and N stages.

2.4. Selection Criteria

2.4.1. Inclusion Criteria

(i) Patients diagnosed with urinary bladder cancer, clinical stage T3a, N0, M0 or less [6], scheduled for radical cystectomy
(ii) 30–80 years of age
(iii) Able to comprehend and sign informed consent

2.4.2. Exclusion Criteria. The following exclusion criteria were predefined:

(i) Patients with nodal and/or distant metastasis
(ii) Patients with severe medical comorbidities contraindicated for major surgery
(iii) Patients with uncorrectable bleeding diathesis
(iv) Patients with previous extensive abdominal surgery/adhesions precluding laparoscopic access
(v) Patients who received preoperative radiation therapy to the pelvis

2.5. Intervention

2.5.1. Surgical Technique (Control Group). A standard lower midline laparotomy was used for either conventional open radical cystoprostatectomy in male patients or anterior pelvic exenteration in females.

2.5.2. Surgical Technique (Study Group). Transperitoneal approach to laparoscopic radical cystectomy was performed as described in literature [7]. A muscle-splitting Pfannenstiel incision was utilized to deliver the specimen and perform the diversion (Figure 2).

2.6. Data Collection and Outcome Measures. Baseline characteristics, operative variables, complications, and pathologic outcomes will be discussed in detail in the "Results" section. All clinical and pathological information was recorded prospectively, with patient datasheets filled out by healthcare personnel. Both groups were matched in terms of preoperative parameters, including preoperative serum creatinine levels, preoperative hemoglobin values, body mass index (BMI), and clinical T and N stages (Table 1).

2.7. Randomization and Blinding. Randomization was generated using the SPSS. Both the patient and the operating surgeon knew the allocated intervention before the surgery. However, the study statistician performing the final analysis was masked to the interventions.

2.8. Statistical Analysis

2.8.1. Sample Size Estimation. This study aims to compare laparoscopic radical cystectomy with open radical cystectomy regarding perioperative outcome. Based on a previous study by Lin and colleagues [8], the mean operative time for LRC was 282 minutes for LRC vs. 235 for ORC. Comparable results were observed in our pilot of 10 patients. Thus, a total sample of 26 patients per group will be sufficient to detect a power of 90%, significance level of 0.05. The number was increased to a total of 30 patients per group to allow for the use of parametric tests and account for possible drop-outs. Sample size estimation was performed by G power sample size program (*Franz Faul, University of Kiel, Germany*).

2.8.2. Statistical Methods. Data were analyzed using SPSS statistical package version 22 (*SPSS Inc., Chicago, IL*). Numerical data were expressed as mean and standard deviation (SD), median, and range as appropriate. Qualitative data were expressed as frequency and percentage. Student *T*-test was used to examine the relation between quantitative variables as appropriate. Chi-square (Fischer's exact) test was used to examine the relation between qualitative variables as appropriate. Tests were two-tailed and *P* values ≤0.05 were considered statistically significant.

2.9. Ethical Standards. The study adhered to the World Medical Association Declaration of Helsinki and the ethical standards of the National Cancer Institute, Cairo University. IRB full approval was obtained prior to the initiation of the study (IRB number: 201819018.3) (Study ID: S01901-31004), as well as written informed consent from all participants.

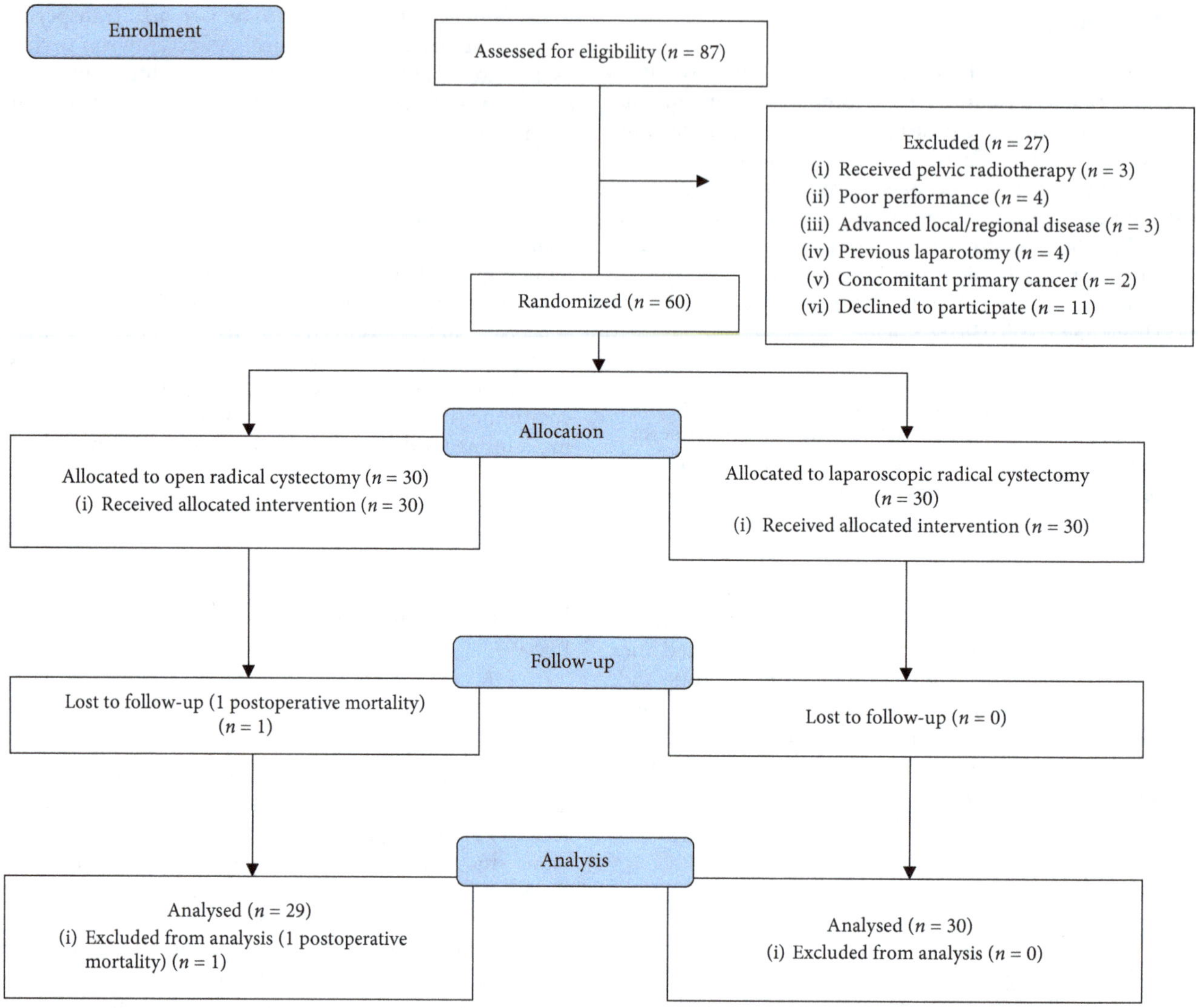

FIGURE 1: Flowchart of the study.

2.10. Follow-Up. Patients were followed for at least 1 year postoperatively. Regular follow-up visits were scheduled at 1 week after discharge, the third month, the sixth month, and the twelfth month unless the patient required closer follow-up for specific complaints.

3. Results

3.1. Baseline Characteristics. At the first postoperative day, no statistically significant change in serum creatinine or hemoglobin levels was detected (Table 1).

3.2. Perioperative Parameters and Complications

3.2.1. Conversion to Open Surgery. No conversions to open surgery were encountered. However, in the prior pilot study, we encountered 3 conversions (3/10 cases, 30%), one due to extensive intra-abdominal adhesions and the other two due to grossly enlarged iliac lymph nodes.

3.2.2. Blood Loss and Transfusion. There was a trend towards decreased blood loss and transfusion requirements in favor of the laparoscopic approach; however, it did not reach statistical significance (Table 2).

3.2.3. Operative Time. In our pilot of 10 patients undergoing laparoscopic radical cystectomy, average operative time was 389 minutes (range: 215–455). In the study itself; difference in operative (OR) time (cystectomy and lymphadenectomy time) was statistically significant, with longer operative times in the laparoscopic cystectomy group (Table 3, Figure 3(a)). The difference in OR time between the first 15 laparoscopic cases and the last 15 cases was statistically significant ($P = 0.0488$) (Figure 3(b)).

3.2.4. Types of Urinary Diversion. There was no difference regarding the trend of urinary reconstruction in either group (Table 1).

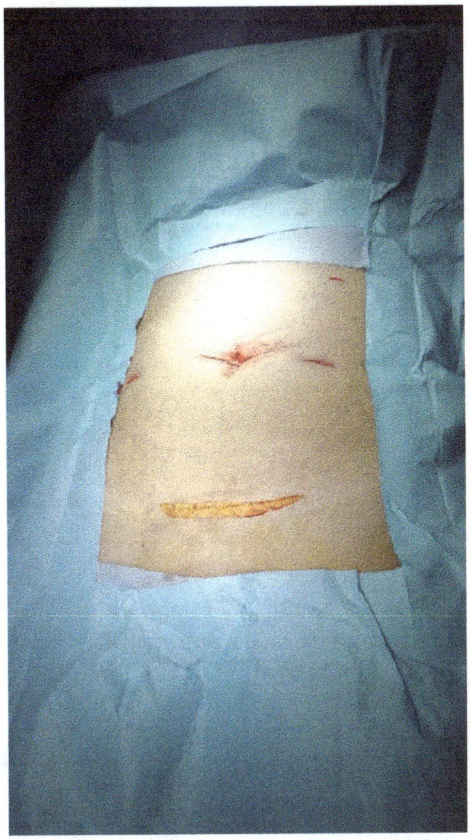

FIGURE 2: Pfannenstiel incision is used to deliver the specimen and perform urinary diversion.

TABLE 1: Baseline patient characteristics.

		Whole cohort N = 60	LRC N = 30	ORC N = 30	P value
Age (years)		59.02 ± 7.55	57.20 ± 8.38	60.83 ± 6.24	0.062
Follow-up (months)		20.5 (16–24)	20.4 (16–24)	20.7 (17–24)	0.6
Sex	Male	47 (78.3%)	22 (73.3%)	25 (83.3%)	0.532
	Female	13 (21.7%)	8 (26.7%)	5 (16.7)	
ASA	1	22 (36.7%)	12 (40%)	10 (33.3%)	0.838
	2	35 (58.3%)	17 (56.7%)	18 (60%)	
	3	3 (5%)	1 (3.3%)	2 (6.7%)	
Body mass index (BMI)		24.9 ± 2 (range: 20–28.5)	24.9 ± 1.8 (range: 20.5–28)	24.8 ± 2.1 (range: 20–28.5)	0.8
Previous abdominal surgery		8 (13.3%)	4 (13.3%)	4 (13.3%)	1.00
Neoadjuvant chemotherapy		22 (36.7%)	14 (46.7%)	8 (26.7%)	0.18
SCr preoperative (mg/dl)		1.12 ± 0.30	1.08 ± 0.25	1.15 ± 0.34	0.323
SCr 1st postoperative day (mg/dl)		1.08 ± 0.19	1.03 ± 0.15	1.14 ± 0.20	0.026
Hb preoperative (gm/dl)		12.00 ± 1.50	12.01 ± 1.46	11.98 ± 1.57	0.932
Hb 1st postoperative day (gm/dl)		10.62 ± 1.25	10.70 ± 1.24	10.53 ± 1.29	0.611
Clinical T stage	cT1	10 (16.7%)	5 (16.7%)	5 (16.7%)	0.920
	cT2	34 (56.7%)	18 (60%)	16 (53.3%)	
	cT3	16 (26.7%)	7 (23.3%)	9 (30%)	
Clinical N stage	cN0	49 (81.7%)	23 (76.7%)	26 (86.7%)	0.488
	cN1-3	11 (18.3%)	7 (23.3%)	4 (13.3%)	
Diversion	Orthotopic	9 (15%)	4 (13.3%)	5 (16.7%)	0.99
	Ileal conduit	51 (85%)	26 (86.7%)	25 (83.3%)	

LRC: laparoscopic radical cystectomy; ORC: open radical cystectomy; ASA: American Society of Anesthesiologists' classification; SCr: serum creatinine; Hb: hemoglobin. P value ≤0.05 is considered significant. Values are given in means ± SD or n (%).

3.2.5. Narcotic Requirements, Time to Solid Intake, and Length of Hospital Stay (LOS). Regarding laparoscopic radical cystectomy, time to oral solid food intake and length of hospital stay were shorter when compared with open radical cystectomy. Postoperative opioid requirement was also significantly lower for laparoscopic radical cystectomy (Table 4).

Table 2: Comparison of intraoperative estimated blood loss and required blood transfusion units between the LRC and ORC groups.

		LRC $N = 30$	ORC $N = 30$	P value
Estimated blood loss (ml)		437.33 ± 374.24	602.67 ± 432.44	0.119
RBCS transfusion (unit)	0	23 (76.7%)	16 (53.3%)	0.207
	1	3 (10%)	3 (10%)	
	2	2 (6.7%)	8 (26.7%)	
	3	1 (3.3%)	2 (6.7%)	
	4	1 (3.3%)	1 (3.3%)	

Table 3: Comparison of cystectomy and lymphadenectomy operative time (minutes) between the LRC and ORC groups.

	Whole cohort $N = 60$	LRC $N = 30$	ORC $N = 30$	P value
Total operative time (min)	311.7 ± 110.5	394.8 ± 94.8	228.6 ± 39.2	<0.001
Cystectomy operative time (min)	129.6 ± 76.2	194.7 ± 51.2	64.5 ± 20.9	<0.001
Lymphadenectomy operative time	61.1 ± 15	66.5 ± 14	55.7 ± 14.2	0.002

3.2.6. Complications. Ileus was more pronounced with ORC ($P = 0.02$). There was no difference regarding any type of complications between both study groups. There was one mortality in the ORC group, from pulmonary embolism secondary to left lower limb deep vein thrombosis. More hospital readmissions were observed in the ORC group, but this was not statistically significant (Table 4).

3.3. Pathologic Outcome. Only one patient developed a positive surgical margin from the ORC group; no patients from the LRC developed positive margins. No statistically significant differences regarding pathologic T stage or lymph node involvement were reported. Lymph node yield was higher in the LRC group. Twelve patients developed recurrence/metastasis during the follow-up period (Table 5).

4. Discussion

Our institute has been one of the main hospitals managing bladder cancer in the country since the seventies; however, we have not adopted laparoscopic surgery until recently, and it was primarily reserved for adrenalectomies and nephrectomy for small renal masses.

4.1. Operative Time. This study showed that the operative time was significantly longer in the LRC group compared to the ORC group (366 vs. 229 min; $P < 0.001$), being consistent with literature, which almost uniformly reports operative time to be longer with minimally invasive approaches [6, 9, 10]. This is our early experience with laparoscopic radical cystectomy, and even though the operative duration difference was significant between the open and laparoscopic approaches, there was a trend towards a reduction of operative time when comparing the first and the last laparoscopic cases (370 minutes for the first case vs. 150 minutes for the last case); that difference was statistically significant and reflects the improvement in operative efficiency as challenges within the learning curve are gradually overcome.

4.2. Conversion to Laparotomy. It is reported that the rate of open conversion of laparoscopic radical cystectomy ranges from 2 to 6% [11–13]. No cases were converted to open surgery in our study; however, three cases were converted in the prior pilot study (3/10 cases, 10%), one due to extensive intra-abdominal adhesions causing lack of progress and the other two due to the presence of grossly enlarged iliac lymph nodes. The pilot study might have helped add to our vigilance in obtaining recent abdominal-pelvic scans before operation. A low threshold for continuing laparoscopy in advanced bladder cancer should be exercised due to concerns about compromising oncologic control as a result of potential pneumoperitoneum-induced circulation of tumor cells. An expert laparoscopic surgeon was present as a mentor in all cases and scrubbed in if required, for any encountered technical difficulty; this might have reduced the conversion rate further.

4.3. Blood Loss and Transfusion Requirements. There was an overall trend towards lower estimated blood loss and lower transfusion rate in LRC group, which is consistent with other studies [7, 8, 14], but this was statistically nonsignificant ($P = 0.119$ and $P = 0.207$, respectively). Additionally the rate of transfusion of more than 1 unit of RBCs was higher in the open cystectomy group (11 cases vs. 4 cases). The lack of a statistically significant difference might be attributed to the fact that the cystectomy cases in the control group were performed by two highly open experienced surgeons well beyond their learning curves. If the laparoscopic interface allows surgeons in their early laparoscopic experience to achieve similar or even slightly more favorable blood loss rates and transfusion requirements to experienced open surgeons, this could be considered an advantage for minimally invasive surgery. Laparoscopy adds certain benefits allowing for lower

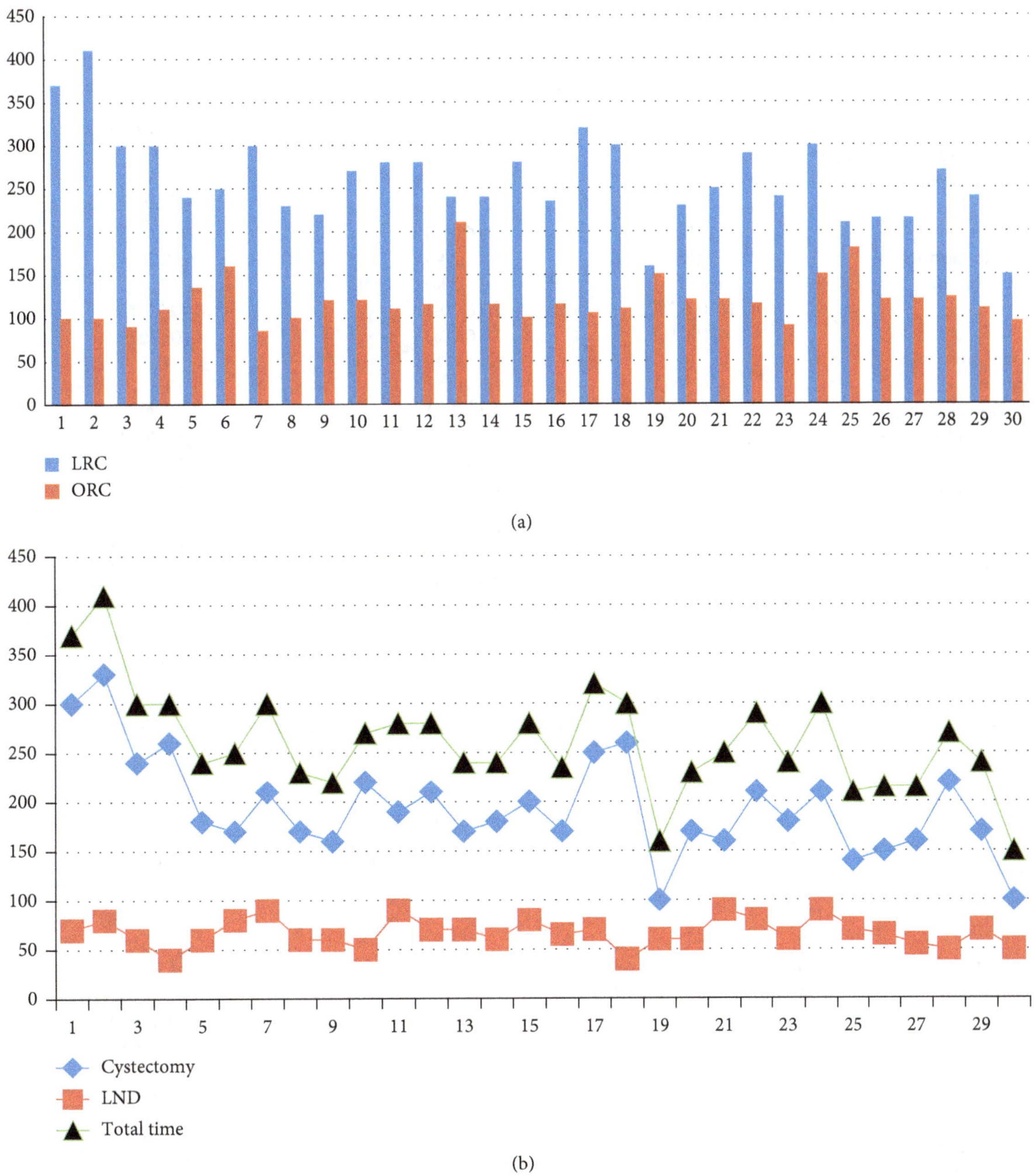

FIGURE 3: (a) Comparison of operative duration between open and laparoscopic cystectomy. (b) The difference in OR time between the first 15 laparoscopic cases (mean: 280 minutes ± 52) and the last 15 laparoscopic cases (mean: 242 minutes ± 49) ($P = 0.0488$).

blood loss: the field is magnified which allows preemptive control of small potential bleeders especially in areas of restricted exposure, pneumoperitoneal pressure allows for control of small venous oozing, and lastly the surgeon is compelled to operate in a bloodless environment to enhance their visualization.

4.4. Opioid Requirements. Lower narcotic requirement is consistently reported with minimally invasive radical cystectomy when compared to open surgery [5, 10]. Our study reports similar results; even though we used a muscle-splitting Pfannenstiel incision for specimen delivery and extracorporeal diversion, the duration of abdominal wall retraction is much less than in a completely open radical cystectomy. Studies suggest that midline laparotomy is more painful than transversely oriented incisions [15], which might be another explanation of the reduced opioid requirements in the LRC group.

4.5. Start of Oral Solids and Length of Hospital Stay. Time to regular oral diet and length of hospital stay were significantly shorter for LRC compared with the ORC group, which was consistent with many reports [7, 8, 16]. Open radical cystectomy involves packing of the intestine which

Table 4: Comparison of postoperative outcomes and complications between LRC and ORC groups.

	Whole cohort ($N=60$)	LRC ($N=30$)	ORC ($N=30$)	P value
Time to solids oral intake (days)	7.35 ± 4.64	6.07 ± 3.62	8.63 ± 5.22	0.031
LOS (days)	11.82 ± 4.83	9.8 ± 4.13	13.83 ± 4.69	0.001
Postoperative opioid requirement	23 (38.3%)	7 (23.3%)	16 (53.3%)	0.033
Conversion from laparoscopy to open	0	0	N/A	
Seroma	7 (11.7%)	2 (6.7%)	5 (16.7%)	0.4
Surgical site infection (SSI)	3 (5%)	1 (3.3%)	2 (6.7%)	0.99
Urinary tract infection	1 (1.7%)	1 (3.3%)	0	0.99
Ileus	10 (16.7%)	2 (6.7%)	8 (26.7%)	0.02
Urine leak	4 (6.7%)	2 (6.7%)	2 (6.7%)	0.99
Small intestinal injury	0	0	0	0.99
Rectal injury	1 (1.7%)	0	1 (3.3%)	0.99
Anastomotic bowel leak	4 (6.7%)	2 (6.7%)	2 (6.7%)	0.47
Abdominal wall dehiscence	3 (5%)	0	3 (10.3%)*	0.24
Pneumonia	2 (3.3%)	0	2 (6.7%)	0.47
Pulmonary embolism	2 (3.3%)	1 (3.3%)	1 (3.3%)	0.99
Hospital readmission	7 (11.7%)	2 (6.7%) (i) Small intestinal leakage (ii) DVT	5 (17.2%)* (i) Small intestinal leakage (2 cases) (ii) Abdominal wall dehiscence (2 cases) (iii) Small bowel obstruction (1 case)	0.4
Mortality	1 (1.7%)	0	1 (3.3%)	0.99
Incisional hernia	3	0	3/29 (10.3%)	0.2
Port-site recurrence	0	0	N/A	

DVT: deep vein thrombosis; LOS: length of stay; LRC: laparoscopic radical cystectomy; ORC: open radical cystectomy; N/A: not applicable; *Total number of cases is 29 due to the presence of one postoperative mortality in the ORC group.

Table 5: Pathologic outcome.

		Whole cohort $N=60$	LRC $N=30$	ORC $N=30$	P value
Pathological T stage	pT0	5 (8.3%)	5 (16.7%)	0	0.098
	pT1	3 (5%)	1 (3.3%)	2 (6.7%)	
	pT2a	4 (6.7%)	1	3 (10%)	
	pT2b	6 (10%)	2 (6.7%)	4 (13.3%)	
	pT3a	10 (16.7%)	7 (23.3%)	3 (10%)	
	pT3b	25 (41.7%)	11 (36.7%)	14 (46.7%)	
	pT4a	7 (11.7)	3 (10%)	4 (13.3%)	
Positive margin		1 (1.7%)	0	1 (3.3%)	0.99
LNs no.		13.82	15.23 ± 4.14	11.97 ± 5.48	0.008
Recurrence		12 (20.3%)*	5 (16.7%)	7 (24.1%)**	0.7

*Total number of cases is 59 due to the presence of one postoperative mortality in the ORC group. **Total number of cases is 29 due to the presence of one postoperative mortality in the ORC group.

potentially exposes them to mechanical trauma for the whole duration of the procedure [17]; this may translate into ileus which is reported in 26% of patients in literature [16].

4.6. Complications. According to Challacombe et al., major complication rates ranged from 10 to 13% in LRC [18]. In our trial, we did not find a high rate of complications specific to the laparoscopic approach. This may be because urinary diversions were constructed extracorporeally in all cases, which is a safe and effective way to decrease operative time and surgical complexity. Mortality after radical cystectomy is reported in under 5% [19]. One case died in our study in the ORC group due to pulmonary embolism complicating DVT, with no significant difference between both study groups.

Wound complications including infection, seroma, and dehiscence were not statistically significant between both groups. Important potential advantages of transverse incisions are that they are cosmetically favorable, less liable to evisceration, and associated with less pain and pulmonary compromise [11, 20–22]. Although this is not a consistent finding in literature [23, 24], in this study the only advantage of the transverse incision was the lower opioid requirement in favor of laparoscopic cystectomy.

Hospital readmission was required in seven patients (11.7%; 2 from the LRC and 5 from the ORC groups, respectively, P = 0.42). This was in line with other studies which reported a relatively high readmission rate of 8.6–28% after radical cystectomy [25, 26]. In a large cohort of 8827 Medicare patients, there was no difference in rates of hospital readmissions between minimally invasive and open radical cystectomy, which suggests that the high readmission rates are inherent to radical cystectomy itself regardless of the approach [27].

4.7. Influence of the Approach on the Choice of Diversion. There were no differences in the trend of urinary tract reconstruction between both groups. A well-performed laparoscopic radical cystectomy can replicate open surgery principles and allow for nerve preservation and urethral complex sparing as prerequisites for orthotopic reconstruction. The Pfannenstiel incision does not hinder the creation of any type of neobladder (performed in 4 cases). While the number of neobladder reconstructions was few in both groups, laparoscopic radical cystectomy did not seem to influence the choice of diversion.

4.8. Pathologic Metrics of Adequate Resection

4.8.1. Surgical Margins. According to Chade et al., the incidence of positive surgical margins ranged from 4 to 5% of ORC cases and from 0 to 5% of the LRC cases [28]. Only one patient from the control arm developed a positive surgical margin in our study with no statistically significant difference. These findings are similar to those of previous studies [9, 29].

4.8.2. Lymph Node Count. LRC showed a statistically significant higher mean lymph node yield 15.67 (LN) than ORC 11.97, which was contradictory to other relevant reports [5, 7]. Most studies reported similar or higher nodal yields with ORC. The CORAL trial showed that lymph node yield was higher with ORC when compared to LRC (18.8 vs. 15.5) [16]. We did not attempt extended lymph node dissection in any case in the ORC group. However, we could not find an explanation for the higher lymph node yield reported for LRC in our study, other than the fact that the laparoscopic arm was performed by experienced open surgeons. Nevertheless, lymph node yield is considered a measure of adequate staging and regional control in radical cystectomy, and the laparoscopic approach did not compromise lymph node yield in our study.

5. Strengths and Limitations

Limitations of our study include short follow-up with lack of oncologic evaluation and the relatively small single institution sample. Both the patients and the surgeon could not be blinded because of the surgical nature of the trial. Strengths include randomized design, all patients adhered to their follow-up schedule with no drop-outs, the open radical cystectomy arm was used by two expert oncosurgeons, and the laparoscopic arm was utilized by the same team throughout the study. This study is also of relevance to other institutes with limited laparoscopic experience aiming to start a laparoscopic cystectomy program.

6. Conclusion

Our results show that laparoscopic radical cystectomy is associated with satisfactory short-term outcome, even in an institute with limited laparoscopic experience. Lower narcotic requirements, less time to oral intake and earlier convalescence, were observed in the current study. Longer follow-up is required to monitor oncologic results. We recommend benefiting from the assistance of an experienced laparoscopic surgeon in early series of advanced laparoscopic surgery.

References

[1] A. S. Ibrahim, H. M. Khaled, N. N. Mikhail, H. Baraka, and H. Kamel, "Cancer incidence in Egypt: results of the national population-based cancer registry program," *Journal of Cancer Epidemiology*, vol. 2014, Article ID 437971, 18 pages, 2014.

[2] J. Kulkarni, "Perioperative morbidity of radical cystectomy: a review," *Indian Journal of Urology*, vol. 27, no. 2, pp. 226–232, 2011.

[3] L. T. Lavallée, D. Schramm, K. Witiuk et al., "Peri-operative morbidity associated with radical cystectomy in a multicenter database of community and academic hospitals," *PLoS One*, vol. 9, no. 10, Article ID e111281, 2014.

[4] R. O. Parra, C. H. Andrus, J. P. Jones, and J. A. Boullier, "Laparoscopic cystectomy: initial report on a new treatment for the retained bladder," *Journal of Urology*, vol. 148, no. 4, pp. 1140–1144, 1992.

[5] K. Matsumoto, K.-i. Tabata, T. Hirayama et al., "Robot-assisted laparoscopic radical cystectomy is a safe and effective procedure for patients with bladder cancer compared to laparoscopic and open surgery: perioperative outcomes of a single-center experience," *Asian Journal of Surgery*, vol. 42, no. 1, pp. 189–196, 2019.

[6] C. Wittekinf, J. D. Brierly, and M. K. Gospodarowicz, *TNM Classification of Malignant Tumors*, John Wiley and Sons, Hoboken, NJ, USA, 8th edition, 2017.

[7] A. M. Abdel-Hakim, F. Bassiouny, M. S. Abdel Azim et al., "Laparoscopic radical cystectomy with orthotopic neobladder," *Journal of Endourology*, vol. 16, no. 6, pp. 377–381, 2002.

[8] T. Lin, X. Fan, C. Zhang et al., "A prospective randomised controlled trial of laparoscopic vs. open radical cystectomy for bladder cancer: perioperative and oncologic outcomes with 5-year follow-upT Lin et al," *British Journal of Cancer*, vol. 110, no. 4, pp. 842–849, 2014.

[9] X. Hu, S.-C. Xiong, W.-C. Dou et al., "Minimally invasive vs. open radical cystectomy in patients with bladder cancer: a systematic review and meta-analysis of randomized

controlled trials," *European Journal of Surgical Oncology*, vol. 46, no. 1, pp. 44–52, 2020.
[10] K. Tang, H. Li, D. Xia et al., "Laparoscopic versus open radical cystectomy in bladder cancer: a systematic review and meta-analysis of comparative studies," *PLoS One*, vol. 9, no. 5, Article ID e95667, 2014.
[11] S. Albisinni, L. Fossion, M. Oderda et al., "Critical analysis of early recurrence after laparoscopic radical cystectomy in a large cohort by the ESUT," *Journal of Urology*, vol. 195, no. 6, pp. 1710–1717, 2016.
[12] O. M. Aboumarzouk, T. Drewa, P. Olejniczak, and P. L. Chlosta, "Laparoscopic radical cystectomy: a 5-year review of a single institute's operative data and complications and a systematic review of the literature," *International Brazilian Journal of Urology*, vol. 38, no. 3, pp. 330–340, 2012.
[13] A. K. Hemal, S. B. Kolla, P. Wadhwa, P. N. Dogra, and N. P. Gupta, "Laparoscopic radical cystectomy and extracorporeal urinary diversion: a single center experience of 48 cases with three years of follow-up," *Urology*, vol. 71, no. 1, pp. 41–46, 2008.
[14] D. Subirá-Ríos, F. Herranz-Amo, M. Moralejo-Gárate et al., "Post-surgical complications in patients with bladder cancer treated with cystectomy: differences between open and laparoscopic approach," *Actas Urológicas Españolas (English Edition)*, vol. 43, no. 6, pp. 305–313, 2019.
[15] S. R. Brown and P. B. Goodfellow, "Transverse verses midline incisions for abdominal surgery," *The Cochrane Database of Systematic Reviews*, no. 4, Article ID CD005199, 2005.
[16] M. Nutt, S. Scaief, D. Dynda, and S. Alanee, "Ileus and small bowel obstruction after radical cystectomy for bladder cancer: analysis from the nationwide inpatient sample," *Surgical Oncology*, vol. 27, no. 3, pp. 341–345, 2018.
[17] M. Sun, P. Ravi, P. I. Karakiewicz et al., "Is there a relationship between leapfrog volume thresholds and perioperative outcomes after radical cystectomy?" *Urologic Oncology*, vol. 32, 2014.
[18] B. J. Challacombe, B. H. Bochner, P. Dasgupta et al., "The role of laparoscopic and robotic cystectomy in the management of muscle-invasive bladder cancer with special emphasis on cancer control and complications," *European Urology*, vol. 60, no. 4, pp. 767–775, 2011.
[19] A. Al-Daghmin, A. Aboumohamed, R. Din et al., "Readmission after robot-assisted radical cystectomy: outcomes and predictors at 90-day follow-up," *Urology*, vol. 83, no. 2, pp. 350–356, 2014.
[20] H. Amer, S. M. Mokhtar, and S. E. Harb, "Burst abdomen: should we change the concept, preliminary study," *Egyptian Journal of Surgery*, vol. 36, pp. 199–207, 2017.
[21] T. P. G. J. Rosenberg and J. Rosenberg, "Vertical compared with transverse incisions in abdominal surgery," *The European Journal of Surgery*, vol. 167, no. 4, pp. 260–267, 2001.
[22] S. T. Orcutt, C. J. Balentine, C. L. Marshall et al., "Use of a Pfannenstiel incision in minimally invasive colorectal cancer surgery is associated with a lower risk of wound complications," *Techniques in Coloproctology*, vol. 16, no. 2, pp. 127–132, 2012.
[23] C. M. Seiler, A. Deckert, M. K. Diener et al., "Midline versus transverse incision in major abdominal surgery: a randomized, double-blind equivalence trial (POVATI: ISRCTN60734227)," *Annals of Surgery*, vol. 249, no. 6, pp. 913–920, 2009.
[24] M. J. Greenall, M. Evans, and A. V. Pollock, "Midline or transverse laparotomy? A random controlled clinical trial. Part I: influence on healing," *British Journal of Surgery*, vol. 67, pp. 188–190, 1980.
[25] I. Berger, L. Xia, C. Wirtalla, P. Dowzicky, T. J. Guzzo, and R. R. Kelz, "30-day readmission after radical cystectomy: identifying targets for improvement using the phases of surgical care," *Canadian Urological Association Journal*, vol. 13, no. 7, pp. E190–E201, 2018.
[26] P. S. Kirk, T. A. Skolarus, B. L. Jacobs et al., "Characterising "bounce-back" readmissions after radical cystectomy," *BJU International*, vol. 124, no. 6, pp. 955–961, 2019.
[27] P. K. Modi, B. K. Hollenbeck, M. Oerline et al., "Real-world impact of minimally invasive versus open radical cystectomy on perioperative outcomes and spending," *Urology*, vol. 125, pp. 86–91, 2019.
[28] D. C. Chade, V. P. Laudone, B. H. Bochner, and R. O. Parra, "Oncological outcomes after radical cystectomy for bladder cancer: open versus minimally invasive approaches," *Journal of Urology*, vol. 183, no. 3, pp. 862–870, 2010.
[29] M. S. Khan, C. Gan, K. Ahmed et al., "A single-centre early phase randomised controlled three-arm trial of open, robotic, and laparoscopic radical cystectomy (CORAL)," *European Urology*, vol. 69, no. 4, pp. 613–621, 2016.

25

Retroperitoneal Lymph Node Dissection as Primary Treatment for Metastatic Seminoma

Brian Hu[1] and **Siamak Daneshmand**[2]

[1]*Department of Urology, Loma Linda University, 11234 Anderson Street Room A-560, Loma Linda, CA 92374, USA*
[2]*University of Southern California Institute of Urology, 1441 Eastlake Avenue, Los Angeles, CA 90033, USA*

Correspondence should be addressed to Brian Hu; brian.hu80@gmail.com

Academic Editor: Aditya Bagrodia

Reducing the long-term morbidity in testicular cancer survivors represents a major area of interest. External beam radiation therapy and systemic chemotherapy are established treatments for seminoma; however, they are associated with late toxicities such as cardiovascular disease, insulin resistance, and secondary malignancy. Retroperitoneal lymph node dissection (RPLND) is a standard treatment for nonseminomatous germ cell tumors (NSGCT) that has minimal long-term morbidity. Given the efficacy of RPLND in management of NSGCT, interest has developed in this surgery as a front-line treatment for seminoma with isolated lymph node metastasis to the retroperitoneum. Four retrospective studies have shown promising results when surgery is performed for seminomas with low-volume retroperitoneal metastases. To better determine if RPLND can be recommended as a primary treatment option, two prospective clinical trials (SEMS and PRIMETEST) are underway. This review will examine the literature, discuss the benefits/limitations of RPLND, and compare the methodologies of the two ongoing clinical trials.

1. Introduction

Seminoma with isolated retroperitoneal lymphadenopathy is typically treated with external beam radiation therapy (XRT) or systemic chemotherapy. There has been little change in these recommendations over the last few decades. However, evidence continues to mount with regard to the long-term morbidities associated with these treatments. The risk of secondary malignancies is approximately twofold higher in patients who have had either chemotherapy or XRT for management of germ cell cancers [1]. The risk of cardiovascular disease is also high with testicular cancer survivors having up to a 2.6-fold increased risk over 20 years. Importantly, these long-term toxicities have been linked to decreases in overall survival [2, 3]. Other side effects can include lung injury, metabolic syndrome, renal toxicity, and decreases in fertility. As most testicular cancer survivors will live many decades, the impact and incidence of these toxicities can be profound.

There has been a concerted emphasis to reduce treatment-related morbidity in testicular cancer. A greater utilization of active surveillance in stage I disease, decrease in radiation dosage, limitations in the fields of radiation, and single-agent chemotherapy are examples of efforts to mitigate long-term toxicities. In line with this philosophy, investigators have looked to surgery for treatment of low stage metastatic seminoma given its effectiveness in treating germ cell tumors.

2. Rationale for Retroperitoneal Lymph Node Dissection

Retroperitoneal lymph node dissection (RPLND) represents an attractive treatment option for metastatic seminoma mainly because of the surgery's well-established efficacy. In seminoma, RPLND is generally recommended for residual retroperitoneal masses >3 cm following risk-adapted chemotherapy. In nonseminomatous germ cell tumors (NSGCT), RPLND is a treatment option for patients with high-risk stage I

Table 1: Series of RPLND as primary treatment for seminoma.

Study	n	Stage	Type of RPLND	Discordant staging	Recurrence rate	Follow-up
Warszawski et al. [8]	63	I ($n=45$) IIA ($n=7$) IIB ($n=6$) IIC ($n=5$)	Open	24% 17.5% upstaged 6.3% downstaged	14% Stage I: 7% Stage IIA: 0% Stage IIB: 67% Stage IIC: 40%	79 mo
Mezvrishvili et al. [10]	14	I ($n=10$) IIA ($n=4$)	Open, nerve sparing	21% (all upstaged)	0%	56 mo
Hu et al. [11]	4	IIA ($n=3$) IIC ($n=1$)	Open, midline extraperitoneal, nerve sparing	50% 25% upstaged 25% downstaged	0%	25 mo
Lusch et al. [13]*	11	IIA and IIB	Open and robotic, nerve sparing	Not described	36%	18 mo

*Abstract.

disease and for residual retroperitoneal masses ≥1 cm following systemic chemotherapy for metastatic disease [4]. Importantly, it can be also the primary treatment for stage IIA NSGCT with negative serum tumor markers. Not only is the surgery therapeutic, but it offers accurate pathologic staging with up to 30% of patients with stage I NSGCT having occult metastases and up to 35% of patients with clinical stage IIA disease being downstaged to stage I disease [5].

There are several other reasons that make RPLND a logical treatment for seminoma. A major reason why the surgery has proven to be effective is because of the predictable pattern of lymphatic spread of germ cell cancers. Given that pure seminoma lacks choriocarcinoma, the histology known to spread hematogenously, this could theoretically make RPLND for seminoma even more efficacious. Additionally, physicians treating testicular cancer are already familiar with the procedure and the surgical morbidity continues to decrease. Template dissections and nerve-sparing approaches are established methods for preventing retrograde ejaculation. Newer techniques with laparoscopy or a midline, extraperitoneal approach can also minimize morbidity including decreases in blood loss and length of hospitalization [6, 7].

Lastly, XRT and chemotherapy have limitations. For example, patients with a horseshoe kidney, inflammatory bowel disease, or a history of radiotherapy are not good candidates for XRT. Those with renal insufficiency or pulmonary disease could be precluded from effective chemotherapy. In these cases, another treatment option could prove invaluable.

3. Retrospective Data

There have been four published studies that evaluate RPLND as a primary treatment for testicular seminoma (Table 1). The first study was reported by Warszawski and Schmucking in 1997 from Germany [8]. This study retrospectively reviewed the results of 63 patients with stage I and II seminoma after RPLND ($n=63$) from 1975 to 1985 and compared the results with patients who received XRT. Most patients had stage I seminoma ($n=45$), though some had stage IIA ($n=7$), IIB ($n=6$), and IIC ($n=5$) disease. Table 2 provides a review of stage II seminoma TNM staging [9].

Table 2: Stage II seminoma.

IIA	Any pT/Tx	N1	M0	S0 or S1
IIB	Any pT/Tx	N2	M0	S0 or S1
IIC	Any pT/Tx	N3	M0	S0 or S1

cN1 = metastases to single or multiple retroperitoneal lymph nodes ≤2 cm in size; cN2 = metastases to single or multiple retroperitoneal lymph nodes 2–5 cm in size; cN3 = metastases to single or multiple retroperitoneal lymph nodes >5 cm in size; pN1 = metastases to single or multiple retroperitoneal lymph nodes ≤2 cm in size, no more than 5 positive lymph nodes; pN2 = metastases to single or multiple retroperitoneal lymph nodes 2–5 cm in size, metastases to >5 lymph nodes with none >5 cm in size, extranodal extension; pN3 = metastases to single or multiple retroperitoneal lymph nodes >5 cm in size. Used with the permission of the American Joint Committee on Cancer (AJCC), Chicago, Illinois. The original source for this material is the AJCC Cancer Staging Manual, seventh edition (2010) published by Springer Science and Business Media LLC, www.springer.com.

In those with clinical stage I seminoma, there was a 17.5% incidence of occult retroperitoneal disease, in line with current relapse rates seen in surveillance series. In patients with stage II seminoma, 6.3% were downstaged. In patients with stage I or IIA seminoma, with a median follow-up of 79 months, there was a 5.7% recurrence rate. The surgery provided excellent regional control with all the recurrences being identified as out of the retroperitoneal field. The efficacy of RPLND with larger nodal disease (>2 cm) decreased, with 6/11 (55%) patients recurring in the retroperitoneum.

Though there was no statistical difference in recurrence rates or actuarial survival when comparing XRT to RPLND, the authors concluded that results of XRT "seem to be superior." One reason the authors cited was that the in-field recurrence rate was lower after XRT. When closely examining this, the recurrence rates varied drastically when stratified by clinical stage. Importantly, there were no in-field recurrences after RPLND for stage I and IIA seminoma, which was the same for XRT.

The first of the three more modern studies was by Mezvrishvili and Managadze [10]. They evaluated the outcomes of ten patients with high-risk stage I seminoma and four patients with stage IIA disease. Of the patients with stage I seminoma, there were three (30%) with retroperitoneal metastases at the time of surgery. All patients with clinical lymph node metastases had confirmation of disease after

TABLE 3: Prospective clinical trials of RPLND in seminoma.

	SEMS (Surgery in Early Metastatic Seminoma)	PRIMETEST (Trial to Evaluate Progression Free Survival with Primary Retroperitoneal Lymph-Node Dissection (pRPLND) Only in Patients with Seminomatous Testicular Germ Cell Tumors with Clinical Stage IIA/B)
Phase	II	II
Inclusion criteria	Testicular seminoma Retroperitoneal *lymph node 1–3 cm in size* No more than two enlarged lymph nodes	Testicular seminoma Inguinal, paraaortic, or retroperitoneal lymph nodes classified as local or regional unilateral metastasis Maximum dimensions of *lymph node metastasis 5 cm* Allow patients who have received single dose carboplatin for stage I seminoma
Exclusion criteria	Second primary malignancy History of radiation/chemotherapy	Prior scrotal or retroperitoneal surgery History of radiation/chemotherapy (other than carboplatin)
Serum tumor markers	Beta-HCG normal Allow LDH and AFP up to 1.5 times upper limit of normal	Exclude AFP elevation suspicious for NSGCT
Primary endpoint	2-year recurrence-free survival	3-year progression-free survival
Secondary endpoints	5-year recurrence-free survival Treatment-free survival (time free from radiotherapy or chemotherapy) Complication rate (long and short term)	Overall survival Quality of life Complication rate Long-term sequelae
Accrual goal	46	30
Start date	August 2015	June 2016
Target completion date	August 2020	June 2021
Number of institutions	9	1
Primary location	University of Southern California	Department of Urology, Heinrich-Heine University, Duesseldorf
Principal investigator	Siamak Daneshmand	Peter Albers

RPLND, and none underwent adjuvant treatment. With a mean follow-up of 56 months, they did not have any cases with local or distant recurrence.

Our group has reported on the outcomes of four patients with pure testicular seminoma after RPLND [11]. Three patients had clinical stage IIA seminoma, and one patient had clinical stage IIC disease, with a lymph node 5.5 cm in size. This patient had a presumed burned out primary tumor with scar with dystrophic calcification on the orchiectomy specimen. Patients underwent an open, modified-template RPLND through a midline, extraperitoneal approach [12]. All patients were discharged home on postoperative day 3. Three patients had pathologic stage IIA disease, and one had stage IIB due to a 2 cm lymph node with extranodal extension. No patients underwent adjuvant therapy. With a median follow-up of 25 months, there were no recurrences or deaths.

Lastly, Lusch et al. from Germany have recently presented a series on open or robotic RPLND in patients with stage IIA/B seminoma [13]. They identified 11 patients who underwent RPLND. Three of these patients (22%) received one cycle of carboplatin prior to RPLND. With a mean follow-up of 18 months, they had a 36% recurrence rate. One of the patients with recurrence had more advanced disease with clinical stage IIC disease, an initial lymph node metastasis >6 cm, and a clinically positive inguinal lymph node. All patients who recurred were salvaged with radiotherapy and chemotherapy, and 3 out of 4 have no evidence of disease.

Taken together, these studies include a total of 92 patients with stage I-IIC seminoma and 14 who experienced recurrence. The overall recurrence rate for all patients was 14% with patients having higher stage disease being at greater risk of recurrence.

4. Clinical Trials

This retrospective data has established promising oncologic benefit of RPLND in early stage seminoma. There are currently two active prospective clinical trials formally evaluating the efficacy of the surgery (Table 3).

4.1. SEMS. Our group has started the SEMS (Surgery in Early Metastatic Seminoma) trial, which is a multiinstitutional phase II trial of primary RPLND to treat testicular seminoma with isolated retroperitoneal metastases [14]. The main inclusion criteria are testicular seminomas with the presence of at least one retroperitoneal lymph node between 1 and 3 cm in size. No more than two lymph nodes can be clinically positive. Serum tumor markers may be mildly elevated. The lymphadenopathy can be identified at diagnosis or can represent recurrence in a patient originally diagnosed with stage I seminoma. The recurrence must be within 3 years of the cancer diagnosis in order to avoid enrolling those with late relapse that may represent a different biology.

The trial is currently open and accruing at 9 sites in the United States (University of Southern California, Loma Linda University, University of California San Francisco, Emory University, University of Chicago, Indiana University, Johns Hopkins, Mayo Clinic, and University of Oklahoma). The study has a primary endpoint of recurrence-free survival at 2 years. Secondary endpoints are recurrence-free survival at 5 years, percent of patients who can avoid XRT or systemic chemotherapy, and the complication rate of RPLND (short and long term). The estimated enrollment is 46 with a planned study completion date in the year 2020.

A clinical correlation in this study is utilization of PET scanning preoperatively. Though the established role of PET scanning in germ cell cancer is in postchemotherapy seminoma, it is often utilized in earlier stage disease. Patients undergoing RPLND will have a PET/CT scan done prior to surgery. These results will be compared with intraoperative lymph node pathology and may determine if this imaging modality has any utility in seminoma prior to chemotherapy.

4.2. PRIMETEST. The second study is PRIMETEST (Trial to Evaluate the Progression Free Survival with Primary Retroperitoneal Lymph-Node Dissection pRPLND Only in Patients with Seminomatous Testicular Germ Cell Tumors with Clinical Stage IIA/B) [15]. This study is based out of Heinrich-Heine University in Duesseldorf, Germany, and includes patients with testicular seminoma and retroperitoneal or inguinal lymphadenopathy with a maximum size of 5 cm. Only patients with unilateral disease are included in the study. The study includes those with multiple metastases as long as none is >5 cm. This trial also includes patients who experienced recurrence after a single dose of carboplatin chemotherapy.

Patients will undergo a modified-template RPLND, which can be done in the open fashion or laparoscopically with robotic assistance. The primary endpoint is progression-free survival at 3 years, and the study was designed to exclude a recurrence rate of >30% compared with standard treatment. Secondary endpoints include overall survival, complication rates, quality of life, long-term sequelae, and the rate of retrograde ejaculation. The study plans to accrue 30 patients with an estimated study completion of June 2021.

5. Limitations and Safety of RPLND

Given that RPLND for germ cell tumors have been performed since the early 1900's, the short- and long-term risks have been well documented [16, 17]. The long-term effects of the surgery include retrograde ejaculation, incisional hernia, and bowel obstruction. Most of the risk of surgery is associated with short-term complications including injury to retroperitoneal or peritoneal structures, ileus, bowel obstruction, chylous ascites, thromboembolism, and infection. We recently reported outcomes of our midline extraperitoneal approach to RPLND with no cases of ileus noted in 68 consecutive cases [6].

Some have expressed concern regarding the surgical planes with seminoma. The desmoplastic reaction after chemotherapy in seminoma can be intense and greatly increase the morbidity and technical difficulty of the surgery. This is secondary to the significant fibrosis that is seen with treatment of metastatic seminoma. However, from personal experience and reports from other surgeons who have performed these surgeries, the surgical planes in a primary RPLND for untreated seminoma are the same as would be encountered in NSGCT.

6. Managing Pathology after RPLND

A major benefit from surgery is that pathology can help inform management decisions. Ideally, RPLND will cure a large majority of patients while identifying those at high risk of recurrence. The high-risk patients can then be directed towards adjuvant treatments to further reduce recurrences. Factors such as lymph node positive count, lymph node size, and extranodal extension could become important in risk stratification.

In general, patients will fall into one of three categories after RPLND: those with more favorable pathology, those with the same pathology, and patients who have worse disease than anticipated. Those who are downstaged (e.g., stage I seminoma) could be placed on a less rigorous surveillance schedule. For the other two scenarios, it is important that the reasoning behind surgery be delineated early. In the SEMS trial, the rationale for RPLND is to give patients the opportunity to completely avoid XRT and chemotherapy, which is one of the secondary endpoints. This is the major reason why a ≤3 cm lymph node size was chosen. In patients with nonbulky lymphadenopathy, the data demonstrates that RPLND has a good chance of cure without adjuvant treatment. Therefore, if the pathology matches with the clinical stage, we feel that surveillance should be encouraged. However, in cases of upstaging, adjuvant treatment with chemotherapy can be considered. Chemotherapy is favored over XRT because chemotherapy can treat systemic disease and is preferred for higher stage disease.

The rationale behind the RPLND in the PRIMETEST trial is slightly different. This study hypothesizes that the 3-4 courses of chemotherapy for stage IIA or IIB seminoma is overtreatment. The investigators have selected a larger lymph node size of up to 5 cm, which will likely result in a higher recurrence rate. However, the investigators also hypothesize that a single, adjuvant dose of chemotherapy will reduce the recurrence risk with minimal long-term morbidity. If the recurrence rate from surgery is less than 30%, the investigators feel justified that RPLND with a short course of adjuvant chemotherapy will reduce morbidity. Additionally, they plan future studies to determine which patients can undergo surveillance and who should preferentially receive chemotherapy.

7. Conclusions

There are many reasons why RPLND represents a logical treatment for seminoma metastatic to the retroperitoneum. To date, there have been four retrospective studies that have shown promising results when RPLND is utilized as a primary treatment for early metastatic seminoma. As would be expected, recurrence rates seem to increase with larger retroperitoneal metastases. There are two active phase II clinical trials evaluating the recurrence-free survival of patients after a primary RPLND. The SEMS trial is multi-institutional effort in the United States that includes patients with lymph nodes 1–3 cm in size. The PRIMETEST trial from Germany includes patients with lymph nodes <5 cm in size. The results of these studies will help determine if patients with metastatic seminoma will have a treatment option with minimal long-term morbidity.

References

[1] J. Beyer, P. Albers, R. Altena et al., "Maintaining success, reducing treatment burden, focusing on survivorship: highlights from the third European consensus conference on diagnosis and treatment of germ-cell cancer," *Annals of Oncology*, vol. 24, no. 4, pp. 878–888, 2013.

[2] G. K. Zagars, M. T. Ballo, A. K. Lee, and S. S. Strom, "Mortality after cure of testicular seminoma," *Journal of Clinical Oncology*, vol. 22, no. 4, pp. 640–647, 2004.

[3] G. E. Hanks, T. Peters, and J. Owen, "Seminoma of the testis: long-term beneficial and deleterious results of radiation," *International Journal of Radiation Oncology, Biology, Physics*, vol. 24, no. 5, pp. 913–919, 1992.

[4] S. Daneshmand, P. Albers, S. D. Fossa et al., "Contemporary management of postchemotherapy testis cancer," *European Urology*, vol. 62, no. 5, pp. 867–876, 2012.

[5] K. Yadav, "Retroperitoneal lymph node dissection: an update in testicular malignancies," *Clinical and Translational Oncology*, vol. 19, no. 7, pp. 793–798, 2017.

[6] S. Syan-Bhanvadia, S. T. Bazargani, T. G. Clifford, J. Cai, G. Miranda, and S. Daneshmand, "Midline extraperitoneal approach to retroperitoneal lymph node dissection in testicular cancer: minimizing surgical morbidity," *European Urology*, vol. 72, no. 5, pp. 814–820, 2017.

[7] T. Kunit and G. Janetschek, "Minimally invasive retroperitoneal lymphadenectomy: current status," *Urologic Clinics of North America*, vol. 42, no. 3, pp. 321–329, 2015.

[8] N. Warszawski and M. Schmucking, "Relapses in early-stage testicular seminoma: radiation therapy versus retroperitoneal lymphadenectomy," *Scandinavian Journal of Urology and Nephrology*, vol. 31, no. 4, pp. 355–359, 1997.

[9] F. L. Greene, D. L. Page, and I. D. Fleming, *AJCC Cancer Staging Manual*, Springer, New York, NY, USA, 7th edition, 2010.

[10] Z. Mezvrishvili and L. Managadze, "Retroperitoneal lymph node dissection for high-risk stage I and stage IIA seminoma," *International Urology and Nephrology*, vol. 38, no. 3-4, pp. 615–619, 2006.

[11] B. Hu, S. Shah, S. Shojaei, and S. Daneshmand, "Retroperitoneal lymph node dissection as first-line treatment of node-positive seminoma," *Clinical Genitourinary Cancer*, vol. 13, no. 4, pp. e265–e269, 2015.

[12] P. Kim, S. Syan-Bhanvadia, H. Djaladat et al., "Midline extraperitoneal approach for retroperitoneal lymph node dissection for testicular germ cell tumor," *Urology*, vol. 80, no. 4, pp. 941–945, 2012.

[13] A. Lusch, L. Gerbaulet, C. Winter, and P. Albers, "Primary retroperitoneal lymph node dissection (RPLND) in stage IIA/B seminoma patients without adjuvant treatment: a phase II trial (PRIMETEST)," *Journal of Urology*, vol. 197, no. 4, pp. e1044–e1045, 2017.

[14] ClinicalTrials.gov, *Retroperitoneal Lymph Node Dissection in Treating Patients With Testicular Seminoma*, National Library of Medicine, Bethesda, MD, USA, 2017, http://www.clinicaltrials.gov/show/NCTNCT02537548.

[15] ClinicalTrials.gov, *Trial to Evaluate Progression Free Survival With Primary Retroperitoneal Lymph-node Dissection (pRPLND) Only in Patients With Seminomatous Testicular Germ Cell Tumors With Clinical Stage IIA/B (PRIMETEST)*, National Library of Medicine, Bethesda, MD, USA, 2017, http://www.clinicaltrials.gov/show/NCTNCT02797626.

[16] J. Baniel, R. S. Foster, R. G. Rowland, R. Bihrle, and J. P. Donohue, "Complications of primary retroperitoneal lymph node dissection," *Journal of Urology*, vol. 152, no. 2, pp. 424–427, 1994.

[17] A. Heidenreich, P. Albers, M. Hartmann et al., "Complications of primary nerve sparing retroperitoneal lymph node dissection for clinical stage I nonseminomatous germ cell tumors of the testis: experience of the German Testicular Cancer Study Group," *Journal of Urology*, vol. 169, no. 5, pp. 1710–1714, 2003.

26

Quality of Health Information on the Internet for Prostate Cancer

Dwayne T. S. Chang,[1] **Robert Abouassaly**,[2,3] **and Nathan Lawrentschuk**[4,5]

[1]*Department of Urology, Sir Charles Gairdner Hospital, WA, Australia*
[2]*Urology Institute, University Hospitals Case Medical Center, Cleveland, OH, USA*
[3]*Department of Surgery, Division of Urology, Louis Stokes Cleveland VA Medical Center, Cleveland, OH, USA*
[4]*Department of Urology, Austin Hospital, VIC, Australia*
[5]*Olivia Newton-John Cancer Research Institute, Austin Hospital, VIC, Australia*

Correspondence should be addressed to Dwayne T. S. Chang; dwayne.chang@health.wa.gov.au

Academic Editor: Kostis Gyftopoulos

Introduction. To compare (1) the quality of prostate cancer health information on the Internet, (2) the difference in quality between websites appearing earlier or later in the search, and (3) the sources of sponsorship for each of these websites. *Materials and methods.* The top 150 listed websites on the Google search engine for each of the 11 search terms related to prostate cancer were analysed. Quality was assessed on whether the website conforms to the principles of the Health On the Net Foundation. Each of these websites was then reviewed to determine the main source of sponsorship. Statistical analysis was performed to determine if the proportion of HON accreditation varied among the different cohorts of listed websites and among the 11 search terms used. *Results.* In total, 1650 websites were analysed. Among these, 10.5% websites were HON-accredited. The proportion of HON-accredited websites for individual search terms ranged from 3.3% to 19.3%. In comparison with the search term of "Prostate cancer," four search terms had statistically significant odds ratio of the rate of HON accreditation. Websites 51–150 were statistically less likely to have HON accreditation than websites 1–50. The top three website sponsors were journal/universities (28.8%), commercial (28.1%), and physician/surgeon (26.9%). *Conclusions.* The lack of validated and unbiased websites for prostate cancer is concerning especially with increasing use of the Internet for health information. Websites sponsored or managed by the government and national departments were most likely to provide impartial health information for prostate cancer. We need to help our patients identify valid and unbiased online health resources.

1. Introduction

Prostate cancer remains a huge burden in Australia and the United States of America (USA). In 2012, the age-standardised incidence rate of prostate cancer in Australia was 162.7 per 100,000 males, an increase from 137.4 per 100,000 in 2002 [1]. Australia also has a higher age-standardised incidence rate of prostate cancer than the World Health Organisation (WHO) world standard population and the USA in 2012 (162.7 vs. 119.5 vs. 108.4 per 100,000 males, respectively) [1, 2]. In the same period of time, the risk of diagnosis of prostate cancer rose from 1 in 10 to 1 in 7 in men before the age of 75 years [1]. Currently, more men are getting diagnosed with prostate cancer, so more will be seeking answers about their disease and the varied treatment options.

Patients are increasingly resorting to the Internet for medical information. An Australian study of nearly 3000 patients found that 63% of them accessed the Internet within the previous month with 28% seeking health information online and 17% obtained information in relation to medical conditions managed by their family practitioner at the time [3]. In that study, patients within the age group of 45–64 years were the second most likely cohort to obtain health information online, whereas those in the 65–74 years cohort were the fourth most likely [3]. In 2012, the highest incidence of prostate cancer diagnosis was in the 60–69 years age group [1]. A survey by Pai et al. on men with prostate cancer showed that not only were most of them knowledgeable with using the Internet, most men and their spouses/partners want to be able to access their health information over the Internet [4]. Better diagnostic tests have led to younger men being diagnosed with prostate cancer, and these men are more likely to use the Internet to obtain health information.

It is important to keep a level head when browsing through the ocean of health information on the Internet. Anyone in the world can easily set up a website and publish any form of data to be accessed by the mass of unknowing Internet users. The amount of unregulated and potentially biased information online may end up confusing lay users of the Internet [5]. Fortunately, services are available to direct Internet users towards trustworthy online health information. One of the earliest examples is the Health On the Net (HON) Foundation, which is a nonprofit and nongovernmental organisation found in 1995 from a collaboration of the WHO and prominent physicians and scientists all over the world [6]. This organisation certifies websites that provide objective and transparent health information and is currently one of the most widely accepted certification tools in use [6].

Our objectives in this study were to compare (1) the quality of health information on the Internet relating to prostate cancer, (2) the difference in quality between websites appearing earlier or later in the search, and (3) the sources of sponsorship for each of these websites.

2. Materials and Methods

We used a tried and tested methodology as previously described in other studies [7–10]. The Google search engine (http://www.google.com) was used to search for 11 keywords related to prostate cancer. These keywords were "Prostate cancer;" "Prostate specific antigen" (PSA); "Transrectal prostate biopsy;" "Transperineal prostate biopsy," "MRI prostate;" "Prostate-specific membrane antigen" (PSMA); "Radical prostatectomy;" "Robotic prostatectomy;" "Prostate radiotherapy;" "Prostate chemotherapy;" and "Prostate cancer hormone therapy." Throughout this entire study, "sponsored links" presented by the Google search engine anywhere on the search page or under a banner were not included in the list of websites analysed.

Sponsorship of each website was analysed and categorised in a similar way to previous studies on the quality of health information on the Internet [7–9]. These categories were (i) journal/university institutions (e.g., scientific journals and University of Oxford), (ii) nonprofit organisations (e.g., Prostate Cancer Foundation of Australia and Cancer Council Australia), (iii) governmental/national institutions (e.g., Healthdirect Australia and World Health Organisation), (iv) commercial (e.g., da Vinci Surgery and GlaxoSmithKline), (v) physician/surgeon (including their corresponding professional organisations, e.g., American Urological Association), (vi) nondoctor health professionals (such as naturopaths), and (vii) others (e.g., personal blogs with no other affiliations). If the source of sponsorship was not obviously apparent, such as a website with multiple types of sponsors, the website was explored by all authors until the primary source of sponsorship could be determined.

The first 150 websites found from each search were selected to be analysed. The HON Foundation's HONcode web browser toolbar (available from http://www.hon.ch/) was used on a personal computer. An indicator on the toolbar lights up automatically if the website viewed is currently accredited by the HON Foundation. The HONcode toolbar was used in several studies and was found to be a valid and reliable tool [7–10].

For quality control, nonaccredited websites found for the search term "Prostate cancer" were individually evaluated to determine HON Foundation principles [11] were adhered to and then compared to the findings from using the automated HONcode web browser toolbar. The HON Foundation reviewed each website according to their published principles [11] which includes authority of the authors, complementarity of the information, privacy of submitted personal data, attribution of information to sources, justifiability of information, transparency, financial disclosure, and advertising policy of websites.

The first 150 websites found for each term were divided into tertiles (first, middle, and last 50 search results). The proportion of HON-accredited websites within each tertile was analysed and compared using the chi-squared test. This analysis determines whether HON-accredited websites were more likely to appear in the first, middle, or last tertile of search results. The proportions of accredited websites were compared across search terms and languages using the chi-squared test (or Fisher exact tests when cell counts were less than five). All statistical tests were two-sided, and statistical significance was defined as $P < 0.05$. Univariate logistic regression analysis was performed using the variables of search terms and tertiles of search results. The referent group for search terms was the word "prostate cancer" as it was the base search term. The referent group for tertiles 2 and 3 was tertile 1 (the first 50 websites) as it had the highest proportion of HON-accredited websites. Odds ratios and 95% confidence intervals were calculated from the logistic regression analysis. Analyses were performed using SAS 9.3 (SAS Institute Inc., Cary, NC, USA).

3. Results

In total, 1650 websites were analysed. Among these, 173 (10.5%) websites were HON-accredited. Less than 10% of search results were made up of HON-accredited websites in six out of the 11 searched terms. The proportion of HON-accredited websites for individual search terms ranged from 3.3% (robotic prostatectomy) to 19.3% (prostate cancer hormone therapy) (Table 1). In comparison with the search term of "Prostate cancer", four search terms had statistically significant odds ratio of the rate of HON accreditation (Table 2). The proportion of HON-accredited websites decreased progressively from tertiles 1 to 3 (Figure 1). Websites in tertiles 2 and 3 were more likely to have lower rates of HON accreditation than websites in tertile 1, and this achieved statistical significance (Table 2). The rates of website sponsors in descending frequency were journal/

Table 1: Rates of HON-accredited websites among the search terms.

Search term	Total websites	HON+	HON−	%HON+ (%)
Prostate cancer	21700000	23	127	15.3
Prostate specific antigen	1580000	23	127	15.3
Transrectal prostate biopsy	177000	12	138	8.0
Transperineal prostate biopsy	38900	14	136	9.3
MRI prostate	7710000	9	141	6.0
Prostate-specific membrane antigen	835000	6	144	4.0
Radical prostatectomy	687000	18	132	12.0
Robotic prostatectomy	437000	5	145	3.3
Prostate radiotherapy	2260000	14	136	9.3
Prostate chemotherapy	23100000	20	130	13.3
Prostate cancer hormone therapy	1710000	29	121	19.3

Note. HON+, HON-accredited; HON−, non-HON-accredited; %HON+, percentage of HON-accredited websites out of a total of 150 websites for each search term.

Table 2: Univariate logistic regression analysis showing odds ratio estimates comparing search terms to "Prostate cancer" and tertiles 2 and 3 against tertile 1.

Odds ratio comparison	Point estimate	95% confidence interval limits	
PSA vs. Prostate cancer	1.00	0.53	1.89
*Transrectal prostate biopsy vs. Prostate cancer	2.12	1.01	4.47
Transperineal prostate biopsy vs. Prostate cancer	1.79	0.87	3.65
*MRI prostate vs. Prostate cancer	2.90	1.29	6.56
*PSMA vs. Prostate cancer	4.47	1.75	11.40
Radical prostatectomy vs. Prostate cancer	1.34	0.68	2.62
*Robotic prostatectomy vs. Prostate cancer	5.41	1.98	14.73
Prostate radiotherapy vs. Prostate cancer	1.79	0.87	3.65
Prostate chemotherapy vs. Prostate cancer	1.18	0.61	2.28
Prostate cancer hormone therapy vs. Prostate cancer	0.75	0.41	1.38
*Tertile 2 vs. tertile 1	2.04	1.36	3.07
*Tertile 3 vs. tertile 1	3.22	2.03	5.11

Note. *Statistically significant difference (95% confidence interval not crossing the value of 1).

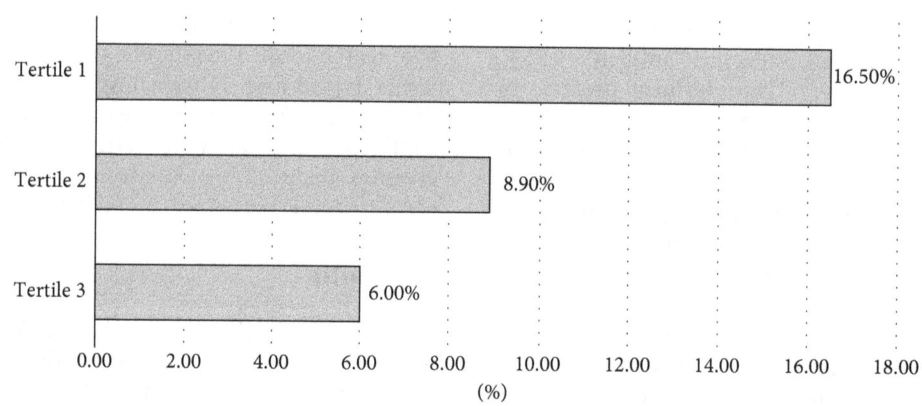

Figure 1: Rates of HON-accredited websites within each tertile group. *Note.* Tertile 1, websites 1–50; Tertile 2, websites 51–100; Tertile 3, websites 101–150.

universities (28.8%), commercial (28.1%), physician/surgeon (26.9%), nonprofit organisations (8.0%), governmental/national institutions (6.7%), others (1.27%), and non-doctor health professionals (0.2%). Among the various sources of sponsorship, websites sponsored by governmental/national department sources had the highest rate of HON accreditation (26.4%) followed by those sponsored by non-doctor health professionals (25.0%), nonprofit organisations (12.9%), and commercial sources (12.3%) (Figure 2). Although websites sponsored by nondoctor health professionals ranked highly, there were a total of only four of such websites found in this search, and only one was HON-accredited. The number of HON-accredited websites found by manually applying the HON Foundation principles correlated with the number found via using the automated HONcode web browser toolbar.

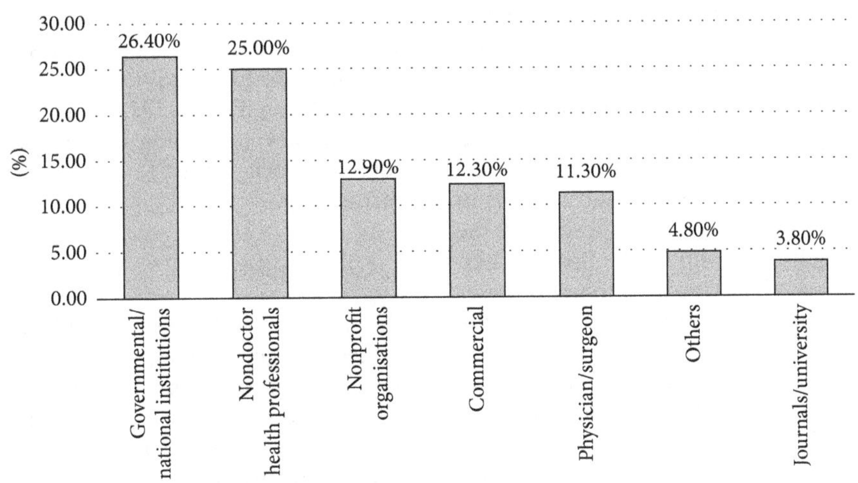

FIGURE 2: Rates of HON accreditation for various types of sponsorship.

4. Discussion

A staggering finding was that even after accounting for overlap of websites that are relevant with more than one search term, there were at least more than 21 million websites relating to prostate cancer (Table 1). It is difficult to imagine that a lay person would be able to keep a level head and critically appraise each website with the vast amount of unfiltered information available. A silver lining is that the proportion of HON-accredited websites is slowly growing. In a similar study done previously [8], the number of HON-accredited websites among the first 150 listed in the search term "prostate cancer" was 13 in 2004, 18 in 2009, and 23 in this study in 2016. This shows a steady growth of approximately one extra HON-accredited website each year in the past 12 years in the first 150 listed websites for the search term "prostate cancer."

Overall, less than one in nine websites found in this study had HON accreditation. Such a low proportion can make it difficult for our patients to safely delineate fact from fiction on these websites and may promote distrust by physicians of cancer resources from the Internet. Previous studies in 2004–2010 found the rate of HON accreditation to range from 10% to 29% [8, 9]. It is interesting that the overall proportion of HON-accredited websites have lessened. Theories for this include growth of new unaccredited websites outpacing the accredited ones, "drop-out" or discontinuation of previously HON-accredited websites, and unaccredited websites achieving higher user traffic than accredited websites. Furthermore, four search terms had statistically different odds ratio of HON accreditation. This means selecting the right search term can result in a list of websites with a greater proportion of HON accreditation, and vice versa.

A reassuring finding was that more than a quarter of all websites sponsored by governmental/national institution sources were accredited by the HON Foundation. Although websites sponsored by commercial sources accounted for more than a quarter of all websites in this study, the rate of HON accreditation among them ranked fourth (less than one in eight). Interestingly, the same applied to websites sponsored by journals/universities which were slightly more common than commercial-type websites but fared much worse in the rate of HON accreditation (less than one in 25 websites). As governmental/national department and journal/university sponsors typically have strong financial backing, the reason for the lower rate of HON accreditation with journal/university-sponsored websites may be related to being unaware of this service and its associated benefits rather than financial cost.

In this study, there were nearly as many commercial websites as journal/university sources, which was the most prevalent. This can be disadvantageous to us as doctors as commercial websites have just as much exposure to the general public on the online search. It is then up to the patient to decide which website to read, and branding of websites may influence this process as readers may opt for articles by familiar sources. It was demonstrated that the general public in Australia were more familiar with simpler brands containing the words, "general practitioner," "research," and "prostate cancer," instead of the one containing "urological" [12]. They also had limited understanding of the role of urologists in prostate cancer and the central organisation that Australian urologists belong to [12]. There may be a role for adding further clarity to the brand names of national urological associations to illustrate the key services we provide [12]. We as doctors should also act as custodians of evidence-based knowledge. One such custodian for urologists is the BJU International journal which centralises quality evidence-based urological knowledge. For example, this journal has key papers in the myriad of localised and systemic [13] treatment of prostate cancer, such as active surveillance [14], robotic prostatectomy [15], brachytherapy [16], and even alternative treatments like phytotherapy [17]. In the same way, reputable organisations can summarise evidence-based knowledge into a centralised online library in simple language so that our patients do not have to sift through the ocean of unsorted information on the Internet.

We used the Google search engine as it is the most widely used search engine; therefore, it is the one most likely to be used by our patients for whom we conducted this study for. There are other Internet search engine services available. Each of them uses different mechanics or algorithms to search for relevant websites; thus, the order of listed websites may differ even if the same study methodology is performed using a different search engine. In addition, specific alterations can be made to the website structure and content to artificially increase the relevance factor in the eye of the search engine thus placing it higher up on the list of search results. Furthermore, the search engine or Internet browser may analyse the history of previous Internet searches on the device and customise future search results to match it. To minimise this effect, we deleted all website and Internet browser information cookies and data cache prior to conducting the Internet search. However, not all patients may take this extra precaution routinely and may end up with search results influenced by their previous use of the search engine and Internet browser. For example, if the user had a significant history of using the device for online shopping, their search for websites relating to prostate cancer may favour commercially oriented websites instead of educational ones.

Several non-modifiable limitations were present in this study. The order of website listing on a search engine result depends on the real-time popularity of each website, and this may change on a daily basis. Theoretically, it is possible for a website ranked 99 today to be ranked 101 tomorrow thus causing movement of websites between tertile groups. There may also be a risk of false negatives as not all websites without HON accreditation provide biased or invalid information. This may simply be due to lack of awareness of the existence of this service or the financial cost of maintaining HON certification. HON accreditation is free of charge for the first year but subsequent to that there is an annual membership fee to renew and extend the HON certification. The type and popularity of each website will determine the amount of fee charged, which usually ranges between EUR50 and EUR325 per year [18]. However, renewal of HON accreditation does not automatically happen after payment of membership fee; essentially, there is no blind renewal of HON certification. Every year, each member website will be reviewed by a team from the HON Foundation and if they find that the website has deviated from the HON principles, the payment will be refunded and certification revoked [18].

To readers from the general population, we advise to use general and less-complicated search terms as from our experience, this may allow the search engine to present a better representation of relevant websites. For example, searching for "prostate cancer test" will result in a lot more search results than searching for "prostate cancer PSA, MRI scan" as websites with PSA-only or MRI-only information may not be listed higher on the search even if they happen to provide valid information. We also advise to select the first 50 websites of the search which, in our study, has a higher proportion of websites with unbiased information. It is also a good idea to focus on websites by educational institutions, governmental organisations, and scientific journals which tend to be unbiased. Websites by doctors need to be critically assessed to determine as some are meant to promote or publicise their services and others have the sincere aim of educating the general public. Another important tip is that most websites have an "About us/this organisation" webpage which is key to finding out whether these websites hold potential bias due to their sponsorship source or partnership.

5. Conclusions

The lack of validated and unbiased websites for prostate cancer is concerning especially with the rise in Internet use for health information by patients and physicians alike. Although there was slow growth in the number of HON-accredited websites in the main search term of "prostate cancer," the overall proportion of HON-accredited websites was still very low. Websites sponsored or managed by the government and national departments were the most likely to provide impartial health information for prostate cancer. We can help our patients identify valid and unbiased health resources. We need to act as custodians of valid information by creating online libraries of valid information or direct our patients to these sources.

References

[1] Australian Institute of Health and Welfare, "Australian cancer incidence and mortality (ACIM) books: prostate cancer," AIHW, Canberra, Australia, June 2017, http://www.aihw.gov.au/acim-books.

[2] U.S. Cancer Statistics Working Group. United States Cancer Statistics, "1999–2013 incidence and mortality web-based report," Atlanta, U.S. Department of Health and Human Services, Centers for Disease Control and Prevention and National Cancer Institute, Atlanta, GA, USA, June 2017, https://nccd.cdc.gov/uscs/toptencancers.aspx.

[3] C. Wong, C. Harrison, H. Britt, and J. Henderson, "Patient use of the internet for health information," *Australian Family Physician*, vol. 43, no. 12, pp. 875–7, 2014.

[4] H. H. Pai and F. Lau, "Web-based electronic health information systems for prostate cancer patients," *Canadian Journal of Urology*, vol. 12, no. 3, pp. 2700–2709, 2005.

[5] L. G. Gomella, "Doctor google and the internet prescription," *Canadian Journal of Urology*, vol. 17, no. 1, p. 4971, 2010.

[6] Health on the Net Foundation, "About HON (internet)," Health on the Net Foundation, Geneva, Switzerland, June 2017, http://www.hon.ch/Global/.

[7] D. T. S. Chang, R. Abouassaly, and N. Lawrentschuk, "Quality of health information on the Internet for urolithiasis on the Google search engine," *Advances in Urology*, vol. 2016, Article ID 8243095, 5 pages, 2016.

[8] N. Lawrentschuk, R. Abouassaly, N. Hackett, R. Groll, and N. E. Fleshner, "Health information quality on the internet in urological oncology: a multilingual longitudinal evaluation," *Urology*, vol. 74, no. 5, pp. 1058–63, 2009.

[9] N. Lawrentschuk, D. Sasges, R. Tasevski, R. Abouassaly, A. M. Scott, and I. D. Davis, "Oncology health information quality on the Internet: a multilingual evaluation," *Annals of Surgical Oncology*, vol. 19, no. 3, pp. 706–713, 2012.

[10] E. C. Chen, R. P. Manecksha, R. Abouassaly, D. M. Bolton, O. Reich, and N. Lawrentschuk, "A multilingual evaluation of current health information on the Internet for the treatments of benign prostatic hyperplasia," *Prostate International*, vol. 2, no. 4, pp. 161–168, 2014.

[11] Health on the Net Foundation, "HONcode," Health on the Net Foundation, Geneva, Switzerland, June 2017, http://www.hon.ch/HONcode/Pro/Conduct.html.

[12] T. R. Gianduzzo, R. A. Gardiner, P. Rashid, R. Young, M. Frydenberg, and S. Kelly, "Impact of branding on public awareness of healthcare-related governing bodies: a pilot study of the Urological Society of Australia and New Zealand brand," *BJU International*, vol. 118, no. 3, pp. 23–29, 2016.

[13] J. Corfield, J. Crozier, A. Joshua, D. Bolton, and N. Lawrentschuck, "Understanding the role of new systemic agents in the treatment of prostate cancer," *BJU International*, vol. 118, no. 3, pp. 8–13, 2016.

[14] S. Liu, S. Lee, P. Rashid et al., "Active surveillance is suitable for intermediate term follow-up of renal oncocytoma diagnosed by percutaneous core biopsy," *BJU International*, vol. 118, no. 3, pp. 30–34, 2016.

[15] M. W. Louie-Johnsun, M. M. Handmer, R. J. Calopedos et al., "The Australian laparoscopic non robotic radical prostatectomy experience—analysis of 2943 cases (USANZ supplement)," *BJU International*, vol. 118, no. 3, pp. 43–48, 2016.

[16] M. W. Chao, P. Grimm, J. Yaxley, R. Jagavkar, M. Ng, and N. Lawrentschuk, "Brachytherapy: state-of-the-art radiotherapy in prostate cancer," *BJU International*, vol. 116, no. 3, pp. 80–88, 2015.

[17] M. D. van Die, K. M. Bone, J. Emery, S. G. Williams, M. V. Pirotta, and C. J. Paller, "Phytotherapeutic interventions in the management of biochemically recurrent prostate cancer: a systematic review of randomised trials," *BJU International*, vol. 117, no. 4, pp. 17–34, 2016.

[18] Health on the Net Foundation, "About the HONcode reassessment payment process," Health on the Net Foundation, Geneva, Switzerland, June 2017, http://www.hon.ch/HONcode/Webmasters/reassessment.html.

Undescended Testes and Laparoscopy: Experience from the Developing World

Shabir Ahmad Dar,[1] Rajandeep Singh Bali,[2] Yawar Zahoor,[3] Arshad Rashid Kema,[4] and Rajni Bhardwaj[2]

[1]MS General Surgery, Resident Surgeon, SKIMS, Jammu and Kashmir, India
[2]MS General Surgery, Consultant Surgeon, GMC-Jammu, Jammu and Kashmir, India
[3]MS General Surgery, Resident Surgeon, MAMC, Delhi, India
[4]MS General Surgery, Consultant Surgeon, DHSK, Jammu and Kashmir, India

Correspondence should be addressed to Rajandeep Singh Bali; rajandeepbali@gmail.com

Academic Editor: Walid A. Farhat

Background. Cryptorchidism or undescended testes is the most common disorder of the male endocrine glands in children. With the advancements in laparoscopic techniques and instruments, laparoscopic orchidopexy has become the standard procedure in the management of nonpalpable undescended testes. *Aim.* To evaluate and determine the therapeutic role, sensitivity, and specificity of laparoscopy in localizing nonpalpable testes and the mean operative time, the conversion rate (and reasons thereof), postoperative wound infection, postoperative stay, and time taken for return to daily activities following laparoscopic orchidopexy or orchidectomy. *Materials and Methods.* This was a prospective study carried out in the Postgraduate Department of Surgery, Government Medical College, Srinagar, J&K, India, from May 2008 to August 2011. All patients who presented to the outpatient department with complaints of absent testes were examined, and the ones with nonpalpable testes were included in the study. *Results.* The mean operative time for bilateral and unilateral nonpalpable testis was 102.76 and 53.67 minutes, respectively. Minor postoperative wound infections were noted in 4 of our patients. Mean duration of hospital stay was 14.23 hrs for unilateral cases and 16.27 hrs for bilateral cases. Patients who underwent laparoscopic orchidopexy resumed their normal activities within 4 ± 1 days. *Conclusion.* Laparoscopy clearly demonstrates the anatomy and provides visual information upon which a definitive decision can be made for further management of the undescended nonpalpable testis.

1. Introduction

Cryptorchidism or undescended testes is the most common disorder of the male endocrine glands in children. Physical examination of the testis can be difficult, and further evaluation should be considered if a normal testis cannot be definitely identified. Reasons for treatment of cryptorchidism are increased infertility, testicular malignancy, testicular torsion, trauma, and psychological stigma of an empty scrotum [1].

About 1% incidence of cryptorchidism is reported by 1 year of age, and about 20% of children with cryptorchidism may have one or both nonpalpable testes. The condition of the nonpalpable testis may fall into one of the following categories: agenesis, vanishing testis, intra-abdominal testes, or inguinal testes [2]. Although there are various imaging studies, i.e., ultrasonography, CT, and MRI, have been used to locate nonpalpable testes in boys, none has been able to provide comparable accuracy to laparoscopy [3]. In experienced hands, laparoscopy is capable of providing 100% accuracy in the diagnosis of the intra-abdominal testis with minimal morbidity. With the advancements in laparoscopic techniques and instruments, laparoscopic orchidopexy has become a standard procedure in the management of nonpalpable undescended testes.

Approximately two-thirds of neonates born with an undescended testis will undergo spontaneous testicular descent, typically by 4 to 6 months postnatally, mediated by postnatal testosterone surge [4]. Approximately 20% of all cryptochoid testes are nonpalpable. Of all childhood testes that are nonpalpable, 50 to 60 percent are intra-abdominal but can also be found in the inguinal canal (canalicular) or just inside the internal ring (peeping) [5].

Majority of the intra-abdominal testes are located less than 2 cm from the internal ring. The intra-abdominal testis may be associated with a closed or an open deep inguinal ring. In the closed ring variant, the processus vaginalis does not develop, the gubernaculum is absent, and the internal ring is closed. In the open ring variant, a patent processus vaginalis exists in the internal inguinal ring and the gubernaculum is present. Vanishing testis is one in which testicular vessels and vas deferens are found on surgical exploration but a testis is absent. Supporting evidence for testicular infarction includes the common finding of hemosiderin, and calcium deposits in testicular remnants found on exploration [6]. One in 600 males has bilateral undescended testes, representing 10 to 25% of patients with cryptorchidism. The finding of bilateral nonpalpable testes however represents a special situation that may warrant further investigations to rule out intersex abnormalities which may have life-threatening implications in the neonatal period, especially associated with severe hypospadias.

2. Aim

This study entailed the following aims and objectives:

(1) To determine the sensitivity and specificity of laparoscopy in localizing nonpalpable testes

(2) To evaluate the therapeutic role of laparoscopy in nonpalpable testes

(3) To determine the mean operative time, the conversion rate (and reasons thereof), postoperative wound infection, postoperative stay, and time taken for return to activities of daily life

3. Materials and Methods

This was a prospective study carried out in the Postgraduate Department of Surgery, Government Medical College, Srinagar, from May 2008 to August 2011. All patients who presented to the outpatient department with complaints of absent testes were examined, and boys with nonpalpable testes were included in the study. These boys were examined as outpatients, at the time of admission and after general anesthesia to exclude palpable testes. Patients with nonpalpable testes were subjected to diagnostic and operative laparoscopy. The primary 5 mm camera port was introduced by open technique (inferior rim of the umbilicus on its internal surface), pneumoperitoneum was created (10 mmHg) with the patient in a 30° head-down Trendelenburg position, the area of the internal inguinal ring was inspected bilaterally, and subsequent trocars (all 5 mm) were placed under laparoscopic (30° telescope) visualization into the right and left lumbar region in line with the umbilical port. Subsequent surgery was planned according to the laparoscopic findings following the algorithm for the management of the nonpalpable testis (Figure 1).

A diagnostic laparoscopy was done for rest of the abdominal quadrants in all cases. The inguinal ring was first examined to evaluate its patency, and then the bilateral iliac areas and pelvis were inspected. If intra-abdominal blind ending cord structures were found, no further exploration was performed, and a diagnosis of intra-abdominal vanishing testes was made.

If an intra-abdominal testis was found, it was classified as high (in the iliac fossa or pelvic inlet or pelvis >2 cm from the internal ring) or low (adjacent to the internal ring/emergent testis <2 cm from the internal ring) depending on its position to the internal ring.

With gentle traction on the testis, the most distal gubernacular attachment was divided with electric hook cautery, and gubernaculum was used as a handle for mobilizing the testis. Once the testis had been adequately mobilized, confirmed by performing stretch maneuver where the testes are stretched to the contralateral deep inguinal ring, the dissection was further carried out medially all around the ipsilateral deep inguinal ring to complete the herniotomy. Peritoneal coverage between the vas deferens and urinary bladder was dissected. Usually, a neotunnel was created between the medial umbilical ligament and the inferior epigastric artery (Prentiss maneuver) to gain extra length for reaching the scrotum. The blunt tip of the laparoscopic dissector was passed over the pubic bone into the ipsilateral hemiscrotum, thus creating a pathway. A dartos pouch was prepared in the hemiscrotum. A suction cannula was passed along the passage which was created transabdominally by laparoscopic dissector, and grasping the tip of the suction cannula, a long curved clamp was passed into the abdominal cavity and stretched in all directions to create adequate passage for bringing the testes down. The gubernacular tissue was grasped and pulled, thus delivering the testes out into the scrotal dartos pouch, and the length was checked by deflating the abdomen. Releasing the pneumoperitoneum gave additional length. Any tension found on the pedicle was released by further mobilization of the peritoneal flaps. Testes were fixed in the scrotum using 5-0 chromic catgut suture. At the end of the procedure, the abdomen was examined for any bleeding, the pneumoperitoneum was released, and trocars were removed. Trocar sites were closed. Children were discharged home next day. All the patients were followed at 6 weeks and 6 months.

4. Results

We used diagnostic and operative laparoscopy in the management of 52 patients with 61 undescended testes. 26 patients had 28 palpable testes (45%), and 26 patients had 33 nonpalpable testes (55%). Boys with the palpable testis at any point were excluded from the study. The study sample size of our series was 26 patients with 33 nonpalpable testes. Ratio of palpable testis to nonpalpable testis was 1:1.17, respectively.

The youngest and the eldest patient in our study group were 1 and 18 years of age, respectively. Majority of patients,

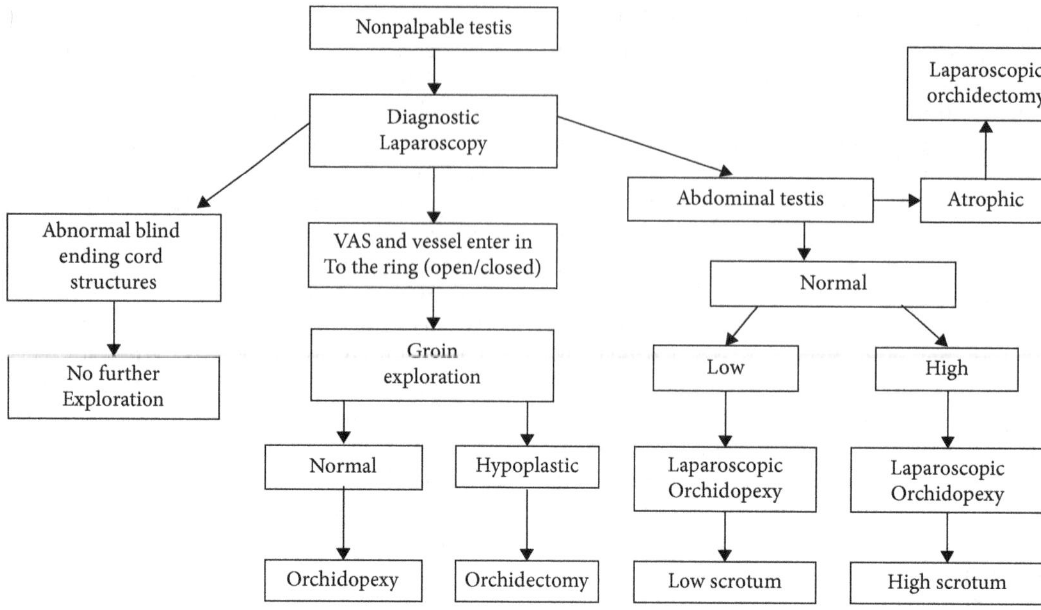

FIGURE 1: Algorithm for the management of nonpalpable undescended testes.

i.e., 12, were in the age group of 4–7 years. Of these 33 nonpalpable testes, 7 (21%) were on the right side, 12 (36%) on the left side, and 14 (42%) bilateral. On ultrasonography, nonpalpable testes were localized at various sites as intra-abdominally (3 cm proximal to deep inguinal ring), near deep inguinal ring, in inguinal canal, and in superficial inguinal pouch and could not be localized in 11 (33.33%), 9 (27.2%), 3 (9%), 3 (9%), and 7 (21.2%) cases, respectively.

Table 1 shows the relation of testis to deep inguinal ring as confirmed on diagnostic laparoscopy (n = 33).

On diagnostic laparoscopy, the deep inguinal ring was found to be open or closed in 30 (90.9%) and 3 (9.1%) cases, respectively. The number of testes found normal on diagnostic laparoscopy was 18 (54.5%) followed by 11 hypoplastic (33.3%) and 3 atrophic (9.09%) testes. Blind ending vas deferens and vessels (vanishing testis) were found in 1 (3.03%) patient only.

Majority of high intra-abdominal testis were hypoplastic (58.8%), highlighting the deleterious effect of increased abdominal temperature on development of the testis.

Table 2 shows the morphology of the undescended nonpalpable testis in relation to its position as determined by diagnostic laparoscopy.

The operative procedures performed were laparoscopic orchidopexy, laparoscopic orchidectomy, open orchidopexy (conversion), open orchidectomy (conversion), and diagnostic laparoscopy in 24 (72.7%), 5 (15.1%), 2 (6.06%), and 1 (3.03%) cases, respectively. All of the patients were managed by single-stage procedure.

Laparoscopy was successful (diagnostic or therapeutic) in 30 (90.90%) cases, and the procedures included laparoscopic orchidopexy, laparoscopic orchidectomy, and diagnostic laparoscopy. Mean operative time for 14 bilateral undescended testes was 102.76 (with SD of 2.37 and SEM of 5.08) minutes while as for 19 unilateral cases, it was 53.67 (with SD of 5.38 and SEM of 4.02) minutes.

TABLE 1

S. No.	Position of testis on diagnostic laparoscopy	Number
1.	<2 cm from deep ring (low intra-abdominal)	17 (51.5%)
2.	>2 cm from deep ring (high intra-abdominal)	12 (36.3%)
3.	Blind ending vas and vessels	1 (3.03%)
4.	Vas and vessels entering deep ring	3 (9.09%)

Postoperative complications included surgical emphysema [2], type 1 surgical site infection [1], and scrotal hematoma [1]. The average postoperative hospital stay was 14.23 hours (SD 2.37 hours) for unilateral undescended nonpalpable testes and 16.27 hours (SD 5.38 hours) for bilateral undescended nonpalpable testes. Most of our patients were discharged on next day because no immediate postoperative surgical complications were seen. Time taken to return to daily activities was more in patients who underwent orchidopexy (4 ± 1 days) as compared to patients who underwent orchidectomy (2 ± 1 days).

5. Discussion

The median age group of our study subjects was 5.2 years with patients from 1 to 18 years of age included in our study. Satar and Hvistendahl have reported similar median age group in their respective studies as 5.4 and 5.7 years [7, 8].

42% of our patients had bilateral undescended testis, and the incidence of bilateral undescended testis was relatively higher as compared to those reported by Ismail (13.5%), Zubair (33%), and Hassan (21%) [9–11]. This could be explained by the fact that our hospital is the main referral

Table 2

Diagnostic laparoscopy findings	Number of testis	Morphology of testis (n)	%
High intra-abdominal testis	17	Normal (4)	23.5
		Hypoplastic (10)	58.8
		Atropic (3)	17.6
Low intra-abdominal testis	12	Normal (11)	91.6
		Hypoplastic(1)	9.4
Blind ending vas and vessels	1	No testis found (1)	100
Vas and vessels entering the deep ring	3	Normal testis (3)	100

centre for laparoscopy and that our patients presented early as compared with other studies.

The USG (abdomen) could localize 78.78% of nonpalpable testes in our study. Ismail reported that USG was helpful in localization of the nonpalpable testis in 100% of his patients, as he used colour Doppler USG in his study [9].

We found the diagnostic yield of laparoscopy was 100% and the therapeutic yield was 96.9%, as we could localize and manage 32 nonpalpable testes while one case was diagnosed as vanishing testes on laparoscopy. El-Gohary has reported 100% accuracy in laparoscopic assessment of the testis [12].

The closed deep inguinal ring with vas deferens and vessels traversing it were found in 28% of our study subjects. The significance of this fact was that these patients had testis in the superficial inguinal pouch (ectopic testis). Godbole (33%) and Masao (35%) have also reported similar findings of the closed deep inguinal ring from their studies [13, 14].

Our study revealed normal testes in 54.5% of cases followed by hypoplastic testes in 33.3% of cases. Morphology of testis was correlated with localization of testis which revealed that features of hypoplasia were high in intra-abdominal testis. Similar findings were noted in the study of Humphery and Boekmann [5, 15]. One patient (3%) in our study had vanishing testis, confirmed upon diagnostic laparoscopy which saved the patient from unnecessary groin exploration, as has been suggested by Koyama et al. [2].

We performed orchidopexy in 26 out of 33 nonpalpable testes (78%) out of which laparoscopic orchidopexy was done in 24 (72.7%) testis, and conversion to open orchidopexy was necessitated in 2 (6.06%). The reasons for conversion were dense adhesions of testis with surrounding structures. Orchidectomy was done in 6 (18%), of which 3 testes were atrophic and 3 testes were hypoplastic (could not be mobilized adequately as determined by the stretch test). Masao and Khan et al. have reported laparoscopic orchidopexy in 33% and 35% cases [14, 16]. The high percentage of successful laparoscopic orchidopexy in our study can be explained by the fact that 96% of testis in our study were intra-abdominal or intracanalicular; moreover, the number of vanishing testis (3%) in our study group was much lower as reported by Humphrey (19%), Ismail (9%), and Hassan (38%) [5, 9, 11].

The mean operative time in our study was 53.67 minutes (SD of 2.37 minutes) for unilateral testis and 102.76 minutes (SD of 5.38 minutes) for bilateral nonpalpable testis. Mark and Davidson reported 15 minutes as average time for laparoscopy in unilateral nonpalpable testis [17]. As our study was the first of its kind at our institution and because of the learning curve of pediatric laparoscopy, operative time was relatively more in our study.

No major surgical complications were observed in our patients. Postoperative surgical emphysema was seen in 2 of our cases, which resolved spontaneously. One of our patients developed superficial surgical site infection, and one patient developed scrotal hematoma. The patients were on regular follow-up. No evidence of testicular atrophy was seen in those patients with follow-up till the study time. Various other authors have also reported similar findings as regards to complications following laparoscopic management of nonpalpable undescended testes [16, 18, 19]. This substantiates the fact that complication rates are markedly reduced in good centres with high expertise.

The average postoperative hospital stay was 14.23 hours (SD of 2.37 hours) for unilateral undescended nonpalpable testes and 16.27 hours (SD of 5.38 hours) for bilateral undescended nonpalpable testes. Most of our patients were discharged on the next day because no immediate postoperative surgical complications were seen. Time taken to return to daily activities was more in patients who underwent orchidopexy (4 ± 1 days) as compared to patients who underwent orchidectomy (2 ± 1 days). Koyama reported a hospital stay of less than one day, and Desai discharged his patients on the next day [2, 20].

In one (3%) of our cases, no testis was found as it was a vanishing testis. The morphology of testes as determined by laparoscopy was 96.9%. Laparoscopic procedures were performed in 90.9% of our cases. Open orchidectomy/orchidopexy was done in 9.1% of cases. Patients with vanishing testis (3%) had the advantage of avoiding unnecessary groin exploration. Zubair and Godbole have reported that unnecessary exploration or negative exploration can be avoided in 20% and 42% cases, respectively [10, 13].

6. Conclusion

Our study showed that patients with intra-abdominal testis and vanishing testes benefited from laparoscopy due to the fact that this technique provided them with a definitive diagnosis, direct surgical approach according to the location of testes, and avoidance of unnecessary abdominal exploration in case of vanishing testis. Laparoscopy clearly demonstrates the anatomy and provides visual information upon which a definitive decision can be made.

References

[1] C. H. Chui and A. S. Jacobson, "Laparoscopy in the evaluation of the non-palpable undescended testes," *Singapore Medical Journal*, vol. 41, no. 5, pp. 206–208, 2008.

[2] T. Koyama, K. Nonomura, K. Ameda et al., "Laparoscopic evaluation and management of the NonpalpableTestis," *Diagnostic and Therapeutic Endoscopy*, vol. 4, no. 2, pp. 69–74, 1997.

[3] A. A. Bakr and M. Kotb, "Laparoscopic orchidopexy: the treatment of choice for the impalpable undescended testis," *JSLS*, vol. 2, no. 3, pp. 259–263, 1999.

[4] I. S. Gill and J. H. Ross, "Needlescopic surgery for cryptorchidism: the initial series," *Journal of Paediatric Surgery*, vol. 35, no. 10, pp. 1426–1430, 2000.

[5] G. M. E. Humphrey, "Laparoscopy in the management of the impalpable undescended testis," *British Journal of Surgery*, vol. 85, no. 7, pp. 983–985, 1998.

[6] S. Corvin, W. Sturm, A. Anastasiadisa, M. Kuczyk, and A. Stenzl, "Laparoscopic management of adult nonpalpabletesticle," *Urologia Internationalis*, vol. 75, no. 4, pp. 337–339, 2005.

[7] N. Satar, Y. Bayazit, and S. Doran, "Laproscopy in management of impalpable testicle," *Acta Chirurgica Belgica*, vol. 105, no. 6, pp. 662–666, 2005.

[8] G. M. Hvistendahl and E. U. Poulsen, "Laparoscopy for impalapable testis-Experience with 80 intra abdominaltestis," *Journal of Pediatric Urology*, vol. 5, no. 5, pp. 389–392, 2009.

[9] K. Ismail, M. Ashour, M. El-Afifi, and A. Hashish, "Laparoscopy in the management of impalpable testis," *World Journal of Surgery*, vol. 33, no. 7, pp. 1514–1519, 2009.

[10] M. Zubair, I. M. Javad, and M. Saleem, "Role of laparoscopy in diagnosis of nonpalpable undescended testis," *The Professional*, vol. 4, no. 4, pp. 80-81, 1998.

[11] M. E. Hassan and A. Mustafawi, "Laproscopic management of impalpable testes in children–new classification; lessons learned and rare anomalies," *Journal of Laparoendoscopic and Advanced Surgical Techniques*, vol. 20, no. 3, pp. 265–269, 2010.

[12] M. A. El-Gohary, "The role of laparoscopy in the management of impalpable testes," *Pediatric Surgery International*, vol. 12, no. 5-6, pp. 463–465, 1997.

[13] P. P. Godbole, J. A. Morecroft, and A. E. Mackinnon, "Laparoscopy for impalpable testis," *British Journal of Surgery*, vol. 84, no. 10, pp. 1430-1432, 2005.

[14] T. Masao, M. Osamu, Y. Kazuhiro, and K. M. KenichiK, "Laparoscopy in diagnosis and treatment of nonpalpable testis," *International Journal of Urology*, vol. 8, no. 12, pp. 692–696, 2001.

[15] W. Boeckmann, A. Brauers, A. Mersdorf, D. Rohrmann, and G. Jakse, "Diagnostic and therapeutic laparoscopy of the non palpable testis," *Scandinavian Journal of Urology and Nephrology*, vol. 30, no. 6, pp. 479–484, 1996.

[16] S. A. Khan, A. A. Laghari, M. R. Abbasi, and S. Bhatti, "Laparoscopic assisted—management of impalpable testis in patients older than 10 years," *Journal of the society of LaproEndoscopic Surgeons*, vol. 14, no. 2, pp. 251–255, 2010.

[17] S. D. Mark and P. J. T. Davidson, "The role of laparoscopy in evaluation of the impalpable undescended testes," *ANZ Journal of Surgery*, vol. 67, no. 6, pp. 332–334, 1997.

[18] B. W. Lindgren, I. Franco, S. Bilick et al., "Laparoscopic fowler Stephens orchidopexy for the high abdominal testis," *Journal of Urology*, vol. 162, no. 3, pp. 990–994, 1999.

[19] K. D. Mehta, S. M. Kacheriwala, R. Y. Jain, B. Pillai, and A. P. Sodhi, "Management of impalapable testis-Laparoscopic approach," *Indian Journal of Surgery*, vol. 65, no. 5, pp. 430–434, 2003.

[20] C. S. Desai, R. Y. Prabhu, and A. N. Supe, "Laparoscopic orchiectomy for undescended testis in adults," *Journal of Postgraduate Medicine*, vol. 48, p. 25, 2002.

28

Supine Percutaneous Nephrolithotripsy in Double-S Position

Giuseppe Giusti and Antonello De Lisa

Department of Urology, University of Cagliari, Via Is Mirrionis 92, 09121 Cagliari, Italy

Correspondence should be addressed to Giuseppe Giusti; giuseppegiusti.med@gmail.com

Academic Editor: Kostis Gyftopoulos

Background. At present, the percutaneous nephrolithotripsy (PCNL) is performed both in supine and in prone position. The aim of this paper is to describe an innovative position during PCNL. *Methods.* We describe a supine position. The patient's legs are slightly abducted at the hips. The thorax is laterally tilted (inclination 30°–35°) and kept in the right position by one or two gel pads placed between the scapula and the vertebrae. External genitalia can be accessed at any time, so that it is always possible to use flexible instruments in the upper urinary tract. We used this position for a period of 12 months to treat with PCNL 45 patients with renal lithiasis. *Results.* All the procedures were successfully completed without complications, using the position we are describing. The following are some of its benefits: an easier positioning of the patient; a better exposure of the flank for an easier access to the posterior renal calyces of the kidney; a lower risk of pressure injuries compared to positions foreseeing the use of knee crutches; the possibility of combined procedures (ECIRS) through the use of flexible instruments; and a good fluoroscopic visualization of the kidney not overlapped by the vertebrae. *Conclusions.* This position is effective, safe, easy, and quick to prepare and allows for combined anterograde/retrograde operations.

1. Background

Percutaneous access to the kidney was first used in 1954 when radiologists dared to puncture the pelvis of hydronephrotic kidneys to perform anterograde pyelography [1]. The techniques to place nephrostomy drainages have been developed over the years, as well as the technique to extract stones from the kidney's cavities (percutaneous nephrolithotripsy (PCNL)) [2].

The traditional prone position has in fact been developed by radiologists, who used to puncture the pelvis directly, and not through the renal parenchyma. In 1987-88, Valdivia et al. [3] reported a safe percutaneous access to the kidney with a supine patient, and 10 years later they reported the *in vivo* experience with 557 patients [4]. The supine position became more popular after 2007 when the Galdakao modification was reported in an international publication [5].

The advantages of percutaneous nephrolithotripsy (PCNL) performed in the supine position are both of an anesthesiological and urological kind. The surgeon does not experience the cardiovascular [6], ventilatory, neuroendocrine, and pharmacokinetic problems of the prone position in the supine ones that grant better access to the airways and the cardiovascular system. Urological advantages include an easier puncture of the kidney which lies closer to the skin; a demonstrated decreased risk of colon injury [7]; a better descending drainage and retrieval of stone fragments, facilitated by the downward position of the Amplatz sheath; and a lower intrarenal pressure leading to smaller pyelovenous back flow and postoperative infectious risk [8].

Authors have suggested many different versions of the supine and prone positions to optimize the technique: the lateral [9], laterally flexed [10], lateral with abducted legs [11], prone split leg [12], prone-reverse lithotomy [13], supine crossed-leg [14], and supine with legs flexed in supports [3] are only some of them.

In our department, we perform an average of 79 percutaneous nephrolithotripsy per year. The need for an easy and quick-to-prepare position, which could at the same time allow for a safe and effective execution of the procedure, led us to develop the supine double-S (Slightly tilted thorax-Slightly split legs) position, which will be described in the following lines.

2. Materials and Methods

This is a preliminary study, carried out by the Department of Urology at the University of Cagliari (Cagliari, Italy) with the purpose to first describe the innovative position we developed.

The objective of the study was explained to all enrolled patients. Informed consents to participate and use personal data and images were signed by all enrolled patients.

For every case study, we recorded the patient's BMI, the dimension and the position of the stones, the operating time, and the complications occurred (using the Clavien-Dindo classification).

2.1. Description of the Position. The patient is placed on the operating table with the glutei at the lower end of the bed and the external genitalia exposed for an easy access.

It is important not to place the patient too close to the metallic side of the table, which is radiopaque and may project on the fluoroscopic field, obscuring the images. The patient's legs are secured independently and slightly abducted at the hips without being flexed (Figure 1). This position of the legs allows for retrograde access to the bladder and the upper urinary tract using flexible instruments. The ipsilateral arm is placed on the thorax and fixed to the contralateral one, by means of a wrist bandage (Figure 2). The contralateral arm is abducted and placed on a support. The thorax is slightly tilted. Its inclination, between 30° and 35°, can be measured by placing a smartphone over the body of the sternum, using Protractor (ExaMobile S.A., Poland—available on Google Play Store), an application which exploits the phone's accelerometers (Figure 2). The position is secured by one or two gel pads placed between the ipsilateral scapula and the spine. The positioning of the anaesthesia screen at the level of the interscapular line prevents the pads from moving. The position offers a good exposure of the flank to be treated. The retrograde access to the urinary tract is always possible through the use of flexible instruments (with or without the use of the ureteral sheath).

The renal puncture and the remaining phases of the surgery do not differ from the traditional procedure in the Valdivia position (Figure 3).

Between March 1, 2016, and March 1, 2017, the double-S position was used to treat 45 patients.

Patients presented an average body mass index (BMI) of 27.4.

In the CT (computed tomography) study, the mean stone size was 2.2 cm. The stones were positioned in the renal pelvis (48.8%), in the inferior calyx (22.2%), and in the medium calyx (8.8%). No staghorn stones were documented. In 9 cases, we treated multicalyceal stones (20%). In these 9 cases, we preferred not to perform a secondary access but a combined anterograde-retrograde procedure using a flexible ureteroscope. When possible, the stone was relocated in a place where lithotripsy could be performed through the percutaneous access; when this maneuver was not feasible, the stone was shattered using laser energy.

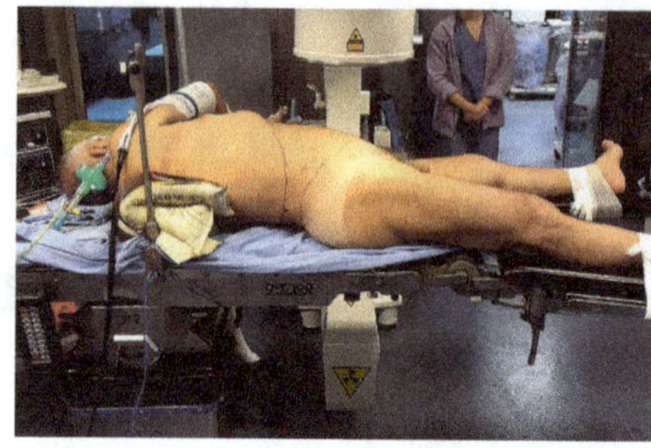

Figure 1: Patient's position on the operating table.

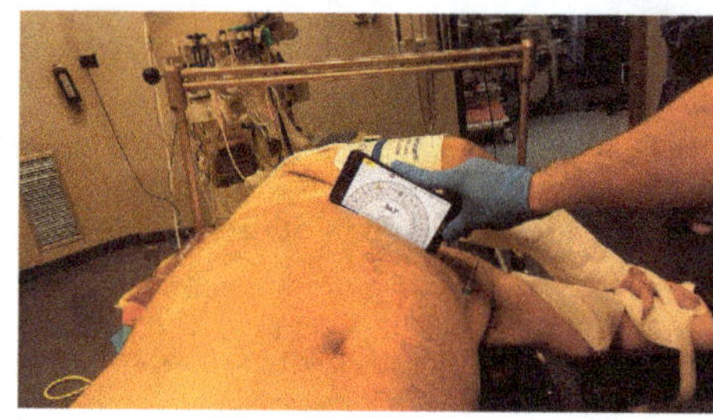

Figure 2: Measurement of the inclination of the patient's thorax through the app Protractor.

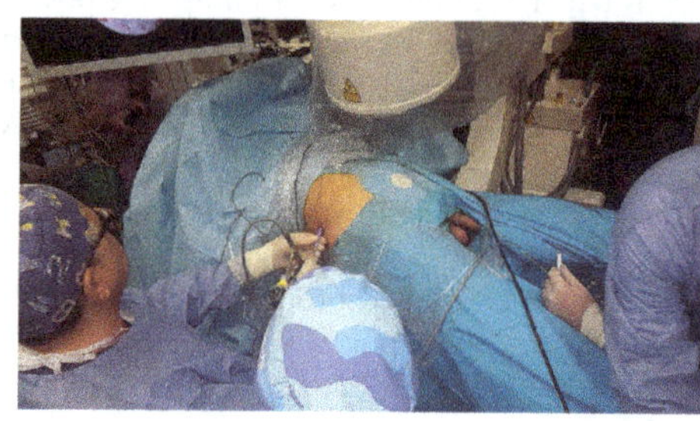

Figure 3: The procedure. The assistant has access to the upper urinary tract by standing between the patient's legs.

Patients were treated with an antibiotic prophylaxis before any procedure.

The effectiveness of all the operations was evaluated on the basis of the stone-free status after one month from the procedure, ascertained with CT abdomen examination without medical contrast medium (stone-free status < 3 mm).

3. Results

All the procedures performed in the described position were successfully completed. The mean operating time was 43.5 minutes.

At the end of each operation, a flexible pyelocalycealscopy and an anterograde pyelogram were performed, and in all cases the patients resulted 100% stone-free. With a CT abdomen without medical contrast medium after one month, we had the confirmation of the stone-free status for all operations.

There were neither high (III–V) nor low level (I-II) complications according to Clavien-Dindo.

4. Discussion

Besides the well-known anesthesiological advantages of the supine position, the double-S position presents other benefits. It indeed combines all the advantages of the several variations of the supine position already described in the scientific literature [15–17]:

(i) A smaller number of nurses in the operating room, who have an easier position to prepare and lighter loads to shift.

(ii) A better exposure of the flank and an increased distance between the last rib and the iliac crest (as reported by Desoky), providing a wider space for puncture, dilatation, and maneuverability of the nephroscope. This is feasible thanks to the fact that a single support is placed under the shoulder, and not under the lumbar region as in the Valdivia position (Figure 1).

(iii) A lower risk of pressure injuries to vascular and nervous structures compared to positions foreseeing the use of knee crutches (e.g., Galdakao position).

(iv) The absence of flank support, which prevents the cephalad sliding of the kidney, making upper-pole puncture more feasible.

(v) A lower degree of thorax rotation, allowing for a better fluoroscopic view of the kidney, which is not overlapped by the vertebrae, as it may happen in semi-supine (more tilted) positions.

(vi) The possibility to always have a retrograde access to the high urinary tract.

Someone could state that the lack of space between the legs, as they are only slightly abducted, could represent an issue for the assistant carrying out the retrograde intrarenal procedure. We, however, did not experience such a drawback. For every retrograde procedure, we chose the use of a ureteral sheath that allowed for an easy access and the possibility, when necessary, of multiple entries and exits. Sometimes, with female patients, we had to ask for the assistance of the scrub nurse to find the urethral meatus. Even in those cases, however, after the positioning of the sheath, the access was always easy.

A similar supine position has been reported by Desoky et al. and published in the *Arab Journal of Urology* in 2012 [18]. Desoky's position differs, however, from the double-S for the positioning of the patient's legs—slightly split in ours, and crossed in the flank-free position he described—and does not allow for the use of retrograde access in the upper urinary tract, which is instead always possible in ours.

Another similar position is the Barts "flank-free" modified supine one [19], which differs from the double-S for the necessary use of stirrups and the placement of a second support under the gluteus. These supplementary requirements take a long time. Our position is quicker to prepare and not as dangerous as those entailing a wider abduction of the legs, especially in patients with hip joint and femur problems.

5. Conclusions

The supine double-S position we describe turned out to be efficient, safe, easy, and quick to prepare. It allows for an easy access to the upper urinary tract and therefore for the performance of combined anterograde/retrograde operations. In our clinical practice, it has become the standard position for PCNL procedures in a supine position. In the age of flexible endoscopy, we believe that this position could be a new valid option and we recommend it both to those with a good experience in percutaneous kidney operations as well as to those who are approaching this technique.

Abbreviations

PCNL: Percutaneous nephrolithotripsy
ECIRS: Endoscopic combined intrarenal surgery.

Consent

Consent to participate and for publication of information was obtained from all the patients.

Authors' Contributions

Antonello De Lisa was the main surgeon in every procedure. Giuseppe Giusti was the major contributor in writing the manuscript and was the first assistant in all the procedures performed. All authors contributed to the development of the position described. All authors read and approved the final manuscript.

References

[1] H. S. Ween and T. J. Florence, "The diagnosis of hydronephrosis by percutaneous renal punctures," *Journal of Urology*, vol. 72, no. 2, pp. 589–595, 1954.

[2] I. Ferstrom and B. Johansson, "Percutaneous pyelolithotomy. A new extraction technique," *Scandinavian Journal of Urology and Nephrology*, vol. 10, no. 3, pp. 257–259, 1976.

[3] J. G. Valdivia, J. Valer, S. Villarroya et al., "Why is percutaneous nephroscopy still performed with the patient prone?," *Journal of Endourology*, vol. 4, no. 3, pp. 269–277, 1990.

[4] J. G. Valdivia Uria, J. Valle Gerhold, J. A. Lopez Lopez et al., "Technique and complications of percutaneous nephroscopy: experience with 557 patients in the supine position," *Journal of Urology*, vol. 160, no. 6, pp. 1975–1978, 1998.

[5] G. Ibarluzea, C. M. Scoffone, C. M. Cracco et al., "Supine Valdivia and modified lithotomy position for simultaneous anterograde and retrograde endourological access," *BJU International*, vol. 100, no. 1, pp. 233–236, 2007.

[6] J. E. Backofen and J. F. Schauble, "Hemodynamic changes with prone position during general anaesthesia," *Anesthesia and Analgesia*, vol. 64, p. 194, 1985.
[7] D. N. Tuttle, B. M. Yeh, M. V. Meng, R. S. Breiman, M. L. Stoller, and F. V. Coakley, "Risk of injury to adjacent organs with lower-pole fluoroscopically guided percutaneous nephrostomy: evaluation with prone, supine, and multiplanar reformatted CT," *Journal of Vascular and Interventional Radiology*, vol. 16, no. 11, pp. 1489–1492, 2005.
[8] C. M. Scoffone and C. M. Cracco, "PCNL supine technique," in *Surgical Management of Urolithiasis, Percutaneous, Shockwave and Ureteroscopy*, S. Y. Nakada and M. S. Pearle, Eds., , Chapter 2, p. 14, Springer, New York, NY, USA, 2013.
[9] K. Kerbl, R. V. Clayman, P. S. Chandhoke, D. A. Urban, B. C. De Leo, and J. M. Carbone, "Percutaneous stone removal with the patient in a flank position," *Journal of Urology*, vol. 151, no. 3, pp. 686–688, 1994.
[10] A. D. Smith, *Smith's Textbook of Endourology*, Wiley, Chichester, UK, 3rd edition, 2012.
[11] A. G. Papatsoris, F. Zaman, A. Panah, J. Masood, T. El-Husseiny, and N. Buchholz, "Simultaneous anterograde and retrograde endourologic access: "the Barts technique"," *Journal of Endourology*, vol. 22, no. 12, pp. 2665-2666, 2008.
[12] R. C.-G. A. Nord, A. Cubler-Goodman, and D. H. Bagley, "Prone split-leg position for simultaneous retrograde ureteroscopic and percutaneous nephroscopic procedures," *Journal of Endourology*, vol. 5, no. 1, pp. 13–16, 1991.
[13] T. Lehman and D. H. Bagley, "Reverse lithotomy. Modified prone position for simultaneous nephroscopic and ureteroscopic procedures in women," *Urology*, vol. 32, no. 6, pp. 529–531, 1988.
[14] E. A. Neto, A. I. Mitre, C. M. Gomes, M. A. Arap, and M. Srougi, "Percutaneous nephrolithotripsy with the patient in a modified supine position," *Journal of Urology*, vol. 178, no. 1, pp. 165–168, 2007.
[15] S. Falahatkar, A. Farzan, and A. Allahkhah, "Is complete supine percutaneous nephrolithotripsy feasible in all patients?," *Urological Research*, vol. 39, no. 2, pp. 99–104, 2011.
[16] S. Falahatkar, A. Allahkhah, and S. Soltanipour, "Supine percutaneous nephrolithotomy: pro," *Urology Journal*, vol. 8, no. 4, pp. 257–264, 2011.
[17] D. Curry, R. Srinivasan, R. Kucheria et al., "Supine percutaneous nephrolithotomy in the galdako-modified Valdivia position: a high-volume single center experience," *Journal of Endourology*, vol. 31, no. 10, pp. 1001–1006, 2017.
[18] E. A. Desoky, M. N. Allam, M. K. Ammar et al., "Flank free modified supine position: a new modification for supine percutaneous nephrolithotomy," *Arab Journal of Urology*, vol. 10, no. 2, pp. 143–148, 2012.
[19] C. Bach, A. Goyal, P. Kumar et al., "The Barts "flank-free" modified supine position for percutaneous nephrolithotomy," *Urologia Internationalis*, vol. 89, no. 3, pp. 365–368, 2012.

29

Analysis of Learning Curve in Robot-Assisted Radical Prostatectomy Performed by a Surgeon

Roman I. Slusarenco,[1] **Konstantin V. Mikheev**,[2] **Artem O. Prostomolotov**,[1] **Roman B. Sukhanov**,[1] **and Evgeny A. Bezrukov**[1]

[1]*Institute for Urology and Reproductive Health, Moscow, Russia*
[2]*International School "Medicine of the Future", FGAOU VO I.M. Sechenov First Moscow State Medical University, Moscow, Russia*

Correspondence should be addressed to Roman I. Slusarenco; slusarenco.roman@gmail.com

Academic Editor: Matthew Rutman

This study aimed to report the learning curve in robot-assisted radical prostatectomy (RARP) performed by one surgeon who is experienced in laparoscopic prostatectomies. The records of 145 RARP cases performed between 2015 and 2017 were evaluated retrospectively. Patients were divided into three groups: group 1 comprised the first 49 cases, group 2 comprised 50–88 cases, and the rest of the cases were assigned to group 3. Continence was defined as the necessity to use at least one pad during a day. Additionally, erectile function recovery was defined as having erection sufficient for sexual intercourse regardless of using a phosphodiesterase type 5 inhibitor. Continence and erectile function recovery were assessed during interviews at 3, 6, and 12 months after surgery. First, all procedures were successfully performed without conversions or blood transfusions. The median follow-up period was 22 months. Moreover, the median skin-to-skin operative time (OT) was 220 minutes. The median blood loss was 150 ml, and the mean hospital stay was 8.9 ± 3.87 days. The median prostate volume was 36 cm^3. The overall positive surgical margin rate was 13.1%. Overall, 38 (26.2%) postoperative complications were observed, and 17.9% of them were graded as minor. Anastomotic leakage decreased significantly from group 1 to group 3 (26.5% and 7%, respectively). The continence recovery (0-1 pad) rates were 60.6%, 75.7%, and 84.9% at 3, 6, and 12 months after surgery, respectively. Subsequently, the erectile function recovery rates were 50.9% and 65.4% at 6 and 12 months after surgery, respectively. In conclusion, there are several types of learning curves for RARP. First, the shallowest learning curve was observed for the OT. Regarding the analysis of "advanced learning curve," demonstrating the improvement of OT and blood loss is considered insufficient. Therefore, additional oncological and functional results that require a longer period of investigation are required.

1. Introduction

Prostate cancer is the second most common type of cancer and is the fifth leading cause of oncological death in men worldwide [1]. Prostatectomy is the gold standard treatment option for patients with localized disease [2]. Previously, this procedure was performed with a retropubic open approach [3]. The main drawbacks of this approach are as follows: long hospitalization, necessity of prescribing additional pain medication, and significant blood loss. Today, mini-invasive methods, such as laparoscopic radical prostatectomy (LRP) and robot-assisted radical prostatectomy (RARP), are becoming significantly more popular compared with the retropubic open approach. In particular, RARP has replaced retropubic radical prostatectomy (RRP) in Europe and the USA, which has been the gold standard surgical treatment of the localized and locally advanced prostate cancer [2]. Clearly, RARP has become the main standard treatment of prostate cancer. Recently, RARP has also demonstrated better outcomes than RRP and LRP. Although RARP has several advantages, adequate equipment and sufficient training programs are still required in this treatment method. Thus, this technique is rarely used in developing countries considering that it lacks financial support [4].

A short learning curve is one of the main advantages of the RARP, which makes it an interesting option for junior doctors. Certainly, surgeons who do not have significant experience in laparoscopic surgery achieve promising results. According to a recent study, doctors perform RARP more quickly compared with laparoscopic techniques [5]. Additionally, decreased intraoperative blood loss and reduced number of complications are observed after performing a total of 25–40 RARPs [6, 7]. Nevertheless, a significant clinical experience is still required to achieve adequate functional and oncological results in terms of negative surgical margins when performing RARP [8]. There are two types of learning curves, which can be used for RARP's assessment [9, 10]. The "basic learning curve" includes 25–50 cases, after which the operative time (OT) decreases to 200–240 minutes [9]. In case of the "advanced learning curve," 100–300 cases are required to achieve stable erectile function and continence recovery [9]. There are several factors that affect the speed of surgical technique mastery including the following: initial surgical skills, type of the learning program, and experience in performing laparoscopic surgeries [11, 12]. This study aimed to identify the pace of mastering RARP by a surgeon with significant clinical experience in performing LRP using the structured "advanced learning curve" method.

2. Materials and Methods

We studied 145 patients who had undergone radical robotic prostatectomy. It is worth mentioning that only one surgeon who is experienced in laparoscopic surgery had been performing RARP between 2015 and 2017. The data were collected retrospectively. All patients were divided into three groups according to the surgery date: group 1 comprised the first 49 cases, group 2 comprised 50–88 cases, and the rest of the cases were assigned to group 3.

All patients underwent standard transperitoneal RARP. Pelvic lymph node dissection (PLND) was performed in case of possible lymph node involvement according to the Briganti nomogram [13]. Moreover, a nerve-sparing technique was performed when prostate cancer was localized according to the D'Amico classification. The postoperative general prostate-specific antigen (PSA) level was measured at 3, 6, 9, and 12 months after surgery. According to the recommendations, biochemical recurrence was considered provided that the general PSA level was higher than 0.2 ng/ml [14]. Positive surgical margin (PSM) was defined as a tumor observed at the inked margin. Patients experiencing the extension of the tumor through the prostatic capsule were considered to experience extracapsular extension (pT3).

We considered our patients continent if they used a maximum of 1 pad per day. Continence was evaluated at 3, 6, and 12 months after surgery. Erectile function was evaluated at 6 and 12 months after surgery using the International Index of Erectile Function-5 (IIEF-5) score. Erectile function recovery was defined as the ability to achieve a sufficient erection for sexual intercourse regardless of using a phosphodiesterase type 5 (PDE 5) inhibitor. The initial results included OT (in minutes), positive surgical margins, blood loss volume, duration of urinary bladder catheterization, and continence and sexual function's recovery. Statistical analysis was performed using the International Business Machines Corporation Statistical for the Social Sciences Statistics version 23. $p < 0.05$ was considered statistically significant.

3. Results

There were no statistically significant differences between the three groups in terms of age, body mass index, IIEF-5 total score, PSA level, prostate volume, Gleason score, clinical stage, D'Amico oncological risk, and possibility of lymph node invasion according to the Briganti nomogram (Table 1).

The median follow-up periods for groups 1, 2, and 3 were 24, 22, and 20 months, respectively ($p < 0.001$). The median age of the patients was 62.18 ± 6.76 years. The mean PSA level was 9.24 ± 6.86 ng/ml. The median OT (defined as the time from creating the first incision to creating the final skin suture, including the time of docking and undocking) was 220 (150–280) minutes. The OT decreased significantly from group 1 to group 3 ($p = 0.0001$) (Figure 1).

Simultaneously, none of the patients required conversion. The median blood loss was 150 (100–250) ml. As the surgeon gained experience, blood loss decreased: group 1, 250 (150–400) ml; group 2, 150 (100–250) ml; and group 3, 100 (100–175) ml ($p = 0.0002$). None of the patients required blood transfusion (Figure 2).

Overall, 38 (26.2%) postoperative complications were observed using the Clavien–Dindo classification, and 26 of them (17.9%) were graded as minor (Clavien I/II) (Table 2).

Clavien IV/V complications were not observed. The incidence rates of anastomotic leakage that required prolonged catheter duration were 26.5%, 23.1%, and 7.0% in groups 1, 2, and 3, respectively ($p < 0.02$). Six major urine extravasations, which required unilateral or bilateral ureteral mono-J stent placement, were observed in the early postoperative period. Six patients required cystoscopy and repeat catheter placement due to major urine extravasation after catheter removal (Table 3).

Extended PLND was performed in only 38 patients (26%). A total of nine patients from group 3 underwent pelvic lymphadenectomy up to the level of the abdominal aorta bifurcation (Table 4).

According to the histological investigation results, the Gleason total score and pT stage were equal in all the three groups ($p > 0.05$). Extracapsular invasion (pT3) and seminal vesicle invasion (pT3b) were observed in 13.79% and 7.6% of patients, respectively. The overall PSM rate was 13.1%, corresponding to 8.2% in pT2 and 19.7% in pT3. A comparison of the pT2 ($p = 0.065$), pT3 ($p = 0.162$), and the overall groups ($p = 0.07$) showed no statistically significant difference (Table 5).

We considered our patients continent if they used a maximum of 1 pad per day. Continence was defined as the

Table 1: Preoperative clinical characteristics of the patients.

Characteristics	Median value	Group 1 (1–49)	Group 2 (50–88)	Group 3 (89–145)	p value
Age (years)					
Mean ± SD	62.18 ± 6.76	61.29 ± 6.73	63.56 ± 6.75	62.00 ± 6.76	0.42
Median (IQR)	62 (57.5–67)	62 (57–67)	63 (60–68)	62 (57–66.5)	
BMI					
Mean ± SD	27.24 ± 3.85	26.76 ± 3.91	27.28 ± 4.71	27.64 ± 3.11	0.52
Median (IQR)	27.0 (25.0–28.7)	27.1 (24.6–28.5)	26.5 (24.6–29.0)	27.0 (25.6–29.0)	
IIEF-5, n (%)					
21–25 points	60 (53.1)	17 (53.1)	13 (46.4)	30 (56.6)	0.35
16–20 points	24 (21.2)	8 (25.0)	4 (14.3)	12 (22.6)	
11–15 points	10 (8.8)	4 (12.5)	2 (7.1)	4 (7.5)	
0–10 points	19 (16.8)	3 (9.4)	9 (32.1)	7 (13.2)	
PSA (ng/ml)					
Mean ± SD	9.24 ± 6.86	8.48 ± 5.97	8.71 ± 5.65	10.25 ± 8.19	0.553
Median (IQR)	7.47 (5.5–9.8)	7.47 (5.6–9.1)	6.97 (5.3–9.9)	8.00 (5.7–10.6)	
Prostate volume (cm^3)					
Mean ± SD	39.84 ± 17.14	38.53 ± 17.57	41.74 ± 20.87	39.58 ± 13.82	0.55
Median (IQR)	36.0 (29.0–47.5)	33.0 (26.5–49.5)	34.00 (29–50)	40 (30.00–45.5)	
Clinical stage, n (%)					
cT1	90 (62.1)	34 (69.4)	23 (59.0)	33 (57.9)	0.8
cT2	40 (27.6)	11 (22.4)	13 (33.3)	16 (28.1)	
cT3	15 (10.3)	4 (8.2)	3 (7.7)	8 (14.0)	
Biopsy Gleason score, n (%)					
≤6	89 (61.4)	32 (65.3)	28 (71.8)	29 (50.9)	0.08
=7	48 (33.1)	17 (34.7)	10 (25.6)	21 (36.8)	
≥8	8 (5.5)	0 (0)	1 (2.6)	7 (12.3)	
D'Amico risk, n (%)					
Low	78 (53.8)	28 (57.1)	29 (74.4)	21 (36.8)	0.128
Median	38 (26.2)	14 (28.6)	5 (12.8)	19 (33.3)	
High	29 (20)	7 (14.3)	5 (12.8)	17 (29.8)	
Briganti lymph node invasion, n (%)					
<5%	92 (63.4)	34 (69.4)	26 (66.7)	32 (56.1)	0.33
≥5%	53 (36.6)	15 (30.6)	13 (33.3)	25 (43.9)	

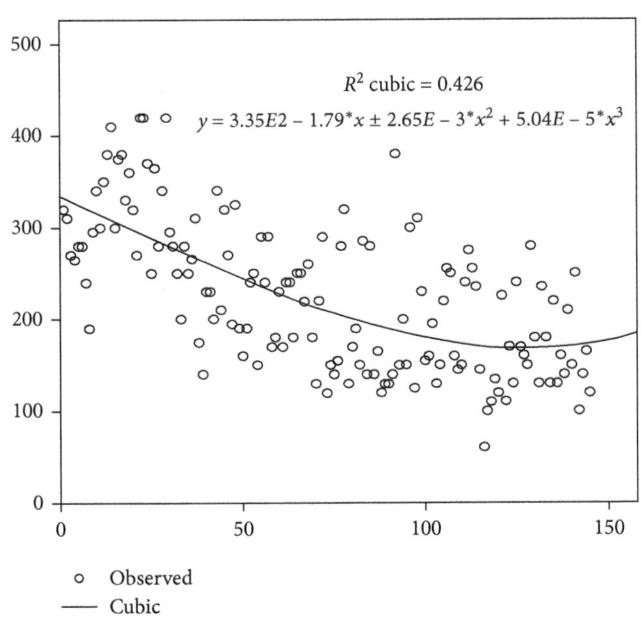

Figure 1: Learning curve for the operative time.

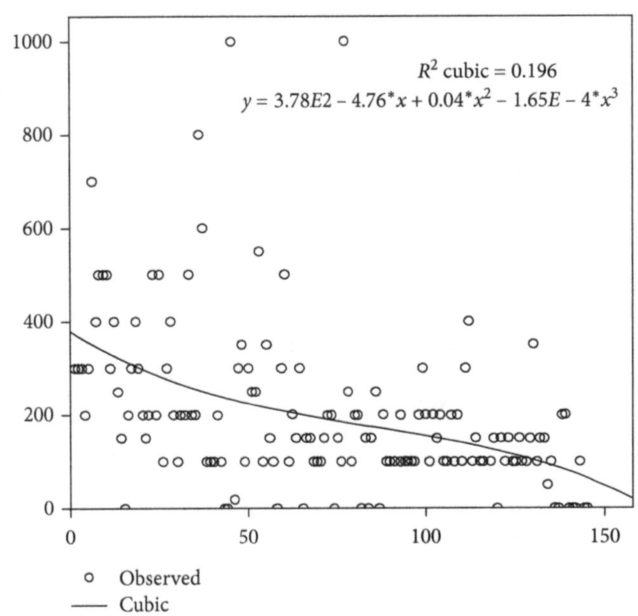

Figure 2: Learning curve for the blood loss.

necessity to use one pad per day. Thus, at 3, 6, and 12 months after surgery, the overall continence rates were 60.6%, 75.7%, and 84.9%, respectively. In comparison with urinary incontinence among the observed groups, at 3 months after surgery, the rates were 64.5%, 66.7%, and 53.5%, respectively ($p = 0.146$), and there was no statistically significant

Table 2: Intraoperative data.

Characteristic	Median (total)	Group 1 (1–49)	Group 2 (50–88)	Group 3 (89–145)	p
Operative time (OT) (min)					
Mean ± SD	224.17 ± 80.87	293.57 ± 68.81	204.23 ± 57.48	178.16 ± 62.22	0.0001
Median (IQR)	220 (150–280)	295 (250–340)	190 (150–250)	160 (130–227.50)	
Console time (min)					
Mean ± SD	120.45 ± 56.40	163.06 ± 58.26	107.44 ± 38.16	92.72 ± 42.35	0.0002
Median (IQR)	100 (80–155)	160 (115–210)	100 (80–130)	80 (70–110)	
Blood loss (mL)					
Mean ± SD	199.10 ± 175.09	290.20 ± 206.8	189.74 ± 182.1	127.19 ± 84.02	0.0002
Median (IQR)	150 (100–250)	250 (150–400)	150 (100–250)	100 (100–175)	
Hospital stay (days)					
Median (IQR)	11 (8.5–14)	12 (9–16)	11 (7–15)	10 (8–12.5)	0.007
Abdominal drains, n (%)					
Placed	69 (47.6)	39 (79.6)*	21 (53.8)	9 (15.8)*	0.0001
Not placed	76 (52.4)	10 (20.4)	18 (46.2)	48 (84.2)	
Complications, n (%)					
Clavien grade I/II	26 (17.9)	13 (26.5)*	9 (23.1)	4 (7.0)*	0.02
Clavien grade III	12 (8.3)	8 (16.3)*	2 (5.1)	2 (3.5)*	0.116

*Statistically significant difference.

Table 3: Complications stratified by the Clavien–Dindo classification system.

Grade	Complications	Group 1 (1–49)	Group 2 (50–88)	Group 3 (89–145)	Management
I/II	Anastomosis leakage	13	9	4	Prolonged catheter duration
IIIA	Major urine extravasation during catheterization	3	1	2	Ureteral stent (mono-J stent)
IIIA	Major urine extravasation after catheter removal	5	1	0	Cystoscopy and catheter placement

Table 4: Operative technique.

Characteristic	Total	Group 1 (1–49)	Group 2 (50–88)	Group 3 (89–145)	p
Nerve sparing, n (%)					
Nonnerve sparing	56 (38.6)	14 (8.6)	17 (43.6)	25 (43.9)	0.035
Bilateral	73 (50.3)	27 (55.1)	15 (38.5)	31 (54.4)	
Unilateral	14 (9.7)	7 (14.3)*	7 (17.9)	0 (0.0)*	
Partial bilateral	2 (1.4)	1 (2.0)	0 (0.0)	1 (1.8)	
Prostatectomy technique, n (%)					
Intrafascial	72 (49.7)	25 (51)	15 (38.5)	32 (56.1)	0.023
Interfascial	8 (5.5)	6 (12.2)*	2 (5.1)	0 (0)*	
Extrafascial	59 (40.7)	15 (30.6)	19 (48.7)	25 (43.9)	
Combined technique	6 (4.1)	3 (6.1)	3 (7.7)*	0 (0)*	
Prostate venous plexus (PVP) suture ligation, n (%)					
No suture ligation	21 (14.5)	3 (6.1)*	10 (25.6)*	8 (14)	0.034
Suture ligation before transection	83 (57.2)	32 (65.3)*	15 (38.5)*	36 (63.2)	
Suture ligation after transection	41 (28.3)	14 (28.6)	14 (35.9)	13 (22.8)	
Anterior reconstruction					
Not performed	66 (45.5)	20 (40.8)	24 (61.5)*	22 (38.6)*	0.045
Performed	79 (54.5)	29 (59.2)	15 (38.5)*	35 (61.4)*	
Posterior reconstruction, n (%)					
Performed	26 (17.9)	12 (24.5)	6 (15.4)	8 (14.0)	0.33
Not performed	119 (82.1)	37 (75.5)	33 (84.6)	49 (86.0)	
Pelvic lymph node dissection (PLND), n (%)					
Not performed	107 (73.8)	36 (73.5)	32 (82.1)	39 (68.4)	0.003
Up to the ureter level	29 (20.0)	13 (26.5)	7 (17.9)	9 (15.8)	
Up to the aorta bifurcation level	9 (6.2)	0 (0)*	0 (0)	9 (15.8)*	

*Statistically significant difference.

Table 5: Histological results.

Characteristics	Total	Group 1 (1–49)	Group 2 (50–88)	Group 3 (89–145)	p
Pathological stage (pT), n (%)					
pT2	125 (86.21)	41 (83.67)	34 (87.18)	50 (87.72)	0.51
Postoperative Gleason score, n (%)					
≤6	65 (44.8)	25 (51.0)	18 (46.2)	22 (38.6)	
7	71 (49.0)	24 (49.0)	17 (43.6)	30 (52.6)	0.2
≥8	9 (6.2)	0 (0.0)	4 (10.3)	5 (8.8)	
Invasion, n (%)					
No invasion (pT2)	102 (70.3)	36 (73.5)	32 (82.1)	34 (59.6)	
Capsular infiltration (pT2)	23 (15.9)	5 (10.2)	3 (7.7)	16 (28.1)	0.097
Extracapsular invasion (pT3)	20 (13.79)	8 (16.33)	5 (12.82)	7 (12.28)	
Seminal vesicle (pT3b)	11 (7.6)	3 (6.1)	3 (7.7)	5 (8.8)	
Surgical margin status, n (%)					
Positive	19 (13.10)	3 (6.12)	9 (23.08)	6 (10.53)	0.07
Negative	126 (86.9)	46 (93.88)	30 (76.92)	51 (89.47)	

difference between the three groups. At 6 months after surgery, continence was completely restored in 77.4%, 86.7%, and 66.7% of patients, respectively ($p = 0.034$). At 12 months after surgery, 83.0%, 89.6%, and 82.1% of patients were continent in groups 1, 2, and 3, respectively ($p = 0.237$), with no statistically significant difference between the three groups. Erectile function was considered to be restored if erection was sufficient for sexual intercourse regardless of using a (PDE 5) inhibitor. Hence, erectile function recovery was achieved in 50.9% (IIEF-5 score, 13.9) and 65.4% (IIEF-5 score 15.3) of patients at 6 and 12 months after surgery, respectively ($p = 0.176$). There were no statistically significant differences in the observed groups.

4. Discussion

RARP has become the most common surgical procedure that is used in the treatment of localized prostate cancer. Surgeons prefer RARP over other surgical methods because of its mini-invasive characteristics and short learning curve. Patel et al. found that only 25 surgeries have to be performed to master RARP [7].

Nevertheless, each surgeon has his/her own learning curve and needs to perform an individual number of surgeries to achieve desirable results.

The main intraoperative index is OT, which is changing as long as the surgeon masters the RARP technique. Long operations are possibly associated with technical difficulties and lack of surgical skills [15]. In our study, the median (skin to skin) OT (interquartile range (IQR)) was 220 (150–280) minutes, which decreased after the 88-th case. According to Doumerc et al., if a surgeon had experience in performing open prostatectomies, 110 cases would be required to achieve the OT of 180 minutes [16]. Our results are consistent with the results of Haglind et al.'s study, which demonstrated that the median OT in the group of RARP was 236 minutes.

The median blood loss was 150 (100–250) ml. Evidently, it decreased after completing a hundred of cases by 100 ml in group 3 (median level, IQR). According to the statistical data, blood loss rates during RARP vary from 142 ml to 230 ml [17], which is considered another advantage of RARP over open radical prostatectomy. According to Tobias-Machado et al., the median blood loss during the first 60 robot-assisted radical prostatectomies was 245.5 ml, as the surgeon had already performed 200 laparoscopic radical prostatectomies [18]. In our investigation, the median hospital stay was 8.9 ± 3.87 days although Rocco et al. mentioned the 3-day hospital stay [19]. Certainly, hospital stay is longer in Russia than that in the recent study considering the differences between the two healthcare systems.

The overall complication rate was 26.2%. Particularly, the complication rates were 17.9% and 8.3% for Clavien I/II and Clavien IIIA complications, respectively. According to Rocco et al., the overall anastomotic leakage rate was 24%, with the anastomoses diagnosed by the postoperative retrograde cystogram. These results could be compared with our data (median rate of 17.9%) [19]. Moreover, the anastomotic leakage rate was evidently lower as the surgeon was gaining experience than that of group 1 (26.5% and 7%, respectively).

Finally, according to Hruza et al., the complication rates were 21.7% for Clavien I/II and 11.5% for Clavien III [20].

Certainly, the main goal of surgical treatment is to achieve the optimal oncological results. Hence, the PSM was the most important rate. According to the systematic review by Yossepowitch et al., the overall PSM rate in different studies varies from 6.5% to 32% [21]. In our investigation, the overall PSM rate was 13.1%, and the PSM rates in pT2 and pT3 were 8.2% and 19.7%, respectively. These results are consistent with the abovementioned results. Interestingly, the PSM rate did not change alongside the learning curve evidently, suggesting that a surgeon should continue to master one's skills after performing 150 surgeries. Some investigators believe that the PSM rate did not change alongside the learning curve because the tipping point might have not been achieved yet [22].

We also believe that the data obtained from Patel et al. should be paid careful attention because they showed that PSM could significantly change after performing 1500 surgeries (e.g., 12.2% for 1–300 cases, 6.6% for 301–600 cases, 13.6% for 601–900 cases, 11% for 901–1.200 cases, and 1.8% for 1201–1500 cases) [23].

Biochemical recurrence was observed in 16.5% of patients at the end of the study period.

Ploussard et al. [24] determined that the overall continence rates (unnecessary use of pads after RARP) were 50.3%, 72%, and 83.6% at 3, 6, and 12 months after surgery, respectively. This result is consistent with the result of our present study (continence rates of 60.6%, 75.7%, and 84.9% at 3, 6, and 12 months after surgery, respectively).

Another important life quality rate is erectile function. Erectile function recovery rates at 6 and 12 months after surgery were 50.9% (IIEF-5 score, 13.9) and 65.4% (IIEF-5 score, 15.3), respectively. In one study (Ploussard et al.), 42% and 57.7% of patients demonstrated adequate erectile function at 6 and 12 months after surgery, respectively [24]. Kim et al. reported that erectile function was restored in 33% and 57.1% of patients at 3 and 6 months, respectively, in the large RARP group ($n = 528$) [25].

Our investigation has a number of limitations. First, this was a nonrandomized and retrospective study. Second, a short period of supervision was observed in this study. The results were assessed throughout the 12-month period after surgery. In RARP, the skills of a surgeon should be developed constantly. Third, small sample sizes were observed in the three groups, decreasing the sample value. Finally, continence and erectile function recovery rates were evaluated through patient interviews without the use of questionnaires.

During the whole learning curve, we observed the considerable improvement of the following rates: OT, blood loss volume, hospital stay duration, anastomotic leak frequency after surgery (according to the cystographic results), and frequency of abdominal cavity draining. Simultaneously, a longer period of investigation and manual practicing are required to evaluate PSM and BCR and urine continence and sexual function recovery.

5. Conclusions

In conclusion, the results of our study have provided evidence that surgeons with previous surgical experience require more than 80 cases to achieve an OT of 180 minutes. The median blood loss, which was approximately 150 ml, was achieved approximately after performing 50 surgeries. Moreover, the PSM had not significantly changed after performing 145 surgeries. Regarding urinary incontinence and erectile function, surgeons started performing simple surgeries and eventually managed to perform nerve-sparing techniques with anterior and posterior reconstructions for better clinical outcomes.

References

[1] J. Ferlay, I. Soerjomataram, R. Dikshit et al., "Cancer incidence and mortality worldwide: sources, methods and major patterns in GLOBOCAN 2012," *International Journal of Cancer*, vol. 136, no. 5, pp. E359–E386, 2015.

[2] N. Mottet, J. Bellmunt, M. Bolla et al., "EAU-ESTRO-SIOG guidelines on prostate cancer. Part 1: screening, diagnosis, and local treatment with curative intent," *European Urology*, vol. 71, no. 4, pp. 618–629, 2017.

[3] P. C. Walsh, A. W. Partin, and J. I. Epstein, "Cancer control and quality of life following anatomical radical retropubic prostatectomy: results at 10 years," *Journal of Urology*, vol. 152, no. 5 Part 2, pp. 1831–1836, 1994.

[4] C. Bolenz, S. J. Freedland, B. K. Hollenbeck et al., "Costs of radical prostatectomy for prostate cancer: a systematic review," *European Urology*, vol. 65, no. 2, pp. 316–324, 2014.

[5] T. E. Ahlering, D. Skarecky, D. Lee, and R. V. Clayman, "Successful transfer of open surgical skills to a laparoscopic environment using a robotic interface: initial experience with laparoscopic radical prostatectomy," *Journal of Urology*, vol. 170, no. 5, pp. 1738–1741, 2003.

[6] J. A. Smith Jr., "Robotically assisted laparoscopic prostatectomy: an assessment of its contemporary role in the surgical management of localized prostate cancer," *The American Journal of Surgery*, vol. 188, no. 4, pp. 63–67, 2004.

[7] V. R. Patel, A. S. Tully, R. Holmes, and J. Lindsay, "Robotic radical prostatectomy in the community setting-the learning curve and beyond: initial 200 cases," *Journal of Urology*, vol. 174, no. 1, pp. 269–272, 2005.

[8] Y. H. Ko, J. H. Ban, S. H. Kang et al., "Does robot-assisted laparoscopic radical prostatectomy enable to obtain adequate oncological and functional outcomes during the learning curve? From the Korean experience," *Asian Journal of Andrology*, vol. 11, no. 2, pp. 167–175, 2009.

[9] H. J. Lavery, D. B. Samadi, R. Thaly et al., "The advanced learning curve in robotic prostatectomy: a multi-institutional survey," *Journal of Robotic Surgery*, vol. 3, no. 3, pp. 165–169, 2009.

[10] T. Hashimoto, K. Yoshioka, T. Gondo et al., "Learning curve and perioperative outcomes of robot-assisted radical prostatectomy in 200 initial Japanese cases by a single surgeon," *Journal of Endourology*, vol. 27, no. 10, pp. 1218–1223, 2013.

[11] A. Volpe, K. Ahmed, P. Dasgupta et al., "Pilot validation study of the European association of urology robotic training curriculum," *European Urology*, vol. 68, no. 2, pp. 292–299, 2015.

[12] C. Lovegrove, G. Novara, A. Mottrie et al., "Structured and modular training pathway for robot-assisted radical prostatectomy (RARP): validation of the RARP assessment score and learning curve assessment," *European Urology*, vol. 69, no. 3, pp. 526–535, 2016.

[13] A. Briganti, A. Larcher, F. Abdollah et al., "Updated nomogram predicting lymph node invasion in patients with prostate cancer undergoing extended pelvic lymph node dissection: the essential importance of percentage of positive cores," *European Urology*, vol. 61, no. 3, pp. 480–487, 2012.

[14] N. Mottet, *EAU—ESTRO—ESUR—SIOG Guidelines on Prostate Cancer 2018 in European Association of Urology Guidelines*, European Association of Urology Guidelines Office, Arnhem, Netherlands, 2018.

[15] A. J. Vickers, C. J. Savage, M. Hruza et al., "The surgical learning curve for laparoscopic radical prostatectomy: a

retrospective cohort study," *The Lancet Oncology*, vol. 10, no. 5, pp. 475–480, 2009.

[16] N. Doumerc, C. Yuen, R. Savdie et al., "Should experienced open prostatic surgeons convert to robotic surgery? The real learning curve for one surgeon over 3 years," *BJU International*, vol. 106, no. 3, pp. 378–384, 2010.

[17] Q.-D. Trinh, J. Sammon, M. Sun et al., "Perioperative outcomes of robot-assisted radical prostatectomy compared with open radical prostatectomy: results from the nationwide inpatient sample," *European Urology*, vol. 61, no. 4, pp. 679–685, 2012.

[18] M. Tobias-Machado, A. I. Mitre, M. Rubinstein, E. F. d. Costa, and A. K. Hidaka, "Roboticssisted radical prostatectomy-learning curve for experienced laparoscopic surgeons: does itreally exist," *International Brazilian Journal of Urology*, vol. 42, no. 1, pp. 83–89, 2016.

[19] B. Rocco, D.-V. Matei, S. Melegari et al., "Robotic vs open prostatectomy in a laparoscopically naive centre: a matched-pair analysis," *BJU International*, vol. 104, no. 7, pp. 991–995, 2009.

[20] M. Hruza, H. O. Weiß, G. Pini et al., "Complications in 2200 consecutive laparoscopic radical prostatectomies: standardised evaluation and analysis of learning curves," *European Urology*, vol. 58, no. 5, pp. 733–741, 2010.

[21] O. Yossepowitch, A. Briganti, J. A. Eastham et al., "Positive surgical margins after radical prostatectomy: a systematic review and contemporary update," *European Urology*, vol. 65, no. 2, pp. 303–313, 2014.

[22] Y. M. Hong, D. E. Sutherland, B. Linder, and J. D. Engel, "Learning curve" may not be enough: assessing the oncological experience curve for robotic radical prostatectomy," *Journal of Endourology*, vol. 24, no. 3, pp. 473–477, 2010.

[23] V. R. Patel, K. J. Palmer, G. Coughlin, and S. Samavedi, "Robot-assisted laparoscopic radical prostatectomy: perioperative outcomes of 1500 cases," *Journal of Endourology*, vol. 22, no. 10, pp. 2299–2306, 2008.

[24] G. Ploussard, A. de la Taille, M. Moulin et al., "Comparisons of the perioperative, functional, and oncologic outcomes after robot-assisted versus pure extraperitoneal laparoscopic radical prostatectomy," *European Urology*, vol. 65, no. 3, pp. 610–619, 2014.

[25] S. C. Kim, C. Song, W. Kim et al., "Factors determining functional outcomes after radical prostatectomy: robot-assisted versus retropubic," *European Urology*, vol. 60, no. 3, pp. 413–419, 2011.

Removal of the Tumor Thrombus from the Right Atrium without Extracorporeal Circulation: Emphasis on the Displacement of the Tumor Apex

D. V. Shchukin,[1,2] V. N. Lesovoy,[1,2] G. G. Khareba,[1,2] A. I. Harahatyi,[1,2] A. V. Maltsev,[1] M. M. Polyakov,[1,2] R. V. Stetsyshyn,[2,3] M. P. Kopytsya,[4] P. V. Mozzhakov,[2] and O. O. Makovozov[5]

[1]*Kharkiv National Medical University, Kharkiv 61022, Ukraine*
[2]*V.I. Shapoval Regional Clinical Center of Urology and Nephrology, Kharkiv 61037, Ukraine*
[3]*Kharkiv Medical Academy of Postgraduate Education, Kharkiv 61176, Ukraine*
[4]*L.T. Malaya Therapy National Institute of the National Academy of Medical Sciences of Ukraine, Kharkiv 61039, Ukraine*
[5]*Dniprovsky Regional Clinical Oncology Dispensary, Dnipro 49055, Ukraine*

Correspondence should be addressed to D. V. Shchukin; shukindv@gmail.com

Academic Editor: Mohammad H. Ather

Objectives. To assess the outcomes of cavoatrial tumor thrombus removal using the liver transplantation technique for thrombectomy, a retrospective study was conducted. *Materials and Methods.* Five patients with atrial tumor thrombi who underwent piggyback mobilization of the liver, surgical access to the right atrium from the abdominal cavity, and external manual repositioning of the thrombus apex below the diaphragm (milking maneuver) were included into the study. Extracorporeal circulation was used in none of the cases. The average length of the atrial component of the tumor was 20.0 ± 11.7 mm (10 to 35 mm), and the width was 14.8 ± 8.5 mm (10 to 30 mm). In this work, the features of patients and surgical interventions as well as perioperative complications and mortality were analyzed. *Results.* External manual repositioning of the tumor thrombus apex below the diaphragm was successfully performed in all patients. Tumor thrombi with the length of the atrial part up to 1.5 cm were removed through the extrapericardial approach. For evacuation of the thrombi with the large atrial part (3.0 cm or more), a transpericardial surgical approach was required. Specific complications associated with the access to the right atrium from the abdominal cavity (paresis of the right phrenic nerve, pneumothorax, and mediastinitis) were not detected in any case. The average clamping time of the supradiaphragmatic inferior vena cava (IVC) was 6.3 ± 4.6 min. The volume of intraoperative blood loss varied from 2500 to 5600 ml (an average of 3675 ± 1398.5 ml). *Conclusion.* Our work represents the initial experience in the liver transplantation technique for thrombectomy in distinct and well-selected patients with atrial tumor thrombi. The effectiveness of this approach needs further study. The video presentation of our research took place in March 2019 at the 34th Annual EAU Congress in Barcelona.

1. Introduction

One of the most important aspects of surgical treatment for renal tumors extending into the inferior vena cava (IVC) is control of the apical part of the tumor thrombus. This stage can be quite challenging in case of "high" localization of the thrombus apex (retrohepatic or intrapericardial IVC and right atrium) and mainly depends on the type of surgical approach selected. Traditionally, for these patients, cardiopulmonary bypass with or without deep hypothermic circulatory arrest is used [1].

However, this surgical technique results in wide opening of several body cavities, significantly increases the duration of surgery, and also can be accompanied by specific postoperative complications such as mediastinitis, sternal pain syndrome, pericardial adhesion scars, coagulopathy, and central nervous system complications [2, 3].

In recent years, there have been more and more reports on alternative surgical approaches without use of cardiopulmonary bypass and circulatory arrest in patients with the tumor thrombi extending above the mouths of the major hepatic veins [4–10]. However, the cases of intraluminal tumor removal from the right atrium with the help of these surgical techniques are quite rare in the world literature [9, 11–15].

We retrospectively evaluated our own experience in the surgical treatment of renal cell carcinoma spreading to the IVC and the right atrium with the use of the liver transplantation technique described by Ciancio et al. [10]. The features of this surgical technique, including access to the right atrium through the diaphragm from the abdominal cavity, and complications were analyzed. Particular attention was paid to the manual repositioning of the tumor thrombus apex below the diaphragm.

2. Materials and Methods

2.1. Characteristics of Patients and Tumors. Between 2002 and 2018, ninety-six nephrectomies with the removal of caval tumor thrombi in patients with renal cell carcinoma (RCC) were performed. The tumors spread above the diaphragm in 16 (16.7%) cases, including 5 (5.2%) patients with atrial thrombi.

The study included only those patients in whom the tumor thrombus apex was located in the lumen of the right atrium. This was confirmed by abdominal and chest multidetector computed tomography (MDCT) with contrast enhancement, as well as abdominal ultrasound examination. Ultrasonography demonstrated free flotation of tumor apex in the atrial lumen in all five patients.

The main characteristics of the patients and the tumors with atrial extension are presented in Table 1.

Among our patients, males predominated (3 : 2). The mean age of the patients was 58.8 ± 11.2 years (from 41 to 72 years). Their Eastern Cooperative Oncology Group (ECOG) score did not exceed 1 in 4 cases. A glomerular filtration rate (GFR) ranged from 36.8 to 76.2 ml/min (an average of 57.2 ± 16.0 ml/min), and a body mass index (BMI) was from 17.8 to 28.9 kg/m^2 (an average of 24.8 ± 4.5 kg/m^2). One patient had developed a significant body mass deficit.

Right-sided tumors were detected in 3 out of 5 patients. The average size of the tumors was 14.9 ± 9.4 cm. The histological examination confirmed RCC in all cases.

Two patients had synchronous lung metastases. In one patient, a giant kidney tumor spread into *m. psoas* and into the wall of the right common iliac artery.

Persistent swelling of the lower extremities was noted only in one patient with the right-sided tumor. Moderate symptoms of heart failure were observed in two patients. Their left ventricular ejection fraction was 44% and 48%. In the whole group, this parameter averaged 52 ± 5.7%.

The length of the atrial part of the tumor thrombus ranged from 10 to 35 mm (20.0 ± 11.7 mm on average) and the width from 10 to 30 mm (14.8 ± 8.5 on average) (Figure 1). The average diameter of the tumor thrombus reached 32.6 ± 19.9 mm (13 to 63 mm). Presence of a blood clot, which was located below the tumor thrombus, was detected in 2 cases. A complete block of blood flow through the IVC by visual diagnosis occurred in three patients. Invasion of the intraluminal tumor into the caval wall was registered in 3 cases.

After surgical treatment, two patients with pulmonary metastases received systemic therapy with pazopanib. The mean follow-up period was 12.4 ± 3.6 months. The follow-up was performed by ultrasound examination every 3 months, as well as abdominal and chest MDCT every 6 months. Statistical analysis was carried out using standard descriptive statistical methods by means of "Statistica 8.0" software.

2.2. Surgical Technique. Patients with tumor extension to the right atrium were operated on with the help of the transplant technique for thrombectomy without extracorporeal circulation [10]. In all cases, "chevron" access was made. The duodenum was kocherized. Afterwards, liver mobilization was performed: the falciform, triangular, and coronal ligaments were transected. The piggy-back liver mobilization was carried out by section and ligation of the small hepatic veins draining into the anterior surface of the retrohepatic vena cava. We passed a tourniquet around the suprahepatic infradiaphragmatic IVC and proceeded to the surgical access to the supradiaphragmatic IVC and the right atrium without opening the pericardium.

Initially, a transverse diaphragmotomy was performed, which included incision of the diaphragm parallel to the anterior semicircle of the inferior vena cava with the margin of 3–5 mm. This access was extended by a perpendicular longitudinal incision within 4-5 cm (T-shaped diaphragmotomy) (Figure 2). Then, a circular diaphragmotomy was performed, which involved total circular isolation of the IVC from the diaphragm, and the tourniquet was passed around the cavoatrial junction. The right semicircle of the supradiaphragmatic IVC was mobilized with extreme precautions. Surgical dissection in this area was made as close as possible to the caval surface to avoid the right phrenic nerve injury.

The right lobe of the liver was turned and moved to the medial side. Subsequently, the subhepatic and retrohepatic parts of the inferior vena cava were isolated. In cases of right-sided tumors, the renal artery was ligated through the interaorta-caval space. In patients with left-sided tumors, the renal artery was controlled posteriorly after mobilization and medial rotation of the kidney.

The next stage of the surgical intervention was the displacement of the tumor thrombus apex ("milking maneuver"). First, intraoperative transabdominal ultrasonography and palpation of the cavoatrial junction with the right atrium were performed. If the apical part of the intraluminal tumor extended to the right atrium by 10–15 mm, then it was covered by the thumb and index fingers of the left hand and displaced below the diaphragm afterwards. Further, a vascular clamp was placed directly above the upper end of the tumor, but below the cavoatrial junction. The pericardium

TABLE 1: Characteristics of patients and tumors with atrial extension.

	Case 1	Case 2	Case 3	Case 4	Case 5
Sex	M	F	M	F	M
Age	59	41	72	60	62
ECOG status	0	2	1	1	0
GFR (mL/min)	68.6	46.4	58.2	36.8	76.2
BMI (kg/m^2)	24.3	17.8	28.9	25.3	28.6
Lesion side	Right	Right	Right	Left	Left
Tumor size (cm)	6.5	30	10	18	10.2
TNM	pT3cN0M1	pT4N0M1	pT3cN0M0	pT3cN0M0	pT3cN0M0
Metastasis localization	Lungs	Lungs	–	–	
Symptoms	Hematuria	Weight loss Weakness Pain	Hematuria Dyspnea Lower extremity swelling	Hematuria Weakness	Hematuria
Heart failure	–	–	+	+	–
LVEF (%)	55	57	48	44	56
Blood clot below tumor thrombus	–	+	+	–	–
Thrombus maximal diameter (mm)	32	38	63	17	13
Thrombus atrial part (mm)	Length-35 Width-30	Length-15 Width-12	Length-10 Width-10	Length-10 Width-12	Length-30 Width-10
Complete blood flow block in the IVC	+	+	+	–	–
Tumor invasion into the IVC wall	–	+	+	+	–
Follow-up (months)	14	15	9	8	16

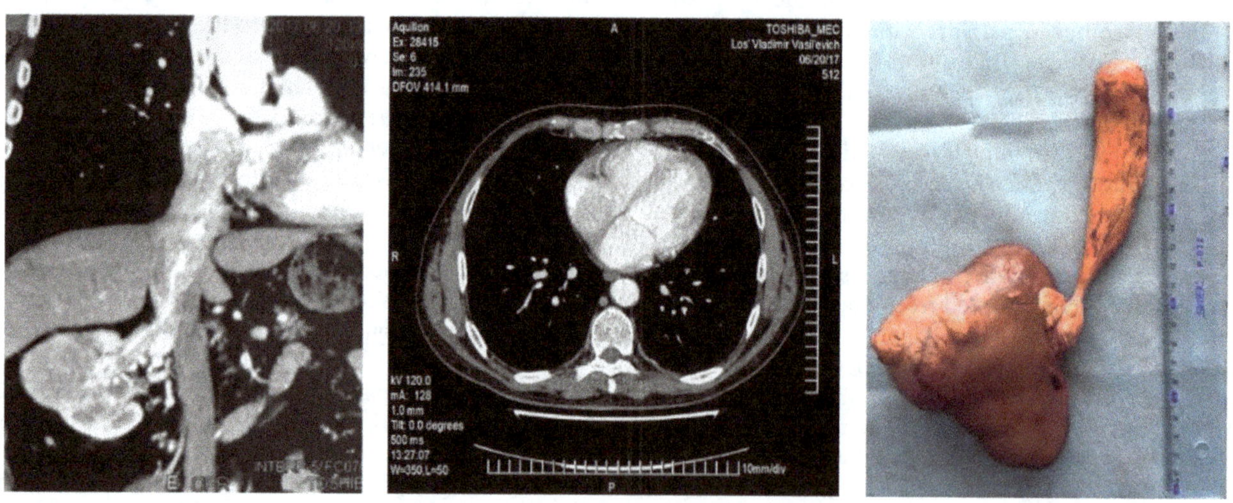

(a) (b) (c)

FIGURE 1: MDCT ((a) frontal reconstruction and (b) axial scan) and surgical specimen (c) of a patient with cavoatrial extension of RCC. The length of the atrial part of the tumor thrombus is 3.5 cm.

was never opened in these patients. The tight fixation of the thrombus apex by fingers through the atrial walls was the main measure for the prevention of the intraluminal tumor fragmentation and pulmonary embolism.

In cases of large thrombi with the length of their intra-atrial part reaching 30–35 mm, transpericardial access to the right atrium was used. For this purpose, the pericardium was opened with a longitudinal incision for a length of 4.0–5.0 cm.

The incision of the pericardium continued around the anterior, right, and posterior sectors of the intrapericardial

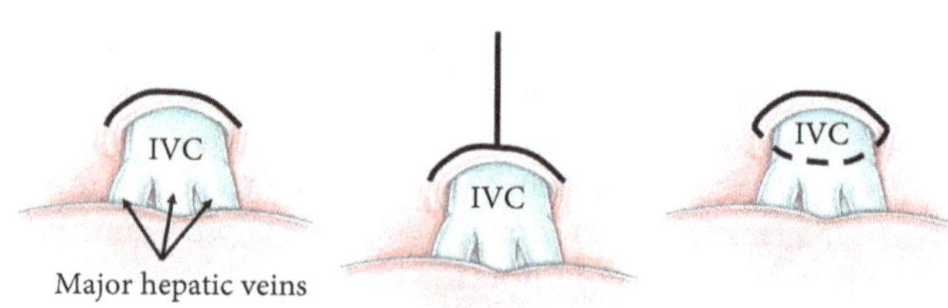

(a) (b) (c)

FIGURE 2: Types of diaphragmotomy: (a) transverse diaphragmotomy, (b) T-shaped diaphragmotomy, and (c) circular diaphragmotomy.

IVC. This maneuver provided wide access to the entire right atrium from the abdominal cavity (Figure 3). The displacement of the thrombus apex was carried out the same way as in the extrapericardial surgical access. Selection of the surgical access to the right atrium for performing the "milking maneuver" (either the extrapericardial access only, or the extended transpericardial access) was made in every patient individually based on palpation of the right atrium after a T-shaped and circular diaphragmotomy.

After the displacement of the thrombus below the diaphragm, a standard technique of three tourniquets was used to remove it. For control of bleeding from the hepatic veins, the Pringle maneuver was performed. The IVC was opened with a longitudinal incision from the level of the renal vein down to the lower edge of the major hepatic vein mouths. Immediately after evacuation of the thrombus, a tourniquet was placed on the IVC directly below the mouths of the major hepatic veins. The clamps were removed from the cavoatrial junction and the hepatoduodenal ligament.

3. Results

In all cases, the renal artery was ligated prior to thrombectomy. Since the right-sided tumors were present in most patients, control of the renal artery was fulfilled most often between the aorta and the IVC. However, in two cases, this stage of surgery was very difficult due to a large diameter and limited mobility of the inferior vena cava. Significant bleeding from the retroperitoneal venous collaterals, during mobilization and medial rotation of the kidney, took place in one of the patients with the left-sided tumor. The main characteristics of surgical interventions and complications are presented in Table 2.

Piggy-back liver mobilization was necessary in all five observations. At this stage of surgery, 4 to 10 short hepatic veins were transected (an average of 6.5 ± 2.6). During the access to the right atrium from the abdominal cavity, in most cases, only the anterior diaphragmatic veins were ligated at their confluence with the IVC (on average 2 ± 0.7 veins). In one case, the posterior diaphragmatic vein draining into the infra-diaphragmatic IVC was identified and transected.

Displacement of the thrombus apex below the diaphragm was successfully carried out in all 5 patients. In three patients with small atrial thrombi (up to 15 mm), it was sufficient to perform extrapericardial access to the right atrium for manual thrombus displacement. In two remaining patients with the thrombus atrial component length of 3.0 cm and 3.5 cm, control of the thrombus apex without opening the pericardium was impossible. Transpericardial access provided an opportunity for adequate palpation and fixation of the atrial component of the tumor thrombus by fingers. Displacement of the thrombus below the diaphragm in these patients passed without any significant difficulties. In all cases, the thrombus apex was moved below the cavoatrial junction and a clamp was placed at this level. The average clamping time of the supradiaphragmatic IVC was comparable to the average time of the Pringle maneuver, which was 5.6 ± 4.3 min. All patients were hemodynamically stable during this period. A

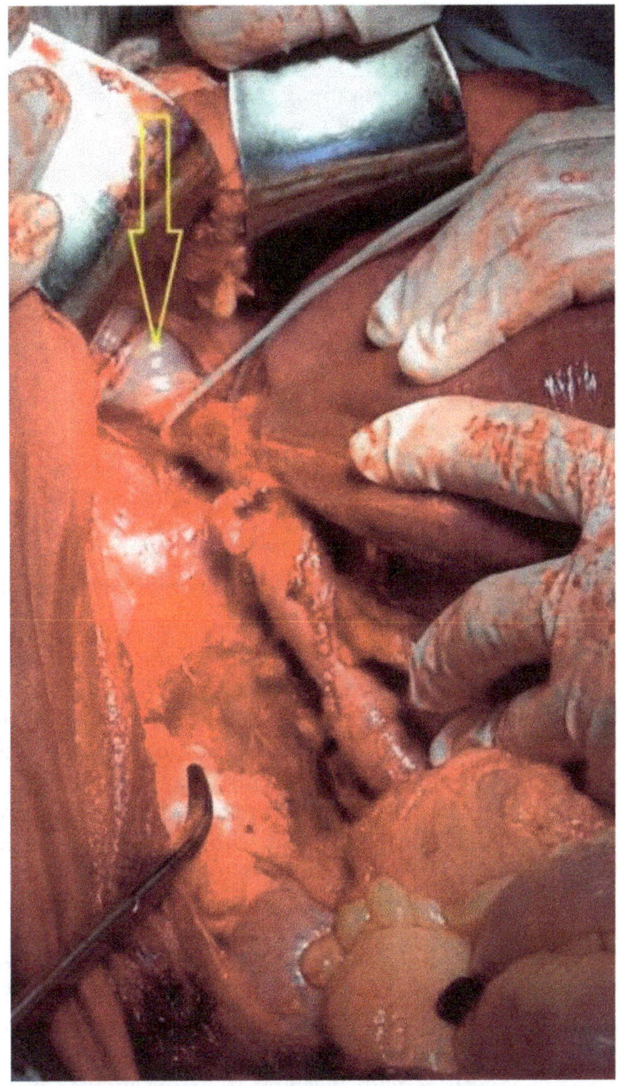

FIGURE 3: Transpericardial access to the right atrium (arrow) through the diaphragm from the abdominal cavity. Mobilization of the retrohepatic and supradiaphragmatic IVC with the liver piggy-back mobilization.

moderate decrease in blood pressure was noted in 4 out of 5 patients (by 14.0 ± 8.9 mmHg on average).

Among intraoperative complications during the access to the right atrium, injuries to the main hepatic veins and the supradiaphragmatic IVC predominated (3 observations). However, these traumatic defects were small, not accompanied by any significant bleeding and easily repaired. Two patients had certain complications associated with liver mobilization—diaphragm and liver injuries, which also did not cause any serious problems. In one case, a giant kidney tumor spread to the right common iliac artery, which led to the need for its resection and placement of a vascular prosthesis.

Lateral resection of the suprarenal component of the IVC was performed in 3 patients due to invasion of the intraluminal tumor into the caval wall. The diameter of the IVC at the level of resection was at least 2/3 of the initial values.

Table 2: Characteristics of surgical procedures and complications.

	Case 1	Case 2	Case 3	Case 4	Case 5
Thrombus atrial part length (mm)	35	15	10	10	30
Piggy-back liver mobilization	+	+	+	+	+
Anterior phrenic veins transection	3	2	2	1	2
Posterior phrenic veins transection	1	–	–	–	–
Transpericardial approach	+	–	–	–	+
Successful external thrombus displacement	+	+	+	+	+
BP reduction during upper IVC clamping (mmHg)	20	–	20	10	20
Supradiaphragmatic IVC clamping time (min)	3	12	3	8	2
Major hepatic veins injury	+	–	–	+	–
Supradiaphragmatic IVC injury	–	–	+	–	–
Liver injury	–	–	+	–	–
Diaphragm injury	–	–	–	+	–
Other intraoperative complications	–	*A. iliaca* injury	–	–	–
Longitudinal IVC resection	–	+	+	+	–
Surgery time (min)	220	320	280	260	280
Blood loss volume (ml)	2500	5600	3800	2800	3000
Packed red blood cell transfusion volume (U)	5	11	9	5	6
Postoperative complications	–	IVC thrombosis	–	Intestinal obstruction	–

In 2 cases, after evacuation of the tumor thrombus, a blood clot was removed from the infrarenal IVC and femoral veins using a Fogarty catheter. Recurrent thrombosis of the inferior vena cava caused by a blood clot was detected subsequently in one of these patients. Another patient had intestinal obstruction, which was managed conservatively. Specific complications associated with access to the right atrium from the abdominal cavity (paresis of the right phrenic nerve, pneumothorax, and mediastinitis) were not detected in any case.

The volume of intraoperative blood loss ranged from 2500 to 5600 ml and averaged 3540 ± 1248.2 ml. Most of the intraoperative blood loss was associated with damage to the massive venous collaterals during mobilization of the liver and IVC as well as with bleeding from the lumbar veins draining into the vascular isolation zone of the tumor thrombus. The average volume of transfused erythrocytes was 7.2 ± 2.7 units. The average operation time did not exceed 272 ± 36.3 min.

The length of ICU stay varied from 2 to 3 days (on average 2.4 ± 0.5 days), and the duration of hospital stay was 10–16 days (12.2 ± 2.3 days on average).

All the patients were still alive at the time of this work preparation. The median overall survival was 14 months. In three nonmetastatic patients, tumor progression was not detected during the entire follow-up period. One of two patients with pulmonary metastases receiving pazopanib in the postoperative period demonstrated bone and new pulmonary metastases, as well as local tumor recurrence in the wall of the inferior vena cava after 10 months. In another observation, there was no increase in size and number of pulmonary lesions within 14 months.

4. Discussion

The use of extracorporeal circulation and circulatory arrest during surgery of caval tumor thrombi extending above the diaphragm may be accompanied by serious complications (coagulopathy, neurological disorders, and multisystem failure) [2, 3]. Such approach significantly increases the trauma level and duration of the operation (the setup time for cardiopulmonary bypass is at least 30 minutes). On the other hand, one should take into account that the use of this technique requires median sternotomy, which also significantly increases the length of surgery and can result in serious postoperative complications. Therefore, many surgeons currently tend to search for alternative approaches for removing the supradiaphragmatic tumor thrombi without sternotomy, cardiopulmonary bypass, and circulatory arrest.

Surgical interventions without the use of extracorporeal circulation include three basic options for displacement of the thrombus apex downwards: the balloon technique, insertion of a finger into the right atrium, and external manual displacement (milking maneuver).

Control of the tumor thrombus apex with a balloon catheter wins by its simplicity and low invasiveness. Ability to remove the tumor masses from the lumen of the right atrium and inferior vena cava without complete liver mobilization, additional access to the mediastinum and opening the atrium, looks very tempting. However, the safety of this technique depends on several important conditions. First of all, the intraluminal tumor masses should not completely fill the caval lumen. The catheter should pass freely between the thrombus and caval wall. The dimensions of the thrombus atrial part should not be large. It is desirable for the thrombus to be of dense consistency. Finally, the tumor thrombus should not invade the caval wall.

The recent paper by Sobczyński et al. has demonstrated good results of using the balloon technique in four patients with cavoatrial tumor thrombi, which completely matches the abovementioned criteria [11]. However, one should take into account that atrial thrombi of a small diameter without signs of invasion into the caval wall are not very common. Considering our patients for possible thrombectomy with the balloon catheter, it should be noted that an average diameter of the tumor thrombus reached 32.6 ± 19.9 mm (13 to 63 mm); the atrial part of the tumor was 3.0 and 3.5 cm in two cases, and in three patients, there were the signs of caval wall invasion. Due to the abovementioned factors, the balloon catheter could be used potentially only in two out of five patients. However, from our point of view, displacement of the tumor thrombus apex with the balloon is a rather risky maneuver, which can be accompanied by thrombus fragmentation, pulmonary artery embolism, and incomplete removal of the intraluminal tumor in the case of its firm fixation to the caval wall. It is also necessary to consider the possibility of arrhythmia and acute hypotension due to the rapid decline of atrial volume during balloon inflation.

In 1989, Skinner et al. proposed displacement of the atrial thrombus with the help of the index finger inserted into the right atrium through a small incision on the beating heart [16]. The main advantages of this approach are direct control of the thrombus apex by tactile sensation of the surgeon, as well as the possibility of rapid displacement of the thrombus below the diaphragm or major hepatic vein mouths. In the study by Schneider et al., who used this surgical technique together with transesophageal echocardiography in 4 patients, the feasibility and safety of this procedure were demonstrated [9]. They noted that the risk of embolism and other complications during this maneuver was extremely low. Nevertheless, one should note the potential problems and limitations of this surgical technique, which include significant trauma (sternotomy or thoracolaparotomy and atriotomy), risk of bleeding, and air embolism. Although the authors have demonstrated minimal risk of thrombus fragmentation and tumor embolism, it still exists. It should also be borne in mind that displacement of the thrombus is carried out by pushing movements, so it is quite difficult to fix the thin and mobile thrombus apex in the lumen of the atrium beating by one finger.

Ciancio et al. introduced a liver transplantation technique for caval thrombectomy which included piggy-back liver mobilization with complete mobilization of the retrohepatic IVC, surgical access to the supradiaphragmatic IVC from the abdominal cavity, and external manual displacement of the thrombus below the diaphragm or major hepatic veins [10]. This surgical technique has become popular and now it is actively used to remove tumor thrombi reaching the retrohepatic and intrapericardial IVC [6, 15, 17, 18]. There are also rare reports on the use of this technique in patients with right atrial tumor thrombi. In particular, Cerwinka et al. described one patient with invasion of an atrial thrombus into the endocardium who was treated by this surgical method [14]. In 2010, Ciancio et al. presented successful results of the liver transplant technique in 7 patients with right atrial thrombi [13]. We also used this technique in our 5 patients with a modified surgical access to the right atrium.

The main advantages of thrombectomy with the help of the liver transplantation technique are the possibility of an easy access to the mediastinum through the diaphragm from the abdominal cavity and the rapid and safe displacement of the thrombus apex below the diaphragm or the mouths of the major hepatic veins. However, with respect to this method, there are several questions that need to be answered. In particular, what kinds of surgical accesses to the right atrium from the abdominal cavity are the most convenient? Are these approaches safe? How feasible and safe is the external displacement of the tumor thrombus from the atrium? What size of the tumor atrial part is acceptable for this technique?

In recent years, several reports have been published regarding the approaches to the intrapericardial part of the inferior vena cava and to the right atrium through the diaphragm from the abdominal cavity [5, 12, 15, 19–22]. All these approaches are divided into longitudinal, transverse, and circular (around the IVC) diaphragmotomy, or they are a combination of several incision types. Also, two other types of these approaches are distinguished as extrapericardial and transpericardial. Undoubtedly, extrapericardial approaches have certain priorities in terms of safety, since opening the pericardium during surgery can be accompanied by a decrease in cardiac output and, in the postoperative period, can lead to the development of constrictive or purulent pericarditis, as well as cardiac tamponade [23, 24].

In our study, in patients with tumor thrombi extending to the right atrium by 1.0 or 1.5 cm, the apex was easily palpated and shifted through the extrapericardial approach. However, in cases of atrial thrombi reaching 3.0 cm or more, it was impossible to perform external manual control of the thrombus apex without opening the pericardium.

Earlier we conducted an anatomical study devoted to the feasibility and safety of various surgical approaches to the supradiaphragmatic IVC from the abdominal cavity [25]. The best results were obtained in the case of extraperipercardial T-shaped diaphragmotomy (a combination of longitudinal and circular incisions of the diaphragm). In our clinical practice, we use this access most often, since it is convenient, not traumatic, and allows reliable manual control of the tumor thrombi located next to the cavoatrial junction. In situations where adequate control of the thrombus apex from T-shaped extrapericardial access was impossible, we performed longitudinal opening of the pericardium and continued incision around the anterior, right, and posterior sectors of the intrapericardial IVC. Such approach affords an opportunity for the successful performance of the "milking maneuver," even when the length of the atrial part of the thrombus reaches 3.5 cm. One of the most important arguments in favor of the transpericardial approach is that the apex of a large thrombus, spreading into the lumen of the right atrium, extends not only upwards, but also to the left, along the course of the blood flow from the right atrium to the right ventricle. Therefore, for reliable fixation of the thrombus, the whole right atrium must be controlled by fingers (Figure 4).

Analysis of the presented surgical approaches to the right atrium, which were used in our clinical work, demonstrated their safety. The diaphragmatic veins drained mostly in the area of the anterior semicircle of the IVC. Only in one case, damage to the posterior surface of the IVC in the place of its confluence with the posterior diaphragmatic vein was identified. However, this damage was not accompanied by any significant bleeding and was easily repaired. In the postoperative period, we did not register any signs of mediastinitis, pericardial tamponade, or injury to the right phrenic nerve.

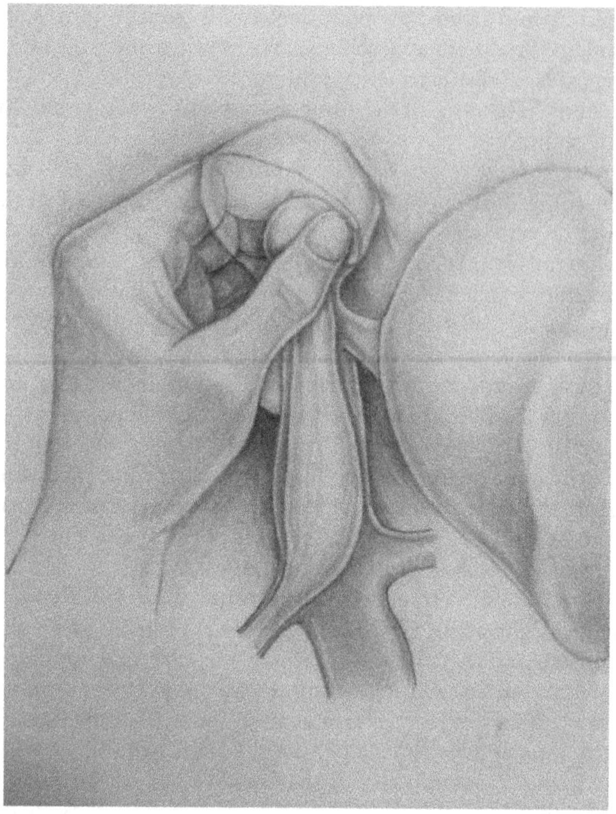

Figure 4: Performing "milking maneuver" in a patient with a large atrial tumor thrombus through the transpericardial access from the abdominal cavity.

Regarding the stage of thrombus displacement from the right atrium, it should be noted that, in all cases, it was performed quickly and was not accompanied by any significant decrease of blood pressure, arrhythmia, or tumor embolism. We encountered moderate technical difficulties during performing this maneuver only in one patient with the largest atrial component of the thrombus (3.5 cm). The problem was associated with active movements of the tumor apex in the atrial lumen, which caused some issues with fixation and shifting of the tumor thrombus.

Considering a very small experience, it is currently difficult to estimate the maximal size of the atrial thrombus, for which the transplant technique for thrombectomy is safe to use. Nevertheless, as our study has demonstrated, these dimensions can be up to 3.5 cm. The liver transplantation technique during the removal of thrombi with the atrial component length up to 1.5 cm is safe and easily achievable. It actually does not differ from the technique used in patients with nonatrial supradiaphragmatic IVC thrombi.

The most serious problems of the transplantation technique in patients with cavoatrial thrombi are the inability to displace the thrombus apex below the diaphragm due to adhesions with the atrial endothelium, as well as hemodynamic instability in the moment of the cavoatrial junction clamping. In these situations, the safest option is to switch to cardiopulmonary bypass, which must be available to the surgical team. Although none of our patients needed extracorporeal circulation, we believe that these operations should be performed in a cardiac surgery operating unit.

Good visualization of the atrial part of the thrombus and identification of its mobility in the atrium are the most important factors for the success of the transplantation technique for thrombectomy. For these purposes, we used MDCT and transabdominal echocardiography before surgery, which were accurate in all patients. Nevertheless, it should be borne in mind that these methods have significant drawbacks. In particular, in patients with the thin cavoatrial thrombi, their atrial part is not clearly visible on MDCT due to high mobility of the intraluminal tumor. Performing transabdominal echocardiography may be difficult due to the constitutional features of patients or chest deformity. For intraoperative identification of the atrial tumor, we used transabdominal ultrasonography. This method is accurate, from our point of view, but not convenient enough. Undoubtedly, the transesophageal echography, which allows monitoring the position of the thrombus at all stages of the operation and makes surgical intervention safer, is the "gold standard" of intraoperative imaging of cavoatrial tumor thrombi.

It should be objectively recognized that surgical methods, including cardiopulmonary bypass with or without deep hypothermic circulatory arrest, are necessary for most atrial tumor thrombus removals. However, in distinct patients, this surgical problem can be solved with the help of the liver transplant technique for thrombectomy. From our point of view, while determining the indications for the use of this method, the leading role belongs to the experience of a surgeon in the operations on patients with retrohepatic and intrapericardial IVC thrombi. Another important aspect is careful selection of patients for performing such surgical interventions, which adhere to two main conditions: during ultrasonography, the thrombus apex should float freely in the atrial lumen and the patient should not have severe heart failure. However, further multicenter randomized studies are needed to determine the feasibility and safety of this surgical approach in comparison with other techniques.

5. Conclusion

Our work represents the initial experience in the use of the transplantation technique in distinct and well-selected patients with the right atrium tumor thrombi. The effectiveness of this approach needs further study.

References

[1] A. A. Glazer and A. C. Novick, "Long-term follow up after surgical treatment for renal cell carcinoma extending into the right atrium," *Journal of Urology*, vol. 155, no. 2, pp. 448–450, 1996.

[2] D. Shchukin and Y. Iliukhin, *Surgery of the Inferior Vena Cava Tumor Thrombi for Renal Cancer Belgorod: OJSC*, Belgorod Regional Printing House, Belgorod, Russia, 2007.

[3] A. C. Novick, M. C. Kaye, D. M. Cosgrove et al., "Experience with cardiopulmonary bypass and deep hypothermic circulatory arrest in the management of retroperitoneal tumors with large vena caval thrombi," *Annals of Surgery*, vol. 212, no. 4, pp. 472–477, 1990.

[4] M. B. Patil, J. Montez, J. Loh-Doyle et al., "Level III-IV inferior vena caval thrombectomy without cardiopulmonary bypass: long-term experience with intrapericardial control," *Journal of Urology*, vol. 192, no. 3, pp. 682–689, 2014.

[5] G. Ciancio and M. S. Soloway, "Renal cell carcinoma with tumor thrombus extending above diaphragm: avoiding cardiopulmonary bypass," *Urology*, vol. 66, no. 2, pp. 266–270, 2005.

[6] T. Taweemonkongsap, C. Nualyong, S. Leewansangtong et al., "Surgical treatment of renal cell carcinoma with inferior vena cava thrombus: using liver mobilization technique to avoid cardiopulmonary bypass," *Asian Journal of Surgery*, vol. 31, no. 2, pp. 75–82, 2008.

[7] L. Zini, S. Haulon, X. Leroy et al., "Endoluminal occlusion of the inferior vena cava in renal cell carcinoma with retro- or suprahepatic caval thrombus," *BJU International*, vol. 97, no. 6, pp. 1216–1220, 2006.

[8] K. Yanaga, T. Yoshizumi, K. Komori, T. Nishizaki, M. Masuda, and K. Sugimachi, "Balloon catheter-assisted inferior vena cava tumor thrombectomy without thoracotomy," *Hepatogastroenterology*, vol. 44, pp. 796-797, 1997.

[9] M. Schneider, B. Hadaschik, P. Hallscheidt et al., "Manual repositioning of intra-atrial kidney cancer tumor thrombus: a technique reducing the need for cardiopulmonary bypass," *Urology*, vol. 81, no. 4, pp. 909–914, 2013.

[10] G. Ciancio, J. Gonzalez, S. P. Shirodkar, J. C. Angulo, and M. S. Soloway, "Liver transplantation techniques for the surgical management of renal cell carcinoma with tumor thrombus in the inferior vena cava: step-by-step description," *European Urology*, vol. 59, no. 3, pp. 401–406, 2011.

[11] R. Sobczyński, T. Golabek, M. Przydacz et al., "Modified technique of cavoatrial tumor thrombectomy without cardiopulmonary by-pass and hypothermic circulatory arrest: a preliminary report," *Central European Journal of Urology*, vol. 68, no. 3, pp. 311–317, 2015.

[12] P. Bassi, F. Dal Moro, M. Ciaccia, F. Rea, and F. Pagano, "Transdiaphragmatic-intrapericardiac approach to supradiaphragmatic vena cava invasion secondary to renal cell carcinoma: a novel surgical approach," *Urology*, vol. 66, no. 5, pp. 1101–1105, 2005.

[13] G. Ciancio, S. P. Shirodkar, M. S. Soloway, A. S. Livingstone, M. Barron, and T. A. Salerno, "Renal carcinoma with supradiaphragmatic tumor thrombus: avoiding sternotomy and cardiopulmonary bypass," *The Annals of Thoracic Surgery*, vol. 89, no. 2, pp. 505–510, 2010.

[14] W. H. Cerwinka, G. Ciancio, T. A. Salerno, and M. S. Soloway, "Renal cell cancer with invasive atrial tumor thrombus excised off-pump," *Urology*, vol. 66, pp. 1319.e9–1319.e11, 2005.

[15] M. E. Facciuto, M. K. Singh, J. P. Rocca et al., "Benefits of liver transplantation surgical techniques in the management of extensive retroperitoneal tumors," *World Journal of Surgery*, vol. 32, no. 11, pp. 2403–2407, 2008.

[16] D. G. Skinner, T. R. Pritchett, G. Lieskovsky, S. D. Boyd, and Q. R. Stiles, "Vena caval involvement by renal cell carcinoma," *Annals of Surgery*, vol. 210, no. 3, pp. 387–394, 1989.

[17] G. Ciancio, C. Hawke, and M. Soloway, "The use of liver transplant techniques to aid in the surgical management of urological tumors," *Journal of Urology*, vol. 164, no. 3, pp. 665–672, 2000.

[18] G. Ciancio, A. Vaidya, M. Savoie, and M. Soloway, "Management of renal cell carcinoma with level III thrombus in the inferior vena cava," *Journal of Urology*, vol. 168, no. 4, pp. 1374–1377, 2002.

[19] M. Miyazaki, H. Ito, and K. Nakagawa, "An approach to intrapericardial inferior vena cava through the abdominal cavity, without median sternotomy, for total hepatic vascular exclusion," *Hepatogastroenterology*, vol. 48, pp. 1443–1446, 2001.

[20] T. W. Chen, C. H. Tsai, S. J. Chou et al., "Intrapericardial isolation of the inferior vena cava through a transdiaphragmatic pericardial window for tumor resection without sternotomy or thoracotomy," *European Journal of Surgical Oncology (EJSO)*, vol. 33, no. 2, pp. 239–242, 2007.

[21] S. Mizuno, H. Kato, Y. Azumi et al., "Total vascular hepatic exclusion for tumor resection: a new approach to the intrathoracic inferior vena cava through the abdominal cavity by cutting the diaphragm vertically without cutting the pericardium," *Journal of Hepato-Biliary-Pancreatic Sciences*, vol. 17, no. 2, pp. 197–202, 2010.

[22] E. Belgrano, C. Trombetta, G. Liguori, S. Siracusano, G. Savoca, and B. Zingone, "Intrahepatic tumor thrombectomy through an abdominal diaphragmatic approach," *Journal of Urology*, vol. 158, no. 6, pp. 2233-2234, 1997.

[23] M. Mathru, B. Kleinman, D. J. Dries, T. Rao, and D. Calandra, "Effect of opening the pericardium on right ventricular hemodynamics during cardiac surgery," *Chest*, vol. 98, no. 1, pp. 120–123, 1990.

[24] F. Sangalli, L. Colagrande, B. Manetti et al., "Hemodynamic instability after cardiac surgery: transesophageal echocardiographic diagnosis of a localized pericardial tamponade," *Journal of Cardiothoracic and Vascular Anesthesia*, vol. 19, no. 6, pp. 775-776, 2005.

[25] D. Shchukin, V. Lesovoy, I. Garagatiy, G. Khareba, and R. Hsaine, "Surgical approaches to supradiaphragmatic segment of IVC and right atrium through abdominal cavity during intravenous tumor thrombus removal," *Advances in Urology*, vol. 2014, Article ID 924269, 9 pages, 2014.

31

Management of Long-Segment and Panurethral Stricture Disease

Francisco E. Martins,[1,2] Sanjay B. Kulkarni,[3] Pankaj Joshi,[3] Jonathan Warner,[4] and Natalia Martins[2]

[1] *Department of Urology, Hospital Santa Maria, University of Lisbon, School of Medicine, 1600-161 Lisbon, Portugal*
[2] *ULSNA-Hospital de Portalegre, 7300-074 Portalegre, Portugal*
[3] *Kulkarni Reconstructive Urology Center, Pune 411038, India*
[4] *City of Hope Medical Center, Duarte, CA 91010, USA*

Correspondence should be addressed to Francisco E. Martins; faemartins@gmail.com

Academic Editor: Kostis Gyftopoulos

Long-segment urethral stricture or panurethral stricture disease, involving the different anatomic segments of anterior urethra, is a relatively less common lesion of the anterior urethra compared to bulbar stricture. However, it is a particularly difficult surgical challenge for the reconstructive urologist. The etiology varies according to age and geographic location, lichen sclerosus being the most prevalent in some regions of the globe. Other common and significant causes are previous endoscopic urethral manipulations (urethral catheterization, cystourethroscopy, and transurethral resection), previous urethral surgery, trauma, inflammation, and idiopathic. The iatrogenic causes are the most predominant in the Western or industrialized countries, and lichen sclerosus is the most common in India. Several surgical procedures and their modifications, including those performed in one or more stages and with the use of adjunct tissue transfer maneuvers, have been developed and used worldwide, with varying long-term success. A one-stage, minimally invasive technique approached through a single perineal incision has gained widespread popularity for its effectiveness and reproducibility. Nonetheless, for a successful result, the reconstructive urologist should be experienced and familiar with the different treatment modalities currently available and select the best procedure for the individual patient.

1. Introduction

Management of long-segment urethral stricture remains a challenge in reconstructive urology. The surgical treatment of urethral strictures varies according to etiology, location, length, and density of the lesion and fibrosis involving surrounding tissues [1–3]. Treatment of strictures involving the bulbar urethra is relatively well defined and, in most cases, is amenable to excision and end-to-end anastomosis or a short patch onlay substitution urethroplasty [4]. However, long-segment urethral stricture or panurethral stricture disease is less common and the literature on the subject is not abundant.

In the treatment of this condition, several issues must be factored in, such as cause of the stricture, previous urethral surgeries, the quality of the urethral plate, availability of different autologous tissues to be used as flaps or grafts, experience, expertise, and preference of the treating urologist, including his familiarity with tissue transfer techniques [5]. Lichen sclerosus (LS), also known as balanitis xerotica obliterans (BXO), raises specific problems related to treatment, prognosis, and prolonged follow-up [6–10]. The complexity of this condition may require a different dynamic treatment paradigm. However, although a multistage reconstruction may be used by some surgeons in certain situations due to hostile urethral tissues, in the majority of cases, LS is amenable to a single-stage reconstruction with highly favorable results. Additionally, reconstruction of long-segment urethral strictures is not only about restoring voiding function but also preserving sexual function in all its aspects, such as erection, ejaculation, and orgasm as well as guaranteeing good penile cosmesis.

Current surgical options employed are associated with reasonable success rates and may include a single- or a multiple-stage reconstruction, with the use of a flap, a graft, or a combination of both, and lastly, in extreme circumstances a perineal urethrostomy may offer the best solution for the patient who does not wish to go the extra (long) mile.

2. Materials and Methods

A review of the international literature was conducted using MEDLINE/PubMed database and Google Search, using keywords as "complex urethral stricture," "long segment urethral stricture," "panurethral," "lichen sclerosus," "oral mucosa," and "urethroplasty." We included in the review only articles published in the English language from 1990 to 2015.

3. Epidemiology, Etiology, and Pathogenesis

Generally speaking, male urethral stricture is a common disease worldwide and has been so for centuries. The first known description of urethral dilatation is credited to Shusruta more than 600 years BC [11]. In the 19th century, expert opinion estimated an incidence of 15–20% in the adult male population [12]. In the 21st century in the UK NHS more than 16,000 men required hospital admission annually due to urethral stricture and more than 12,000 of these admissions ended up necessitating surgical treatment with more than £10,000 million [12]. The estimated prevalence in the UK averages 10/100,000 young males doubling this figure by the age of 55 years and rising to over 100/100,000 in males over 65 years. In the USA male urethral stricture accounted for about 5,000 inpatient visits and 1.5 million office visits annually between 1992 and 2000. The incidence was estimated to be approximately 0.6% in susceptible populations [13]. The estimated costs to the medical system for male urethral disease in the USA surpassed US$ 190 million in 2000 [13]. However, there are no direct measures to assess the true incidence of urethral stricture disease worldwide, much less so for panurethral stricture disease in particular. A recent study, including 268 patients, reported panurethral or multifocal anterior urethral stricture in a total of 36 patients (13.4%). However, in a more recent retrospective analysis of all strictures that had been treated surgically at a single institution, the vast majority of strictures were anterior (92.2%) with panurethral strictures totalling 4.9% [14].

Urethral stricture disease can have a profound impact on quality of life, including sexual life, as a result of a number of complications associated with urinary obstruction, such as infection, bladder calculi, urethral diverticulum, fistulation, sepsis, and ultimately chronic renal failure.

The etiology of long-segment or panurethral strictures may vary in industrialized and developing countries. Today, in industrialized countries, most urethral strictures in general have iatrogenic or idiopathic origin [2, 3]. Iatrogenic causes include urethral catheterization, cystourethroscopy, transurethral resection, and previous urethral surgeries. Other causes include idiopathic, trauma, infection/inflammation, and lichen sclerosus. In the developing world, the most common cause of panurethral stricture is genital lichen sclerosus (LS) [6]. Although less frequent, gonorrhea still remains an important cause of long-segment strictures in the developing world.

The pathogenesis of long-segment or panurethral stricture disease has not been widely studied. Historically, and although it is an important cause in some regions of the developing world, infection was blamed as the main cause of urethral stricture [15]. However, it must follow a similar pathogenic process as other types of urethral stricture, that is, injury to the epithelium of the urethra and underlying corpus spongiosum, ultimately leading to fibrosis during the healing process. Excepting a traumatic cause when the urethral lumen is obliterated, corpus spongiosum deep to the urethral epithelium is replaced by dense fibrous tissue and the normal urethral pseudostratified columnar epithelium being replaced by squamous metaplasia [16–18]. Metaplastic change can also occur proximal to a stricture, due to chronic distension under pressure of voiding [12]. Small tears occurring repeatedly in the metaplastic tissue result in focal urinary extravasation, which in turn leads to a fibrotic reaction within the spongiosum. Initially, this fibrosis can be asymptomatic, but, over time, the scar or fibrotic plaque produced can enhance the narrowing of the urethral lumen, resulting in symptomatic urinary obstruction.

The pathology of a urethral stricture is characterized by changes in the extracellular matrix of the spongiosal tissue and replacement of the normal connective tissue by dense fibrosis associated with a decrease in the ratio of type III to type I collagen and a significant decrease in the smooth muscle and nitric oxide content in the strictured urethral tissue [19, 20].

The pathology of lichen sclerosus in inducing urethral stricture is different. LS is a chronic, progressive, inflammatory process which in the male can involve foreskin, glans, and anterior urethra. The etiology is for the most part unclear, although it has been associated with an autoimmune reaction and a genetic pattern. However, an infectious cause has been suggested [21]. This is an atrophic rather than a proliferative process that usually originates in the foreskin or glans as diffuse or patchy plaques of white discoloration giving the glans a characteristically mottled appearance (Figure 1). It can progress further to include the meatus, fossa navicularis, penile urethra, and eventually the bulbar urethra, resulting in a long-segment or panurethral stricture disease [7, 8]. It remains unclear whether LS-induced urethral strictures develop as a consequence of extension of glandular disease into the penile urethra or whether they result from chronically obstructed voiding or instrumentation, or both [22]. Long-segment urethral strictures, as any anterior urethral stricture, typically occur following trauma or infection, but mostly from iatrogenic causes, especially urethral catheterization, dilatation, and endoscopic manipulation, or may be idiopathic. Nonetheless, LS has been reported as the most frequent cause of this type of stricture, especially in India [6, 8, 9].

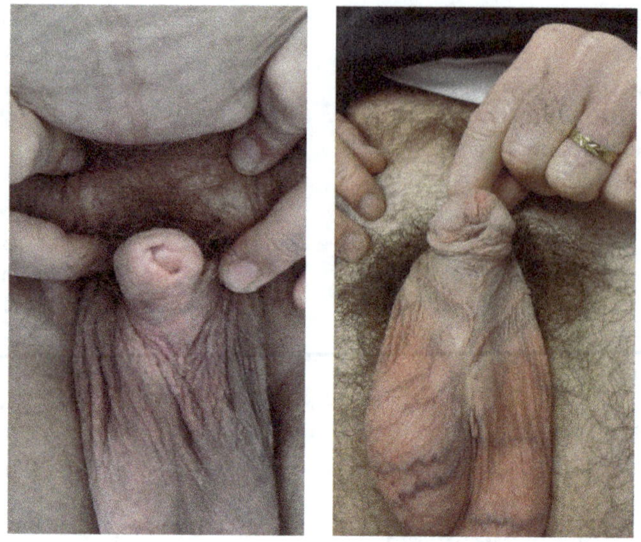

(a) (b)

FIGURE 1: Lichen sclerosus of the glans and prepuce (a) and hypospadias cripple (b). Both patients with panurethral stricture.

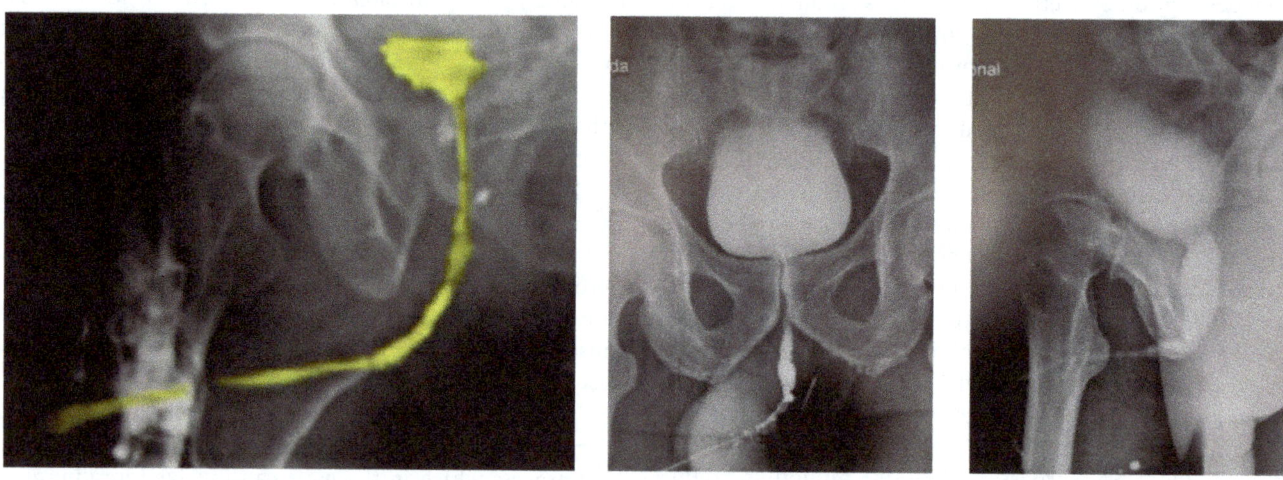

FIGURE 2: Retrograde and voiding urethrogram of panurethral stricture disease.

4. Diagnostic Evaluation

A critical initial pitfall in the diagnostic evaluation is not to fully understand and properly diagnose the stricture as being panurethral. Symptomatic stricture disease typically presents with progressive obstructive voiding complaints, such as a weak stream, frequency, incomplete emptying, terminal dribbling and straining, or complications of an obstructive voiding syndrome, such as recurrent tract infections, epididymitis, haematuria, and bladder stones. Symptomatic evaluation should be best formalized using a validated questionnaire, such as the AUA symptom index [24, 25].

Physical examination may be vague and uneventful in some cases. Nonetheless, the penis should always be carefully examined for scars related to previous surgery, penile malformations, signs of LS, or associated penile cancer. Careful attention should also be drawn to palpation of the spongiosum and genital area in general. The mouth should also be carefully inspected, particularly if an oral mucosa graft is planned.

Uroflowmetry, ultrasonography, and cystourethroscopy may be important adjuncts in the diagnosis of panurethral stricture disease, but the most critical is retrograde urethrography (RUG) and voiding cystourethrography (VCUG). The latter tests determine the location, length, and severity of the stricture in great detail (Figure 2). Endoscopy can give an idea of the elasticity and appearance of the urethra, especially following previous urethroplasty(ies). Ultrasonography can be used to determine the length and degree of fibrosis and eventually influence the operative approach [26]. Although ultrasonography seems to provide important additional information during preoperative evaluation, it has not gained the expected widespread popularity. This may be due to its relatively limited usefulness in the more proximal bulbar urethra, where the distance between the ultrasound probe and the target area surpasses its resolution accuracy.

It is of paramount importance that these imaging modalities ensure that all diseased portions of the urethra are included in the repair. Often, the narrowing of the lumen can be fairly uniform, with spots of more severe reduction in caliber. Thus, a panurethral stricture can be erroneously interpreted as just a short stricture and the other less severe areas underestimated as being of "normal" caliber. To avoid this diagnostic error, some authors have suggested that if the urethral lumen does not expand to ≥ 8 mm in diameter on imaging, then it is probably stenosed. Sometimes, it may be necessary to proceed to a full examination under anesthesia with endoscopy and bougienage and retrograde urethral imaging [27].

5. Surgical Reconstruction

In rare instances, where symptoms are not particularly troublesome, surgical treatment may not be necessary. In the majority of patients, both urethral dilatation and direct vision internal urethrotomy are inappropriate and, therefore, have no place in the treatment of panurethral stricture disease. At the other extreme end of the spectrum of this disease, typically patients who have undergone multiple failed surgical attempts, particularly when associated with significant comorbidity, might prefer a definitive perineal urethrostomy or even opt a simple suprapubic cystostomy catheter.

Panurethral stricture disease is definitely a complex subset of urethral stricture disease. Defining "panurethral" has been a matter of debate. This has implications in the interpretation of the literature as there is no homogeneity in the study populations. In a recent multi-institution study including 466 patients, long-segment or panurethral stricture was defined as any single stricture or multifocal diseased areas of the penile and bulbar (anterior) urethra measuring ≥ 8 cm in length [23]. Several surgical reconstructive procedures have been described to address this full-length anterior urethral strictures (Table 1). When planning the surgical treatment of panurethral stricture disease, some surgeons have concerns of whether to select a one- or two-stage operation and, if a one-stage operation is chosen, whether adequate transfer tissue for reconstruction is available. Panurethral stricture disease associated with LS has been successfully treated with a single-stage repair and OM onlay grafting. Indeed, the authors' experience has clearly shown that it should be preferred over a multistage approach, which in their opinion has no role in the surgical treatment of genitourethral LS [6, 23]. The main arguments are the high failure rate; the fact that genitourethral LS is a penile skin disease and, lastly, that staged operations will allow ingrowth of the disease into the urethra. In less common instances, where there is significant urethral narrowing with an unsalvageable plate, after multiple failed previous repairs, or if the stricture disease is associated with infection, abscess or calculi, a two-stage marsupializing procedure, like the Johanson procedure, may be preferable. In the majority of cases, substitution urethroplasty is the rule. Substitution urethroplasty can be performed using a flap, a graft, or sometimes a combination of both.

Table 1: Options for surgical reconstruction of long-segment and panurethral strictures.

Options
Flaps
Circular fasciocutaneous penile flap (McAninch flap)
Q-flap and variants (Quartey and Jordan)
Biaxial epilated scrotal flap (Gil-Vernet)
Grafts
Oral mucosa (cheek, tongue, and lower lip)—Kulkarni technique
Postauricular skin (Wolf)
Penile and preputial skin
Bladder mucosa
Colonic mucosa
Combination of flaps and grafts
Staged procedures
Johanson technique and variants
Schreiter's mesh graft technique
Tunica albuginea (Monseur) urethroplasty
Perineal urethrostomy

5.1. Flaps. Several flaps have been described and used in panurethral stricture reconstruction. In 1993, McAninch described the *circular fasciocutaneous penile flap* for the reconstruction of extensive urethral stricture [28]. Circular fasciocutaneous penile flap originates on the distal penis and uses Buck's fascia as the major vascular supply. He reported his results with the use of this flap for 1-stage reconstruction of complex anterior urethral strictures involving long penile and also bulbar urethral strictures in 66 men [29]. The stricture length measured up to 24 cm (average 9.08 cm). The flap was used as an onlay procedure and tubularized flap for urethral substitution. In some cases, additional adjunctive tissue transfer and proximal graft placement were required. Initial success rate was 79%, rising up to 95% after an additional procedure. Recurrent strictures occurred usually at the proximal and distal anastomotic sites. The penile circular fasciocutaneous flap reliably provided 12–15 cm of length for reconstruction in most patients, although approximately 90% had been previously circumcised. The less favorable results were seen in patients after flap tubularization for urethral replacement. The McAninch technique is worldwide considered as a reliable surgical option for panurethral strictures and numerous publications are available in the literature about its use. A major advantage of the McAninch flap is its versatility, as it can be utilized in all areas of the urethra, from the membranous area to the external meatus [29, 30]. Because of compartment syndrome noted in 2 different cases due to prolonged exaggerated lithotomy position that usually occurs if the patient remains in this position more than 5 hours, the authors begin the operation with flap harvesting with the patient in the supine position, thereby reducing exposure to the lithotomy position by 2-3 hours.

The *Q-flap* is a modification of the McAninch circular penile fasciocutaneous skin flap. It is so called because it incorporates an additional midline ventral longitudinal penile extension, thus resembling the letter Q. Similar "hockey-stick" flap configurations have also been described by Quartey [31]. Morey et al. reported their experience with the Q-flap in 15 patients with a mean stricture length of 15.5 cm (range 12–21) who underwent single-stage urethral reconstruction. All patients had a prepuce and the flap was harvested with the patient initially supine to avoid compartment syndrome [32]. The flap is outlined with the penis on stretch and the penis degloved, meticulously preserving the blood supply on the tunica dartos pedicle. The Q-flap is sewn into place after ventral urethrotomy as an onlay flap with running 4-0 absorbable suture, similar to the McAninch flap procedure. The fossa navicularis is typically reconstructed through a glans-wings or a glans-preserving technique. Once the pendulous portion of the onlay flap is sewn in, the patient is repositioned into the lithotomy position and the flap is transferred to the perineum through a scrotal tunnel wide enough to accommodate loose passage of the flap. The potential major advantage of these flap procedures is to allow a single-stage reconstruction of long-segment and complex strictures and to avoid the need for additional, morbid, time-consuming tissue transfer techniques.

These two procedures are extremely labor-intensive and are among the most difficult and tedious in reconstructive urology. A common complication with the above two flaps, particularly with unexperienced surgeons, is necrosis of penile skin proximal to the flap [29, 30]. In some instances, this penile skin necrosis may lead to wound infection and ultimately to disruption of the flap and necrosis.

In 1997, Gil-Vernet et al. described another type of flap for urethroplasty, the *biaxial epilated scrotal flap* [33]. They used this flap, which measured up to 20 × 2.5 cm, to reconstruct the entire anterior urethra from the bulbomembranous urethra to the external meatus. This flap consists of scrotal skin, dartos, external spermatic fascia, cremasteric fibers and fascia, internal spermatic fascia, and scrotal septum. Tunica vaginalis is not included. Vascular anastomoses between cremasteric (deep) and scrotal (superficial) blood supply plexuses are included in the flap and hence biaxial flap. The authors used this technique in 37 men including 10 with panurethral stricture disease. Two of these 10 patients failed due to graft shrinkage, necessitating perineal urethrostomy. There were also problems with incorrect scrotal skin epilation leading to sclerosis, vascular lesions, and penile ventral curvature. Nonetheless, the authors considered this flap technique ideal for urethral reconstruction from the penoscrotal angle to the prostatic apex. Because of anatomical proximity, good tissue availability, and potentially good tolerance to contact with urine due to abundance of sebaceous glands, this is always the authors' first option for bulbomembranous urethroplasty. They also believe that scrotal skin flap is less likely to develop lichen sclerosus as compared to penile skin. Despite all the potential advantages mentioned by the authors, epilation, deepithelialization, and flap mobilization may not be so straightforward. Epilation is an extremely time-consuming process. Although flaps with their own blood supply would be more appropriate in severely fibrotic urethral beds, such as after previously failed urethroplasties, several problems with postvoid dribbling of urine, ejaculatory dysfunction, and flap outpouching or pseudodiverticulum formation are truly troublesome and impact on quality of life [30]. It should be kept in mind that, in general, the use of skin flaps for urethral reconstruction is more technically demanding than substitution urethroplasty. In a study by McAninch and Morey, for patients with an average stricture length of 9 cm, the initial overall success rate of the fasciocutaneous flap reconstruction was 79%. Recurrent stricture rate was noted in 13% of onlay grafts and in 58% of tubularized repairs [29].

5.2. Grafts. The use of grafts in urethral reconstruction has become a more popularized surgical option worldwide. Theoretically, grafts in general are inherently less reliable because they need to be vascularized. However, they are quick and relatively easier to harvest and deploy. There are several studies of both flaps and grafts showing similar restricture rates [34]. Therefore, in the authors' opinion, a graft should be the procedure of choice due to its simplicity and speed by which it can be harvested and deployed, since the restricture rate is similar. There may be specific indications favoring a flap rather than a graft: revision surgery following multiple failed attempts, any cause of local devascularization such as irradiation or severe peripheral vascular insufficiency, and local infection, all of which hamper the ability of a graft to take. In summary, a graft repair is preferred due to the reasons mentioned above. Both grafts and flaps contract, although full-thickness flaps tend to contract less than split-thickness flaps and grafts, and patch grafts do better than tubed grafts, which may imply a two-stage procedure if a circumferential reconstruction of the urethra is necessary.

The widespread popularity of *oral mucosa* in urethral reconstruction has similarly allowed the introduction of new techniques in long-segment and panurethral stricture repair. In 2000, Kulkarni et al. first described the use of long oral mucosa grafts to repair the entire anterior urethra through a simple perineal incision in a single stage, thus preserving the penile components, their anatomy, function, and cosmesis [35] (Figure 3). In 2009, the same authors described a modification of their original technique, suggesting a minimally invasive procedure with dissection of the urethra from the corpora cavernosa along one side only, thus preserving the entire neurovascular supply to the urethra [36] (Figure 4). Buccal mucosa graft urethroplasty has been used for long anterior urethral strictures by several authors following the initial report by Kulkarni et al. in 2000 [37–40]. All these authors have reported favorable results at short- and medium-term follow-up with acceptable complication rates. In 2004, Gupta et al. described a technique of dorsal graft placement by ventral sagittal urethrotomy and minimal-access perineal approach and used this technique in patients with anterior urethral stricture, including 2 with panurethral stricture disease [40]. In the Kulkarni technique, the whole anterior urethra is repaired by a single perineal incision, single technique, and single substitute material (Figure 4). In a retrospective study including 117 patients with panurethral stricture disease treated from June 1998 to December 2010, the overall success rate was 83.7%. Mean stricture length was 14 cm and median follow-up was 59 months. Most recurrent

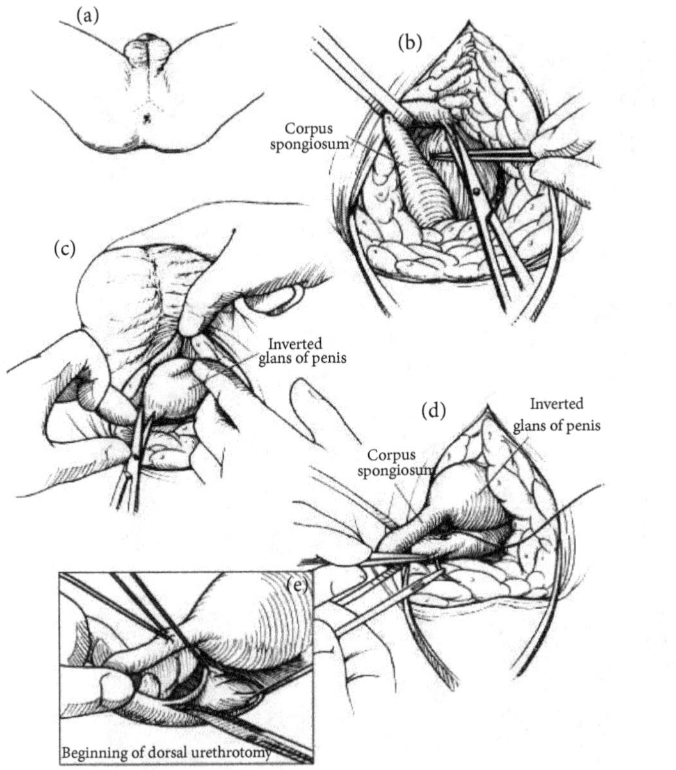

(a) A midline perineal incision bifurcated posteriorly which is used for its excellent access to the proximal bulbar urethra
(b) Full mobilization of the anterior urethra through the perineum as for a total urethrectomy. A Gelpi retractor which is used
(c) The glans penis which is inverted and delivered to the perineal wound for dissection of the distalmost segment of the urethra
(d) Placement of stay sutures in preparation for dorsal external urethrotomy
(e) Dorsal external urethrotomy which is begun in the proximal bulbar urethra

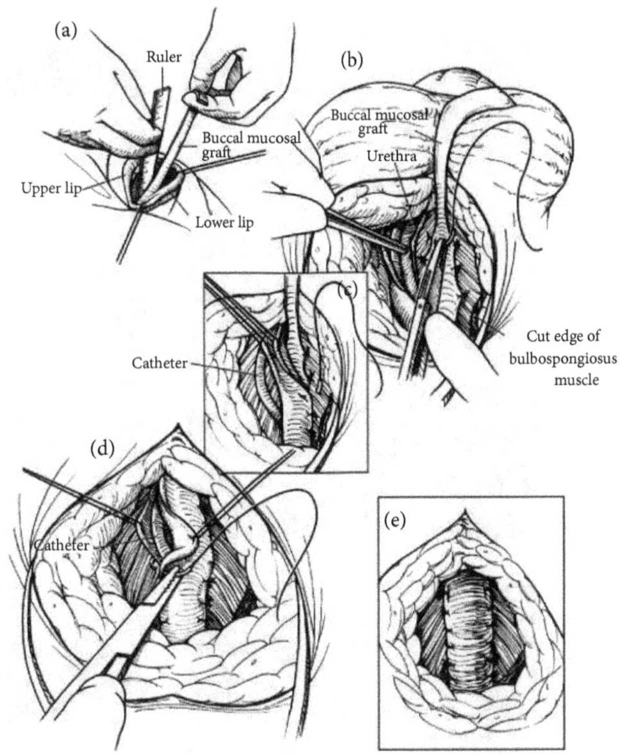

(a) Harvesting of buccal mucosa graft involving lower lip and both inner cheeks
(b) The urethra which is fully mobilized and rotated 180° for external urethrotomy along its dorsal surface. A single strip of BM which is spread and sutured to the tunica albuginea of the corpora cavernosa. Quilting sutures which are applied along the graft
(c) The right urethral margin which is sutured to the ipsilateral side of the patch
(d) Suturing of the left side of the urethra-graft anastomosis
(e) Suturing which is completed and the grafted area which is covered by urethral plate

FIGURE 3: Schematic representation of the Kulkarni operation.

strictures occurred at the proximal anastomotic site and none of these was a full-length recurrence [6]. The major advantage of this technique is that it is minimally invasive and performed in one stage. It also avoids the psychological trauma of 2 (or more) operations and the need of living for 6 months with bifid scrotum after staged procedures. Additionally, because it is a one-side dissection the risk of injury to the neurovascular bundles to the penis and urethra is minimal. This procedure is carried out through the perineum, avoiding a penile scar, and does not lead to a hypospadiac meatus.

More recently, some authors have described the use of *lingual mucosa* in urethroplasty [41–45]. The graft characteristics of lingual mucosa are similar to those of buccal mucosa (cheek and lip) [41, 42]. Lingual mucosal graft was used as the sole graft in 18 men with long anterior urethral strictures by Das et al. [41]. Most cases were etiologically associated with LS or infection. Overall success rate was 83.3%. However, separate results regarding panurethral strictures were not given. A particular advantage of lingual mucosa is that it can be harvested in continuity across the midline with the opposite side of the tongue, allowing a graft of sufficient length for panurethral strictures.

Prepuce and penile skin in the form of flaps or grafts are recognized alternatives for this type of reconstruction and are mentioned in the Table 1. In experienced hands, oral mucosal grafts measuring 10×1.5 cm can routinely be harvested from each inner cheek. If necessary, lingual grafts can be harvested in addition. A great number of our patients who have LS have scarred prepuce and glans and already had circumcision. In LS, no form of genital skin can or should be used. Preputial/distal penile skin graft was described for dorsal onlay anterior urethroplasty. In most studies, panurethral stricture patients were a minority [46, 47]. Most failures occurred if the skin graft was placed onto the penile urethra. Although previous circumcision did not preclude the use of penile skin, buccal mucosa was recommended as the best choice if the shaft skin was not abundant [46].

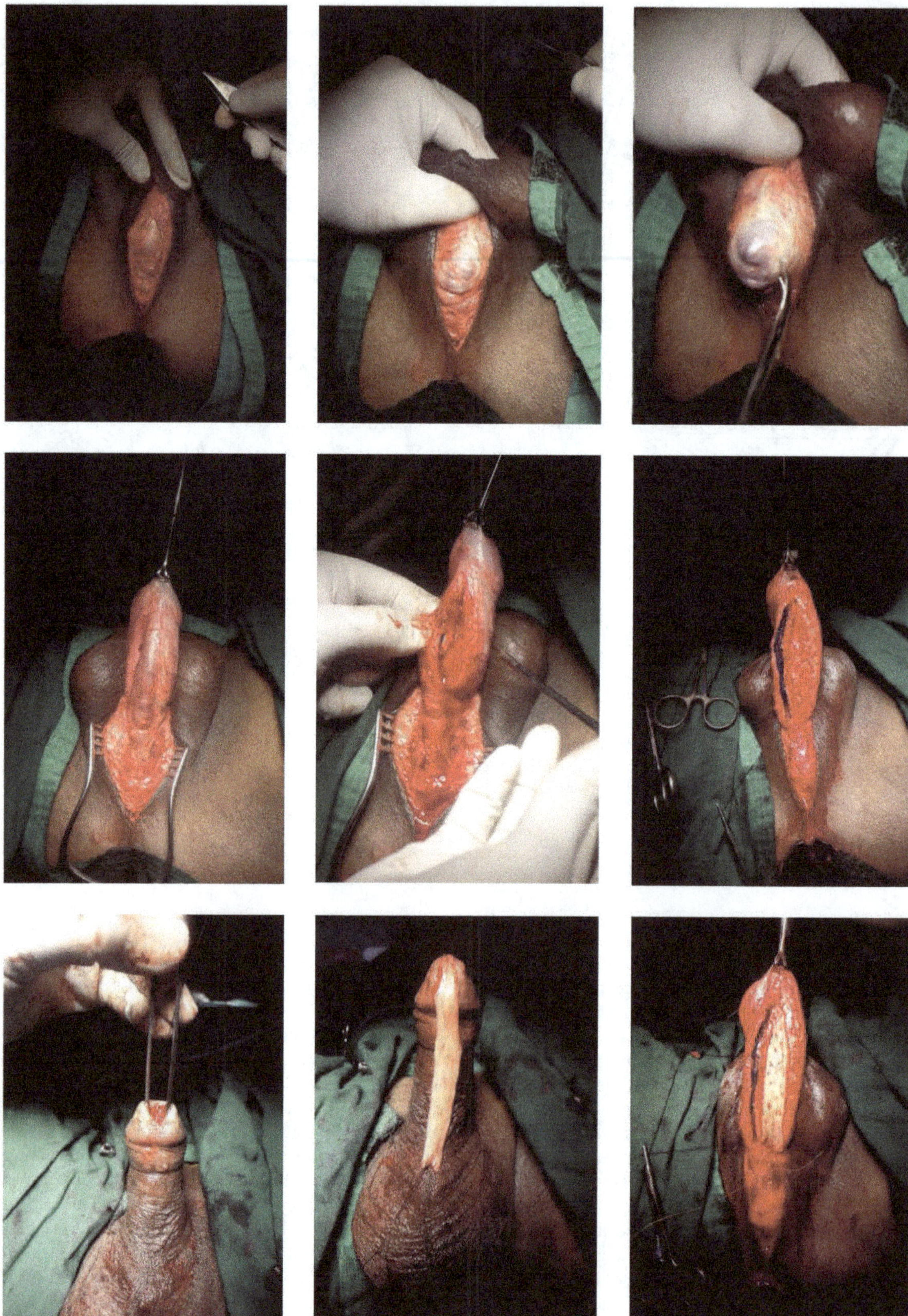

Figure 4: Kulkarni operation.

Postauricular skin has also been used as a good alternative for men with panurethral strictures with high success rate [48–50]. Postauricular skin is thin and has a dense subdermal plexus, and, therefore, graft take and functional outcomes are superior to other nongenital skin grafts. However, Andrich and Mundy cautioned that no skin graft should be used for urethroplasty in LS patients. LS is a skin disease and can also affect any skin graft in due course [49].

Another subject of controversy is the location for graft placement. Ventral graft placement, particularly in the pendulous urethra, is usually associated with poorer results. In the bulbar urethra, similar results can be expected, as long as ventral grafting is not used for long and complex strictures. A flap or a two-stage procedure is advocated by some authors for these strictures [46]. Dorsal graft placement usually produces the best outcomes and, therefore, is the method of choice in panurethral strictures [6, 23, 51–53]. Although doubled-sided dorsal plus ventral oral mucosa grafting has also been suggested for bulbar urethroplasty, the authors did not recommend its use for strictures measuring more than 4 cm in length [54]. Therefore, this technique is not indicated in long-segment or panurethral stricture disease.

Colonic mucosa has been employed for the reconstruction of panurethral stricture disease [55]. This graft is harvested from sigmoid colon using a laparoscopic approach or by a lower abdominal paramedian incision. Full-thickness grafts of 12 to 15 cm in length of sigmoid colon mucosa can be obtained and the colon continuity is immediately restored by an end-to-end anastomosis. An unstretched colonic mucosa graft is trimmed and sized to an appropriate individual need (ranging from 15 to 22 cm in length and 3 cm in width) and is tubularized over a 16 to 18 Fr fenestrated or fluted silicone catheter with interrupted 5-0 absorbable suture to create a neourethra. An end-to-end anastomosis is performed between the neourethra and the proximal end of the native urethra. The distal end of the neourethra is pulled through the glans tunnel to form the neomeatus. Xu et al. reported their experience with 35 patients who underwent colonic mucosal graft urethroplasty for complex, long-segment urethral strictures, ranging from 11 to 21 cm in length (mean 15.1). Five (14.2%) of these patients developed recurrent strictures. However, 3 of the recurrences were not related to the urethroplasty. Therefore, they concluded that tubularized urethroplasty using colonic mucosa grafts was successful and had a lower recurrence rate than patch urethroplasty. Nonetheless, this procedure needs further investigation and confirmation and, therefore, should be reserved as an alternative in complex patients where other options are not available or possible.

5.3. Combination of Flaps and Grafts. The exclusive use of long flaps for complex or panurethral strictures may be a technically challenging ordeal and are usually associated with long operating times and morbidity due to positioning and the surgical procedure itself. Furthermore, sufficient length of skin flaps may not be available, particularly in circumcised men or if LS is present. In such cases, a reasonable treatment option is to combine a shorter flap with a graft, and the graft placed proximally in the bulbar urethra [51]. A penile circular fasciocutaneous flap combined with an oral mucosa graft placed proximally was used by Wessells et al. in 7 patients with a mean stricture length of 18.3 cm [56]. The mean flap length was 12.6 cm (range 10–15) and mean graft length was 6.2 cm (range 3–9). The overall success rate was 88% at 16 months follow-up. Unfortunately, the authors did not mention results specific to panurethral strictures separately. The authors emphasized the importance of avoiding tubed reconstructions as these are associated with high risk of restricture and other flap-related complications.

Oral mucosa has become the graft material of choice for substitution urethroplasty, but at times it may be insufficient to completely reconstruct a long-segment or panurethral stricture. The combined use of oral mucosa and a genital skin flap has proved to be a reliable and durable alternative for single-stage reconstruction of long-segment or panurethral stricture disease [51].

5.4. Staged Procedures. At present, the majority of uncomplicated anterior urethral strictures can be successfully managed with a single-stage procedure. However, complex strictures associated with adverse local conditions, such as extensive scarred tissue formation of the urethra, infection, fistulation, prior multiple failed urethral reconstruction attempts, totally obliterated residual urethra, graft or flap-related factors, or following heavy irradiation, represent a challenge and are more appropriately treated with a staged procedure. A staged reconstruction may also be indicated in some long urethral strictures. All these situations are associated with unhealthy, poorly vascularized, and inelastic urethral and neighbouring tissues for urethral reconstruction. Although LS can be managed with a single-stage reconstruction, in some cases a staged procedure may be a reasonable option, as it may have a beneficial impact on the natural history of the disease [57–60]. A perineal urethrostomy for urinary diversion avoids continuous extravasation into the corpus spongiosum and promotes quicker and better urethral tissue healing.

The classical two-stage method was developed in the 1950s by Johanson [61]. The Johanson procedure is based on marsupialization of the strictured urethra, followed by a second surgical stage approximately 4–6 months after the first stage has healed (Figures 5 and 6). In the past, scrotal or perineal skin was used for urethral reconstruction. The great achievement of Johanson's technique was its use in all types of strictures, apart from initiating an era of urethral reconstructive surgery. The drawbacks of this technique resulted from the use of hair-growing scrotal and perineal skin, which lead to chronic urinary tract infection, abscesses, lithogenesis, fistulation, sacculation, and diverticula formation in the reconstructed urethra.

In the 1980s, Schreiter reported a two-stage mesh graft procedure in an attempt to avoid the use of scrotal or perineal skin by using a hairless skin graft which is transferred to a two-stage procedure [62, 63]. Although this technique can be employed in every type of stricture, apparently its best indication is in complex strictures, especially associated with severe tissue scarring and absence of healthy penile skin for urethral reconstruction.

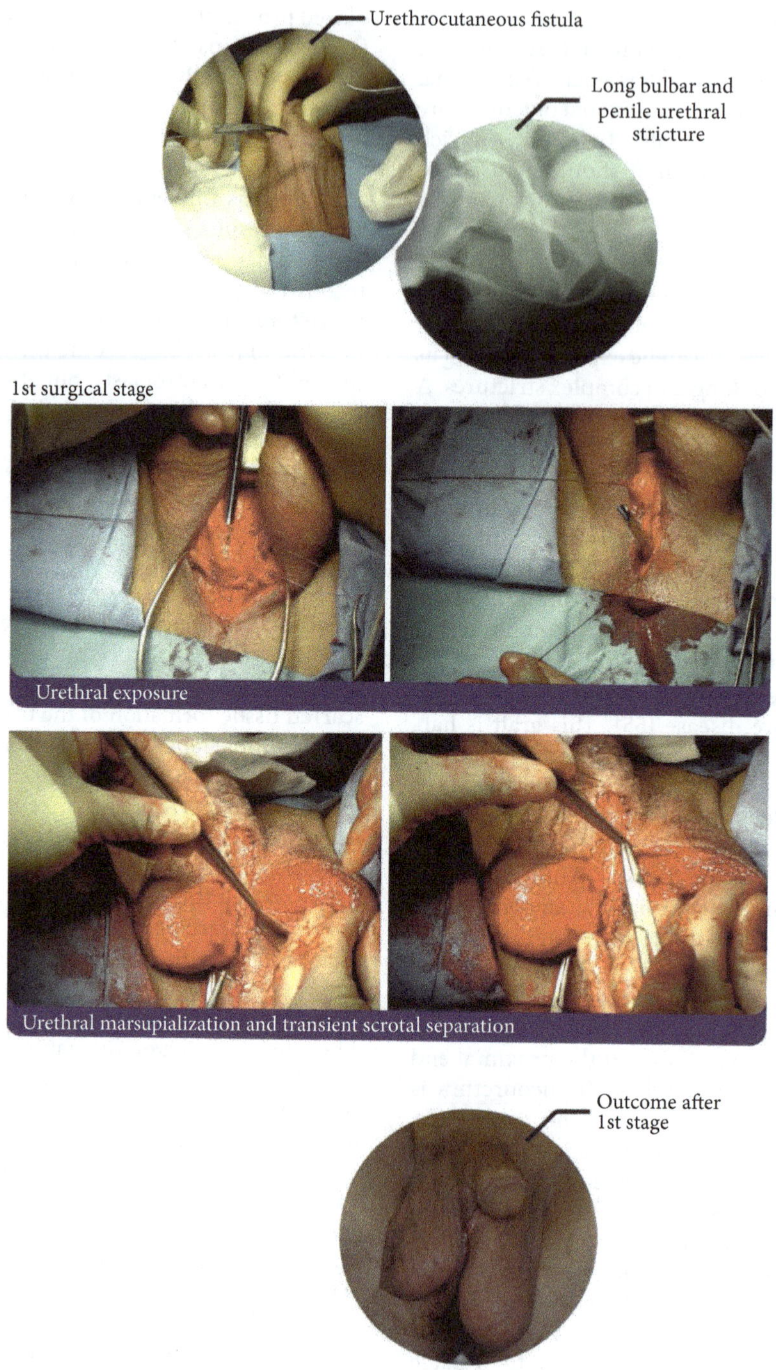

FIGURE 5: First stage of Johanson reconstruction with OMG inlay of panurethral stricture.

More recently, other authors have reported on a two-stage Johanson-type urethroplasty with oral mucosa grafting for anterior urethral strictures. For penile urethral strictures, Patterson and Chapple favor a two-stage procedure with dorsal onlay oral mucosa grafting after complete excision of the scarred urethra [64].

Staged reconstructions are associated with significant inconvenience to some patients, exposing them to an increased risk of morbidity due to multiple general anesthetics. Additionally, revision is common after two-stage operations and in one series half of the patients ended up needing a three-stage repair [65].

5.5. Tunica Albuginea (Monseur) Urethroplasty. In 1969, Monseur described a procedure by which a neourethra was created and its lumen continuity was maintained by the tunica albuginea through a supraurethral or subcavernosal groove without the need of a graft or flap [66]. Recently, there has been some renewed interest in this technique and various

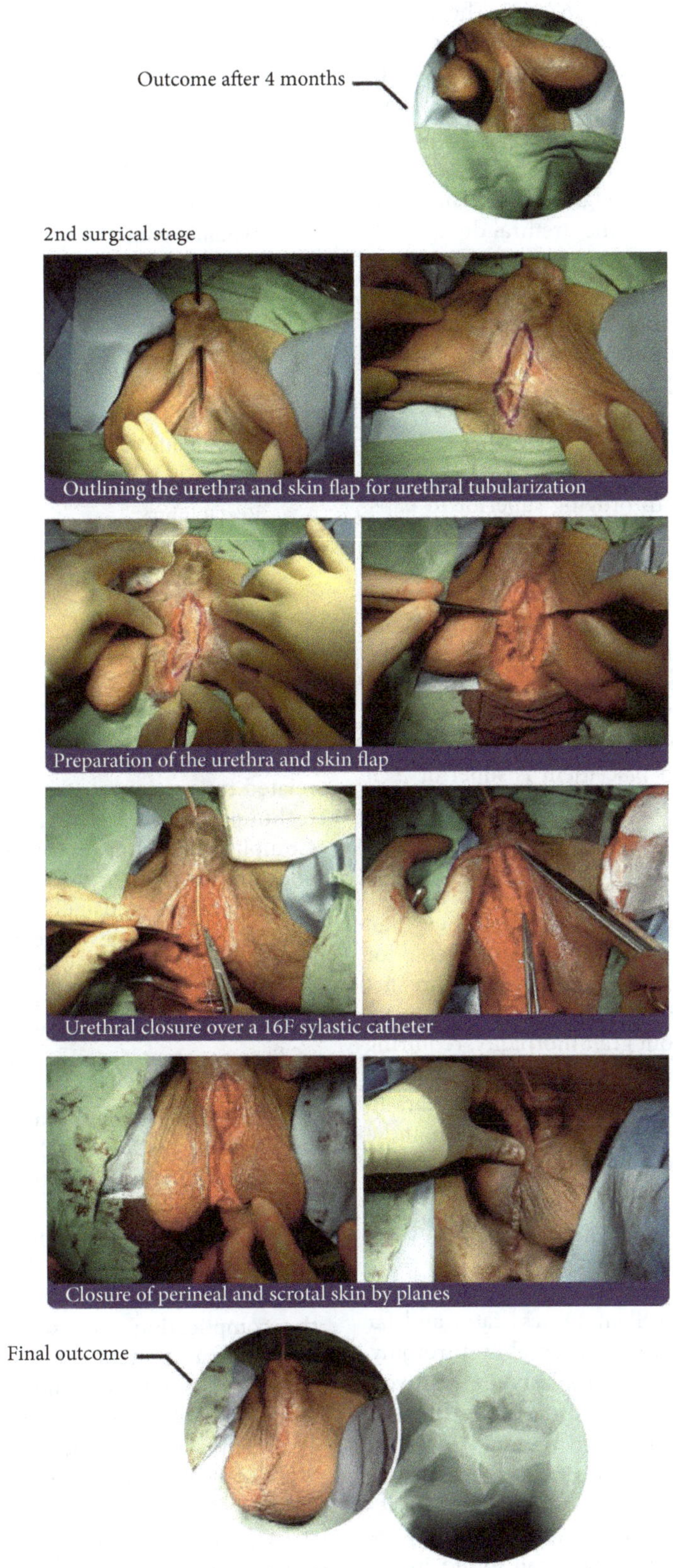

FIGURE 6: Second stage and closure.

reports have been published on the use of Monseur's tunica albuginea urethroplasty for short- and long-segment urethral strictures with acceptable success rates [67, 68]. The authors reported on the utility of this technique in cases where oral mucosa urethroplasty is not feasible due to lack of healthy oral mucosa associated with tobacco chewing or need of very long grafts to bridge panurethral strictures [69]. The authors described some similarity with the tubularized incised plate (TIP) urethroplasty described by Snodgrass and Bush, where the tunica exposed after incision of the urethral dorsal plate forms the roof of the neourethra and has stood the test of time for that purpose [70]. The authors argue that flap procedures are considered extremely labor-intensive, tedious, and among the most difficult in reconstructive urology [32]. Oral mucosa graft procedures, although very successful in medium-sized strictures, may not be feasible in very long strictures. Because some studies have shown that, even in dorsal onlay grafting, oral mucosa and penile skin grafts have shown similar results, while both proving superior to flaps, these authors concluded that it is not the type of graft, but rather the site of graft that is ultimately responsible for the success of the procedure [71]. Other studies have reported that a ventral onlay graft has a significant disadvantage over a dorsal onlay. It is claimed that complications are decreased if the graft is placed dorsally over the urethral groove [72]. Based on the concept advocated by Monseur, Barbagli et al. introduced the dorsally placed (onlay) graft technique and postulated that dorsal graft placement is superior as it allows better mechanical support for the graft and a richer and predictable vascular blood supply for the graft from the underlying corpora cavernosa [73, 74]. So if it is assumed that dorsal onlay grafts yield results better than ventral, then it must be the site of graft placement rather than the type of graft material that is ultimately responsible for the better success rates [75]. Lastly, the authors claim that Monseur's tunica albuginea urethroplasty is easy to perform, with short learning curve, without graft morbidity, requiring less time and resources, and success rates are comparable to oral mucosa urethroplasty. Tunica albuginea appears to be sufficient to allow regrowth of urethral epithelium and a patent distensible lumen if proved by urethrosccopic biopsy. However, we think that further studies are necessary.

6. Success and Complications

Generally, urethroplasty has excellent success rates and far exceed those found with direct vision internal urethrotomy. Serious complications following urethroplasty are relatively uncommon, 3% of them occurring in the early postoperative period and 18% in a late follow-up period [76]. Most reports in the literature contain heterogeneous data, that is, different types of strictures treated by different modalities and surgeons. When complications are mentioned, they are mixed for all the procedures. Another pitfall found in the literature is in comparing success rates in different series, as these have variable definitions of treatment failure. Therefore, consensus in reconstructive urology needs to be established in the future.

TABLE 2: Major and minor complications of "panurethroplasty"*.

Major	Minor
Early	Early
Hematuria	Oral numbness
RUG leak	Drooling when eating or Speaking
Oral discomfort	Speech impairment
Wound dehiscence	Perineal hypoesthesia
Wound tightness	Scrotal hyperesthesia
Epididymitis	Stensen's duct squirting
Penile ecchymosis	Penile pain
Penile swelling	Penile shortening
Penile skin ischemia/necrosis	Postvoid dribbling
UTI	Stress incontinence
Wound infection	Urine splaying
Late	Late
Rectal injury	Recurrent stricture
Urosepsis	Sexual dysfunction
	Chordee
	Fistulation

*Generally, similar and common to any urethroplasty.

Generally, complications of urethroplasty are directly related to location of stricture, length of stricture, operative technique, and type of transfer tissue employed (Table 2). Complications after urethroplasty can be divided into major and minor groups, occurring early or late. Most minor complications are usually mild and temporary and may be amenable to simple corrective procedures. Major complications are usually severe and complicated and result in failure of urethroplasty. In this review we will focus on complications associated with the reconstructive procedures of long-segment anterior urethral or panurethral strictures (Table 3).

Oral mucosal grafts are now considered the standard substitution material for urethral surgery. Surgical procedures involving oral mucosa onlay have better success rates and less morbidity compared with fasciocutaneous flaps [23, 46, 73, 74, 76]. One report has mentioned complication rates of fasciocutaneous flaps between 3% and 56% [77]. In a multi-institutional study, Warner et al. reported on the complication rates of different surgical techniques to repair long-segment and panurethral strictures [23]. The complication rate was higher in the fasciocutaneous cohort compared with those without a flap (32% versus 14%, resp.; $P = 0.02$). In this review, a 2-stage Johanson urethroplasty was not as successful as the buccal mucosal graft procedure (BMG) (64% versus 82.5%, resp.). It was found that 2-stage Johanson urethroplasties performed with skin had a higher failure rate than those performed with a BMG (66.7% recurrence rate versus 28.3%, resp.). Meticulous follow-up of patients after long-segment or "panurethroplasty" may show an important percentage of early and late complications. Perineal neuralgia or neuropraxia is a well-known

TABLE 3: Complications by most common techniques for pan-urethroplasty.

Type of surgery	Early	Late	Recurrence
FC flap	Transient pain and numbness Fistula (resolved)	Fistula	37.5%
OMG	UTI Penile edema Bleeding	Chordee Fistula ED Oral and lip discomfort numbness Cold glans	17.5%
Second-stage Johanson	Wound dehiscence UTI Scrotal abscess Penile numbness Epididymitis	ED Graft contracture Fistula Chordee Cold glans	35.7%
PU and definitive 1st-stage Johanson	Wound dehiscence UTI Transient pain and numbness	Chordee Fistula	24.1%
FC flap + graft	Wound hematoma PE Penile skin ischemia	Fistula Chordee	23.5%

FC: fasciocutaneous; OMG: oral mucosal graft; UTI: urinary tract infection; ED: erectile dysfunction; PU: perineal urethrostomy; PE: pulmonary embolism. Adapted from [23].

complication of bulbar and posterior urethroplasty, or any surgery performed in the exaggerated lithotomy position (i.e., radical perineal prostatectomy and urorectal fistula repair) [78–80]. The most common position-related complications of complex urethroplasty include superficial peroneal nerve neuropraxia, rhabdomyolysis, and lower extremity compartment syndrome. Although several causes of neuropraxia have been identified, the mechanical nerve compression seems to be the most common. It usually resolves spontaneously within 6–8 weeks. Recent studies have reported much lower position-related complication rates not exceeding 3% due to shortening of overall lithotomy position and meticulous protocol of patient protection during this type of surgery. In the authors' personal series, the severe neuropraxia rate has been in accordance with these reports.

Although most complications are minor, with little impact, and easily corrected, they seem to occur in a higher number than previously published (40%) [76]. These complications are important to the patient and should be discussed in the counseling before surgery.

7. Impact on Sexual Function

Impairment of male sexual function (penile sensation, erectile, and ejaculatory dysfunctions) are usually underreported. However, this scenario has been changed recently. In 2001, Coursey et al. reported a study on erectile function after anterior urethroplasty based on a questionnaire evaluation of erectile dysfunction. ED occurred in 19% of patients after OMG and 27% after anastomotic urethroplasty. Although he postulated that men with a long stricture might be at increased risk for transient erectile changes, the overall postoperative sexual dysfunction rate was no higher than circumcision [81]. Based on validated inventory questionnaires, such as the International Index of Erectile Function (IIEF-5) or the O'Leary Brief Male Sexual Function Inventory (BMSFI), the majority of the studies published recently have not shown that urethral reconstructive surgery impairs erectile function and sexual drive. Ejaculatory function was even improved in the younger ages [82–86]. Although erectile dysfunction has been associated with urethroplasty operations, its incidence is largely unknown. A 1% incidence of *de novo* erectile dysfunction after anterior urethroplasty was found in a meta-analysis study by Blaschko et al. However, in most cases the erectile dysfunction was transient and resolved within the first 12 months [85]. Another study reported an incidence of transient erectile dysfunction after anterior urethroplasty in approximately 40%, although recovery was observed in most by 6 months [83]. In 2006, the same authors had described a relationship between older age and a higher incidence of erectile dysfunction after surgery. Nonetheless, overall, men had not reported a decline in erectile dysfunction or sexual drive after urethroplasty [82]. In 2015, Xu et al. published a study dealing specifically with the impact of erectile dysfunction on complex panurethral stricture disease. They concluded that the surgical reconstruction with the use of grafts (buccal, lingual, and colonic mucosa) had limited effect on erectile function. The only adverse factor was extension of the stricture to posterior urethra, in which case an impairment was observed [86]. Ejaculatory dysfunction was reported in patients after ventrally placed flaps or grafts, possibly due to urethrocele formation [87]. However, no ejaculatory dysfunction has been reported in patients after dorsal onlays [77, 87].

8. Conclusion

One-stage repairs with BMG offer an excellent option for patients with long-segment and panurethral stricture disease. In cases with obliterative or absent urethral plate, a 2-stage

Johanson urethroplasty with BMG offers a viable alternative. In cases of LS, 1-stage BMG has better outcomes than a 2-stage repair. If BMGs are not available, FC flaps offer similar success; however, these are associated with higher rates of complications. Skin grafts should be avoided, unless no alternatives exist. Finally, the valuable role of PU cannot be understated in the setting of multiple failed urethroplasties.

The options currently available to reconstruct the urethra are in permanent development and attention should be focused on both old and new concepts. No surgical technique should compromise penile length, cause chordee, and affect cosmesis. Oral morbidity should be given attention after OMG to avoid permanent late sequelae in mouth function. Critical attention should also be given to sexual function as any urethral reconstructive method can eventually cause its occurrence.

References

[1] A. C. Peterson and G. D. Webster, "Management of urethral stricture disease: developing options for surgical intervention," *BJU International*, vol. 94, no. 7, pp. 971–976, 2004.

[2] A. S. Fenton, A. F. Morey, R. Aviles, and C. R. Garcia, "Anterior urethral strictures: etiology and characteristics," *Urology*, vol. 65, no. 6, pp. 1055–1058, 2005.

[3] N. Lumen, P. Hoebeke, P. Willemsen, B. De Troyer, R. Pieters, and W. Oosterlinck, "Etiology of urethral stricture disease in the 21st century," *Journal of Urology*, vol. 182, no. 3, pp. 983–987, 2009.

[4] E. A. Eltahawy, R. Virasoro, S. M. Schlossberg, K. A. McCammon, and G. H. Jordan, "Long-term follow-up for excision and primary anastomosis for anterior urethral strictures," *Journal of Urology*, vol. 177, no. 5, pp. 1803–1806, 2007.

[5] A. Goel, A. Goel, A. Jain, and B. P. Singh, "Management of panurethral strictures," *Indian Journal of Urology*, vol. 27, no. 3, pp. 378–384, 2011.

[6] S. B. Kulkarni, P. M. Joshi, and K. Venkatesan, "Management of panurethral stricture disease in India," *Journal of Urology*, vol. 188, no. 3, pp. 824–830, 2012.

[7] I. Depasquale, A. J. Park, and A. Bracka, "The treatment of balanitis xerotica obliterans," *BJU International*, vol. 86, no. 4, pp. 459–465, 2000.

[8] G. Barbagli, F. Mirri, M. Gallucci, S. Sansalone, G. Romano, and M. Lazzeri, "Histological evidence of urethral involvement in male patients with genital lichen sclerosus: a preliminary report," *Journal of Urology*, vol. 185, no. 6, pp. 2171–2176, 2011.

[9] S. B. Kulkarni, G. Barbagli, D. Kirpekar, F. Mirri, and M. Lazzeri, "Lichen sclerosus of the male genitalia and urethra: surgical options and results in a multicenter international experience with 215 patients," *European Urology*, vol. 55, no. 4, pp. 945–956, 2009.

[10] E. Palminteri, E. Berdondini, M. Lazzeri, F. Mirri, and G. Barbagli, "Resurfacing and reconstruction of the glans penis," *European Urology*, vol. 52, no. 3, pp. 893–900, 2007.

[11] S. Das, "Shusruta of India, the pioneer in the treatment of urethral stricture," *Surgery Gynecology and Obstetrics*, vol. 157, no. 6, pp. 581–582, 1983.

[12] A. R. Mundy and D. E. Andrich, "Urethral strictures," *BJU International*, vol. 107, no. 1, pp. 6–26, 2011.

[13] R. A. Santucci, G. F. Joyce, and M. Wise, "Male urethral stricture disease," *Journal of Urology*, vol. 177, no. 5, pp. 1667–1674, 2007.

[14] E. Palminteri, E. Berdondini, P. Verze, C. De Nunzio, A. Vitarelli, and L. Carmignani, "Contemporary urethral stricture characteristics in the developed world," *Urology*, vol. 81, no. 1, pp. 191–197, 2013.

[15] M. Wassermann and N. Hakke, "Uréthite chronique et rétrécissments, nouvelle contribution a l'anatomie pathologique des rétrécissments de l'uréthre," *Annales des Maladies des Organes Génito-Urinaires*, vol. 12, pp. 241–263, 1884.

[16] D. E. Beard and W. E. Goodyear, "Urethral stricture: a pathological study," *The Journal of Urology*, vol. 59, pp. 619–626, 1948.

[17] R. M. Chambers and B. Baitera, "The anatomy of the urethral stricture," *British Journal of Urology*, vol. 49, no. 6, pp. 545–551, 1977.

[18] B. N. Breyer, J. W. McAninch, J. M. Whitson et al., "Multivariate analysis of risk factors for long-term urethroplasty outcome," *Journal of Urology*, vol. 183, no. 2, pp. 613–617, 2010.

[19] L. S. Baskin, S. C. Constantinescu, P. S. Howard et al., "Biochemical characterization and quantitation of the collagenous components of urethral stricture tissue," *Journal of Urology*, vol. 150, no. 2, pp. 642–647, 1993.

[20] A. G. Cavalcanti, S. Yucel, D. Y. Deng, J. W. McAninch, and L. S. Baskin, "The distribution of neuronal and inducible nitric oxide synthase in urethral stricture formation," *Journal of Urology*, vol. 171, no. 5, pp. 1943–1947, 2004.

[21] G. Kaya, M. Berset, C. Prins, P. Chavaz, and J.-H. Saurat, "Chronic borreliosis presenting with morphea- and lichen sclerosus et atrophicus-like cutaneous lesions: a case report," *Dermatology*, vol. 202, no. 4, pp. 373–375, 2001.

[22] E. Palminteri, "Penile urethroplasty," in *Atlas of Penile Reconstructive Surgery*, E. Austoni, Ed., pp. 137–148, Pacini Editore Medicine SpA, 2010.

[23] J. N. Warner, I. Malkawi, M. Dhradkeh et al., "A multi-institutional evaluation of the management and outcomes of long-segment urethral strictures," *Urology*, vol. 85, no. 6, pp. 1483–1488, 2015.

[24] M. J. Barry, F. J. Foweler, M. P. O'Leary, R. C. Bruskewitz, H. L. Holtgrewe, and W. K. Mebust, "Correlation of the American Urological Association symptom index with self-administered versions of the Marsden-Iversen, Boyarsky and Maine Medical Assessment Program symptom indexes. Measurement Committee of the American Urological Association," *The Journal of Urology*, vol. 148, no. 5, pp. 1558–1564, 1992.

[25] M. J. Jackson, J. N'Dow, and R. Pickard, "The importance of patient-reported outcome measures in reconstructive urology," *Current Opinion in Urology*, vol. 20, no. 6, pp. 495–499, 2010.

[26] J. C. Buckley, A. K. Wu, and J. W. McAninch, "Impact of urethral ultrasonography on decision-making in anterior urethroplasty," *BJU International*, vol. 109, no. 3, pp. 438–442, 2012.

[27] S. B. Brandes, "Panurethral strictures," in *Urethral Reconstructive Surgery*, S. B. Brandes, Ed., Current Clinical Urology, pp. 165–170, Humana Press, 2008.

[28] J. W. McAninch, "Reconstruction of extensive urethral strictures: circular fasciocutaneous penile flap," *The Journal of Urology*, vol. 149, no. 3, pp. 488–491, 1993.

[29] J. W. McAninch and A. F. Morey, "Penile circular fasciocutaneous skin flap in 1-stage reconstruction of complex anterior urethral strictures," *Journal of Urology*, vol. 159, no. 4, pp. 1209–1213, 1998.

[30] D. Dubey, A. Kumar, P. Bansal et al., "Substitution urethroplasty for anterior urethral strictures: a critical appraisal of various techniques," *BJU International*, vol. 91, no. 3, pp. 215–218, 2003.

[31] J. K. M. Quartey, "Quartey flap reconstruction of urethral strictures," in *Traumatic and Reconstructive Urology*, J. W. McAninch, Ed., WB Saunders, Philadelphia, Pa, USA, 1996.

[32] A. F. Morey, L. K. Tran, and L. M. Zinman, "Q-flap reconstruction of panurethral strictures," *BJU International*, vol. 86, no. 9, pp. 1039–1042, 2000.

[33] J. Gil-Vernet, O. Arango, A. Gil-Vernet, J. Gil-Vernet Jr., and A. Gelabert-Mas, "A new biaxial epilated scrotal flap for reconstructive urethral surgery," *Journal of Urology*, vol. 158, no. 2, pp. 412–420, 1997.

[34] H. Wessells and J. W. McAninch, "Current controversies in anterior urethral stricture repair: free-graft versus pedicled skin-flap reconstruction," *World Journal of Urology*, vol. 16, no. 3, pp. 175–180, 1998.

[35] S. B. Kulkarni, J. S. Kulkarni, and D. V. Kirpekar, "A new technique for urethroplasty for balanitis xerotica obliterans," *The Journal of Urology*, vol. 163, article 352, abstract V 31, 2000.

[36] S. Kulkarni, G. Barbagli, S. Sansalone, and M. Lazzeri, "One-sided anterior urethroplasty: a new dorsal onlay graft technique," *BJU International*, vol. 104, no. 8, pp. 1150–1155, 2009.

[37] D. Dubey, A. Kumar, A. Mandhani, A. Srivastava, R. Kapoor, and M. Bhandari, "Buccal mucosal urethroplasty: a versatile technique for all urethral segments," *BJU International*, vol. 95, no. 4, pp. 625–629, 2005.

[38] Y.-M. Xu, Y.-L. Sa, Q. Fu, J. Zhang, J.-M. Si, and Z.-S. Liu, "Oral mucosal grafts urethroplasty for the treatment of long segmented anterior urethral strictures," *World Journal of Urology*, vol. 27, no. 4, pp. 565–571, 2009.

[39] B. Datta, M. P. Rao, R. L. Acharya et al., "Dorsal onlay buccal mucosal graft urethroplasty in long anterior urethral stricture," *International Brazilian Journal of Urology*, vol. 33, no. 2, pp. 181–187, 2007.

[40] N. P. Gupta, M. S. Ansari, P. N. Dogra, and S. Tandon, "Dorsal buccal mucosal graft urethroplasty by a ventral sagittal urethrotomy and minimal-access perineal approach for anterior urethral stricture," *BJU International*, vol. 93, no. 9, pp. 1287–1290, 2004.

[41] S. K. Das, A. Kumar, G. K. Sharma et al., "Lingual mucosal graft urethroplasty for anterior urethral strictures," *Urology*, vol. 73, no. 1, pp. 105–108, 2009.

[42] G. Barbagli, M. De Angelis, G. Romano, P. G. Ciabatti, and M. Lazzeri, "The use of lingual mucosal graft in adult anterior urethroplasty: surgical steps and short-term outcome," *European Urology*, vol. 54, no. 3, pp. 671–676, 2008.

[43] A. Simonato, A. Gregori, C. Ambruosi et al., "Lingual mucosal graft urethroplasty for anterior urethral reconstruction," *European Urology*, vol. 54, no. 1, pp. 79–87, 2008.

[44] A. Srivastava, A. Dutta, and D. K. Jain, "Initial experience with lingual mucosal graft urethroplasty for anterior urethral strictures," *Medical Journal Armed Forces India*, vol. 69, no. 1, pp. 16–20, 2013.

[45] N. Lumen, S. Vierstraete-Verlinde, W. Oosterlinck et al., "Buccal versus lingual mucosa graft anterior urethroplasty: a prospective comparison of surgical outcome and donor site morbidity," *The Journal of Urology*, 2015.

[46] H. Wessells and J. W. Mcaninch, "Use of free grafts in urethral stricture reconstruction," *Journal of Urology*, vol. 155, no. 6, pp. 1912–1915, 1996.

[47] S. S. Bapat, A. S. Padhye, P. B. Yadav, and A. A. Bhave, "Preputial skin free graft as dorsal onlay urethroplasty: our experience of 73 patients," *Indian Journal of Urology*, vol. 23, no. 4, pp. 366–368, 2007.

[48] B. Manoj, N. Sanjeev, P. N. Pandurang, M. Jaideep, and M. Ravi, "Postauricular skin as an alternative to oral mucosa for anterior onlay graft urethroplasty: a preliminary experience in patients with oral mucosa changes," *Urology*, vol. 74, no. 2, pp. 345–348, 2009.

[49] D. E. Andrich and A. R. Mundy, "Surgical treatment of urethral stricture disease," *Contemporary Urology*, vol. 13, pp. 32–44, 2001.

[50] T. Nitkunan, N. Johal, K. O'Malley, and P. Cuckow, "Secondary hypospadias repair in two stages," *Journal of Pediatric Urology*, vol. 2, no. 6, pp. 559–563, 2006.

[51] R. K. Berglund and K. W. Angermeier, "Combined buccal mucosa graft and genital skin flap for reconstruction of extensive anterior urethral strictures," *Urology*, vol. 68, no. 4, pp. 707–710, 2006.

[52] W. B. Zimmerman and R. A. Santucci, "Buccal mucosa urethroplasty for adult urethral strictures," *Indian Journal of Urology*, vol. 27, no. 3, pp. 364–370, 2011.

[53] G. Barbagli, S. Sansalone, R. Djinovic, G. Romano, and M. Lazzeri, "Current controversies in reconstructive surgery of the anterior urethra: a clinical overview," *The International Brazilian Journal of Urology*, vol. 38, no. 3, pp. 307–316, 2012.

[54] E. Palminteri, N. Lumen, E. Berdondini et al., "Two-sided dorsal plus ventral oral graft bulbar urethroplasty: long-term results and predictive factors," *Urology*, vol. 85, no. 4, pp. 942–947, 2015.

[55] Y.-M. Xu, Y. Qiao, Y.-L. Sa, J. Zhang, Q. Fu, and L.-J. Song, "Urethral reconstruction using colonic mucosa graft for complex strictures," *Journal of Urology*, vol. 182, no. 3, pp. 1040–1043, 2009.

[56] H. Wessells, A. F. Morey, and J. W. McAninch, "Single stage reconstruction of complex anterior urethral strictures: combined tissue transfer techniques," *Journal of Urology*, vol. 157, no. 4, pp. 1271–1274, 1997.

[57] G. Barbagli, M. Lazzeri, E. Palminteri, and D. Turini, "Lichen sclerosis of male genitalia involving anterior urethra," *The Lancet*, vol. 354, no. 9176, p. 429, 1999.

[58] I. Depasquale, A. J. Park, and A. Bracka, "The treatment of balanitis xerotica obliterans," *BJU International*, vol. 86, no. 4, pp. 459–465, 2000.

[59] D. E. Andrich and A. R. Mundy, "Substitution urethroplasty with buccal mucosal-free grafts," *Journal of Urology*, vol. 165, no. 4, pp. 1131–1133, 2001.

[60] G. Barbagli, E. Palminteri, and M. Lazzeri, "Lichen sclerosus of male genitalia," *Contemporary Urology*, vol. 13, pp. 47–58, 2001.

[61] B. Johanson, "Reconstruction of the male urethra in strictures," *Acta Chirurgica Scandinavica*, vol. 167, supplement, article 1, 1953.

[62] F. Schreiter and F. Noll, "Meshgraft urethroplasty," *World Journal of Urology*, vol. 5, no. 1, pp. 41–46, 1987.

[63] F. Schreiter and F. Noll, "Mesh graft urethroplasty using split thickness skin graft or foreskin," *The Journal of Urology*, vol. 142, no. 5, pp. 1223–1226, 1989.

[64] J. M. Patterson and C. R. Chapple, "Surgical techniques in substitution urethroplasty using buccal mucosa for the treatment

of anterior urethral strictures," *European Urology*, vol. 53, no. 6, pp. 1162–1171, 2008.

[65] D. E. Andrich, T. J. Greenwell, and A. R. Mundy, "The problems of penile urethroplasty with particular reference to 2-stage reconstructions," *Journal of Urology*, vol. 170, no. 1, pp. 87–89, 2003.

[66] J. Monseur, "A new procedure for urethroplasty for urethral stricture: reconstruction of the urethral canal by means of subu-rethral strips and the subcavernous groove," *Journal d"Urologie et de Nephrologie*, vol. 75, no. 3, pp. 201–209, 1969.

[67] R. K. Mathur, A. Himanshu, and O. Sudarshan, "Technique of anterior urethra urethroplasty using tunica albuginea of corpora cavernosa," *International Journal of Urology*, vol. 14, no. 3, pp. 209–213, 2007.

[68] R. K. Mathur, A. K. Sharma, and S. Odiya, "Tunica albuginea urethroplasty for anterior urethral strictures: a urethroscopic analysis," *International Journal of Urology*, vol. 16, no. 9, pp. 751–755, 2009.

[69] R. K. Mathur and A. Sharma, "Tunica albuginea urethroplasty for panurethral strictures," *Urology Journal*, vol. 7, no. 2, pp. 120–124, 2010.

[70] W. Snodgrass and N. Bush, "Tubularized incised plate proximal hypospadias repair: continued evolution and extended applications," *Journal of Pediatric Urology*, vol. 7, no. 1, pp. 2–9, 2011.

[71] G. Barbagli, G. Morgia, and M. Lazzeri, "Retrospective outcome analysis of one-stage penile urethroplasty using a flap or graft in a homogeneous series of patients," *BJU International*, vol. 102, no. 7, pp. 853–860, 2008.

[72] C. E. Iselin and G. D. Webster, "Dorsal onlay graft urethroplasty for repair of bulbar urethral stricture," *Journal of Urology*, vol. 161, no. 3, pp. 815–818, 1999.

[73] G. Barbagli, E. Palminteri, and M. Rizzo, "Dorsal onlay graft urethroplasty using penile skin or buccal mucosa in adult bulbourethral strictures," *Journal of Urology*, vol. 160, no. 4, pp. 1307–1309, 1998.

[74] D. E. Andrich, C. J. Leach, and A. R. Mundy, "The Barbagli procedure gives the best results for patch urethroplasty of the bulbar urethra," *BJU International*, vol. 88, no. 4, pp. 385–389, 2001.

[75] A. K. Sharma, C. S. Ratkal, M. Shivlingaiah, G. N. Girish, R. P. Sanjay, and G. K. Venkatesh, "Analysis of short-term results of monsieur's tunica albuginea urethroplasty as a definitive procedure for pan-anterior urethral stricture," *Urology Annals*, vol. 5, no. 4, pp. 228–231, 2013.

[76] H. S. Al-Qudah and R. A. Santucci, "Extended complications of urethroplasty," *The International Brazilian Journal of Urology*, vol. 31, no. 4, pp. 315–325, 2005.

[77] G. Barbagli, C. Selli, A. Tosto, and E. Palminteri, "Dorsal free graft urethroplasty," *Journal of Urology*, vol. 155, no. 1, pp. 123–126, 1996.

[78] J. G. Anema, A. F. Morey, J. W. Mcaninch, L. A. Mario, and H. Wessells, "Complications related to the high lithotomy position during urethral reconstruction," *Journal of Urology*, vol. 164, no. 2, pp. 360–363, 2000.

[79] D. T. Price, J. Vieweg, F. Roland et al., "Transient lower extremity neurapraxia associated with radical perineal prostatectomy: a complication of the exaggerated lithotomy position," *Journal of Urology*, vol. 160, no. 4, pp. 1376–1378, 1998.

[80] K. W. Angermeier and G. H. Jordan, "Complications of the exaggerated lithotomy position: a review of 177 cases," *The Journal of Urology*, vol. 151, no. 4, pp. 866–868, 1994.

[81] J. W. Coursey, A. F. Morey, J. W. McAninch et al., "Erectile function after anterior urethroplasty," *Journal of Urology*, vol. 166, no. 6, pp. 2273–2276, 2001.

[82] B. A. Erickson, J. S. Wysock, K. T. McVary, and C. M. Gonzalez, "Erectile function, sexual drive, and ejaculatory function after reconstructive surgery for anterior urethral stricture disease," *BJU International*, vol. 99, no. 3, pp. 607–611, 2007.

[83] B. A. Erickson, M. A. Granieri, J. J. Meeks, J. P. Cashy, and C. M. Gonzalez, "Prospective analysis of erectile dysfunction after anterior urethroplasty: incidence and recovery of function," *Journal of Urology*, vol. 183, no. 2, pp. 657–661, 2010.

[84] U. P. Singh, R. Maheshwari, V. Kumar, A. Srivastava, and R. Kapoor, "Impact on sexual function after reconstructive surgery for anterior urethral stricture disease," *Indian Journal of Urology*, vol. 26, no. 2, pp. 188–192, 2010.

[85] S. D. Blaschko, M. T. Sanford, N. M. Cinman, J. W. McAninch, and B. N. Breyer, "*De novo* erectile dysfunction after anterior urethroplasty: a systematic review and meta-analysis," *BJU International*, vol. 112, no. 5, pp. 655–663, 2013.

[86] Y. Xu, Q. Fu, Y. Sa, Y. Qiao, and H. Xie, "The relationship between erectile function and complex panurethral stricture: a preliminary investigative and descriptive study," *Asian Journal of Andrology*, vol. 17, no. 2, pp. 315–318, 2015.

[87] M. Bhandari, D. Dubey, and B. S. Verma, "Dorsal or ventral placement of the preputial/penile skin onlay flap for anterior urethral strictures: does it make a difference?" *BJU International*, vol. 88, no. 1, pp. 39–43, 2001.

Permissions

All chapters in this book were first published by Hindawi Publishing Corporation; hereby published with permission under the Creative Commons Attribution License or equivalent. Every chapter published in this book has been scrutinized by our experts. Their significance has been extensively debated. The topics covered herein carry significant findings which will fuel the growth of the discipline. They may even be implemented as practical applications or may be referred to as a beginning point for another development.

The contributors of this book come from diverse backgrounds, making this book a truly international effort. This book will bring forth new frontiers with its revolutionizing research information and detailed analysis of the nascent developments around the world.

We would like to thank all the contributing authors for lending their expertise to make the book truly unique. They have played a crucial role in the development of this book. Without their invaluable contributions this book wouldn't have been possible. They have made vital efforts to compile up to date information on the varied aspects of this subject to make this book a valuable addition to the collection of many professionals and students.

This book was conceptualized with the vision of imparting up-to-date information and advanced data in this field. To ensure the same, a matchless editorial board was set up. Every individual on the board went through rigorous rounds of assessment to prove their worth. After which they invested a large part of their time researching and compiling the most relevant data for our readers.

The editorial board has been involved in producing this book since its inception. They have spent rigorous hours researching and exploring the diverse topics which have resulted in the successful publishing of this book. They have passed on their knowledge of decades through this book. To expedite this challenging task, the publisher supported the team at every step. A small team of assistant editors was also appointed to further simplify the editing procedure and attain best results for the readers.

Apart from the editorial board, the designing team has also invested a significant amount of their time in understanding the subject and creating the most relevant covers. They scrutinized every image to scout for the most suitable representation of the subject and create an appropriate cover for the book.

The publishing team has been an ardent support to the editorial, designing and production team. Their endless efforts to recruit the best for this project, has resulted in the accomplishment of this book. They are a veteran in the field of academics and their pool of knowledge is as vast as their experience in printing. Their expertise and guidance has proved useful at every step. Their uncompromising quality standards have made this book an exceptional effort. Their encouragement from time to time has been an inspiration for everyone.

The publisher and the editorial board hope that this book will prove to be a valuable piece of knowledge for researchers, students, practitioners and scholars across the globe.

List of Contributors

Zeyad R. Schwen, Mohit Gupta and Phillip M. Pierorazio
Department of Urology, James Buchanan Brady Urological Institute, Johns Hopkins University School of Medicine, Baltimore, MD, USA

Salahaddin Delshad
Department of Pediatric Surgery, School of Medicine, Iran University of Medical Sciences, Tehran, Iran
Department of Pediatric Surgery, Maryam Hospital, Karaj, Iran

Hadith Rastad
Non-Communicable Diseases Research Center, Alborz University of Medical Sciences, Karaj, Iran

Parham Mardi
Student Research Committee, Alborz University of Medical Sciences, Karaj, Iran

Beyene Petros
Department of Microbial, Cellular and Molecular Biology, College of Natural Sciences, Addis Ababa University, Addis Ababa, Ethiopia

Tilahun Alelign
Department of Microbial, Cellular and Molecular Biology, College of Natural Sciences, Addis Ababa University, Addis Ababa, Ethiopia
Department of Biology, Debre Birhan University, Debre Birhan, Ethiopia

Fiorina Kyritsi, Christopher A. Loffredo, Yun-Ling Zheng and George Philips
Lombardi Comprehensive Cancer Center, Georgetown University, Washington, DC, USA

Sania Amr
University of Maryland School of Medicine, Baltimore, MD, USA
Marlene and Stewart Greenebaum Comprehensive Cancer Center, University of Maryland, Baltimore, MD, USA

Diwas Gnyawali, Manish Man Pradhan, Prem Raj Sigdel, Purushottam Parajuli, Sampanna Chudal, Sujeet Poudyal, Suman Chapagain, Bhoj Raj Luitel, Pawan Raj Chalise, Uttam Sharma and Prem Raj Gyawali
Department of Urology and Kidney Transplant Surgery, Tribhuvan University Teaching Hospital, Institute of Medicine, Maharajgung, Kathmandu 44600, Nepal

O. A. Voylenko, O. E. Stakhovsky and I. V. Vitruk
Senior Researcher of Department of Plastic and Reconstructive Oncological Urology, National Cancer Institute, 33/43 Lomonosova Str., Kyiv 03022, Ukraine

O. A. Kononenko
Researcher of Department of Plastic and Reconstructive Oncological Urology, National Cancer Institute, 33/43 Lomonosova Str, Kyiv 03022, Ukraine

M. V. Pikul and S. L. Semko
Urologist of Department of Plastic and Reconstructive Oncological Urology, National Cancer Institute, 33/43 Lomonosova Str., Kyiv 03022, Ukraine

E. O. Stakhovsky
Head of Department of Plastic and Reconstructive Oncological Urology, National Cancer Institute, 33/43 Lomonosova Str, Kyiv 03022, Ukraine

Timothy A. Masterson and Clint Cary
Department of Urology, Indiana University School of Medicine, Indianapolis, IN 46202, USA

Chunkit Fung and Kerry Schaffer
James P. Wilmot Cancer Institute, University of Rochester Medical Center, Rochester, NY, USA

Paul Dinh Jr, Shirin Ardeshir-Rouhani-Fard and Lois B. Travis
Melvin and Bren Simon Cancer Center, Indiana University, Indianapolis, IN, USA

Sophie D. Fossa
Department of Oncology, Oslo University Hospital, Radium Hospital, Oslo, Norway

Aino Fianu Jonasson
Division of Obstetrics and Gynaecology, Karolinska University Hospital, Huddinge, 141 86, Stockholm, Sweden

Karin Bryder and Elisabeth Sthengel
Invent Medic Sweden AB, Medicon Village, 223 81, Lund, Sweden

Clíodhna Browne, Catherine M. Dowling, Patrick O'Malley, Nadeem Nusrat, Kilian Walsh, Syed Jaffry, Eamonn Rogers, Garrett C. Durkan and Frank T. D'Arcy
Department of Urology, University College Hospital Galway, Newcastle Road, Galway, Ireland

A. BhalaguruIyyan and P. Puvai Murugan
Department of Urology, PSG Institute of Medical Sciences and Research, Coimbatore, Tamil Nadu, India

Chandranaath C. Alakhananda
Department of Surgery, PSG Institute of Medical Sciences and Research, Coimbatore, Tamil Nadu, India

B. M. Zeeshan Hameed
Department of Urology, Kasturba Medical College Manipal, Manipal Academy of Higher Education, Manipal, Karnataka, India

Gampo A. Irdam, Bobby Sutojo and Putu A. R. Raharja
Department of Urology, Faculty of Medicine Universitas Indonesia, Cipto Mangunkusumo Hospital, Jakarta 10430, Indonesia

Desmond O. Acheampong, Isaac K. Barffour, Ernest A. Asiamah, Francis A. Armah, Christian K. Adokoh, Joy F. Oluyemi, Benjamin Adrah, Richard Opoku and Emmanuel Adakudugu
Department of Biomedical Sciences, School of Allied Health Sciences, University of Cape Coast, Cape Coast, Ghana

Alex Boye
Department of Medical Laboratory Science, School of Allied Health Sciences, University of Cape Coast, Cape Coast, Ghana

Donald Fedrigon III, Kareem Alazem, Sri Sivalingam, Manoj Monga and Juan Calle
Cleveland Clinic, Glickman Urological & Kidney Institute, 9500 Euclid Avenue, Cleveland, OH 44195, USA

Gianni Paulis
Regina Apostolorum Hospital, Andrology Center, Albano Laziale, Rome, Italy
Castelfidardo Medical Team, Peyronie's Disease Care Center, Rome, Italy

Gennaro Romano
Italian League against Cancer, Department of Urologic Oncology, Section of Avellino, Avellino, Italy

Luca Paulis
Faculty of Pharmacy, University of Rome "La Sapienza", Rome, Italy

Davide Barletta
Department of Urology, Andrology Center, San Matteo Hospital, Pavia, Italy

Mahmoudreza Moradi
Professor in Pediatric Urology, Chairman of Urology Department in Imam Reza Hospital, Chairman of Regenerative Medicine Research Center (RMRC), Kermanshah University of Medical Sciences, Kermanshah, Iran

Abolhassan Seyedzadeh
Professor in Pediatric Nephrology, Kermanshah University of Medical Sciences, Kermanshah, Iran

Saeed Gharakhloo, Aref Teymourinezhad, Kaveh Kaseb and Haress Rezaee
Urology Resident in Kermanshah University of Medical Sciences, Kermanshah, Iran

José Pablo Saffon Cuartas, Carolina Sandoval-Salinas, Juan M. Martínez and Héctor A. Corredor
Clinical Research Group, Boston Medical Group, Bogotá 110111, Colombia

Youssef Kadouri, Salim Lachkar, Hamza Dergamoun, Hachem El Sayegh, Lounis Benslimane and Yassine Nouini
Mohammed V University, Faculty of Medicine and Pharmacy of Rabat, Ibn Sina Hospital, Department of Urology A, Rabat, Morocco

Robert A. Huddart and Alison M. Reid
Institute of Cancer Research and Royal Marsden Hospital FT, Sutton, Surrey, UK

John Barnard, Ali Hajiran, Chad Crigger, Morris Jessop and Chad Morley
West Virginia University Hospitals, Department of Urology, Morgantown, USA

Tyler Overholt
West Virginia University, School of Medicine, Morgantown, USA

Jennifer Knight
West Virginia University Hospitals, Department of Surgery, Morgantown, USA

Seyed Hassan Inanloo, Mohammad Reza Nikoobakht and Hamed Akhavizadegan
Department of Urology, Sina Hospital, Tehran University of Medical Sciences, Tehran, Iran

Mojgan Karbakhsh
Department of Community Medicine, Tehran University of Medical Sciences, Tehran, Iran

Syed Ali Ehsanullah, Brian Kelly, Charlotte Dunford and Zaheer Shah
Worcestershire Acute Hospitals NHS Trust, Redditch, UK

Abida Sultana
University Hospitals Birmingham NHS Foundation Trust, Birmingham, UK

Felipe Monnerat Lott, Deborah Siqueira, Hermano Argolo, Bernardo Lindberg Nóbrega and Franz Santos Campos
Brazilian National Cancer Institute, Rio de Janeiro, Brazil

Luciano Alves Favorito
Urogenital Research Unit, State University of Rio de Janeiro (UERJ), Rio de Janeiro-RJ, Brazil

Waleed Mohamed Fadlalla, Ayman Hanafy, Hatem Aboulkassem, El Sayed Ashraf and Ahmed Abdelbary
National Cancer Institute, Cairo University, Department of Surgical Oncology, Cairo, Egypt

Mahmoud Abdelhakim
Department of Urology, Faculty of Medicine, Cairo University, Cairo, Egypt

Brian Hu
Department of Urology, Loma Linda University, 11234 Anderson Street Room A-560, Loma Linda, CA 92374, USA

Siamak Daneshmand
University of Southern California Institute of Urology, 1441 Eastlake Avenue, Los Angeles, CA 90033, USA

Dwayne T. S. Chang
Department of Urology, Sir Charles Gairdner Hospital, WA, Australia

Robert Abouassaly
Urology Institute, University Hospitals Case Medical Center, Cleveland, OH, USA
Department of Surgery, Division of Urology, Louis Stokes Cleveland VA Medical Center, Cleveland, OH, USA

Nathan Lawrentschuk
Department of Urology, Austin Hospital, VIC, Australia
Olivia Newton-John Cancer Research Institute, Austin Hospital, VIC, Australia

Shabir Ahmad Dar
MS General Surgery, Resident Surgeon, SKIMS, Jammu and Kashmir, India

Rajandeep Singh Bali and Rajni Bhardwaj
MS General Surgery, Consultant Surgeon, GMC-Jammu, Jammu and Kashmir, India

Yawar Zahoor
MS General Surgery, Resident Surgeon, MAMC, Delhi, India

Arshad Rashid Kema
MS General Surgery, Consultant Surgeon, DHSK, Jammu and Kashmir, India

Giuseppe Giusti and Antonello De Lisa
Department of Urology, University of Cagliari, Via Is Mirrionis 92, 09121 Cagliari, Italy

Roman I. Slusarenco, Artem O. Prostomolotov, Roman B. Sukhanov and Evgeny A. Bezrukov
Institute for Urology and Reproductive Health, Moscow, Russia

Konstantin V. Mikheev
International School "Medicine of the Future", FGAOU VO I.M. Sechenov First Moscow State Medical University, Moscow, Russia

A. V. Maltsev
Kharkiv National Medical University, Kharkiv 61022, Ukraine

D. V. Shchukin, V. N. Lesovoy, G. G. Khareba, A. I. Harahatyi and M. M. Polyakov
Kharkiv National Medical University, Kharkiv 61022, Ukraine
V.I. Shapoval Regional Clinical Center of Urology and Nephrology, Kharkiv 61037, Ukraine

P. V. Mozzhakov
V.I. Shapoval Regional Clinical Center of Urology and Nephrology, Kharkiv 61037, Ukraine

R. V. Stetsyshyn
V.I. Shapoval Regional Clinical Center of Urology and Nephrology, Kharkiv 61037, Ukraine
Kharkiv Medical Academy of Postgraduate Education, Kharkiv 61176, Ukraine

M. P. Kopytsya
L.T. Malaya ,erapy National Institute of the National Academy of Medical Sciences of Ukraine, Kharkiv 61039, Ukraine

O. O. Makovozov
Dniprovsky Regional Clinical Oncology Dispensary, Dnipro 49055, Ukraine

Francisco E. Martins
Department of Urology, Hospital Santa Maria, University of Lisbon, School of Medicine, 1600-161 Lisbon, Portugal
ULSNA-Hospital de Portalegre, 7300-074 Portalegre, Portugal

Natalia Martins
ULSNA-Hospital de Portalegre, 7300-074 Portalegre, Portugal

Sanjay B. Kulkarni and Pankaj Joshi
Kulkarni Reconstructive Urology Center, Pune 411038, India

Jonathan Warner
City of Hope Medical Center, Duarte, CA 91010, USA

Index

www.ingramcontent.com/pod-product-compliance
Lightning Source LLC
LaVergne TN
LVHW060520210926
848485LV00005B/1113
* 9 7 8 1 6 3 9 2 7 9 9 4 4 *